Cambridge Handbook of Anesthesiology

Cambridge Handbook of Anesthesiology

Edited by

Richard D. Urman, MD, MBA

Jay J. Jacoby Professor and Chair, Department of Anesthesiology, The Ohio State University and Wexner Medical Center, Columbus, OH

Alan David Kaye, MD PhD, DABA, DABPM, DABIPP, FASA

Professor of Anesthesiology and Pharmacology, Toxicology, and Neurosciences; Vice Chairman of Research, Pain Fellowship Director, Provost, Chief Academic Officer and Vice Chancellor, Louisiana State University Health Sciences Center, Ochsner-LSU Hospital System, Shreveport, Louisiana

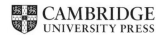
CAMBRIDGE
UNIVERSITY PRESS

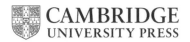

Shaftesbury Road, Cambridge CB2 8EA, United Kingdom

One Liberty Plaza, 20th Floor, New York, NY 10006, USA

477 Williamstown Road, Port Melbourne, VIC 3207, Australia

314–321, 3rd Floor, Plot 3, Splendor Forum, Jasola District Centre,
New Delhi – 110025, India

103 Penang Road, #05–06/07, Visioncrest Commercial, Singapore 238467

Cambridge University Press is part of Cambridge University Press & Assessment,
a department of the University of Cambridge.

We share the University's mission to contribute to society through the pursuit of
education, learning and research at the highest international levels of excellence.

www.cambridge.org
Information on this title: www.cambridge.org/9781108947657

DOI: 10.1017/9781108936941

First published 2023

Printed in the United Kingdom by TJ Books Limited, Padstow Cornwall

A catalogue record for this publication is available from the British Library.

A Cataloging-in-Publication data record for this book is available from the Library of Congress.

ISBN 978-1-108-94765-7 Paperback

....

I would like to dedicate this book to my colleagues, mentors and patients from whom I learn something new every day. I also would like to dedicate this book to my wife Dr. Zina Matlyuk and my two children and thank them for their patience and support during my work on this important project.

Richard D. Urman

-To my wife Dr. Kim Kaye for being the best spouse a man could ask for in his life.

-To my mother Florence Feldman who taught me tremendous things about life, to accomplish tasks with the highest of quality, and to reach my dreams and goals.

-To my good friend James V. Johnson, for his loving support and help over the past 45 plus years.

-To all my teachers and colleagues at the University of Arizona in Tucson, Ochsner Clinic in New Orleans, Massachusetts General Hospital/Harvard School of Medicine in Boston, Tulane School of Medicine in New Orleans, Texas Tech Health Sciences Center in Lubbock, LSU School of Medicine in New Orleans, and LSU School of Medicine in Shreveport.

Alan David Kaye

Contents

Contributors

Edward S. Alpaugh MD
Department of Anesthesiology,
Louisiana State University Health
Sciences Center, New Orleans,
LA, USA

Peter Amato MD
Department of Anesthesiology,
University of Virginia,
Charlottesville, VA, USA

Boris C. Anyama MD
Department of Anesthesiology and
Perioperative Medicine, University
of Pittsburgh Medical Center,
Pittsburgh, PA, USA

Franchesca Arias PhD
Perioperative Cognitive Anesthesia
Network (PeCAN), University of
Florida, Gainesville, FL, USA; Aging
Brain Center, Hebrew SeniorLife,
Beth Israel Deaconess Medical
Center, Harvard Medical School,
Boston, MA, USA

Katherine C. Babin
Louisiana State University Health
Shreveport, Shreveport,
LA, USA

Ankit Bhatia DO
Jackson Memorial Hospital,
University of Miami, Miller School
of Medicine, Miami, FL, USA

Meghan Brennan MD
Department of Anesthesiology,
University of Florida College of
Medicine, Gainesville, FL, USA

Kimberley C. Brondeel BS
University of Texas Medical Branch,
Galveston, TX, USA

Stuart H. Brown MD MD
Department of Anesthesiology,
Louisiana State University Health
Sciences Center, New Orleans,
LA, USA

Garrett W. Burnett MD
Department of Anesthesiology,
Perioperative and Pain Medicine,
Icahn School of Medicine at Mount
Sinai, New York, NY, USA

Ken Candido MD
UCLA Health, Santa Monica,
CA, USA

Oren Cohen MD
Department of Anesthesiology,
Louisiana State University Health
Sciences Center, New Orleans,
LA, USA

Matthew M. Colontonio MD
Department of Anesthesiology,
Louisiana State University Health
Shreveport, Shreveport, LA, USA

Elyse M. Cornett PhD
Department of Anesthesiology,
Louisiana State University Health
Shreveport, Shreveport, LA, USA

Madelyn K. Craig MD
Department of Anesthesiology,
Louisiana State University Health
Sciences Center, New Orleans,
LA, USA

Brittany Deiling MD
Department of Anesthesiology,
University of Virginia,
Charlottesville, VA, USA

Paul C. DeMarco MD
Department of Anesthesiology,
UVA Health System, Charlottesville,
VA, USA

Ricardo Diaz Milian MD, FASE
Mayo Clinic, Jacksonville, FL, USA

James L. Dillon MD
Department of Anesthesiology,
Louisiana State University Health
Sciences Center, New Orleans,
LA, USA

Catherine Dion MS
Clinical and Health Psychology,
Perioperative Cognitive Anesthesia
Network (PeCAN), Anesthesiology,
University of Florida College of
Medicine, Gainesville, FL, USA

Frederick R. Ditmars BA
University of Texas Medical Branch,
Galveston, TX, USA

Jeffrey Dobyns DO MSHA MSHQS FASA
University of Alabama at
Birmingham, Heersink School of

Medicine, Department of
Anesthesiology and Perioperative
Medicine, Birmingham,
AL, USA

Anterpreet Dua
Department of Anesthesiology and
Perioperative Medicine, Augusta
University Medical Center,
Medical College of Georgia at
Augusta University,
Augusta, GA, USA

Ken P. Ehrhardt MD
Beth Israel Deaconess Medical
Center, Harvard Medical School,
Boston, MA, USA

Austin Erney DO
University of North Carolina,
Chapel Hill, NC, USA

Erica Fagelman MD
Department of Anesthesiology,
Icahn School of Medicine at Mount
Sinai, New York, NY, USA

Kenneth Flax MD
Mount Sinai Queens, The Mount
Sinai Hospital Mount Sinai
Morningside and Mount Sinai West,
New York, NY, USA

Amanda Frantz MD
Department of Anesthesiology,
University of Florida College of
Medicine, Gainesville,
FL, USA

Eric Fried MD
Department of Anesthesiology,
Perioperative, and Pain Medicine,
Icahn School of Medicine at Mount
Sinai, New York, NY, USA

Mitchell C. Fuller BS
Medical College of Wisconsin, Wauwatosa, WI, USA

Julie A. Gayle MD
Louisiana State University Health Sciences Center, School of Medicine, New Orleans, LA, USA

Sonja A. Gennuso MD
Department of Anesthesiology, Louisiana State University Health Shreveport, Shreveport, LA, USA

Rhian E. Germany BS MS
Louisiana State University Health Shreveport, Shreveport, LA, USA

Brook Girma MD
Department of Anesthesiology, Louisiana State University Health Shreveport, Shreveport, LA, USA

Sandra N. Gonzalez MD
Department of Anesthesiology, University of Florida College of Medicine, Gainesville, FL, USA

Matthew Graves MD
Department of Anesthesia and Perioperative Medicine, Medical University of South Carolina, Charleston, SC, USA

Logan Gray DO
Department of Anesthesiology, University of North Carolina, Chapel Hill, NC, USA

Karina Gritsenko MD
Montefiore Medical Center, Bronx, NY, USA

Kristin Hamlet PhD
Clinical and Health Psychology, Perioperative Cognitive Anesthesia Network (PeCAN), Anesthesiology, University of Florida, Gainesville, FL, USA

Erik Helander MBBS
US Anesthesia Partners, Denver, CO, USA

John Helmstetter MD DABA
Louisiana State University Health Sciences Center, New Orleans, LA, USA

Carlos Hernaiz Alonso BS
Clinical and Health Psychology, Perioperative Cognitive Anesthesia Network (PeCAN), Anesthesiology, University of Florida, Gainesville, FL, USA

Joshua J. Hurley MD
Department of Anesthesiology, Louisiana State University Health Sciences Center, New Orleans, LA, USA

Sheriza L. Hussain MD MS
MedStar Georgetown University Hospital, Washington, DC, USA

Farees Hyatali MD
Montefiore Medical Center, Bronx, NY, USA

Christina Jeng MD FASA
Department of Anesthesiology, Perioperative and Pain Medicine; Department of Orthopaedics; Department of Medical Education, Icahn School of Medicine at Mount Sinai, New York, NY, USA

Mark R. Jones MD
Department of Anesthesia, Weill Cornell Medical School, New York, NY, USA

Leah A. Kaplan BFA
Louisiana State University Health Shreveport, Shreveport, LA, USA

Vijay Kata MD (expected)
Department of Anesthesiology, Louisiana State University Health Shreveport, Shreveport, LA, USA

Alan David Kaye MD PhD
Department of Anesthesiology, Louisiana State University Health Shreveport, Shreveport, LA, USA

Julia Kendrick MD
Department of Adult Cardiothoracic Anesthesiology, Medical University of South Carolina, Charleston, SC, USA

Ryan J. Kline MD
Department of Anesthesiology, Louisiana State University Health Sciences Center, New Orleans, LA, USA

Gopal Kodumudi MD
Department of Anesthesiology, Louisiana State University Health Sciences Center, New Orleans, LA, USA

Lakshmi N. Kurnutala MD MSc
University of Mississippi Medical Center, Jackson, MS, USA

Brittni M. Lanoux MD
Department of Anesthesiology, Louisiana State University Health Sciences Center, New Orleans, LA, USA

Victoria L. Lassiegne MD (expected)
Louisiana State University Health Sciences Center, School of Medicine, New Orleans, LA, USA

Tamara Lawson MD MPH
Virginia Commonwealth University Health System, Richmond, VA, USA

Kay Lee MD
Montefiore Medical Center, Bronx, NY, USA

William Lee MD
Department of Anesthesiology, Perioperative and Pain Medicine; Icahn School of Medicine at Mount Sinai, New York, NY, USA

Jinlei Li MD PhD FASA
Department of Anesthesiology, Yale University, New Haven, CT

Graham T. Lubinsky MD
Anesthesiology and Critical Care Medicine, MedStar Georgetown University Hospital, Washington, DC, USA

Austin Ly BS
University of Tennessee Health Science Center College of Medicine, Memphis, TN, USA

Eric Ly MD
University of Tennessee Health Science Center College of Medicine, Memphis, TN, USA

Franciscka Macieiski MD
Louisiana State University Health
Shreveport Medical Center,
Shreveport, LA, USA

Timothy Martin MD MBA FASA
Division of Pediatric Anesthesia,
University of Florida College of
Medicine, Gainesville, FL, USA

Sarah McCraney MD
Anesthesiology, University of
Florida, Gainesville, FL, USA

Michael McManus MD
Department of Anesthesiology,
University of Virginia,
Charlottesville, VA, USA

Sonia D. Mehta MD
Department of Anesthesiology,
University of Florida College of
Medicine, Gainesville, FL, USA

Adrienne Mejia MD
Department of Anesthesiology,
Yale University, New Haven,
CT, USA

Bethany Menard MD
Louisiana State University Health
Sciences Center, New Orleans,
LA, USA

Sumitra Miriyala PhD
Department of Cellular Biology and
Anatomy, Louisiana State
University Health Shreveport,
Shreveport, LA, USA

Mark Motejunas MD
UCLA Health, Santa Monica,
CA, USA

George Mychaskiw DO
Department of Anesthesiology,
Louisiana State University Health
Shreveport, Shreveport, LA, USA

Olga C. Nin MD
University of Florida College of
Medicine, Gainesville, FL, USA

Chikezie N. Okeagu MD
Department of Anesthesiology,
Louisiana State University Health
Sciences Center, New Orleans,
LA, USA

Sher-Lu Pai MD
Department of Anesthesiology and
Perioperative Medicine, Mayo
Clinic College of Medicine,
Jacksonville, FL, USA

Chang H. Park MD
Department of Anesthesiology,
Perioperative and Pain Medicine,
Icahn School of Medicine at Mount
Sinai, New York, NY, USA

Jeffrey Park MD
Department of Anesthesiology,
University of North Carolina at
Chapel Hill, Chapel Hill, NC, USA

Nihir Patel MD
Department of Anesthesiology,
Perioperative and Pain Medicine;
Icahn School of Medicine at Mount
Sinai, New York, NY, USA

Shilpa Patil MD
Department of Anesthesiology,
Louisiana State University Health
Shreveport, Shreveport,
LA, USA

Shilpadevi S. Patil MD
Department of Anesthesiology
Louisiana State University Health
Sciences Center, New Orleans,
LA, USA

Stephen Patin MPH MD (expected)
Louisiana State University Health
Shreveport, Shreveport, LA, USA

Alex D. Pham MD
Department of Anesthesiology,
Louisiana State University Health
Sciences Center, New Orleans,
LA, USA

Catherine Price PhD
Clinical and Health Psychology,
Perioperative Cognitive Anesthesia
Network (PeCAN), Anesthesiology,
University of Florida, Gainesville,
FL, USA

Iliana Ramirez-Saldana MD
University of Mississippi Medical
Center, Jackson, MS, USA

Aaron Reagan MD
Department of Anesthesiology and
Perioperative Pain Medicine, The
Mount Sinai Hospital, New York,
NY, USA

Devin S. Reed MD
Louisiana State University Health
Sciences Center, New Orleans,
LA, USA

Pamela R. Roberts MD FCCM FCCP
Department of Anesthesiology,
University of Oklahoma College of
Medicine, Oklahoma City,
OK, USA

Kelsey Rooney BS
Louisiana State University Health
Shreveport, Shreveport, LA, USA

Corey Scher MD
Department of Anesthesiology,
Perioperative Care, and Pain
Medicine, NYU Grossman School of
Medicine, New York, NY, USA

Annemarie Senekal MBChB MMed FCA
Department of Anesthesiology and
Critical Care, University of
Stellenbosch, Tygerberg
Hospital, Cape Town, South Africa

Christopher M. Sharrow MD
Department of Anesthesiology,
University of Virginia,
Charlottesville, VA, USA

Meredith K. Shaw MD
Department of Anesthesiology,
Louisiana State University Health
Sciences Center, New Orleans,
LA, USA

Matthew Sherrer MD MBA FASA
University of Alabama at
Birmingham, Heersink School of
Medicine, Department of
Anesthesiology and Perioperative
Medicine, Birmingham, AL, USA

Meeta M. Sheth MD
Department of Anesthesiology,
Louisiana State University Health
Shreveport, Shreveport, LA, USA

Ashley Shilling MD
Department of Anesthesiology,
University of Virginia,
Charlottesville, VA, USA

Naina Singh MD
Department of Anesthesiology,
Louisiana State University
Health Shreveport, Shreveport,
LA, USA

Harish Bangalore Siddaiah MD
Department of Anesthesiology
Louisiana State University Health
Sciences Center, Shreveport,
LA, USA

Alan M. Smeltz MD
University of North Carolina
Hospital, Chapel Hill, NC,
USA

Zhuo Sun
Department of Anesthesiology and
Perioperative Medicine, Augusta
University Medical Center,
Medical College of Georgia at
Augusta University, Augusta,
GA, USA

Pankaj Thakur MD
Department of Anesthesiology,
Louisiana State University Health
Sciences Center, Shreveport,
LA, USA

George Thomas BS
George Washington School of
Medicine and Health Sciences,
Washington, DC, USA

Patrick Tighe MD
Clinical and Health Psychology,
Perioperative Cognitive Anesthesia
Network (PeCAN), Anesthesiology,
University of Florida, Gainesville,
FL, USA

Sridhar R. Tirumala MD
Department of Anesthesiology,
Louisiana State University Health
Shreveport, Shreveport, LA, USA

Gregory M. Tortorich MD
Department of Anesthesiology,
Louisiana State University Health
Sciences Center, New Orleans,
LA, USA

Christine T. Vo MD
Department of Anesthesiology,
University of Oklahoma College of
Medicine, Oklahoma City, OK, USA

Michael P. Webb MBChB MSc
Counties Manukau Health
Department of Anaesthesia and Pain
Medicine, Auckland, New Zealand

Margaret E. Wiggins MS
Clinical and Health Psychology,
Perioperative Cognitive Anesthesia
Network (PeCAN), Anesthesiology,
University of Florida, Gainesville,
FL, USA

Vishal Yajnik MD MS
Anesthesiology Division of Critical
Care, Virginia Commonwealth
University, Richmond, VA, USA

Erin Yen DO
University of Florida College of
Medicine, Gainesville, FL, USA

Reine Zbeidy MD
Division of Obstetric
Anesthesiology, University of
Miami, Miller School of Medicine,
Miami, FL, USA

Introduction

Douglas R. Bacon

The pages that unfold behind this introduction are full of information for providers of anesthesia services. In some ways, this is a "how to" manual for one of the most misunderstood and difficult practices in medicine. For some, this book will unlock new knowledge and improve clinical practice. For others, it will confirm already acquired information or update knowledge to ensure practice at the forefront of anesthesiology. The transfer of the expertise is seamless, simple, and, by the nature of the publication, created and reviewed by experts.

It was not always so straightforward to find this information in one place. Think for a moment about how the information about the discovery of the anesthetic properties of diethyl ether spread across the world. On October 16, 1846, William Thomas Green Morton anesthetized Gilbert Abbott for the removal of a tumor of the jaw at the Massachusetts General Hospital by the surgeon John Collins Warren. By December, 1846, ether anesthesia was being used in London, several thousand miles across the Atlantic Ocean [1]. The question of how this knowledge crossed the ocean in a time when electronic communication did not exist continues to fascinate historians of medicine.

A letter from Jacob Bigelow, a physician and botanist to Francis Boot, and an expatriate American physician practicing in London, conveyed news of Morton's work. Boot proceeded to anesthetize Miss Lonsdale for the extraction of a tooth by Mr. James Robinson, a dentist, on December 19, 1846. Two days later, Dr. Boot would anesthetize Frederick Churchill for the amputation of his leg by the famous surgeon Robert Liston [1]. All of this occurred due a letter from one physician to another, carried by steamship across the Atlantic! Gwen Wilson has likewise chronicled the arrival of the news of surgical anesthesia in Australia, half a world away from Boston. On June 7, 1847, just shy of eight months later, ether anesthesia was given in Sydney, Australia [2]. Almost a full year later, on October 4, 1847, the physician and missionary Peter Parker gave the first ether anesthetics in China [3].

It would be almost another thirty-five years before a textbook of anesthesia would be published. Henry M. Lyman, Professor of Physiology and Diseases of the Nervous System at Rush Medical College and Professor of Theory and Practice of Medicine at the Woman's College, both in Chicago, would be the sole author of a book entitled *Artificial Anaesthesia and Anaesthetics* [4]. It is a comprehensive text, with many subjects that are recognizable today. Dr. Lyman wrote about medical legal considerations, administration of anesthetics, and several chapters on anesthetic agents. Two things stand out in the book. First, in the chapter on the history of anesthesia is the first recitation of the anesthetic given by William E. Clarke in January, 1842. The other is his section on local anesthesia before the discovery of the anesthetic properties of cocaine by Carl Koller in 1884.

One of the next major and popular textbooks prior to World War I was written by New York City physician James Tayloe Gwathmey. Published in 1914, *Anesthesia* [5], with almost 950 pages, is a summary of anesthetic knowledge of the time. The book may well have been published in response to the need of members of the newly established American Association of Anesthetists, the first truly national association of physician specialists in the United States. Both the textbook and the Association demonstrate the slow-growing trend of physician specialization in anesthesia. The textbook especially demonstrates the growth in knowledge of anesthetics and the techniques for administration in the thirty-three years since Lyman's book was published.

Shortly thereafter, textbooks of anesthesia proliferated. One interesting text was published by Paluel Flagg. In the preface to the second edition [6] in 1919, Flagg wrote that the "purpose of this little volume 'as a groundwork upon which the student, interne, and general practitioner may acquire a more comprehensive knowledge of the Art of Anaesthesia' has been strictly adhered to ..." in the almost 370 pages. A scant three years later, Gaston Labat would publish one of the first comprehensive American textbooks on an anesthetic subspecialty with *Regional Anesthesia* [7]. The book is based largely on the much smaller and less comprehensive text produced by Victor Pauchet, Paul Sourdat, and Gaston Labat entitled *L'Anesthésie Régionale*. In point of fact, much of the text and many of the illustrations are taken almost directly from Pauchet's work, except for a long section on techniques that emphasized the anesthetist's interaction with and approach to the patient [8].

While the emergence of textbooks on the subject of anesthesia, essentially in the early years of the twentieth century, may seem unimportant to the modern reader used to the massive thousand-page or multivolume tome, it remains interesting to understand the growth of information in these books. For the development of the specialty, the core knowledge that constitutes anesthesiology is defined within the bindery of the edition. Reading through the following pages of this volume reconstructs what students of the art and science of anesthesiology have been doing for more than a century. May the insights gained within this book allow the reader to improve care for the most important aspect of our shared specialty – the patient.

References

1. Rushman GB, Davies NJH, Atkinson RS. *A Short History of Anaesthesia*. Oxford: Butterworth-Heinemann; 1996.

2. Wilson G. *One Grand Chain*, Vol. I. Melbourne: The Australian and New Zealand College of Anaesthetists; 1995.

3. Sim P, Du B, Bacon DR. Pioneer Chinese anesthesiologists: American influence on the development of anesthesiology in China. *Anesthesiology*. 2000;93:256–64.

4. Lyman HM. *Artificial Anaesthesia and Anaesthetics*. New York, NY: William Wood and Company; 1881.

5. Gwathmey JT. *Anesthesia*. New York, NY: D. Appleton and Company; 1914.

6. Flagg PJ. *The Art of Anaesthesia*. Philadelphia, PA: J. B. Lippincott Company; 1919.

7. Labat G. *Regional Anesthesia Its Technic and Clinical Application*. Philadelphia, PA: W. B. Saunders Company; 1922.

8. Cote AV, Vachon CA, Horlocker TT, Bacon DR. From Victor Pauchet to Gaston Labat: the transformation of regional anesthesia from a surgeon's practice to the physician anesthetist. *Anesth Analg*. 2003;96:1193–200.

Preoperative Evaluation and Coexisting Disease

Matthew Sherrer, Sher-Lu Pai, and Jeffrey Dobyns

Preoperative Evaluation

The preoperative evaluation is a review of a patient's physical condition in preparation for surgery. The history and physical examination are the foundation of this assessment and focus on identifying predisposing factors for cardiac and pulmonary complications and on determining a patient's functional capacity to define fitness for surgery. The history and physical examination findings determine the need for additional laboratory or diagnostic testing if such evaluation changes the course of action or improves patient health and outcomes. Presurgical medical optimization, including proper subspecialty consultation, improves surgical outcomes in patients with coexisting diseases. Preoperative preparation and optimization efforts focus on identifying and mitigating modifiable risk factors to improve surgical and longitudinal outcomes while reducing healthcare costs.

Elements of Preoperative Evaluation

The essential component of the preoperative evaluation is the history, which details past and current medical and surgical status, family and genetic history, and documentation of tobacco, alcohol, and substance use. A detailed list of allergies and reactions, as well as previous anesthetic experiences, helps formulate the anesthetic plan. A complete 12-point review of systems identifies any undiagnosed or inadequately optimized disease. Cardiovascular and pulmonary diseases are the primary drivers of adverse perioperative outcomes and are the most relevant in determining fitness for anesthesia and surgery [1].

A focused preoperative physical examination includes, at a minimum, documentation of vital signs, including height and weight, with body mass index (BMI) calculation, and an assessment of the airway, lungs, and heart, and a basic neurologic examination. Unexpected abnormal findings on the physical examination, such as a new heart murmur or an unexplained decline in functional capacity, compel investigation before elective surgery.

Medication Reconciliation

A complete medication history, including current and new drug therapy and unusual reactions or responses to drugs, ensures safe perioperative care. Medications that provide physiologic homeostasis should be continued preoperatively. The decision to continue, discontinue, or modify chronic medication regimens requires thoughtful risk–benefit analysis. Polypharmacy is common in elderly patients, and the preoperative evaluation is an opportunity to identify and mitigate duplicated medications and those with cross-reactivity. This encounter is also an opportunity to ensure that appropriate stroke and cardiovascular risk reduction strategies, such as statin therapy, are in place.

Risk Stratification

Perioperative risk is determined by healthcare, patient, and socio-economic factors [2]. Healthcare factors include elements specific to the type and magnitude of the surgical procedure and those encompassing anesthesia type and management techniques employed, such as goal-directed fluid therapy. Patient characteristics include fixed risk factors, such as age and genetics, and modifiable risk factors, such as smoking, nutrition status, and anemia. Perioperative outcomes are directly affected by social determinants of health, such as economic stability, physical environment, and level of education.

Deciding to have surgery is a complex consideration of risks, short- and long-term benefits, alternatives, and effects on longitudinal health. A primary goal of the preoperative evaluation is to make surgery safer by estimating the total risk relative to the benefits of proceeding with surgery and reducing modifiable risk. Communicating the risk to the patient, along with risk reduction strategies in the interest of shared decision-making, affects whether or not to proceed with surgery.

ASA Physical Status Classification

Originally intended to assess and communicate a patient's preanesthesia medical comorbidities, the American Society of Anesthesiologists (ASA) physical status classification is a current standard of risk assessment and a mandated element of the preanesthetic evaluation by the Joint Commission. The ASA scoring system alone does not predict perioperative risks. When combined with other factors such as frailty and functional status, it demonstrates excellent risk prediction, and higher scores correlate with increased postoperative morbidity and mortality [3]. This scale is based solely on the presence of existing disease and does not consider the risk of the surgical procedure.

Cardiac

Cardiac functional status or capacity, expressed as metabolic equivalents (METs), is determined subjectively by assessment with a brief set of questions and has been thought to be positively associated with postoperative outcomes. Many risk models rely on this assessment. Achieving four METs of activity without symptoms is a good prognostic indicator of perioperative outcomes [4]. A subjective assessment of functional status does not accurately identify patients with inadequate functional capacity or predict postoperative morbidity or mortality [5]. The Duke Activity Status Index (DASI) provides an objective assessment of functional capacity. Compared with cardiopulmonary exercise testing and subjective assessment of functional capacity, only DASI scores successfully predicted the primary outcomes of myocardial injury or death at 30 days. A DASI score of <34 is associated with an increased risk of 30-day death, myocardial infarction (MI), and moderate to severe complications [6].

All patients scheduled for noncardiac surgery should have an initial assessment of the percentage risk of a major adverse cardiac event (MACE) using validated models that include information from the history and physical examination, objective functional capacity score, electrocardiogram, laboratory studies, and planned procedure. The calculated risk aids the patient and perioperative specialists in weighing the risks and benefits and determining the optimal timing of surgery. The risk score guides decision-making as to whether the planned surgery should proceed without further preoperative cardiovascular testing or whether postponement for additional testing is indicated. Preoperative risk stratification is also instrumental in determining if a patient would benefit from preoperative coronary revascularization or consideration of a lesser-risk or nonsurgical alternative. The risk assessment occasionally uncovers undiagnosed problems or inadequately managed chronic conditions requiring optimization. The decision to pursue further cardiovascular testing considers both short- and long-term risk reductions.

The Revised Cardiac Risk Index (RCRI) or the American College of Surgeons National Surgical Quality Improvement Program (NSQIP) risk prediction tool are two commonly used risk indices. The RCRI is simpler and has been widely used and validated for many years. The NSQIP calculator is more complex, requiring calculation through an online algorithm. A more straightforward tool derived from the NSQIP database is the Gupta myocardial infarction or cardiac arrest (MICA) calculator. The newer Cardiovascular Risk Index (CVRI) is a validated model with higher discriminatory power than the RCRI [7]. For patients at low MACE risk (<1%), no further testing is indicated. For patients with higher MACE risk (>1%) and inadequate functional capacity (<4 METs), the question becomes whether further cardiovascular testing will change management and improve the outcome.

Pulmonary

Postoperative pulmonary complications adversely influence a patient's postoperative course. They are a significant source of postoperative morbidity and mortality, resulting in substantial increases in healthcare resource utilization. Table 1.1 details the patient and surgical risk factors associated with postoperative pulmonary complications. The ARISCAT Risk Index is a commonly used risk prediction tool to identify patients at risk of postoperative pulmonary complications and likely to benefit from presurgical risk reduction interventions, such as increased physical activity and preoperative incentive spirometry. All available risk indices provide a reliable estimation of postoperative pulmonary complication risk, but the ARISCAT Risk Index is the most practical for preoperative assessment. The strongest predictor for postoperative pulmonary complications is poor functional capacity. Any history suggesting unrecognized chronic lung disease or heart failure, such as reduced functional capacity, unexplained dyspnea, or cough, requires further evaluation. Pulmonary function tests and routine chest X-rays do not appreciably add to risk stratification.

Table 1.1 Predictive risk factors for postoperative pulmonary complications

Patient risk factors	Surgical risk factors
• Age >50 years[a] • Preexisting pulmonary disease • Obstructive sleep apnea • ASA physical status of 3 or higher • Current smoking • Heart failure • Poor functional capacity/frailty • Malnutrition • Diabetes with hyperglycemia/elevated hemoglobin A1c • Preoperative anemia[a] • Morbid obesity • Preoperative oxygen saturation below 95%[a] • Respiratory infection within preceding month[a]	• Upper abdominal or thoracic surgery[a] • Emergency surgery[a] • Surgery lasting longer than 2 hours[a] • General versus combined general and regional anesthesia • Intraoperative fluid management strategy • Blood transfusion • Neuromuscular blockade

[a] Factors assessed by the ARISCAT Risk Index.

Preoperative Optimization and Prehabilitation

Safe and efficient surgical and anesthesia practice requires a fit and medically optimized patient. Numerous epidemiological studies indicate that inadequate preoperative preparation is a significant contributory factor to the primary causes of perioperative morbidity and mortality. Postoperative morbidity is a significant surgical outcome in terms of economic consequences to healthcare institutions. Preoperative comorbidities, coupled with surgical complexity, predict adverse outcomes and increased healthcare resource utilization. Given preoperative time and resource limitations, it is reasonable to focus these efforts on patients at high risk of postoperative morbidity and mortality. Preoperative optimization and prehabilitation represent prudent economic strategies for reducing short- and long-term healthcare expenses and improving longitudinal population health.

Preoperative optimization is a process of clinician-managed interventions not directly involving patient effort or behavior modification, such as medication adjustment, glucose management, or anemia correction, designed to prepare the patient psychologically and physiologically to handle the stress of surgery. Prehabilitation differs from optimization and is the active preoperative process of enhancing a patient's functional capacity to allow better tolerance of the stressors of surgery and recovery. Prehabilitation efforts implemented to improve postoperative outcomes involve lifestyle interventions, such as nutritional supplementation, physical exercise, stress reduction, and smoking cessation.

Coexisting Disease

Cardiac

Ischemic Heart Disease

Patients with coronary stents undergoing noncardiac surgery are at high MACE risk even when receiving perioperative antiplatelet therapy, and withholding one or both antiplatelet medications increases the risk of thrombosis. They are also at high risk of significant bleeding when one or both medications are continued. MACEs, including stroke, are mainly related to previous medical conditions and perioperative blood loss, and not to the surgery itself. In patients undergoing noncardiac surgery after a percutaneous coronary intervention (PCI) with second-generation drug-eluting stents, the incidence of MACEs, including death, MI, stent thrombosis, and the need for repeat revascularization, was highest in the first 6 months after the PCI [8]. Elective procedures should be delayed for at least 6 months in patients with drug-eluting stents, at least 30 days for those with bare-metal stents, and 14 days following balloon angioplasty to allow for uninterrupted dual antiplatelet therapy.

Hypertension

Perioperative hypertension is primarily a manifestation of acute or acute-on-chronic hypertension. Perioperative hypertension occurs mainly for two reasons: (1) worsening of chronic hypertension; or (2) a response to transient factors, such as pain, anxiety, or withholding of blood pressure medications. Hypertension is not a significant factor for determining perioperative cardiac risk, but it does contribute to several conditions that are, such as chronic renal disease and diastolic dysfunction. In the absence of acute end-organ dysfunction, there is little justification for case cancellation for blood pressures below 180/110 mmHg.

Isolated systolic hypertension (ISH) is the most common type of hypertension in the elderly. It is associated with a two- to fourfold increase in the risk of MI, left ventricular hypertrophy (LVH), renal dysfunction, stroke, and cardiovascular mortality. Characteristics of ISH include a widened pulse pressure and a systolic blood pressure of ≥ 140 mmHg, with a diastolic blood pressure of <90 mmHg. Elderly patients benefit significantly from therapies to reduce systolic blood pressure. The preoperative treatment of ISH risks diastolic hypotension and compromise of perfusion to vascular beds, and requires careful consideration.

Bioprosthetic and Mechanical Heart Valves

Anticoagulation management in the patient with a bioprosthetic or mechanical valve undergoing surgery considers the type, location, and number of prosthetic heart valves, planned surgical procedure and bleeding risk, and other patient risk factors for thromboembolism, and the planned procedure. The primary concern with interrupting anticoagulation is thromboembolism, which carries a 20% mortality rate and a 40% rate of significant disability [9]. The decision to interrupt anticoagulation and whether or not to bridge with low-molecular-weight heparin requires stratification of a patient's risk of thromboembolism versus significant bleeding. Thromboembolism risk stratification tools, such as the BleedMAP and HAS-BLED scores, are useful in clinical decision-making. Patients undergoing procedures with associated low bleeding risk should be continued on their regular anticoagulation regimen. The thromboembolic risk is highest within the first three months of bioprosthetic or mechanical mitral valve replacement or repair. Noncardiac surgery should be deferred to avoid interruption of anticoagulation.

Heart Failure

Heart failure represents a spectrum of disease, and perioperative risk varies depending on where the patient is along the continuum. Risk is lowest for those patients with asymptomatic diastolic dysfunction where ejection fraction is preserved, and highest for those at the end-stage with reduced ejection fraction.

The postoperative mortality risk is higher in patients with heart failure than in those with coronary artery disease, and elderly patients with heart failure have substantially higher risks of postoperative mortality and hospital readmission. The preoperative assessment goals for heart failure patients before noncardiac surgery include: assessing functional status; identifying asymptomatic patients who are at risk of developing heart failure in the postoperative period; determining whether heart failure patients are stable and optimally managed or showing signs and symptoms of decompensation; recognizing high-risk heart failure syndromes, including new-onset heart failure; and identifying comorbidities that impact the stability of heart failure in the postoperative period. The inability to achieve 4 METs functional capacity by walking four average-length city blocks and climbing two flights of stairs without experiencing symptomatic limitation was 71% sensitive and 47% specific for predicting severe postoperative complications. Given the critical prognostic implications of functional capacity to surgical outcomes, the New York Heart Association (NYHA) functional classification (see Table 1.2) categorizes heart failure patients based on functional capacity limitations and symptom development. Postoperative mortality increases with severity of the preoperative functional impairment, from 4% in NYHA class 1 to 67% in class IV.

Asymptomatic diastolic dysfunction is common in elderly and hypertensive patients and presents considerable perioperative challenges. Diastolic dysfunction is an underestimated disease and is independently associated with major adverse outcomes in patients undergoing both cardiac or noncardiac surgery. The most straightforward approach to recognizing asymptomatic left ventricular dysfunction is maintaining a high index of suspicion

Table 1.2 New York Heart Association functional classification

NYHA class	Symptoms
I	No limitations of physical activity. Ordinary activity does not cause dyspnea, palpitations, or fatigue
II	Slight limitation of physical activity. Comfortable at rest, but ordinary physical activity results in dyspnea, palpitations, or fatigue
III	Pronounced limitation of physical activity. Comfortable at rest, but less-than-ordinary physical activity results in dyspnea, palpitations, or fatigue
IV	Unable to carry on any physical activity without discomfort. Symptoms of heart failure at rest. Discomfort increases with any physical activity

when a patient provides a history of risk factors or presents with particular physical signs, such as resting tachycardia or the presence of a fourth heart sound. Identification of suspicious signs and symptoms warrants prompt cardiology referral. A risk stratification model, such as the RCRI or NSQIP calculator, including heart failure as a procedural risk factor provides an accurate MACE risk assessment. Both models offer an estimation of MACEs, but the NSQIP calculator also provides estimates of several other adverse outcomes, such as postoperative pulmonary complications (PPCs) and expected length of stay.

Pulmonary

The ARISCAT index identifies patients at risk of PPC and guides preoperative optimization strategies, as described in Table 1.3. Those at low risk of PPCs benefit from simple recommendations, such as practicing good oral hygiene and early mobilization. Those patients at intermediate and high risk of PPCs benefit from preoperative incentive spirometry and increased activity and advanced lung-protective ventilation maneuvers. All patients undergoing general anesthesia benefit from low-tidal-volume ventilation strategies. The use of inhaled bronchodilators more than three times a day in patients with chronic lung disease warrants the preoperative addition of maintenance medications.

Table 1.3 Perioperative pulmonary risk mitigation strategies

Low risk of PPC	Intermediate risk of PPC	High risk of PPC
Early mobilization	All of low maneuvers, plus:	All of low and intermediate maneuvers, plus:
Good oral hygiene	Postoperative incentive spirometry	1–2 weeks of preoperative incentive spirometry
Optimization of chronic lung disease	Identification and communication of "increased risk" status	Increased postoperative surveillance
Smoking cessation counseling and resources	Regional anesthesia/analgesia, if applicable	
	Lung-protective ventilation	

Source: Used with permission from Pfeifer, K. *Guide to Preoperative Evaluation.* www .preopevalguide.com, 2020.

Tobacco, Marijuana, and Vaping Use

Smoking within 1 year of surgery is associated with increased postoperative complications, including poor wound healing, increased healthcare costs, increased hospitalization, and higher utilization of healthcare resources. Preoperative smoking cessation reduces the incidence of these complications and, when maintained long term, improves population health in general. Each week of smoking cessation before surgery decreases the complication risk by 19%, and cessation of one year or more reduces PPC risk to that of a nonsmoker [10]. Preoperative smoking cessation counseling and nicotine replacement therapy increase the likelihood of long-term abstinence. Like the use of traditional tobacco, chronic marijuana use results in similar long-term effects to cigarette use. Preoperative abstinence, comparable to that seen with smoking cessation, leads to a reduction in the risk of adverse outcomes.

There has been an increase in the usage of electronic (e-)cigarettes in recent years. While e-cigarettes do not contain the harmful combustion by-products of traditional cigarettes, they contain toxic solvents, such as glycerol and propylene glycol, and chemical flavorings. Vaping by patients undergoing plastic surgery exhibited an increased risk of skin flap necrosis and death. Perioperative vaping instructions and cessation efforts are identical to those for tobacco users.

Pulmonary Hypertension

The preoperative preparation of patients with pulmonary hypertension is a multidisciplinary effort critical to a good outcome for these patients. It focuses on determining the severity of the disease and the adequacy of physiologic and pharmacologic compensation. All pulmonary hypertension medications continue throughout the day of surgery, including diuretics, angiotensin-converting enzyme inhibitors (ACEIs), and sildenafil, to prevent acute decompensation. Laboratory studies are indicated, based on patient physical status and medication management. An electrocardiogram identifies right ventricular hypertrophy and evidence of right heart strain, and recent echocardiography assesses right ventricular function and pulmonary artery pressures. Evidence of right ventricular failure warrants case delay for further medical management.

Obstructive Sleep Apnea

Patients with obstructive sleep apnea (OSA) have a two- to fourfold higher risk of perioperative complications than patients without OSA. Respiratory complications, such as desaturation and respiratory failure, are the most common. Undiagnosed severe OSA is significantly associated with an increased risk of 30-day postoperative cardiovascular complications [11]. Other perioperative complications include difficulty with airway management, cardiovascular complications, and postoperative delirium, all leading to higher resource utilization. Given the increasing prevalence and associated perioperative risks of OSA, the Society of Anesthesia and Sleep Medicine recommends screening all presurgical patients for OSA.

The STOP-Bang questionnaire is the best-validated tool for preoperative screening for OSA. Patients with zero to two positive responses are considered low risk; those with three or four are at intermediate risk, and those with ≥5 positive responses are at high risk of having OSA. An elevated serum bicarbonate increases the specificity of intermediate STOP-Bang scores. A high risk score of 5–8 was associated with an increased cardiovascular risk following surgery and intensive care unit (ICU) readmission. In contrast, a moderate risk score of 3 or 4 was associated with an increased risk of ICU readmission and wound infection. Most patients with known or suspected OSA may proceed to surgery without additional testing or treatment for OSA. However, select patients benefit from surgical delay for formal diagnosis by sleep study and for initiation of therapy or treatment optimization. Patients requiring further testing or treatment optimization are delayed at least one week for acclimation to the continuous positive airway pressure (CPAP) device or adjusted settings. Patients on CPAP therapy for OSA should continue treatment up to the day of surgery and bring their CPAP or other treatment devices on the day of surgery, including controllers for hypoglossal nerve stimulators.

Frailty

Although frailty is independent of chronological age, it is more prevalent in the geriatric population. Frailty is defined as a decrease in physiologic reserve exceeding that expected from advanced age alone and presents with an increased vulnerability to stressors. Sarcopenia, characterized by a decline in functional capacity with low muscle mass and strength, is a significant component of frailty. Sarcopenia measurement by preoperative grip strength, gait speed, or chair stand test provides an accurate diagnosis of the severity of frailty [12]. Frailty predicts postoperative mortality and morbidity, including delirium, increased hospital stay, discharge to a skilled nursing facility, cognitive impairment, and functional decline [13]. The preoperative evaluation of elderly patients requiring elective major surgery should include a frailty screen. Most assessment tools involve scoring based on specific comorbidities, dependence on others for daily living activities, malnutrition, and dementia, rather than on physical assessment alone. There are several validated frailty screening tools, such as the FRAIL scale (detailed in Table 1.4), but few methods of objective measurement. FRAIL scale scores range from zero to 5, and a score of zero represents robust health status and 1–2 a prefrail state, and 3–5 is consistent with frailty. A positive frailty screen is an indication for a comprehensive evaluation and

Table 1.4 The FRAIL scale

Description	Question	Score
Fatigue	"Have you felt fatigued for most or all of the time over the past month?"	Yes = 1 No = 0
Resistance	"Do you have difficulty climbing a flight of stairs?"	Yes = 1 No = 0
Ambulation	"Do you have difficulty walking one block?"	Yes = 1 No = 0
Illness	"Do you have any of these illnesses: hypertension, diabetes, cancer, chronic lung disease, heart attack, congestive heart failure, angina, asthma, arthritis, stroke, and kidney disease?"	≥5 illnesses = 1 <5 illnesses = 0
Loss of weight	"Have you lost more than 5% of your weight in the past year?"	Yes = 1 No = 0

Source: Morely, JE, Malmstrom, TK, Miller, DK. A simple frailty questionnaire (FRAIL) predicted outcomes in middle aged African Americans. *J Nutr Health Aging*. 2012;16(7):-601–8.

intervention by a geriatric medicine specialist. Identification of preoperative frailty informs patient and family discussions and decision-making regarding surgical techniques and alternative treatments, postoperative recovery strategies, and expected outcomes. The prognosis of frail patients improves with shared decision-making, prehabilitation, and interdisciplinary geriatric co-management [14].

Malnutrition

Preoperative malnutrition leads to immune system dysfunction and contributes to several adverse surgical outcomes, including increased susceptibility to wound infection, cognitive dysfunction, and poor wound healing. Patients with preoperative hypoalbuminemia, either alone or associated with chronic liver disease or congestive heart failure, are more likely to have postoperative complications such as infections, organ dysfunction, increased duration of mechanical ventilation and ICU stay, and mortality. BMI is not an accurate assessment of nutritional status.

Various screening tools exist to identify malnutrition preoperatively. The Nestlé Mini Nutritional Assessment Short Form (MNA-SF) is a validated screening tool which evaluates predictive parameters such as recent oral intake, weight loss, mobility, psychological stress, and neuropsychological problems, in addition to BMI or calf circumference. The sensitivity and specificity of the MNA-SF is 97.9% and 100%, with a diagnostic accuracy of 99% for predicting undernutrition [15]. The MNA-SF is easy to use and efficient, and minimally impacts workflow. A numerical score identifies patients as malnourished, at risk of malnutrition, or of normal nutritional status. Preoperative nutritional optimization includes supplementation with protein or immunonutrient solutions containing arginine and omega fatty acids. Benefits of preoperative dietary supplementation include reduced hospital stays, reduced need for critical care, and reduced postoperative infections, including pulmonary and surgical site infections in patients undergoing gastrointestinal cancer surgery [16]. The Enhanced Recovery After Surgery (ERAS) Society strongly encourages complex carbohydrate loading before surgery, which reduces postoperative insulin resistance and length of stay.

Anemia

Anemia is not merely an independent predictor of adverse perioperative outcomes; it is a potent risk multiplier. The preoperative presence of anemia augments the inherent mortality risk of coexisting diseases, such as chronic kidney disease (CKD) and congestive heart failure. Anemia is widespread in surgical patients, with a reported incidence of up to 76%. Frequently, the anemia is undiagnosed. Consequently, anemia identified on preoperative evaluation is often ignored and accepted as a harmless deviation. Not only is anemia a modifiable preoperative condition, but it is also associated with decreased survival and higher rates of hospitalization, and is one of the strongest predictors of perioperative blood transfusions, an individual risk profile. A preoperative hemoglobin level <6 g/dL increases the risk of death at 30 days 26-fold, compared to a hemoglobin level of 12 g/dL [17].

Iron deficiency is the most common cause of anemia and results from malabsorption or nutritional deficiency, or is medication-related. Oral iron supplementation initiated 4–6 weeks before a scheduled surgery generally results in an increase in reticulocyte count within 7–14 days and an increase in hemoglobin level of about 2 g/dL within 3 weeks. Patients who do not respond to oral iron or who are noncompliant due to gastrointestinal disturbance are candidates for intravenous iron therapy. Intravenous iron results in hemoglobin increases of $0.5–1.0$ g dL^{-1} per week. The use of erythrocyte-stimulating factors concurrently with intravenous iron results in an even greater response, but has an increased incidence of venous thromboembolism. Other nutritional causes of anemia, such as vitamin B12 and folate deficiencies, are easily correctable with over-the-counter supplementation. Preoperative consultation with a hematologist helps manage other identified forms of anemia, such as hemolytic or anemia of chronic inflammation. Intravenous iron initiated after surgery does not reduce the incidence of a perioperative blood transfusion but does reduce the 30-day transfusion incidence.

Cognitive Dysfunction

Many geriatric patients present for surgery with cognitive impairment predisposing them to preventable adverse outcomes, such as delirium, falls, pneumonia, urinary tract infections, functional decline, and increased mortality. Cognitive impairment describes a patient's current state, and usually presents as confusion, memory loss, decreased attention, disorientation, and mood changes. Dementia and delirium are the two most common forms of cognitive impairment, and Table 1.5 differentiates one from the other. Patients with preexisting dementia have an increased incidence of early postoperative mortality.

Approximately one-third of hospitalized elderly patients experience delirium. Routine preoperative screening for cognitive impairment identifies at-risk patients and allows appropriate referral to a neurologist or geriatric medicine specialist. The six-item screen, noted in Table 1.6, is a brief screening tool for identifying patients with cognitive impairment by testing attention, short-term memory, and orientation. Its reliability is comparable to the full Mini-Mental State Examination. A score of 2 or higher suggests cognitive impairment and the need for further evaluation.

Table 1.5 Characteristics of dementia and delirium

	Dementia	Delirium
Duration	Chronic, progressive condition	Hours to weeks
Onset	Chronic onset	Acute onset
Attention	Generally normal	Impaired or fluctuating
Memory	Long- and short-term memory impairment	Recent and immediate memory impairment
Alertness	Generally normal	Lethargic to hypervigilant
Thought pattern	Word-finding difficulty; poor judgment	Disorganized thinking; slow or accelerated thoughts

Source: Adapted from: Agency for Clinical Innovation 2018. www.ausmed.com/cpd/articles/cognitive-impairment.

Table 1.6 Six-item screen for cognitive impairment

Did the patient correctly answer the questions below?	Yes	No
	Correct	Incorrect
What year is this?	0	1
What month is this?	0	1
What day of the week is this?	0	1
What were the three objects you were asked to remember?		
Apple	0	1
Table	0	1
Car	0	1
Total		

Diabetes

An overwhelming quantity of literature establishes a clear correlation between perioperative hyperglycemia and adverse surgical outcomes, including increased surgical site infections and mortality. The risk of postoperative complications and death is a function of both long-term glycemic control and the short-term severity of hyperglycemia on admission. Diabetic patients, particularly those requiring insulin management, undergoing major vascular surgery have a higher incidence of perioperative death and cardiovascular complications. Neither diabetes managed with insulin nor that managed with oral medications independently predicts mortality. Significant risk factors for death include several diabetes comorbidities, such as proteinuria, elevated creatinine level, history of congestive heart failure, and stroke. After adjusting for comorbidities, diabetic patients have a 38% or higher increase in hospital length of stay [18]. Preoperative risk stratification involves a basic metabolic panel within 6 months of the scheduled surgery, or more recent, depending on patient status. A hemoglobin A1c (Hgb A1c) level indicates long-term glucose control over the preceding 2–3 months, but there is no clear delineation of the level above which elective surgery should not occur. The ability of a preoperative Hgb A1c to predict surgical site infections remains controversial, but many orthopedic departments utilize a 7.0–8.5% range, above which elective surgery is delayed. Fructosamine levels are an alternative to Hgb A1c and provide an indication of glucose control over the past 2–3 weeks. Some literature suggests that fructosamine levels are a more significant predictor of adverse outcomes in orthopedic surgery than Hgb A1c. Fructosamine is useful for assessing glucose control in conditions where Hgb A1c is unreliable, such as end-stage renal disease (ESRD) and chronic hemolytic anemia.

Chronic Kidney Disease

The preoperative management of the spectrum of CKD, further detailed in Table 1.7, requires consideration of the disease process and comorbidities, such as cardiovascular dysfunction, anemia, and electrolyte disorders. These coexisting diseases confer significant perioperative risk. Of primary concern is the independent association with underlying coronary artery disease. Objective assessment of functional capacity with DASI and adherence to the American College of Cardiology (ACC)/American Heart Association (AHA) perioperative guidelines aid in risk assessment. ACEIs, angiotensin receptor blockers (ARBs), and diuretics are customarily held before surgery unless indicated for heart failure or volume

Table 1.7 Stages of chronic kidney disease

Stage of chronic kidney disease	Signs and symptoms	Percentage of normal kidney function (estimated GFR)
1	No symptoms, but coexisting disease present (diabetes, hypertension, obesity)	≥90% (normal or increased GFR)
2	No symptoms, but proteinuria present	60–89% (mildly reduced GFR)
3	Edema, fatigue, microalbuminuria, back pain	30–59% (moderately reduced GFR)
4	Stage 3 symptoms plus nausea, vomiting, neuropathy, and loss of appetite	15–29% (severely reduced GFR)
5	Stage 4 symptoms plus fatigue, weakness, anemia, thirst, cramps, skin discoloration, little to no urine output, and easy bruising/bleeding	<15% (kidney failure; dialysis dependent)

GFR, glomerular filtration rate.

overload. All other cardiovascular medications should continue as usual. ESRD patients have a high incidence of coexisting structural heart disease, and both right and left ventricular dysfunction are associated with poor outcomes and death. An echocardiogram obtained within the previous year is useful for risk stratification. Despite a high prevalence of coronary artery disease, many CKD patients are asymptomatic and have adequate functional capacity. An objective assessment of cardiac function, such as dobutamine stress echocardiography, identifies undiagnosed cardiovascular disease and allows for preoperative risk mitigation. CKD is associated with excess surgical morbidity, including acute renal failure, hyperkalemia, volume overload, and infections. Patients with ESRD have an adjusted all-cause mortality rate at least 10-fold higher than that of nonESRD patients.

Decreased renal production of erythropoietin leads to anemia. The National Kidney Foundation suggests optimizing preoperative hemoglobin level to $11–12$ g dL^{-1} with oral or intravenous iron and erythropoietin-stimulating agents. Hemodialysis, preferably on the day before surgery, corrects electrolyte abnormalities and platelet dysfunction. While there is no established upper limit for hyperkalemia, with differences in institutional policy and patient tolerance, a preoperative basic or comprehensive metabolic profile detects potassium and other electrolyte abnormalities.

Summary and Conclusion

Preoperative evaluation and optimization are an opportunity for anesthesia providers to enhance patient safety and outcomes and to create value in healthcare through the identification, risk stratification, and mitigation of modifiable risk factors. A systems-based, collaborative approach and application of high-yield preoperative interventions on modifiable risk factors integrate the quadruple aim of improved outcomes, improved clinical and patient experiences, and reduction in healthcare costs.

Review Questions

1. Which New York Heart Association (NYHA) class is assigned a patient with a history of heart failure who has slight limitation of physical activity and is comfortable at rest, but experiences dyspnea, palpitations, or fatigue with ordinary physical activity?

    (a) Class I
    (b) Class II
    (c) Class III
    (d) Class IV

2. Which of the following is a risk prediction tool commonly used to identify patients at risk of postoperative pulmonary complications?

   (a) Six-item screen
   (b) NSQIP surgical risk calculator
   (c) ARISCAT Risk Index
   (d) FRAIL scale

3. Which of the following is a patient risk factor for the development of postoperative pulmonary complications?

   (a) Poor functional capacity/frailty
   (b) Emergency surgical procedure
   (c) Surgery lasting >2 hours
   (d) Receipt of a perioperative blood transfusion

4. Which of the following laboratory tests is useful for assessing glycemic control over the preceding 2–3 weeks in end-stage renal disease (ESRD) patients?

   (a) Hemoglobin A1c
   (b) Comprehensive metabolic profile
   (c) Fructosamine
   (d) Phenylpropanolamine

Answers

1 (b)   A patient with a history of heart failure who experiences slight limitation of physical activity with dyspnea, palpitations, or fatigue on ordinary activity is assigned NYHA class II.

2 (c)   The ARISCAT Risk Index is a risk prediction tool used to identify patients at risk of postoperative pulmonary complications and to guide perioperative optimization strategies.

3 (a)   Poor functional capacity/frailty is a patient risk factor for postoperative pulmonary complications. The other choices are surgical risk factors.

4 (c)   Fructosamine levels assess glycemic control over the preceding 2–3 weeks, whereas hemoglobin A1c assesses glycemic control over the previous 2–3 months. Fructosamine levels give a more reliable estimation in patients with conditions such as ESRD and chronic hemolytic anemia.

References

1. Gupta S, Fernandes RJ, Rao JS, Dhanpal R. Perioperative risk factors for pulmonary complications after non-cardiac surgery. *J Anaesthesiol Clin Pharmacol*. 2020;36 (1):88–93.

2. Aronson S, Murray S, Martin G, *et al*. Roadmap for transforming preoperative assessment to preoperative optimization. *Anes Analg*. 2020;130(4):811–19.

3. Knuf KM, Maani CV, Cummings AK. Clinical agreement in the American Society of Anesthesiologists physical status classification. *Perioper Med*. 2018;7(14):1–6.

4. Fleisher LA, Fleischmann KE, Auerbach AD, *et al*. 2014 ACC/AHA guideline on perioperative cardiovascular evaluation and management of patients undergoing noncardiac surgery: a report of the American College of Cardiology/American Heart Association Task Force on Practice Guidelines. *Circulation*. 2014;130(24): e278.

5. Wijeysundera DN, Pearse RM, Shulman MA, *et al*. Assessment of functional capacity before major non-cardiac surgery: an international, prospective cohort study. *Lancet*. 2018;391(10140):2631.

6. Wijeysundera DN, Beattie WS, Hillis GS, *et al*. Integration of the Duke Activity Status Index into preoperative risk evaluation: a multicentre prospective cohort study. *Br J Anaesth*. 2020;124(3):261.

7. Dakik HA, Chehab O, Eldirani M, *et al*. A new index for preoperative cardiovascular evaluation. *J Am Coll Cardiol*. 2019;73(24):3067–78.

8. Smith BB, Warner MA, Warner NS, *et al*. Cardiac risk of noncardiac surgery after percutaneous coronary intervention with second-generation drug-eluting stents. *Anesth Analg*. 2019;128(4):621.

9. Tan CW, Wall M, Rosengart TK, *et al*. How to bridge? Management of anti-coagulation in patients with mechanical heart valves undergoing noncardiac surgical procedures. *J Thorac Cardiovasc Surg*.2019;158:200–3.

10. Quan H, Ouyang L, Zhou H, *et al*. The effect of preoperative smoking cessation and smoking dose on postoperative complications following radical gastrectomy for gastric cancer: a retrospective study of 2469 patients. *World J Surg Oncol*. 2019;17(61):1–11.

11. Chan MTV, Wang CY, Seet E, *et al*. Association of unrecognized obstructive sleep apnea with postoperative cardiovascular events in patients undergoing major noncardiac surgery. *JAMA*. 2019;321(18):1788–98.

12. Dalton A, Zafirova Z. Preoperative management of the geriatric patient: fralty and cognitive impairment assessment. *Anesthesiol Clin*. 2018;36(4):599–614.

13. Kim SW, Han HS, Jung HW, *et al*. Multidimensional frailty score for the prediction of postoperative mortality risk. *JAMA Surg*. 2014;149(7):633–40.

14. Alvarez-Nebreda ML, Bentov N, Urman RD, *et al*. Recommendations for preoperative management of frailty from the Society for Perioperative Assessment and Quality Improvement (SPAQI). *J Clin Anesth*. 2018;47:33–42.

15. Mays LC, Drummonds JW, Powers S, *et al*. Identifying geriatric patients at risk for malnutrition: a quality improvement project. *J Nutr Gerontol Geriatr*. 2019;38 (2):115–29.

16. Zhang B, Najarali Z, Ruo L, *et al*. Effect of perioperative nutritional supplementation on postoperative complications – systematic review and meta-analysis. *J Gastrointest Surg*. 2019;23:1682–93.

17. Kumar A. Perioperative management of anemia: limits of blood transfusion and alternatives. *Cleve Clin J Med*. 2009;76(4):S112–18.

18. Axelrod DA, Upchurch GA, DeMonner S, *et al*. Perioperative cardiovascular risk stratification of patients with diabetes who undergo elective major vascular surgery. *J Vasc Surg*. 2002;35:894–901.

Chapter

2

Airway Management

Chikezie N. Okeagu, Madelyn K. Craig,
Brook Girma, Sumitra Miriyala, Meeta
M. Sheth, Sridhar R. Tirumala, Rhian E.
Germany, and Alan David Kaye

Introduction

Airway management is a vital component of administering anesthesia, allowing for the exchange of gases between the patient and the surrounding atmosphere. Difficult or unsuccessful management of the airway is a significant source of anesthesia-related morbidity and mortality [1]. As such, it is important for anesthesia providers to be adept at all aspects of managing the airway. A thorough understanding of the pertinent anatomy and physiology, the ability to use clinical evaluation to identify potential difficulties, and a mastery of interventional techniques and procedures are crucial to safe and effective airway management. This chapter presents a comprehensive overview of the elements related to effective airway management.

Airway Anatomy

Respiration is a complex process that involves the exchange of gases and the breakdown of glucose to yield energy [1]. Understanding the anatomy of the airway is important when performing intubation. The airway can be divided into multiple subsections: the nasal cavity, oral cavity, and pharynx. The pharynx is further divided into the nasopharynx, oral pharynx, and hypopharynx, running from superior to inferior. The nasal cavity consists of the nares, septum, and turbinates (superior, middle, and cheap). It is bound superiorly by the ethmoid bone. It is continuous posteriorly with the nasopharynx (the most prominent portion of the pharynx). The oral cavity consists of the upper/lower rows of teeth, the tongue, hard palate, and soft palate, and is continuous posteriorly with the oropharynx. The oropharynx stretches down to the epiglottis (the cartilaginous structure that serves as a flap to cover the trachea or esophagus). The hypopharynx runs from the epiglottis down to the superior edge of the trachea. This is the region where the vocal cords will be visualized (along with the larynx region). These lie at around the level of the thyroid cartilage. Breathing, or ventilation, is the process of conducting air to and from the lungs. Simultaneously, gaseous exchange is the diffusion of oxygen into the blood vessels and the removal of carbon dioxide and other gases into the air [2]. The respiratory tract organs form a continuous passage for air, and they are divided into upper and lower airways.

The lower airways include the trachea, bronchi, bronchioles, and alveoli. Their primary function is to facilitate the movement of air between the lungs and the atmosphere. The *trachea* is a hollow tube supported by cartilage. It begins from the larynx and branches into the bronchi. The cartilage helps to ensure that it does not collapse or overexpand. The *bronchi* branch from the trachea and subdivide into bronchioles. They serve as passages for bringing air in and out of the lungs. Unlike the trachea and bronchi, the *bronchioles* do not have cartilage and their diameter is much smaller [3]. They are ciliated and have a simple epithelium with mucus-secreting cells. The final portion of the lower airway is made of the alveoli, single-cell layered and near the capillaries. They facilitate the actual exchange of gases in the lungs. The general function of the airway is to allow for airflow to facilitate gaseous exchange, which is essential for respiration. However, they perform other functions to maintain adequate protection and homeostasis. They serve as moisture barriers to prevent loss of excessive moisture through humidification of air. They work as temperature barriers by warming the air from the environment as it gets into the airways. Finally, they work as barriers to infection, primarily through the mucosa-associated lymphoid tissue (MALT).

From the base of the trachea, the airways branch into the right and left sides. Two bronchi further divide into lobar (secondary) bronchi, which in turn divide into segmental (tertiary) bronchi that eventually form the bronchioles [4]. The right- and left-sided airways connect to the respective lungs. The branching of the airways into the left and right sides forms an extensive pulmonary tree. The right lung is broader and shorter, whereas the left lung is thinner and longer. The reason why the right lung is shorter is because the liver rests beneath it. On the other hand, the left lung has to make room for the heart, hence is narrower.

The right lung refers to the right side of the pair of lungs at the front of the thoracic cavity, whereas the left side is known as the left lung. One of the key differences is the number of lobes, with the right lung having three (superior, middle, and inferior). By contrast, the left lung has only two lobes (upper and lower). There is a thick cardiac notch at the left lung, making it distinct, although it does not serve any role in the right lung. Finally, the left lung has a horizontal and an oblique fissure, whereas the left has only the oblique fissure.

These different upper airway areas are innervated differently by branches and terminal ends of some cranial nerves. The primary nerves that give sensation to the airway are the trigeminal nerve (CN V), the glossopharyngeal nerve (CN IX), and the vagus nerve (CN X). The trigeminal nerve is almost exclusively a cranial sensory nerve and gives off three main branches: ophthalmic (V1), maxillary (V2), and mandibular (V3). The ophthalmic nerve and its smaller branches provide sensory innervation to the superior region of the internal nasal cavity. Many internal components supply the medial and lateral parts of the ethmoidal area and the superior nares. The maxillary nerve provides sensory innervation to the inferior nasal region, nasal septum, and soft palate in the oral cavity. It also provides some innervation to the external nasal area via the infraorbital nerve (one of the terminal branches of the maxillary nerve). The pterygopalatine ganglion lies in between the palatine and maxilla bones, receives fibers from the maxillary nerve, and then sends smaller components out (nasopalatine, greater/lesser palatine, etc.). Remember, the nasopalatine nerve comes from the pterygo-palatine ganglion, runs along inside the nasal septum mucosa, dives through the incisive canal, and terminates in the anterior hard palate. Finally, the mandibular nerve gives sensation to the anterior two-thirds via the lingual nerve [5].

The posterior one-third of the tongue and posterior pharyngeal mucosa (down to the aryepiglottic fold level) receive sensory innervation from the glossopharyngeal nerve. This nerve also provides fibers to the dense pharyn geal nerve plexus, which innervates the palatopharyngeal arch. The pharyn-geal nerve plexus receives some glossopharyngeal nerve fibers. However, the plexus is mainly made up of motor fibers from the vagus nerve. The vagus nerve mediates sensory innervation to the larynx and laryngopharynx, and gives rise to the superior laryngeal nerve. The superior laryngeal nerve branches into the internal and external. The inner laryngeal nerves provide sensory innervation to the epiglottic region's mucosa, extending to the level of the vocal folds. Below the vocal folds, sensory *and* motor innervation is supplied by the left and right recurrent laryngeal nerves (also branches of the vagus). Therefore, they innervate all the larynx's intrinsic muscles (sparing the cricothyroid muscle, which is innervated by the external laryngeal nerve). All of these innervations are important for airway management when per-forming intubation because the endotracheal (ET) tube will pass through most, if not all, of these regions to end up in the trachea to provide oxygena-tion to the lungs [5].

During routine intubation, the blade should move the patient's tongue out of the visual field to directly see the vocal cords. The vocal cords are the most medial. They connect to the cricoid cartilage anteriorly, and posteriorly to the arytenoid cartilage on the larynx's posterior edge. Visualization of the ET tube moving midline through the cords should give successful intubation. The ET tube was kept in place just superior to the carina level (e.g., bifurcation of the trachea into the two primary bronchi). Although adult and pediatric patients have all of the same airway structures, there can be differences in length, size, and width. In pediatric patients, note the prominent occiput will cause neck flexion in the supine position, so a towel should be placed under the shoulders to keep a direct airway ready for intubation. The hypopharynx will also be shorter and narrower than in an adult – the cricoid cartilage resting higher at the C4 vertebra (the adult cricoid cartilage is at C6).

Additionally, the pediatric vocal cords are not at a 90-degree angle to the larynx wall as the adult vocal cords are. The pediatric cords slope downwards anteriorly, providing difficulty with the tube rubbing against the cords and possibly causing trauma. Lastly, the epiglottis in a pediatric patient is not as flat as in an adult, presenting problems with using a Macintosh blade instead of a Miller blade. Some physicians prefer the Miller blade during pediatric intubation because it has a better shape to move the pediatric epiglottis out of the visual field, compared to a curved Macintosh blade [5].

Airway Assessment

Airway Assessment

A thorough assessment of the patient's airway should be conducted in the preoperative setting. This consists of obtaining a history of any previous airway instrumentation, reviewing the patient's medical record, with particular attention to previous anesthesia and/or intubations, and noting any disease states that may have implications on airway management. Typically, patients who have presented difficulties with airway management have been informed of this and/or documentation of such can be found in the patient's medical record. The medical record may also contain information regarding which techniques were used in order to successfully manage the airway [6].

A comprehensive history should be accompanied by a physical examination, with the aim of identifying features that may portend difficulty with airway management. Examination of the mouth opening, dentition, oropharyngeal space, submandibular compliance, cervical spine mobility, and body habitus can all help stratify the risk of difficult airway management, and several tools exist to assist in this assessment. The sensitivity and specificity of any single one of these tools are low. However, when used in combination, they can be helpful in predicting which patients may present difficulty in airway management. The Mallampati test is used to evaluate the oropharyngeal space. It consists of visual examination of the oropharyngeal space. A "Mallampati score" is derived based upon which structures are visible in the patient's mouth. To properly administer the test, the observer should be at eye level, with the patient holding the head in a neutral position, opening the mouth maximally, and protruding the tongue without phonating. The Mallampati classification is as follows:

- I: The soft palate, fauces, uvula, and tonsillar pillars are visible.
- II: The soft palate, fauces, and uvula are visible.

- III: The soft palate and base of the uvula are visible.
- IV: The soft palate is not visible [6].

The mnemonic *PUSH* (tonsillar *P*illars, *U*vula, *S*oft palate, *H*ard palate) is often used to remember the Mallampati score. A patient with a Mallampati score of I has all four elements of PUSH visible on examination, whereas a patient with a Mallampati score of IV has only the hard palate visible. A Mallampati score of III or IV correlates with difficult laryngoscopy. Mouth opening is assessed by measurement of the interincisor distance – that is, the distance between the upper and lower incisors. An interincisor distance of <3–4.5 cm correlates with difficult laryngoscopy. Patients with overbites have a reduced effective interincisor distance and therefore may present difficulties with laryngoscopy. The upper lip bite test (ULBT) is also used to predict ease of laryngoscopy and intubation. The ULBT assesses an individual's mandibular prognathic ability. The ULBT is broken down into three classes. Patients who fall in Class III of the ULBT may present difficulty with laryngoscopy and intubation:

- Class I: The lower incisors can bite above the vermilion border of the upper lip.
- Class II: The lower incisors cannot reach the vermilion border.
- Class III: The lower incisors cannot bite the upper lip.

As the soft tissues of the pharynx are displaced into the submandibular space during laryngoscopy, anything that limits the size or compliance of the submandibular space can make laryngoscopy and intubation more challenging. The thyromental distance, which is the distance between the tip of the jaw and the thyroid cartilage, can also be informative. A distance less than three fingerbreadths or of 6–7 cm correlates with difficult laryngoscopy. Difficulty with neck extension and certain physical features, such as obesity and increased neck circumference, also indicate a potential difficult airway [6].

Predictors of Difficult Intubation/Ventilation

The purpose of conducting a thorough preoperative history and physical examination is to identify patients with potential difficult airways and formulate a plan for successful management. The unanticipated difficult airway must be avoided at all costs. A number of congenital and acquired conditions are associated with difficult airway management. Table 2.1 outlines factors that are associated with difficult ventilation and/or intubation. It should be noted that factors that are associated with difficult intubation are not always also associated with difficult ventilation. The reverse is also true.

Table 2.1 Factors associated with difficult ventilation and intubation

Predictors of difficult ventilation	Predictors of difficult intubation
Edentulous	History of difficult intubation
History of snoring	Prognathic inability
Macroglossia	Limited neck range of motion
Micrognathia	Long incisors
Uvula not visible	Mallampati class III or IV
Obesity	Mandibular space stiff, indurated, or occupied
Obstructive sleep apnea	Mouth opening <3–4 cm
Presence of beard	Uvula not visible
Short neck	Obesity
Thick neck	Prominent overbite
	Thyromental distance <6 cm
	Short neck
	Thick neck

Physiology of Airway Management

Preoxygenation

Prior to any intubation, it is important to practice clinical fundamentals of management of the airway with preoxygenation. If possible, preoxygenation with oxygen via face mask should be initiated prior to all airway management interventions or anesthetic induction. Nitrogen makes up about 80% of the concentration in the lung. During preoxygenation, or denitrogenation, the functional residual capacity (FRC) is purged of nitrogen and filled with oxygen, increasing the duration of apnea without desaturation. The four maximal breath technique of preoxygenation was found to be associated with a statistically significant shorter time to onset of oxygen desaturation of blood, when compared to normal breathing of 100% oxygen for 3 minutes [7]. A healthy patient breathing room air will experience desaturation of <90%, with apnea within 1–2 minutes versus up to 8 minutes following preoxygenation. Goals for preoxygenation include: bringing the patient's saturation as close to 100% as possible; denitrogenating the residual capacity of the lungs (maximizing oxygen storage in the lungs); and denitrogenating and maximally oxygenating the bloodstream [8]. Utilizing this technique to achieve the goals mentioned will increase the duration of safe apnea, as oxygen is poorly soluble, and can provide preferable conditions for intubation.

Apneic Preoxygenation

The process by which gases are entrained into the alveolar space during apnea is referred to as apneic preoxygenation. Since oxygen enters blood from the alveoli at a faster rate than carbon dioxide leaving blood, a negative pressure is generated in the alveolus, driving oxygen into the lungs. This method extends the duration of safe apnea after the use of sedatives and muscle relaxants.

Airway Reflexes

Laryngoscopy and tracheal intubation directly stimulate airway reflexes that may elicit protective responses to this stimulation, leading to hypertension and tachycardia. This is commonly seen in a pediatric setting or "light" planes of anesthesia. In the larynx, glottic stimulation, innervated by the superior laryngeal nerve, causes closure of the distal airways, leading to glottic closure to prevent aspiration. When exaggerated, this response can lead to complete glottic closure, and consequently impending respiratory collapse. If laryngospasm occurs and persists, positive pressure ventilation or small doses of succinylcholine may be required to abate this response. However, in certain cases, the spasm is sustained as long as the stimulus continues, and morbidity, such as cardiac arrest, arrhythmia, pulmonary edema, bronchospasm, or gastric aspiration, may occur [9]. Bronchospasm, a reflex more commonly seen in asthmatics, tends to also occur in pediatric patients and those under "light" planes of anesthesia. This response may also be an indicator of bronchial intubation. Aside from respiratory reflexes, intubation may cause an increase in intracranial or intraocular pressure, primarily due to a sympathetic surge.

Aspiration Risk and Ways to Minimize the Risk

Intraoperative pulmonary aspiration, a rare anesthesia-related complication, is associated with potentially fatal complications with significant associated morbidity. Awareness of the risk factors, predisposing conditions, maneuvers to decrease risk, and immediate management options by both the surgeon and the anesthesia team is imperative to reducing risk and optimizing patient outcomes associated with acute intraoperative pulmonary aspiration [10].

Risk factors include, but are not limited to: obesity; medications that reduce lower esophageal tone; gastrointestinal (GI) obstruction; need for emergency surgery; nasogastric tube placement; meal within 8 hours prior to surgery; previous esophageal surgery; lack of coordination of swallowing or respiration; esophageal cancer; hiatal hernia; patient positioning; and provider factors. Assessing preoperative risk factors may assist in planning preventative measures and minimize the risk of intraoperative pulmonary aspiration. The first step in successful management of an intraoperative aspiration is immediate recognition of gastric content in the oropharynx or airways [10]. Signs of aspiration include persistent hypoxia, high airway pressures, bronchospasm, and abnormal breath sounds following intubation. It is important to suction the airway prior to positive pressure ventilation and to position the patient with the head down and rotated laterally if possible. If the patient is not intubated, it is recommended that the airway be secured as rapidly as possible to prevent further aspiration and facilitate airway clearance.

Airway Management Techniques

Mask Ventilation

Mask ventilation is fundamental to the practice of anesthesia. This most basic skill is one of the most important tools in airway management. It is performed prior to ET intubation and used as a rescue maneuver if intubation is difficult or fails. Obtaining a tight seal with the face mask is an important aspect of successful mask ventilation. The face mask should fit over the bridge of the nose and enclose the mouth, with the bottom positioned between the lower lip and the chin. Leaks may develop if the mask is not of the correct size, the cushion is improperly inflated, or the patient has a beard or an abnormal anatomy. Risk factors for difficult mask ventilation include presence of a beard, increased body mass index (BMI), edentulousness, limited mandibular protrusion, Mallampati score III or IV, history of snoring or obstructive sleep apnea (OSA), airway masses or tumors, history of neck radiation, male gender, and age >55. In order to maximize pharyngeal patency, the triple maneuver (jaw thrust, head extension, and chin lift) should be used. Once the triple maneuver is performed, the left hand holds this position, with the mask sealed tightly to the face, while the right hand squeezes the reservoir bag. If maintaining the triple maneuver position or an adequate seal with one hand proves difficult, the two-handed mask ventilation technique should be utilized and a second provider assists ventilation with the bag. An oral or nasal airway may be required to overcome obstruction resulting from the tongue falling back to the posterior pharyngeal wall. It is important to note that using an oral airway may elicit a gag reflex or cause laryngospasm if the depth of anesthesia is inadequate. A nasal airway is better tolerated in these situations. Ventilating pressure should not exceed 20 cmH$_2$O to avoid gastric distension, regurgitation, and aspiration. If mask ventilation proves difficult or impossible, alternative strategies to ventilate the patient must be attempted, such as intubation or placement of a supraglottic airway [11, 12].

Supraglottic Airways

Supraglottic airway (SGA) devices are an alternative method to mask ventilation and ET intubation, and have made their way into the difficult airway algorithm with their ease of use and rescue ventilation ability. Quick placement, less sympathetic stimulation, avoidance of neuromuscular blockers, and maintenance of spontaneous ventilation are a few advantages of using SGAs over ET tubes. SGAs may be used as primary airway devices for selected patients and surgeries, in emergency situations in and out of the hospital, to facilitate ET intubation, and most importantly for airway rescue in the unable-to-ventilate-or-intubate situation. Nonfasting status, morbid obesity, and pregnancy are contraindications for laryngeal mask airway (LMA) use as the primary airway. OSA, gastro-esophageal reflux disease (GERD), gastroparesis, and position other than supine are factors that increase the risk of complications when using SGAs [13].

The LMA Classic, one of the first SGAs, is a reusable device made of silicone. A disposable, single-use version of the LMA Classic is the LMA Unique. Designed for intraoral procedures, the LMA Flexible has a wire-reinforced shaft to allow flexible positioning away from the surgical site. The LMA Fastrach, an intubating LMA, has a rigid, curved shaft and handle that facilitates placement of an ET tube through its ventilating tube, with or without the assistance of a fiberoptic scope. The reusable LMA ProSeal was the first LMA designed with a drainage tube to reduce the risk of aspiration. This drainage tube also facilitates placement of an orogastric tube. The LMA ProSeal's design creates an improved airway seal without adding pressure to the oropharyngeal tissue. A disposable alternative to the LMA ProSeal is the LMA Supreme. In addition to the gastric drainage tube, such as the LMA ProSeal, the LMA Supreme has a curved shaft similar to the LMA Fastrach. The LMA Classic Excel is an intubating version of the LMA Classic. The AirQ (disposable) and Intubating Laryngeal Airway (reusable) were designed with unique features to assist ET intubation but may also be used as a primary airway. The Cobra Perilaryngeal Airway (PLA) differs from the previously discussed SGAs with its high-volume, low-pressure pharyngeal cuff that sits just proximal to the cuffless mask. It also allows passage of an ETT. The Gnana Laryngeal Airway, a novel SGA device, is similar to the LMA Classic in basic design, but with an additional suction port on the convex portion of the laryngeal mask to remove saliva. The Esophageal-Tracheal Combitube and the King Laryngeal Tube have been designed to be able to achieve ventilation after blind insertion, making them useful for prehospital use or by unskilled operators. Their double cuff design allows ventilation via the larynx by inflating the distal cuff in the esophagus and the proximal cuff in the hypopharynx. The uniquely designed I-GEL device uses a cuffless mask made of a gel material that conforms to the larynx. It also has a gastric drainage tube that allows passage of an orogastric tube [14].

Endotracheal Intubation

ET intubation is achieved with an ET tube via an orotracheal or nasotracheal approach. There are several types of ET tubes used to achieve ET intubation. The standard cuffed ET tube is single lumen and comes in a variety of sizes, based on the internal diameter of the tube. Specialty single-lumen tubes include oral and nasal Ring–Adair–Elwyn (RAE) tubes, wire-reinforced tubes, laser-resistant tubes, and electromyogram (EMG) tubes. Oral and nasal RAE tubes have a preformed bend to allow positioning of the tube and circuit away from the surgical field for facial, oral, or dental surgeries or neurosurgeries. Wire-reinforced tubes contain a metal wire that is spiraled along its length to minimize kinking or allow positioning away from the surgical field. Laser-resistant tubes are used during laser surgery of the upper airway to decrease the risk of airway fire. EMG monitoring tubes, such as the neural integrity monitor (NIM) tube, allow monitoring of the recurrent laryngeal nerve during thyroid and other neck surgeries [15, 16].

Several techniques are available for ET intubation. Orotracheal intubation is most commonly performed via direct laryngoscopy using a Macintosh (curved) or Miller (straight) blade to directly visualize the glottic opening and insert the ET tube. Indirect visualization using a video laryngoscope may be chosen for patients with suspected difficult airway or immobilization of the cervical spine. Video laryngoscopes are categorized as either channeled or nonchanneled. Nonchanneled videoscopes include the more commonly used Glidescope, C-MAC, and McGrath. While these devices provide improved glottic visualization, there can still be difficulty in directing the ET tube into the glottis. Channeled videoscopes have a guide channel into which the ET tube is preloaded and which directs the tube towards the glottic opening. Airtraq and King Vision Video Laryngoscope are types of channeled devices. A disadvantage of these devices is that the thicker blades require a greater interincisor distance. Fiberoptic intubation is another option for the management of a known or suspected difficult airway. It allows intubation in an awake patient; however, this technique requires airway anesthesia. Nasotracheal intubation is typically chosen for intraoral and mandibular surgeries. It can be performed blindly, with the assistance of direct or video laryngoscopy or a fiberoptic scope [17, 18]. Table 2.2 summarizes intubation techniques and their indications and contraindications.

Table 2.2 Intubation techniques

Technique	Indications	Contraindications	Equipment
Oral route	Airway protection Prolonged mechanical ventilation General anesthesia for surgery	Penetrating trauma of upper airway	Laryngoscope/fiberoptic Stylet Bougie/Eschmann Airway exchange catheter Intubation introducer/catheter
Nasal route	Intraoral surgery Mandibular surgery Poor mouth opening	Basilar skull fracture Nasal fractures Epistaxis Nasal polyps Coagulopathy	Laryngoscope/fiberoptic McGills Red rubber
Direct laryngoscopy	Airway protection Prolonged mechanical ventilation General anesthesia for surgery	Poor mouth opening Documented difficult airway Airway mass/tumor	Light handle Blade
Video laryngoscopy	History of difficult intubation Suspected difficult intubation Inability to extend the neck Cervical instability	Severe bleeding of upper airway	Videoscope handle and screen

Table 2.2 (cont.)

Technique	Indications	Contraindications	Equipment
Flexible fiberoptic	History of difficult intubation	High-grade stenosis of airway	Fiberoptic scope
	Suspected difficult intubation	Severe bleeding of upper airway	
	Compromised airway	Pharyngeal abscess	
	Inability to extend the neck		
	Cervical instability		
	Trauma to upper airway		

See references [17–19].

Management of Difficult Airway

Difficult Airway Algorithm

At present, there is no standard definition that defines a difficult airway. Rather, a difficult airway may be related to a clinical situation in which there is difficulty with patient cooperation, difficulty ventilating, inability to visualize any portion of the vocal cords after multiple attempts with direct laryngoscopy, difficulty with ET intubation requiring multiple attempts, or difficulty with surgical access. These complex situations place an emphasis on the skills of the practitioner, as well as on careful preoperative risk analysis to overcome the situation. Guidelines have been created to provide a sequential series of plans to be used when tracheal intubation fails and are designed to prioritize oxygenation while limiting the number of airway interventions in order to minimize trauma and complications [20]. A special task force was created by the American Society of Anesthesiologists (ASA) to evaluate several published research studies from peer-reviewed journals and to reach a consensus on the most effective recommendations on approaches to manage a difficult airway once the primary plan fails, with the most updated version seen in Figure 2.1. Basic preparation for difficult airway management includes: (1) availability of equipment for management of a difficult airway (i.e., portable storage unit); (2) informing the patient with a known or suspected difficult airway; (3) assigning an individual to provide assistance when a difficult airway is encountered; (4) preanesthetic preoxygenation by mask; and (5) administration of supplemental oxygen throughout the process of difficult airway management [21]. Noninvasive methods of intubation, also mentioned in the "Airway Management Techniques" section, include: awake intubation; video-assisted laryngoscopy; intubating stylets or tube changers; SGA for ventilation or intubation; rigid laryngoscopic blades of varying designs; fiberoptic-guided intubation; and lighted stylets.

Emergency Airway Procedures

Cricothyrotomy

As seen in the difficult airway algorithm, a cricothyrotomy may be invasive but can be a lifesaving procedure once all approaches have been exhausted. Factors that indicate this procedure include a patient who is difficult to ventilate or intubate, but also those with severe facial trauma or upper airway bleeding or obstruction. Common techniques are the Seldinger or surgical technique. The Seldinger technique involves locating the cricothyroid membrane (CTM), puncturing the membrane with an 18-gauge wall needle, and aspirating air once a pop is felt as the needle enters the trachea. A guidewire is then advanced

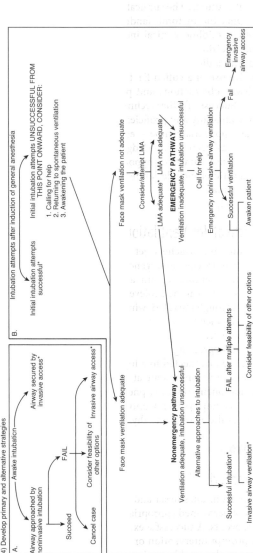

DIFFICULT AIRWAY ALGORITHM

1) Assess the likelihood and clinical impact of basic management problems
   A. Difficult ventilation
   B. Difficult intubation
   C. Difficulty with patient cooperation or consent
   D. Difficult tracheostomy

2) Actively pursue opportunities to deliver supplemental oxygen throughout the process of difficult airway management

3) Consider the relative merits and feasibility of basic management choices
   A. Awake intubation versus intubation attempts after induction of general anesthesia
   B. Noninvasive technique for initial approach to intubation versus invasive technique for initial approach to intubation
   C. Preservation of spontaneous ventilation versus ablation of spontaneous ventilation

4) Develop primary and alternative strategies

A.

Airway approached by noninvasive intubation

Awake intubation

Airway secured by invasive access*

FAIL

Succeed

Consider feasibility of Invasive airway access* other options

Cancel case

Face mask ventilation adequate

Nonemergency pathway
Ventilation adequate, intubation unsuccessful

Alternative approaches to intubation

Successful intubation*

Invasive airway ventilation*

FAIL after multiple attempts

Consider feasibility of other options

B.

Intubation attempts after induction of general anesthesia

Initial intubation attempts successful*

Initial intubation attempts UNSUCCESSFUL FROM THIS POINT ONWARD, CONSIDER:
1. Calling for help
2. Returning to spontaneous ventilation
3. Awakening the patient

Face mask ventilation not adequate

Consider/attempt LMA

LMA adequate*   LMA not adequate

EMERGENCY PATHWAY
Ventilation inadequate, intubation unsuccessful

Call for help

Emergency noninvasive airway ventilation

Successful ventilation   Fail   Emergency invasive airway access

Awaken patient

Figure 2.1 Updated guidelines for difficult airway placement with end-tidal carbon dioxide. * Denotes tracheal intubation or laryngeal mask airway placement with end-tidal carbon dioxide.

through the needle, followed by removal of the needle. A small incision is made at the guidewire and a combined dilator and airway is placed. Finally, the wire and dilator are removed, leaving the airway in place, which is then secured with sutures. The surgical technique involves a vertical and transverse incision. Once the anatomic landmarks of the larynx and CTM are identified, a 3- to 4-cm midline vertical incision is made, followed by a 1.5- to 2-cm horizontal incision at the inferior third of the CTM. The resulting hole is enlarged with a dilator and a cuffed tracheal cannula is inserted. Both techniques involve use of a cuffed ET tube or cannula, which provides a bypass to upper airway obstructions and provides ventilation and protection against aspiration. Success of either technique is determined on the provider's knowledge of the anatomy and proficiency in technique and performing the procedure at an appropriate time – early in a difficult airway situation. Lack of experience has been acknowledged as the main source of cricothyrotomy failure, because practice opportunities of any kind are scarce [22]. Contraindications include laryngeal or tracheal disruption, coagulopathies, and thyroid masses. Complications include: bleeding; injury to the larynx, trachea, or esophagus; infection to the site; and subglottic stenosis.

Transtracheal Jet Ventilation

Percutaneous transtracheal jet ventilation (PTTJV) is another invasive method which provides emergency ventilatory support in patients who cannot be adequately ventilated with a face mask or SGA, or are unable to be intubated. PTTJV can be achieved by placing an over-the-needle catheter in the trachea through the CTM, which is then connected to a syringe. The needle should be advanced at a 90-degree angle until air is aspirated, signifying the needle is in the trachea. The catheter should then be advanced into the trachea at a 30- to 45-degree angle caudally. After reconfirming proper placement, the catheter is then connected to a high-pressure oxygen source with specialized tubing that can accommodate at least 50 psi. Risks involved with this procedure include pneumothorax, pneumomediastinum, bleeding, infection, and subcutaneous emphysema. Contraindications are upper airway obstruction, disruption of the airway, and thyroid masses.

Extubation

Extubation Criteria and Considerations

Emergence from anesthesia and extubation are critical points in anesthesia which, if not performed appropriately, can be associated with an increased risk of adverse events. A successful extubation is defined as extubation without the need for prompt intervention or reintubation. Prior to extubation, the pharynx should be thoroughly suctioned to decrease the risk of aspiration of blood and/or secretions. The patient should also be ventilated with 100% oxygen in case of complications preventing maintenance of the airway following extubation. Most often, extubation is performed when the patient is either deeply anesthetized or awake. In either case, recovery from paralytics should be achieved and the patient should have a period of spontaneous breathing with adequate tidal volumes before extubation can occur. Commonly used criteria for awake extubation in children include: eye opening; facial grimace; movement other than coughing; purposeful movement; conjugate gaze; and end-tidal anesthetic concentration below a predetermined level [23]. In adults, extubation is traditionally based on global patient status. Global patient factors consist of return of consciousness, ability to protect the airway, normal body temperature, absence of residual neuromuscular blockade, and normal metabolic parameters (e.g., absence of clinically significant anemia, acidosis, major electrolyte abnormality) [24]. Although many criteria rely on patient status, an objective criterion that may assist in determining whether a patient is ready for extubation is the negative inspiratory force (NIF). The NIF is defined as the maximum pressure that can be generated against an occluded airway for 20 seconds from the FRC. In this sense, it can be considered as a direct marker of inspiratory muscle function and, in particular, of diaphragmatic force [25]. A NIF ≥-20 or -25 cmH$_2$O is adequate to begin weaning and eventually extubating a patient. Studies have shown that patients with a NIF >-30 cmH$_2$O have a 90% or more chance of successful ventilation weaning and extubation. In patients with difficult intubations, extubation should be carefully considered because reintubation can be more difficult than the initial intubation.

Complications

Extubation during a light plane, especially during stage 2, is avoided due to an increased risk of laryngospasm, which is the most common cause of airway obstruction after tracheal extubation. It is precipitated by local irritation of the vocal cords by secretions or blood, when the plane of anesthesia is insufficient to prevent the laryngospasm reflex, but too deep to allow coordinated cough [26]. Laryngospasm should be first managed by administering 100% oxygen by positive pressure ventilation until the patient awakens and laryngospasm disappears. The provider may also deepen the plane of anesthesia by using intravenous (IV) or inhalational anesthetics until laryngospasm and airway reflexes are abolished. If this fails, it may be necessary to utilize short-acting neuromuscular blocking agents, such as succinylcholine, to enable oxygenation and, if required, reintubation. Patients with prolonged, sustained laryngospasm may develop negative pressure pulmonary edema. Extubating with an ET tube my also cause coughing (bucking), which may lead to increased heart rate, blood pressure, intracranial pressure, and abdominal pressure. If a patient begins to cough, this may also cause wound dehiscence and increased bleeding. In asthmatics, there should be careful observation during tracheal extubation as they are associated with a higher risk of bronchospasm. Administering IV lidocaine 1–2 minutes before extubation or extubating deep may mitigate coughing. Upper airway edema may also be seen during extubation where patients develop stridor and respiratory distress, typically within 6 hours of tracheal extubation. Those patients in acute distress may require nebulized epinepherine in combination with nebulized corticosteroids. The value of systemic steroids is less clear, but IV dexamethasone at 0.25 mg kg^{-1}, immediately followed by 0.1 mg kg^{-1} every 6 hours for 24 hours has been recommended. Other complications include trauma to the airway, tracheal collapse, and vocal cord paralysis, which may be related to the procedure performed.

References

1. Klinger K, Infosino A. Airway management. In: M Pardo, R Miller, eds. *Basics of Anesthesia*, 7th ed. Philadelphia, PA: Elsevier, 2018; pp. 239–72.

2. Ward JPT, Ward J, Leach RM. *The Respiratory System at a Glance*, 3rd ed. Oxford: John Wiley & Sons; 2010.

3. Davies A, Moores C. *The Respiratory System*, 2nd ed. Oxford: Elsevier; 2010.

4. Ball M, Hossain M, Padalia D. Airway anatomy. In: *StatPearls*. Treasure Island, FL: StatPearls Publishing; 2020. Available from: www.ncbi.nlm.nih.gov/books/NB K459258/.

5. Bates JHT. Systems physiology of the airways in health and obstructive pulmonary disease. *Wiley Interdisc Rev Syst Biol Med*. 2016;8(5):423–37.

6. Harless J, Ramaiah R, Bhananker SM. Pediatric airway management. *Int J Crit Illn Inj Sci*. 2014;4(1):65–70.

7. Nimmagadda U, Salem MR, Crystal GJ. Preoxygenation: physiologic basis, benefits, and potential risks. *Anesth Analg*. 2017;124(2):507–17.

8. Weingart SD, Levitan RM. Preoxygenation and prevention of desaturation during emergency airway management. *Ann Emerg Med*. 2012;59(3):165–75.e1.

9. Alalami AA, Ayoub CM, Baraka AS. Laryngospasm: review of different prevention and treatment modalities. *Pediatr Anesth*. 2008;18(4):281–8.

10. Nason KS. Acute intraoperative pulmonary aspiration. *Thorac Surg Clin*. 2015;25 (3):301–7.

11. El-Orbany M, Woehlck HJ. Difficult mask ventilation. *Anesth Analg*. 2009;109 (6):1870–80.

12. Apfelbaum JL, Hagberg CA, Caplan RA, *et al.* Practice guidelines for management of the difficult airway: an updated report by the American Society of

Anesthesiologists Task Force on Management of the Difficult Airway. *Anesthesiology*. 2013;118(2):251–70.

13. Gordon J, Cooper RM, Parotto M. Supraglottic airway devices: indications, contraindications and management. *Minerva Anestesiol*. 2018;84(3):389–97.

14. Hernandez MR, Klock PA, Ovassapian A. Evolution of the extraglottic airway: a review of its history, applications, and practical tips for success. *Anesth Analg*. 2012;114(2):349–68.

15. Haas CF, Eakin RM, Konkle MA, Blank R. Endotracheal tubes: old and new. *Respir Care*. 2014;59(6):933–55.

16. Gray AW. Endotracheal tubes. *Clin Chest Med*. 2003;24(3):379–87.

17. Hurford WE. Techniques for endotracheal intubation. *Int Anesthesiol Clin*. 2000;38 (3):1–28.

18. Cooper RM. Strengths and limitations of airway techniques. *Anesthesiol Clin*. 2015;33(2):241–55.

19. Koerner IP, Brambrink AM. Fiberoptic techniques. *Best Pract Res Clin Anaesthesiol*. 2005;19(4):611–21.

20. Frerk C, Mitchell VS, McNarry AF, *et al*. Difficult Airway Society 2015 guidelines for management of unanticipated difficult intubation in adults. *Br J Anaesth*. 2015;115(6):827–48.

21. Apfelbaum JL, Hagberg CA, Caplan RA, *et al*. Practice guidelines for management of the difficult airway: an updated report by the American Society of Anesthesiologists Task Force on Management of the Difficult Airway. *Anesthesiology*. 2013;118(2):251–70.

22. Eisenburger P, Laczika K, List M, *et al*. Comparison of conventional surgical versus Seldinger technique emergency cricothyrotomy performed by inexperienced clinicians. *Anesthesiology*. 2000;92(3):687–90.

23. Templeton TW, Goenaga-Díaz EJ, Downard MG, *et al*. Assessment of common criteria for awake extubation in infants and young children. *Anesthesiology*. 2019;131(4):801–8.

24. Howie WO, Dutton RP. Implementation of an evidence-based extubation checklist to reduce extubation failure in patients with trauma: a pilot study. *AANA J*. 2012;80 (3);179–84.

25. Cortés E, Parrado BK, Arango F. Negative inspiratory pressure as a predictor of weaning mechanical ventilation. *J Anaesth Intensive Care Med*. 2017;3(1). DOI: 10.19080/JAICM.2017.03.555602.

26. Hartley M, Vaughan RS. Problems associated with tracheal extubation. *Br J Anaesth*. 1993;71(4);561–8.

Chapter

3

Anesthesia Equipment: Clinical Considerations

George Mychaskiw, Eric Ly, Austin Ly, Kelsey Rooney, Leah A. Kaplan, Stephen Patin, Victoria L. Lassiegne, Katherine C. Babin, George Thomas, Elyse M. Cornett, and Alan David Kaye

Introduction

The anesthesia workstation, commonly referred to as the "anesthesia machine," is a complex and very specialized piece of equipment that is relatively unique in medical practice. It is, in essence, a device to control the delivery of medical gases to patients, including oxygen, air, nitrous oxide, and volatile anesthetics, along with a specialized ventilator adapted to operating room conditions. The safe use of the anesthesia workstation requires proper training, preuse checkout, and continuous monitoring of its function. The medical literature is replete with examples of patient harm from inappropriate use of the anesthesia workstation and from mechanical or electrical failure of its components. Additionally, volatile anesthetics, while valuable in medical practice, have a very low therapeutic index and manifest severe, and even fatal, side effects when administered improperly. Finally, many patients under general anesthesia are paralyzed for surgery and ventilated through an endotracheal tube. Their safety is completely dependent on the anesthesia professional's use of the anesthesia workstation to deliver breathing gases, remove carbon dioxide from exhaled gas, and precise administration of volatile anesthetics. Obviously, mechanical or operator error can be catastrophic and the design and functionality of the contemporary anesthesia workstation represent an evolution of numerous safety features and engineering to decrease the incidence of mechanical and human error.

Overview of Gas Flow from Pipeline and Cylinder Supply Gas Flow through the Anesthesia Workstation

The anesthesia workstation receives, processes, and administers medical gases and volatile anesthetics. The delivery of volatile anesthetics to the patient breathing circuit, which connects to the patient's airway, requires medical gases such as oxygen, nitrous oxide, and air. The anesthesia workstation receives the gas source from facility pipelines (e.g., intermediate pressure system) in the walls that eventually link to the operating room and from cylinder inlets (e.g., high-pressure system) that attach to the anesthesia work-station [1, 2]. The wall gas conduits in an operating room are color-coded and fitted via a specific tube diameter to the workstation by gas type. Yellow represents air; green signifies oxygen, and blue denotes nitrous oxide. The diameter–index safety system (DISS) provides gas-specific outlet fastening and helps prevent accidental gas mixing and attachment. The required pipe-line gas pressure supplied to the workstation is around 50 psi [3–5].

Cylinders offer gas supply if the central source fails or is unavailable. Gas flows through a fail-safe device called a hanger–yoke assembly, which fastens to workstations and ensures unidirectional flow. The apparatus incorporates gas-specific pins and holes (e.g., pin index safety system (PISS)), and gas travels past a filter to prevent debris from accumulating in the cylinder and machine [3, 6]. Gas cylinders also carry the same color-coded features to help prevent inappropriate assembly and gas mixing.

The high-pressure cylinder gas then flows through an initial pressure regu-lator, consisting of a diaphragm and a spring, to form a reduced, constant pressure of 45–60 psi. For nitric oxide, gas flows through a nitric oxide pressure regulator and an additional valve, called the fail-safe valve, that closes nitric oxide flow when oxygen from the pipeline or cylinder pressures reach low levels (<20 psi) [4]. This helps to prevent a hypoxic gas mixture, in the event of failure or depletion of oxygen supply. For the intermediate-pressure system, the gas source facility pipelines enter the gas flow circuit immediately after bypassing the initial pressure regulator, as the gas pressure is already reduced at approximately 50 psi [7].

After nitric oxide and oxygen pass through second-stage pressure regulators, both gases reach their respective flow control valves (e.g., needle valve), which control the rate of gas flow to the breathing circuit. Color-coded, specifically sized, and textured flow control knobs turn counterclockwise or clockwise to increase or decrease the flow rate, respectively. Gas enters flowmeter glass tubes where measurement of pressure occurs based on the principle that, among other factors, flow through a resistance (e.g., glass tube diameter) corresponds to pressure [3]. The bobbin (e.g., float or ball) within the flowmeter glass tube rises in height with increasing flow and lowers in height with decreasing flow. Increasingly, medical gases in newer systems are electronically metered into the breathing circuit and animated flowmeter tubes/displays are replacing glass tubes, with the control dials mimicking the dials on older, mechanical systems.

Following flow and pressure measurements, gases mix in a chamber called the manifold at the top of the flowmeter, according to specific sequences in gas flowmeters. Gas flow exits the flowmeter in a sequence that requires oxygen flowing out first [6]. Arranging oxygen downstream reduces the risk of hypoxic mixtures should a leak emerge from an upstream gas flowmeter tube. Again, this is true only in mechanical, nonelectronic systems. Following gas mixing, gas travels to the common gas outlet and breathing circuit [8, 9]. Table 3.1 describes a summary of the pipeline supply gas flow.

Table 3.1 Pipeline supply gas flow

Steps	Nitrous oxide pipeline	Oxygen pipeline
1	"Fail-safe" valve	
2	Nitrous oxide/oxygen pressure regulator	
3	Flow control valve	
4	Flowmeter glass tube	
5	Manifold	
6	Common gas outlet	
7	Breathing circuit	

Overview of Air and Oxygen Flush Flow

Air may also flow through the anesthesia workstation. Air can travel through the low-pressure circuit (e.g., components after the flowmeters) of the anesthesia workstation, and it also encounters a secondary pressure regulator. Air may also flow to the flowmeter assembly for measuring and ultimately delivery to the breathing circuit and patient, even without sufficient oxygen pressure present.

A direct link from the first oxygen pressure regulator to the common gas outlet is an additional oxygen circuit within the anesthesia workstation that a provider may use with the oxygen flush button (e.g., valve). By circumventing the flowmeter, manifold, and vaporizer, the circuit flows through an oxygen flush regulator to deliver 100% oxygen and supply an oxygen pressure starting from 50 psi [10, 11]. Functions of the oxygen flush button include diluting anesthetic gases or mixtures in the breathing circuit with oxygen, inflating the patient breathing bag, and supporting situations in which the patient requires high-flow oxygen at 35–75 L min^{-1}, such as with mask ventilation [4, 9]. In newer, fully electronic, and computerized gas delivery systems, there is a mechanical backup/override that can provide oxygen to the breathing circuit in the event of an electrical or software failure.

Overview of Volatile Anesthetic Gas Flow

Volatile anesthetics enter the anesthetic workstation gas flow in the low-pressure system, which consists of the components after the flowmeters (e.g., vaporizers) and lies slightly above atmospheric pressure. Injection and mixing of volatile anesthetics with the combined gas flow occur immediately after the flowmeters. Since volatile anesthetics exist as liquids in room temperature and atmospheric pressure (with the exception of desflurane), vaporization, the transforming of liquid to vapor, must occur before delivery to the common gas outlet and breathing circuit [9, 12]. Since desflurane's vapor pressure is close to atmospheric pressure, it must be delivered through a specialized "vaporizer" that heats and pressurizes its vapor, which is then electronically metered into the fresh gas flow. Modifications of the flowmeters and vaporizers influence respective gas compositions before gas flows through the anesthetic workstation's common gas outlet, which attaches to the anesthetic breathing system (e.g., circuit) [6].

Overview of Anesthetic Breathing System Gas Flow

The anesthetic breathing system serves to distribute gases, including oxygen and anesthetic gases, and remove carbon dioxide from the patient. Three commonly used anesthetic breathing systems include the Mapleson F (Jackson-Rees) system, Bain circuit, and circle system. Based on a number of factors, classifications of anesthetic breathing systems include open, semi-open, semi-closed, and closed [13].

The most commonly utilized anesthetic breathing system is the circle system, which employs an inspiratory and expiratory limb made up of tubular arrangements to create a circular gas flow. Gas flows from the common gas outlet to the inspiratory limb and travels through a series of tubular extensions that include corrugated tubes, tracheal tube connectors, and endotracheal tubes to reach the patient's lung. On exhalation, gases, including carbon dioxide generated by cellular respiration, flow through the expiratory limb to reach a carbon dioxide processor [3, 12, 13]. Gas flows through a Y-piece, which connects the inspiratory and expiratory limbs to the tracheal tube connector, on inhalation and exhalation to complete the circular gas flow. The design also includes check valves to create unidirectional gas flow through the inspiratory and expiratory limbs. Some systems apply rebreathing of exhaled gases, which function to reduce overall anesthetic use and maximize humidification of inhaled gases [12].

Workstation Components

Gas Inlets and Safety Systems

Anesthesia machines typically have multiple gas inlets, with pressure gauges for each inlet [14]. Pipeline inlets are those that supply gas from pipelines that run throughout the healthcare facility [14]. These inlets usually provide oxygen and nitrous oxide from the facility's central supply [14]. The pipeline inlets utilize tubing that connects to the anesthesia machine via a noninterchangeable DISS fitting that mitigates the risk of incorrect hose attachment [14]. A second gas inlet provides gas from a secondary source stored as either compressed gas (air, oxygen, helium) or liquefied under pressure (nitrous oxide, carbon dioxide) in the cylinders [14]. This gas supply is typically used as a backup supply if the primary pipeline source were to fail [15]. A hanger–yoke assembly attaches these gas cylinders to the anesthesia machine by utilizing a PISS [15]. This safety system is crucial in ensuring correct connection of gases when needed. The yoke assembly safety system consists of index pins, a washer, a gas filter, and a check valve [15]. The check valve prevents retrograde gas flow through the gas inlet back into the attached cylinder [15]. To ensure additional safety, the cylinders are thoroughly checked and tested by manufacturers regularly to ensure the safety of both patients and healthcare professionals operating the machinery [14]. There is also a consistent color-coded labeling system to safely differentiate between the different gases stored in these cylinders [14].

Gauges and Sensors

The pipeline inlet consistently provides gases to the anesthesia machine at approximately 50 psig [15]. The pressure at which a cylinder source provides gases is more variable but is usually downregulated to approximately 45 psig [15].

Pressure Regulators

While the pipeline gas supply maintains relatively constant pressure, variable gas pressure in cylinders complicates flow control [15]. In order to utilize cylinder gas sources more safely, anesthesia machines feature a pressure regulator that keeps the pressure between 45 and 47 psig [15].

Oxygen Flush Valve

The oxygen flush valve provides additional safety to the anesthesia machine by allowing high-flow, high-pressure oxygen to flow directly from the source into the breathing circuit [16]. In this way, oxygen bypasses the vaporizers and flowmeters [16]. Malfunction of this feature is rare but can cause significant harm to the patient if this occurs, resulting in barotraumas or intraanesthetic awareness [16].

Pressure Sensors, Fail-Safe, and Alarms

When oxygen pipeline pressure drops, a fail-safe device senses this drop and ensures that the set oxygen concentration is maintained despite the loss of oxygen pressure [17]. The fail-safe system maintains the oxygen concentration by promptly shutting off the flow of nitrous oxide [17]. The drop in pressure of oxygen sets off both audible and visual alarms that draw attention to the issue [18].

Oxygen Ratio Proportioning Systems

Most modern machines use a proportioning safety device, in addition to the "fail-safe" pressure threshold shutoff valve [19]. Depending on the manufacturer of the anesthesia machine, these devices either mechanically link the oxygen and nitrous oxide flow controls or reduce the flow of nitrous oxide and other gases via pressure feedback from the oxygen supply, so that the proportion of nitrous oxide to oxygen results in a minimum oxygen concentration at the common gas outlet of between 23% and 25% [19].

Fresh Gas Controllers and Flowmeters

In a circle system, fresh gas flow is typically set to minute ventilation [10]. If fresh gas flow exceeds the patient's alveolar minute ventilation, then the fresh gas will force out the remaining exhaled alveolar gas in the breathing circuit before the next inspiration [10]. If the exhaled carbon dioxide volume is equal to or greater than the patient's tidal volume, then the next inspiration will only contain fresh gas [10]. Fresh gas decoupling is an element in newer workstation models that prevents high volumes and pressures from being transported to the patient during inspiration, resulting in a more precise delivery of tidal volume [20]. Flowmeters measure each individual gas before they mix together with other gases and enter into the vaporizer [20]. As noted previously, the oxygen flowmeter is positioned the furthest downstream, which helps maintain flow to the patient in the event of an upstream leak [20]. Electronic flow meters are less likely to develop leaks and breakages since there are fewer mechanical parts [10]. The electronic numerical display allows for inspection of gas flow even in a dimmed operating room, and data will be electronically sent to an information system, making it an advantageous choice for many surgeries and procedures [10].

Workstation Ventilators: Bellows versus Piston

Traditionally, anesthesia ventilator bellows are driven either pneumatically by oxygen or by pressurized air [10]. Some newer ventilators use electronically driven pistons to generate gas flow and do not require oxygen or pressurized gas consumption, an economical feature [10]. Ventilator bellows in nonpiston machines can be ascending or descending, based on whether the bellow ascends or descends during the inspiratory phase [10]. A descending bellow is generally safer since it will not fill during a circuit leak [10]. An advantage of a piston ventilator is the ability to deliver accurate tidal volumes to the patient, regardless of patient size or poor lung compliance [10].

Vaporizers and Manifold

Vaporizers are located between the flowmeters and the common gas outlet [14]. They receive gas flow from the flowmeter and add a concentration-calibrated amount of volatile anesthetic agent to the gas [14]. Vaporizers are temperature-corrected for the specific anesthetic agent supplied, allowing for the transport of a constant concentration of agent, irrespective of temperature or flow [14]. This temperature correction is significant because high temperatures cause increased amounts of gas to be elaborated from the volatile, liquid state [14]. Oxygen enters the manifold downstream to the other gases, which prevents hypoxia in case there is a gas leak upstream [14]. Unidirectional valve malfunction has occurred in older anesthesia machines because of condensation from water vapor [10]. Condensation can be reduced by heating the manifold and using water traps to collect the liquid [10].

Common Gas Outlet and Check Valve

The common gas outlet is the single connection between the vaporized volatile anesthetic and the patient's airway [14]. The common gas outlet supplies the tidal volume delivered to the patient during inspiration [14]. Gas composition in the gas outlet is affected by different elements, compared to gas composition in the breathing circuit [14]. In the gas outlet, the composition of the gas is affected by alterations in flowmeters and vaporizers [14]. Additionally, a one-way check valve is positioned between the vaporizers and the oxygen flush [14]. The purpose of the check valve is to prevent retrograde gas flow into the pipeline supplies, which can occur from variations in positive pressure ventilation in older anesthesia machines [14].

Waste Gas Scavenging

Waste gas scavenging is important to the safety of operating room personnel, as excess pollutants may lead to spontaneous abortion, birth defects, and various organ system disorders [21]. Scavenging consists of collecting exhaled anesthetic gas from the equipment and venting it outside of the operating room or bringing it to a reservoir for safe disposal [21]. Vacuum exhaust is a principal component of the medical gas system by scavenging the waste anesthetic [22]. The waste disposal reservoir may use a suction regulator [22]. The amount of suction used should be maintained in a delicate balance [22]. Excess suction could result in insufficient ventilation, and an inadequate amount of suction could result in leftover anesthetic gas entering the operating room atmosphere [22]. Positive pressure should be maintained in the operating room to drive away escaped gas [22].

Electrical Systems

There are four main parts in the electrical system: a master switch, an alternating current source, monitoring equipment, and an oxygen analyzer [21]. The first step is to turn on the workstation with the master switch, then confirm the machine is connected to the alternating current source [21]. The alternating current source battery should be charging during workstation use and should have at least a 30-minute reserve supply before use [21]. The monitoring equipment should be checked for appropriate functioning, leaks, or kinks, with appropriate alarm settings adjusted for the patient [21]. The oxygen analyzer should be connected to the specified point in the circuit and calibrated to at least 95% [21]. Safety when working with electrical systems is greatly emphasized, and the first step is to ensure the workstation is in a safe area, with electrical wiring secured [21]. Next, malfunctions with electrical systems and other components of the workstation do occur, so it is very important to have a backup functioning self-inflating bag to fit the patient's size [21]. Electrical shock or electrocution can occur if bodily contact is made with two conductive materials at different voltage potentials; however, if a person is grounded, then only one live conductor is needed to receive a shock [22] (see Table 3.2).

Gas Flow through the Anesthesia Machine

Delivery of Oxygen and Inhalational Agents to the Patient

Nitrous Oxide

Nitrous oxide is the most rapid-onset inhalational anesthetic agent and is transported in blood as free gas. It is considered relatively safe because of its low potency and inability to impact vital physiologic function unless it is combined with other, more potent inhalational agents [25]. Nitrous oxide is also considered useful for its analgesic properties and reduced perioperative pain management requirements, which can possibly reduce the use of opioids for pain [26, 27].

Other Inhalational Agents/Medical Gases

Medical air serves various purposes in anesthesia, including serving as a power source for ventilators, mixing with delivered oxygen, or as a driving gas for chemotherapy and/or aerosolized drugs [15]. It can be used in three main forms, including compressed air, synthetic air, and cylinder manifolds. Although it is not sterile, it is considered clean at the right temperature and pressure. Compressed medical air, used to power ventilators, is formed by drawing ambient air into the compressor. From there, the compressed air is moved through a series of filter driers for separating condensed water, as well as separators to remove other contaminants and particulate matter from the compressed air. Synthetic air, on the other hand, is prepared by blending liquid nitrogen and liquid oxygen in the gaseous state [7]. This form of medical air is advantageous in that it does not require a power supply and there are few, if any, contamination considerations [15].

Table 3.2 Workstation component findings

Workstation component	Author (year)	Type of resource	Findings
Gas inlets	Das et al., 2013 [15] Butterworth et al., 2018 [14, 20]	Review article Textbook chapter	Pipeline inlets are those that supply gas from pipelines that run throughout the healthcare facility. A second gas inlet provides gas from a secondary source, stored as either compressed gas (air, oxygen, helium) or liquefied under pressure (nitrous oxide, carbon dioxide) in the cylinders

This second gas supply is typically used as a backup supply if the primary pipeline source were to fail |
Gauges and sensors	Das et al., 2013 [15]	Review article	The pipeline inlet consistently provides gases to the anesthesia machine at approximately 50 psig. The pressure at which a cylinder source provides gases is more variable but is usually approximately 45 psig
Pressure regulators	Das et al., 2013 [15]	Review article	While the pipeline gas supply maintains relatively constant pressure, variable gas pressure in cylinders complicates flow control. In order to utilize cylinder gas sources more safely, anesthesia machines feature a pressure regulator that keeps the pressure between 45 and 47 psig
Oxygen flush valve	Petty, 1993 [16]	Journal article	The oxygen flush valve provides additional safety to the anesthesia machine by allowing high-flow, high-pressure oxygen to flow directly from the source into the breathing circuit. In this way, oxygen bypasses the vaporizers and flowmeters. Malfunction of this feature is rare but can cause significant harm to the patient if this occurs, resulting in barotraumas or intraanesthetic awareness

Table 3.2 (cont.)

Workstation component	Author (year)	Type of resource	Findings
Pressure sensors	Mun and No, 2013 [17] Dosch and Tharp, 2018 [18]	Review article Website	When oxygen pipeline pressure drops, a fail-safe device senses this drop and ensures that the set oxygen concentration is maintained despite loss of oxygen pressure. The fail-safe system maintains the oxygen concentration by promptly shutting off
			The drop in pressure of oxygen sets off both audible and visual alarms that draw attention to the issue
Oxygen ration proportioning systems	Anesthesia Key [19]	Website	Most modern machines use a proportioning safety device instead of a "fail-safe" threshold shutoff valve. These devices reduce the pressure of nitrous oxide and other gases, so that the proportion of nitrous oxide to oxygen results in a minimum oxygen concentration at the common gas outlet between 23% and 25%, depending on the manufacturer of the anesthesia machine
Fresh gas controllers and flowmeters	Patil et al., 2013 [10] Butterworth et al., 2018 [14, 20]	Review article Textbook chapter	Flowmeters measure each individual gas before they mix together with other gases and enter into the vaporizer
			Fresh gas decoupling is an element on newer workstation models that prevents high volumes and pressures from being transported to the patient during inspiration, resulting in a more precise delivery of tidal volume
			To achieve spontaneous ventilation, fresh gas flow is set to minute ventilation. If fresh gas flow exceeds the patient's alveolar minute ventilation, then the fresh gas will force out the remaining alveolar gas before the next inspiration. If the exhaled carbon dioxide volume is equal to or greater than the

			patient's tidal volume, then the next inspiration will only contain fresh gas
Workstation ventilators: bellows versus pistons	Patil et al., 2013 [10]	Review article	Newer ventilators use electronically driven pistons to generate airflow and do not require oxygen or pressurized gas consumption, an economical feature. An advantage of a piston ventilator is the ability to deliver accurate tidal volumes to the patient, regardless of patient size or poor lung compliance
Vaporizers and manifold	Patil et al., 2013 [10] Butterworth et al., 2018 [14, 20]	Review article Textbook chapter	Vaporizers are temperature-corrected for the specific anesthetic agent supplied, allowing for the transport of a constant concentration of agent, irrespective of temperature or flow. This temperature correction is significant because high temperatures cause gas to precipitate out as liquid
			Unidirectional valve malfunction has occurred in older anesthesia machines because of condensation from water vapor. Condensation can be reduced by heating the manifold and using water traps to collect the liquid
Common gas outlets and check valve	Butterworth et al., 2018 [14, 20]	Textbook chapter	The gas outlet is the single connection between the vaporized volatile anesthetic and the patient's airway. The gas outlet supplies the tidal volume delivered to the patient during inspiration
			The purpose of the check valve is to prevent retrograde gas flow into the pipeline supplies, which can occur from variations in positive pressure ventilation in older anesthesia machines
Waste gas scavenging	Goneppanavar et al., 2013 [21]	Review article Textbook chapter	Scavenging consists of collecting exhaled anesthetic from the equipment and bringing it to a reservoir for safe disposal

Table 3.2 (cont.)

Workstation component	Author (year)	Type of resource	Findings
	Cowles *et al.,* 2018 [22]		The amount of suction used should be maintained in a delicate balance. Excess suction could result in insufficient ventilation, and an inadequate amount of suction could result in leftover anesthetic gas
Electrical systems	Goneppanavar *et al.,* 2013 [21] Cowles *et al.,* 2018 [22]	Review article Textbook chapter	There are four main parts in the electrical system: a master switch, an alternating current source, monitoring equipment, and an oxygen analyzer
			Electrical shock or electrocution can occur if bodily contact is made with two conductive materials at different voltage potentials, or one conductive material if the person is grounded

Medical air is considered a safe, versatile substitute for nitrous oxide in the setting of anesthesia. A mixture of medical air and oxygen is often used as a carrier gas, leaving the anesthesiologist to choose the oxygen concentration and allowing greater control of the oxygen delivered to the patient [28]. Medical gas mixed with oxygen has been shown to improve the PaO_2/FiO_2 ratio, when compared with nitrous oxide and air, in young, healthy patients during general anesthesia [29]. Likewise, medical gas is not known to carry the same side effect profile that nitrous oxide may carry, namely hypoxic properties, postoperative nausea and vomiting, and environmental effects (although it should be noted that this is a minor source of atmospheric greenhouse gas) [27, 30, 31].

Other gases used in anesthesia include Entonox, carbon dioxide, and heliox [15]. Entonox, a 50:50 combination of oxygen and nitrous oxide, is used as an analgesic agent most often on maternity wards, chiefly in labor and delivery suites. It does carry certain risks, such as bolus delivery of hypoxic 100% nitrous oxide gas; however, if handled correctly, this risk can be mitigated. Carbon dioxide, used for insufflation during laparoscopy, is a commonly utilized gas, especially as robotic-assisted techniques become more common in the operating room. A colorless, odorless, and nonflammable gas, it is a readily available by-product of hydrogen manufacturing, as well as a by-product from a number of petroleum or natural gas reactions after purification. Heliox is another gas mixture (21% oxygen and helium), particularly of interest in recent times. Helium's lower density allows easy delivery to the patient as it is more readily breathed in, reducing the overall work of breathing for the patient undergoing general anesthesia. Helium is also an abundant element and can be produced in the fractional distillation of natural gas.

Anesthesia Workstation Checkout

It is important that the operator has a methodical way to ensure the proper functioning of the machine before its use [22]. This is encouraged by the use of a machine "checkout" or "checklist" performed preoperatively by the operator. By promoting machine inspection before use, it ensures proper functioning and increases the familiarity of the operators with the machine itself [14]. Failing to ensure the proper functioning of the anesthesia workplace equipment can lead to malfunction that results in "near misses" or even patient injury [32]. By checking the equipment before the procedure, there is a decreased risk of severe postoperative morbidity and mortality [33]. With wide variations in anesthetic equipment used by differing institutions, creating a universal checklist has proven difficult to achieve. The more recently developed guidelines have kept this in mind, with the goal of creating steps that are applicable to all institutions.

The Food and Drug Administration (FDA) has created a general checklist to be used by all operators of an anesthesia workspace. The first thing that should be checked is the machine's location and wiring. The machine should be placed in a safe area with wiring that is secure [34, 35]. Beyond this, the checkout is divided into a variety of different categories, including verification of the functionality of the high-pressure system, low-pressure system, scavenging system, breathing system, ventilation systems, and monitors. For the high-pressure system, it is important to check the oxygen cylinder supply, along with the central pipeline supplies, hose connections, and gauges. The low-pressure system checklist should include verifying the status of flow control valves and fill level, performing the leak check with a suction bulb, and testing flowmeters through their full range of output. For the scavenging system, it is important to adjust and confirm the connections between the system and the adjustable pressure-limiting (APL) valve, along with the ventilator relief valves. The waste gas vacuum should also be adjusted accordingly. The breathing system should have the oxygen monitor calibrated, along with checking the initial status of the breathing system for a complete circuit, installing the breathing circuit accessory equipment, and verification of no leaks in the system. The unidirectional valves of the ventilation system should also be properly functioning. All monitors should be calibrated, with alarms set for the capnograph, pulse oximeter, oxygen analyzer, respiratory volume monitor, and pressure monitor with high and low airway pressure alarms. Other miscellaneous items should also be checked, such as proper functioning of suction, for instance [14].

Following these protocols should theoretically take <10 minutes, and this time is reduced in the event that an institution has a self-checking machine. In the case of a change of anesthesiologist during a procedure, the handoff should include checking that the machine and its components are properly functioning. Long procedures should involve periodic checks for volatile anesthetic liquid and carbon dioxide absorbent [22].

Comparison of Modern Anesthesia Workstations

Modern anesthetic workstations consist of six specific subsystems. These subsystems include gas supplies, flow meters, vaporizers, gas delivery systems, scavenging systems, and monitoring systems [2]. Advantages of these workstations include improved accuracy of vaporizers, included software for improved control of gas flow and vaporizer output, increased sophistication of electronic alarms, advanced modes of ventilation, self-testing capabilities, lower dead space, sleeker and more efficient design, and automated records. Modernized anesthesia workstations have improved on the "bag-in-bottle" ventilation system to ascending and descending bellows. The most obvious improvement in design is perhaps in the improved monitoring systems displayed on user-friendly and easily configured to preference monitors. Many workstations offer increased real-time communications between the station and other departments such as the laboratory, pharmacy, and radiology [10].

Drager Medical, GE Healthcare, Maquet Getinge Group, Mindray North America, and Penlon create the most popular anesthesia workstations today. Table 3.3 details the differences between Drager Medical's and GE Healthcare's machines, two of the most popular workstations today [36]. Many of the dimensions of these workstations are very similar, and user preference should dictate purchase and trust in the respective manufacturer. A recent 2017 study investigated the error rates of the workstations of Drager Medical, GE Healthcare, and Maquet. Workstations by all three manufacturers exhibited low overall user error rates. Operators in the study most commonly rated the usability of Drager Medical's workstations higher than that of workstations of the other companies. However, these operators had routinely worked with Drager Medical's workstations in their practice and were more accustomed to its user interface. Inherent differences exist between the workstations in the user interface for accomplishing routine anesthesia tasks, but different operators may come to prefer different interfaces. Limitations in usability exist across the different manufacturers, but the study found experienced operators to accomplish tasks efficiently regardless [37].

For hospitals, provider-owned distributors, private practices, and other physician groups, inevitably the decision of anesthesia workstations will come to user preference. Proper training of personnel is first and foremost. While modernized anesthetic workstations have many advantages, certain limitations still persist in the design for certain workstations. These limitations include power supply dependence on electricity, no carbon monoxide production detection, a descending bellows system that delivers some positive end-expiratory pressure (PEEP) during ventilation, and movement of the ascending bellows regardless of a faulty leak [10] (see Table 3.3).

Conclusion

The modern anesthesia workstation is an important tool for the delivery of anesthesia care. Throughout the history of anesthesia, it has evolved from a simple gas delivery system of a few metal tubes and valves to a sophisticated and complex apparatus for the precise measurement and delivery of medical gases and volatile anesthetics, along with multiple modes of mechanical ventilation. Contemporary anesthesia workstations incorporate numerous safety features that have resulted in the practice of anesthesiology being a far safer and more precise science than in the premodern era of open-drop ether and flammable anesthetic agents. Increasingly, anesthesia workstations are electronically and computer-controlled. As with any complex piece of medical equipment, patient injury can result from operator error or equipment failure, so it is important that the anesthesia practitioner is thoroughly familiar with

Table 3.3 Comparison of Drager Medical and GE Healthcare anesthesia machines by dimensions and specifics

	Drager Medical	GE Healthcare
Flow control method	Electronic	Conventional flowmeters
Anesthetic gas-driving mechanisms	Piston	Bellows
Ventilation modes	VCV, PSV, PCV, volume mode autoflow	VCV, SIMV-PC, PSV, PSVPro, PCV, PCV-VG
Ventilator display	Color, flat screen	Color SVGA LCD
Dimensions	59 × 33.5 × 31.5 in	53.5 × 29.5 × 29.1 cm
Weight	365 lb	300 lb
Drawers	Two drawers, one lockable	Two drawers
Vaporizer mount type	Auto or manual exclusion	Select-a-Tec
Vaporizer positions	Two or three vaporizers	Two vaporizers
Battery backup	Yes	Yes
Gas types	Oxygen, nitrous oxide, air	Oxygen, nitrous oxide, air
Carbon dioxide absorber capacity	1.5 L	1.76 L

VCV, volume-controlled ventilation; PSV, pressure support ventilation; PCV, pressure-controlled ventilation; SIMV-PC, synchronized intermittent mandatory ventilation pressure control; PSVPro, pressure support ventilation with ventilator backup if spontaneous respirations stop; PCV-VG, pressure-controlled ventilation–volume guaranteed.
See reference [36].

the proper checkout and functioning of the anesthesia workstation. Additionally, backup safety equipment, outside of the anesthesia workstation (e.g., self-inflating ventilation bag/mask, suction, oxygen cylinder, and flowmeter) should be immediately available, in the event of workstation failure or breakdown. A program of regular preventative maintenance, by either the manufacturer or other qualified professional, is also essential for safe and reliable functioning of the anesthesia workstation.

References

1. Davey AJ, Diba A, Ward CS, eds. *Ward's Anaesthetic Equipment*, 6th ed. Edinburgh: Elsevier; 2011.

2. Sinclair CM, Thadsad MK, Barker I. Modern anaesthetic machines. *Contin Educ Anaesth Crit Care Pain*. 2006;6(2):75–8.

3. Dorsch JA, Dorsch SE. *Understanding Anesthesia Equipment*, 5th ed. Philadelphia, PA: Lippincott Williams & Wilkins; 2008.

4. Ehrenwerth J, Eisenkraft J, Berry J. *Anesthesia Equipment: Principles and Applications*, 3rd ed. Philadelphia, PA: Elsevier; 2020.

5. Gurudatt C. The basic anaesthesia machine. *Indian J Anaesth*. 2013;57(5):438.

6. Butterworth JF, Mackey DC, Wasnick JD. Chapter 4. The anesthesia machine. In: JF Butterworth, DC Mackey, JD Wasnick, eds. *Morgan & Mikhail's Clinical Anesthesiology*, 5th ed. New York, NY: McGraw Hill; 2013. Available from: https://accessmedicine.mhmedical.com/content.aspx?aid=57230318.

7. Cowles CE. Chapter 2. The operating room environment. In: JF Butterworth, DC Mackey, JD Wasnick, eds. *Morgan & Mikhail's Clinical Anesthesiology*, 5th ed. New York, NY: McGraw Hill; 2013. Available from: https://accessmedicine.mhmedical.com/content.aspx?aid=57230046.

8. Caplan RA, Vistica MF, Posner KL, Cheney FW. Adverse anesthetic outcomes arising from gas delivery equipment. *Anesthesiology*. 1997;87(4):741–8.

9. Brockwell RC, Andrews JJ. Complications of inhaled anesthesia delivery systems. *Anesthesiol Clin North Am*. 2002;20(3):539–54.

10. Patil VP, Shetmahajan MG, Divatla JV. The modern integrated anaesthesia workstation. *Indian J Anaesth*. 2013;57(5):446–54.

11. Thompson PW, Wilkinson DJ. Development of anaesthetic machines. *Br J Anaesth*. 1985;57(7):640–8.

12. Hendrickx JFA, De Wolf AM. The anesthesia workstation: quo vadis? *Anesth Analg*. 2018;127(3):671–5.

13. Butterworth JF, Mackey DC, Wasnick JD. Chapter 3. Breathing systems. In: JF Butterworth, DC Mackey, JD Wasnick, eds. *Morgan & Mikhail's Clinical Anesthesiology*, 5th ed. New York, NY: McGraw Hill; 2013. Available from: https://accessmedicine.mhmedical.com/content.aspx?aid=57230207.

14. Butterworth JF, Mackey DC, Wasnick JD. Chapter 4. The anesthesia workstation. In: JF Butterworth, DC Mackey, JD Wasnick, eds. *Morgan & Mikhail's Clinical Anesthesiology*, 6th ed. New York, NY: McGraw Hill; 2018. Available from: https://accessmedicine.mhmedical.com/content.aspx?aid=1161425729.

15. Das S, Chattopadhyay S, Bose P. The anaesthesia gas supply system. *Indian J Anaesth*. 2013;57(5):489–99.

16. Petty C. Understanding your machine: O2 flush valve key to safety. Anesthesia Patient Safety Foundation. 1993. Available from: www.apsf.org/article/understanding-your-machine-o2-flush-valve-key-to-safety/.

17. Mun SH, No MY. Internal leakage of oxygen flush valve. *Korean J Anesthesiol.* 2013;64(6):550–1.

18. Dosch MP, Tharp D. The anesthesia gas machine. 2021. Available from: https://healthprofessions.udmercy.edu/academics/na/agm/04.htm.

19. Anesthesia Key. The anesthesia machine. 2017. Available from: https://aneskey.com/the-anesthesia-machine-5/.

20. Butterworth JF, Mackey DC, Wasnick JD. Chapter 3. Breathing systems. In: JF Butterworth, DC Mackey, JD Wasnick, eds. *Morgan & Mikhail's Clinical Anesthesiology*, 6th ed. New York, NY: McGraw Hill; 2018. Available from: https://accessmedicine.mhmedical.com/content.aspx?aid=1161425570.

21. Goneppanavar U, Prabhu M. Anaesthesia machine: checklist, hazards, scavenging. *Indian J Anaesth.* 2013;57(5):533–40.

22. Cowles CE Jr. The operating room environment. In: JF Butterworth, DC Mackey, JD Wasnick, eds. *Morgan & Mikhail's Clinical Anesthesiology*, 6th ed. New York, NY: McGraw Hill; 2018. Available from: https://accessmedicine.mhmedical.com/content.aspx?aid=1161425482.

23. Parthasarathy S. The closed circuit and the low flow systems. *Indian J Anaesth.* 2013;57(5):516–24.

24. Kim J, Kang D, Lee H, Ryu S, Ryu S, Kim D. Change of inspired oxygen concentration in low flow anesthesia. *Anesth Pain Med (Seoul).* 2020;15(4):434–40.

25. Becker DE, Rosenberg M. Nitrous oxide and the inhalation anesthetics. *Anesth Progr.* 2008;55(4):124–31.

26. Venkatachalapathy R, Cherian A, Panneerselvam S. Changes in gas composition during low flow anaesthesia without nitrous oxide. *J Clin Diagn Res.* 2017;11(7):UC29–33.

27. Banks A, Hardman JG. Nitrous oxide. *Contin Educ Anaesth Crit Care Pain.* 2005;5(5):145–8.

28. Baum JA. The carrier gas in anaesthesia: nitrous oxide/oxygen, medical air/oxygen and pure oxygen. *Curr Opin Anaesthesiol.* 2004;17(6):513–16.

29. Agarwal A, Singh PK, Dhiraj S, Pandey CM, Singh U. Oxygen in air (FiO$_2$ 0.4) improves gas exchange in young healthy patients during general anesthesia. *Can J Anesth.* 2002;49(10):1040–3.

30. Young ER. Sedation: a guide to patient management, 4th edition. *Anesth Prog.* 2005;52(1):43–4.

31. Schlesinger WH. On the fate of anthropogenic nitrogen. *Proc Natl Acad Sci U S A.* 2009;106(1):203–8.

32. Cooper JB, Newbower RS, Kitz RJ. An analysis of major errors and equipment failures in anesthesia management: considerations for prevention and detection. *Anesthesiology.* 1984;60(1):34–42.

33. Arbous MS, Meursing AEE, van Kleef JW, *et al.* Impact of anesthesia management characteristics on severe morbidity and mortality. *Anesthesiology.* 2005;102(2):257–68; quiz 491–2.

34. Merchant R, Chartrand D, Dain S, *et al.* Guidelines to the practice of anesthesia revised edition 2013. *Can J Anaesth.* 2013;60(1):60–84.

35. Association of Anaesthetists of Great Britain and Ireland (AAGBI); Hartle A, Anderson E, Bythell V, *et al.* Checking anaesthetic equipment 2012: Association of Anaesthetists of Great Britain and Ireland. *Anaesthesia.* 2012;67(6):660–8.

36. Avante Health Solutions. GE and Drager anesthesia machines: how do they measure up? 2018. Available from: https://avantehs.com/learn/buying-guides/ge-drager-anesthesia-comparison.

37. Spaeth J, Schweizer T, Schmutz A, Buerkle H, Schumann S. Comparative usability of modern anaesthesia ventilators: a human factors study. *Br J Anaesth.* 2017;119(5):1000–8.

Patient Monitoring

William Lee, Nihir Patel, and Christina Jeng

Introduction

Patient monitoring is fundamental to the job of the anesthesiologist. Anesthetic drugs and surgical procedures can produce rapid changes in patient physiology and these changes may last throughout the perioperative period. It is essential that anesthesiologists have the capability to monitor these changes in real time to optimize patient safety and care throughout the perioperative period. The information acquired via various monitoring devices can be used to maintain quality patient care, but it does not guarantee any particular outcome. Multiple medical societies, including the preeminent anesthesiology society, the American Society of Anesthesiologists (ASA), have agreed upon a standard set of monitoring devices referred to as the ASA standard monitors. Other monitoring devices and invasive monitoring methods may be used, in addition to the standard ASA monitors, depending on specific patient and intraoperative surgical concerns. It is important that anesthesiologists are aware of the variety of devices at their disposal, so that they may appropriately utilize those monitors to optimize and ensure quality patient care.

Standard Intraoperative Patient Monitoring

A basic standard of monitoring has been recommended by various societies, including the ASA, for any procedures performed with an anesthetic administered by an anesthesiologist. The common theme among these standard requirements is their ability to monitor a patient's *oxygenation*, *ventilation*, *circulation*, and *temperature*. These four components provide a thorough, albeit not comprehensive, physiologic snapshot of a patient. During most procedures, these four components can be monitored via the standard ASA monitors. These include *pulse oximetry* to ensure adequate oxygenation, arterial *blood pressure* monitoring usually with a noninvasive blood pressure (NIBP) cuff and *electrocardiography* (ECG) to ensure adequate circulation, *capnography* to ensure adequate ventilation, and a thermometer to measure temperature. While these monitors are incredibly useful, they do not replace a vigilant clinician closely observing the patient throughout the procedure.

Pulse Oximetry

Pulse oximetry provides a significant amount of information with regard to oxygenation and circulation. The oximeter utilizes the differing light absorptions of oxyhemoglobin and deoxyhemoglobin to determine the overall oxygen saturation of the patient's hemoglobin. Oxygenated hemoglobin absorbs more infrared light at approximately 940 nm, and deoxyhemoglobin absorbs red light at 660 nm. The oximeter is typically placed on a single digit or earlobe, the nasal septum, or another part of the patient's body in which the oximeter can pulse light through the tissue and subsequently register it on the other side. As oxygenated blood pulses through the tissue between the oximeter, a ratio is generated via these differing absorptions to determine an approximation of the partial pressure of oxygen in the patient's blood and the resulting oxygen saturation (see Table 4.1). The oxygen saturation is measured during arterial pulsations of blood, which also allows for a relatively accurate measurement of the pulse rate and rhythm.

Most pulse oximeters generate a plethysmographic waveform and emit a pitched tone with each pulsation that correlates with various levels of oxygenation. The waveform can demonstrate whether or not the probe is positioned appropriately, and a change in waveform may indicate decreased perfusion. A change in the pitch with a proper waveform may represent decreased oxygenation. This audiovisual tool helps anesthesiologists to both see and hear the patient's rate, rhythm, and oxygenation while performing other tasks to address multiple patient care issues.

Table 4.1 Partial pressure of arterial oxygen (PaO_2) with blood oxygen saturation (SaO_2) estimations

PaO_2 (mmHg)	SaO_2 (%)
100	100
95	97
85	96
75	95
60	90
50	85
40	75
30	60

Of note, pulse oximetry may not always be accurate. Significant patient movement can disrupt wavelength monitoring and make it difficult for the oximeter to determine pulsations. Additionally, if the patient has altered forms of hemoglobin (that is, methemoglobin and carboxyhemoglobin), the oximeter will not provide a reliable representation of oxygen saturation. Carboxyhemoglobin will result in a falsely high reading, as it absorbs infrared light similarly to oxyhemoglobin. Methemoglobin will absorb light closer to 640 nm and consequently may decrease the average oxygenated hemoglobin reading registered by the oximeter. Thus, while pulse oximetry has enormous utility, its limitations and possibility for error should be kept in mind, so as to avoid misinterpretations of the patient's physiology.

Blood Pressure Monitoring

Blood pressure monitoring is a direct measurement of circulation, and a blood pressure measurement within normal range typically represents adequate perfusion. For the vast majority of cases, NIBP monitoring every 3–5 minutes is adequate to ensure hemodynamic stability. There are multiple techniques for NIBP monitoring. The most common method is via oscillometry, which measures oscillations that occur with arterial pulsations after compression with a pressure cuff. Maximum oscillations occur at the point of the mean arterial pressure (MAP), and systolic and diastolic blood pressures are subsequently calculated based on the measured MAP and the measured oscillations. Oscillometry can be inaccurate if the patient does not have a sinus rhythm, if an inappropriate cuff size is used, or in cases of extreme hypertension or hypotension. Other forms of NIBP monitoring can be utilized and should be readily available if the automated oscillometer malfunctions or is unavailable. These include pulse palpation of the extremities with or without cuff occlusion to estimate systolic pressure and auscultation via a stethoscope while using a sphygmomanometer or a Doppler probe which measures sound waves from the traveling pressure wave in the artery.

During procedures that require beat-to-beat blood pressure monitoring, such as procedures that could result in significant blood loss or rapid blood pressure changes or procedures that require multiple instances of intraoperative blood sampling, intraarterial blood pressure monitoring can be utilized. The risks of placing an intraarterial catheter include bleeding, nerve damage, thrombosis, arterial dissection, aneurysm, hematoma, infection, and vascular compromise at the puncture site. The procedure is performed in a sterile fashion by use of a small-gauge catheter. Common sites of arterial cannulation are the radial, axillary, femoral, and dorsalis pedis arteries, secondary to their ease of access and ease of securing the catheter externally without dampening of the arterial pressure waveform. Other sites for cannulation include the brachial or ulnar arteries. The brachial artery is often avoided secondary to its proximity to the median nerve, as well as the lack of collateral blood flow should thrombosis or other injury to the artery occur. The ulnar artery has also historically been avoided, as it is considered the primary arterial supply to the hand and is often deeper and more tortuous than the radial artery, making it more difficult to access.

When intraarterial blood pressure monitoring is used, pressure transducers utilize mechanical energy from pressure changes within the artery to generate electrical energy and a digital signal that is then transferred to the computer monitor observed by the anesthesiologist. When the patient is in the supine position, the transducer should be placed at the level of the heart for an accurate MAP reading that determines cardiac perfusion and cerebral perfusion at the level of the circle of Willis. In cases where the patient's position is altered, the transducer should be maintained in a position that allows for accurate measurement of the vital organs. Most commonly, when a patient is placed in an upright or sitting position, the level of the transducer should be elevated to coincide with the level of the circle of Willis to ensure adequate cerebral perfusion.

The appearance of the arterial waveform may vary with the different vessel sites, but the waveform has some standard components. As shown in Figure 4.1, the initial spike is the systolic upstroke and is a surrogate for left ventricular contractility. This spike is followed by a small dip and then a dicrotic notch, representing the end of systole and closure of the aortic valve. Lastly, a second drop in the waveform back to baseline is representative of the diastolic pressure and peripheral vascular resistance. Significant variability in the waveform with respirations or intraabdominal pressure changes can be indicative of decreased intravascular volume.

Capnography, Gas Analysis, and End-Tidal Carbon Dioxide

While delivering any anesthetic, the ability to perform real-time inhalational gas analysis can be an important tool to monitor a patient's ventilation, level of sedation, adequacy of analgesia, and airway patency while simultaneously indicating possible pathologies. Exhaled gas analysis is typically performed via infrared spectroscopy and is available with most anesthesia machines. Exhaled gas from a sidestream port passes through infrared light and the different components of that gas reflect or absorb infrared at different rates. This allows the sensor to determine what concentrations of gases are present. The composition of the expired air is then displayed as various percentages, which can inform the anesthesiologist how much nitrous oxide, volatile anesthetic gas, and carbon dioxide the patient is exhaling.

An oxygen analyzer is available with every anesthesia machine and is paramount to ensure that a patient does not receive a hypoxic gas mixture. Modern-day oxygen analysis occurs either via a galvanic fuel cell or, most

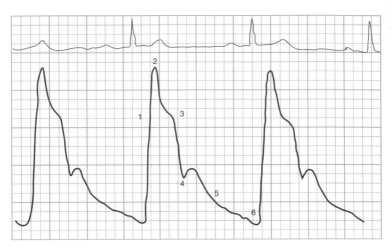

Figure 4.1 Standard intra-arterial blood pressure waveform and its correlation with electrocardiography. (1) Systolic upstroke followed by (2) the systolic peak pressure; (3) the systolic decline leading to the dicrotic notch (4); (5) represents the diastolic runoff ending at (6), the end-diastolic pressure. *Source:* Reproduced from Mark JB. *Atlas of Cardiovascular Monitoring.* Chapter 8, Fig. 8–1, page 94. New York, Copyright Elsevier and Churchill Livingstone,1998.

commonly, via a paramagnetic oxygen analyzer, which takes advantage of the electron imbalance in the oxygen molecule to create a magnetic field. While most anesthesia machines will perform an oxygen calibration with an automated check, it is important to ensure that the machine is appropriately calibrated to the atmospheric oxygen level (normal 21%) prior to any procedure to ensure adequate measurements during the delivery of anesthetic.

Carbon dioxide analysis in the form of end-tidal carbon dioxide ($ETCO_2$) can provide valuable information regarding the patient's metabolic status, respiratory pattern, and ventilation. The gas analyzer can generate a waveform based on the quantity of carbon dioxide exhaled, known as a capnograph. Additionally, the $ETCO_2$ can be used to monitor a patient's respiratory pattern and assess clinical changes.

In a spontaneously ventilating patient, an increase in the number of respirations, as measured by $ETCO_2$, can represent inadequate sedation or increased analgesic requirement. Similarly, a decrease in $ETCO_2$ can represent oversedation or decreased ventilatory drive. In an intubated patient who is mechanically ventilated, the $ETCO_2$ pattern can provide information regarding the adequacy of ventilation based on the waveform of the capnograph. For example, a "shark fin" waveform (see Figure 4.2) is indicative of an obstructive respiratory disorder, including acute bronchospastic disease or chronic obstructive pulmonary disease. Abrupt decreases in the capnograph waveform may be indicative of: a circuit disconnect or circuit leak; decreased perfusion in the setting of new-onset pulmonary embolism, heart failure, anaphylaxis, or cardiac arrest; or severe airway obstruction (that is, mucus plugging or severe multifocal bronchospasm). Changes in capnography, coupled with clinical observations, can guide and improve management.

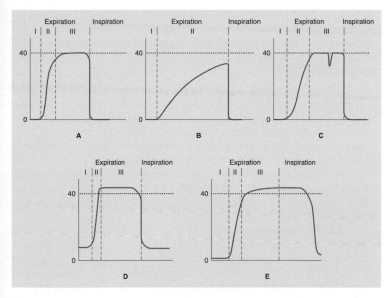

Figure 4.2 End-tidal carbon dioxide: example patterns of capnography. (A) Normal capnograph demonstrating the three phases of expiration: phase I – dead space; phase II – mixture of dead space and alveolar gas; phase III – alveolar gas plateau. (B) Capnograph of a patient with severe chronic obstructive pulmonary disease. No plateau is reached before the next inspiration. The gradient between end-tidal carbon dioxide and arterial carbon dioxide is increased. (C) Depression during phase III indicates spontaneous respiratory effort. (D) Failure of inspired carbon dioxide to return to zero may represent an incompetent expiratory valve or exhausted carbon dioxide absorbent. (E) Persistence of exhaled gas during part of the inspiratory cycle signals the presence of an incompetent inspiratory valve. *Source:* Reproduced with permission from *Morgan and Mikhail's Clinical Anesthesiology*: Chapter 6 Noncardiovascular monitoring. New York, Copyright Mcgraw-Hill, 2013.

Temperature Monitoring

The temperature of a patient can dramatically impact physiology, especially during general and neuraxial anesthetics. When general or neuraxial anesthesia is induced, the patient's vasculature undergoes significant vasodilation. This allows heat to move from the body's core to the periphery, causing hypothermia. Hypothermia can lead to decreased drug metabolism, coagulopathy, and poor perfusion, whereas hyperthermia can lead to tachycardia and neurologic injury. Core temperature can be monitored by placing a thermometer on the tympanic membrane or in the nasopharyngeal space, distal esophagus, or pulmonary artery. Often, direct measurement of core temperature is not always feasible and other appropriate sites such as the bladder, rectum, proximal esophagus, and axilla can also be used to provide a reliable and continuous measurement of a patient's temperature.

Electrocardiography

Standard intraoperative ECG monitoring for adults consists of a five-lead ECG, including the right arm, left arm, right leg, and left leg and V5 precordial leads. This allows the anesthesiologist to monitor the three limb leads, as well as the V5 waveform, for myocardial rhythm, ischemia, and electrolyte imbalances. Most commonly, leads II and V5 are displayed on the monitor. Lead II is utilized to analyze rhythm, as it often has the most prominent P wave and it can also indicate inferior wall ischemia. Lead V5 is one of the most sensitive indicators for ischemia, as it can best display lateral wall ischemia and is a proxy for observing the perfusion area of the left anterior descending artery or left circumflex coronary artery.

Importantly, lead placement may need to be adjusted based on the procedure, patient position, or anatomy, so that a patient can be appropriately monitored. Modifying the lead placement can allow for flexibility in what portion of the heart electrical activity is observed. If a patient has a known area of ischemia, lead placement should be adjusted accordingly to observe this area of perfusion.

While most healthy patients are unlikely to have a major perioperative adverse cardiac event, patients with preexisting coronary artery disease (CAD) or risk factors for CAD (i.e., smoking, diabetes, poor exercise tolerance, obesity, etc.) have a higher risk of an intraoperative and perioperative cardiac event, and therefore, continuous ECG should be monitored in order to detect changes in electrical activity that may indicate an ischemic event. New-onset conduction blocks, arrhythmias, and ST segment elevations or depressions can be indicative of ischemia (see Figure 4.3). Lastly, ECG can help the anesthesiologist suspect and detect electrolyte imbalances. Most prominently, the more extreme values of potassium, calcium, and magnesium can be identified within ECG changes and prompt further testing to guide specific treatments to avoid possible fatal cardiac arrhythmias.

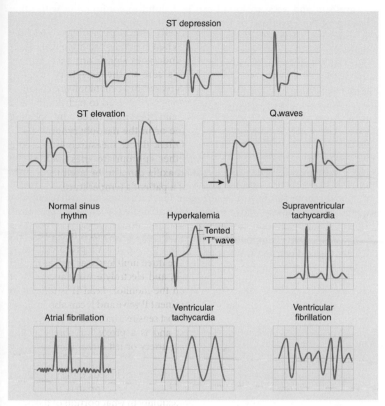

ST depression

ST elevation

Q.waves

Normal sinus rhythm

Hyperkalemia
—Tented "T" wave

Supraventricular tachycardia

Atrial fibrillation

Ventricular tachycardia

Ventricular fibrillation

Figure 4.3 Common ECG waves and their implications. *Source:* Reproduced with permission from *Cardiac Anesthesia and Transesophageal Echocardiography:* Chapter 3. Perioperative rhythm abnormalities. New York, Copyright McGraw-Hill, 2011.

Advanced Cardiovascular Monitoring Devices

Central Venous Pressure

In the past, central venous pressure (CVP) monitoring was commonly used for many high-risk surgeries, given its ease of measurement after placement of a central venous catheter. It was considered a surrogate for intravascular volume status and a predictor of fluid overload. While this has been disproven, the waveform and pressure trend can be helpful in conjunction with other indicators of fluid overload or hypovolemia. It is important to be acquainted with a normal CVP waveform (see Figure 4.4) in order to recognize the changes that can be indicative of pathology. For example, a new-onset large *a* wave, also known as a cannon *a* wave, can be indicative of improper conduction and pressure being transmitted from atrial contraction against a closed tricuspid valve, while fused *c* and *v* waves can be indicative of regurgitation or right ventricular failure.

Pulmonary Artery Catheter

Pulmonary artery catheters (PACs) are invasive monitoring devices that can be used to assess a patient's hemodynamic status. A PAC can provide measurements of a patient's cardiac output, pulmonary pressures, core temperature, mixed venous saturation (a surrogate for perfusion and cardiac output), and pulmonary capillary wedge pressure (a surrogate for left atrial pressure). Although this information can help direct clinical management of complex patients, PACs have not been proven to decrease mortality and are not routinely used. When the CVP is measured and a PAC is in place, multiple calculations can be performed to determine cardiac and physiologic

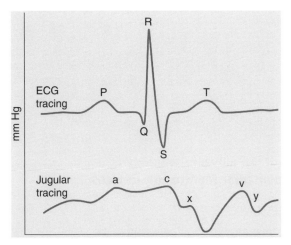

Figure 4.4 CVP waveform and its correlation to electrocardiography. *Source:* Reproduced with permission from Morgan and Mikhail's *Clinical Anesthesiology*: Chapter 5 Cardiovascular monitoring. New York, Copyright McGraw-Hill, 2013.

Table 4.2 Useful formulae for perioperative hemodynamic calculations

Variable	Formula	Normal	Units
Cardiac index	$\dfrac{\text{Cardiac output (L/min)}}{\text{Body surface area (m}^2)}$	2.2–4.2	L/min/m^2
Total peripheral resistance	$\dfrac{(\text{MAP} - \text{CVP}) \times 80}{\text{Cardiac output (L/min)}}$	1200–1500	dynes·s cm^{-5}
Pulmonary vascular resistance	$\dfrac{(\overline{\text{PA}} - \text{PAOP}) \times 80}{\text{Cardiac output (L/min)}}$	100–300	dynes·s cm^{-5}
Stroke volume	$\text{Cardiac output} \left(\dfrac{\text{L/min}) \times 1000}{\text{Heart rate(beats/min)}} \right)$	60–90	mL/bear
Stroke index (SI)	$\dfrac{\text{Stroke volume(mL/beat)}}{\text{Body surface area(m}^2)}$	20–65	ml/beat/m^2
Right ventricular stroke-work index	$0.0136(\overline{\text{PA}} - \text{CVP}) \times \text{SI}$	30–65	g-m/beat/m^2
Left ventricular stroke-work index	$0.0136(\text{MAP} - \text{PAOP}) \times \text{SI}$	46–60	g-m/beat/m^2

Source: Reproduced with permission from *Morgan and Mikhail's Clinical Anesthesiology*: Chapter 5 Cardiovascular monitoring. New York, Copyright McGraw-Hill, 2013.

parameters of the patient (see Table 4.2) that can be helpful in making a thorough assessment of the patient at any given time.

Transthoracic and Transesophageal Echocardiography

Transthoracic echocardiography (TTE) is an important tool that is simple and noninvasive, and can be easily performed to provide real-time analysis of basic cardiac function. While it is beyond the scope of this chapter, TTE will likely become more widely used intraoperatively and postoperatively to help monitor a patient's general cardiac function, valvular abnormalities, and wall ischemia, especially by clinicians who are trained in focus-assessed transthoracic echocardiography (FATE) (see below). Similarly, transesophageal echocardiography (TEE) is a relatively low-risk, informative tool that can provide a full scope of cardiac function. Some relative contraindications to TEE include gastric or esophageal surgery, gastric or esophageal pathology, arteriovenous malformations, portal hypertension with esophageal varices, perforated viscus, or patients who have recently ingested, particularly with an unprotected airway. While not all anesthesiologists are certified to perform TEE, if available, it can provide even more accurate and comprehensive information than TTE. During an acute event, it can provide rapid, high-quality information that may help guide treatment.

Other Monitoring Devices

Point-of-Care Ultrasound (POCUS)

As ultrasound technology has become more widely available, the anesthesiologist's ability to observe and diagnose physiologic changes in real time has improved. Anesthesiologists should be well versed in several standard ultrasound examinations, including focused assessment with sonography in trauma (FAST) and FATE. With an experienced operator, the FAST examination has high utility for both trauma and perioperative patients, especially if they are hemodynamically unstable or if there is concern for hemorrhage. A FAST examination is performed with a curvilinear probe and includes four views: subxiphoid to visualize the pericardium and retrocardiac space; the hepatorenal and splenorenal recesses to visualize retroperitoneal fluid or bleeding; and lastly the suprapubic view to visualize pelvic fluid or blood. If any of the sites demonstrate significant fluid, it is possible the patient is bleeding and may need interventional hemostasis, blood transfusion, or vasoactive support to ensure hemodynamic stability. The FATE examination can be helpful in obtaining an overview of a patient's cardiac function. The four views – parasternal long and short axes, apical four-chamber, and subcostal – are best identified with a phased-array probe and can allow the operator to visualize left ventricular function, right ventricular strain or failure, vascular prolapse, valvular stenosis, and pericardial fluid. While quantification of these pathologies may be difficult with standard ultrasound, visualizing the anatomy and possible cardiac pathology can help guide management perioperatively.

Urine Output

Urine output is often considered a proxy measurement for renal perfusion. Adequate urine output is defined as 0.5–1 ml/(kg hr) and is a fairly reliable surrogate for perfusion of the kidneys, though it does not guarantee adequate kidney function. Moreover, monitoring urine output can help guide fluid management. While other cardiovascular monitoring devices can be utilized, urine output alone may be a good indicator of adequate fluid resuscitation.

Neuromuscular Blockade Monitoring

Neuromuscular blocking (NMB) agents are often utilized to optimize surgical conditions and prevent patient movement during surgical procedures. A nerve stimulator or an accelerometer are tools to measure the level of neuromuscular blockade and recovery. Nerve stimulators can be applied to various sites to stimulate different nerves and subsequent muscle contraction (see Table 4.3). Reactions to tetanus, dual-burst stimulation, and train-of-four (TOF) stimulation can give the anesthesiologist information about the degree of neuromuscular blockade. TOF stimulation is performed by stimulating the nerve with an electrical signal four times in automatic, rapid succession and then observing for muscle twitches in the distribution of the nerve stimulated. When NMB agents are in full effect, stimulation of nerves will likely result in no twitches, but as recovery occurs, more twitches will be visible. When four twitches are present, a TOF ratio can be performed via an accelerometer, a device that measures the amplitude of each twitch and provides a ratio of the last twitch, compared to the first. Full recovery from neuromuscular blockade is commonly defined as a TOF ratio >0.9. It is important to note that in order to achieve adequate recovery, medications to reverse neuromuscular blockade should only be administered when there is at least one twitch present.

Table 4.3 Approximate electrode placement for neuromuscular blockade monitoring

Nerve	Muscle(s) stimulated	Proximal electrode placement	Distal electrode placement
Ulnar nerve	Adductor pollicis	Flexor and medial surface of the forearm, 3–5 cm proximal to distal placement	Flexor and medial surface of the forearm, just proximal to the palm
Facial nerve	Orbicularis oculi	Next to the tragus of the ear on the face	1–2 cm superior and ipsilateral to the eyebrow on the lateral portion
Common peroneal nerve	Tibialis anterior	1–2 cm distal and parallel to the fibular head	1–2 cm distal and parallel to the fibular head
Tibial nerve	Flexor hallucis brevis	3–5 cm superior and 1–2 cm posterior to the medial malleolus	1–2 cm inferior and posterior to the medial malleolus

Consciousness Monitoring

Patients are often most concerned about awareness while under general anesthesia. Previously, monitoring of consciousness and the plane of anesthesia was performed exclusively by clinical observation of pupil size, ocular movement, cranial nerve reflexes, and vital signs. Advances in electroencephalography (EEG) technology have allowed for the advent of consciousness monitoring that is convenient and can be utilized by the anesthesiologist intraoperatively. The most common of these technologies is the bispectral index (BIS). The BIS processes EEG signals obtained from a probe placed on the patient's forehead to generate a unitless number that helps anesthesiologists estimate consciousness. A BIS value of 40–60 has been used as an indicator of adequate depth of general anesthesia. While it can potentially indicate less likelihood of awareness, the BIS can be affected by motor activity and electrocautery. Additionally, there have been case reports of awareness occurring even when BIS monitoring was applied and maintained below a value of 60. Clinical signs of awareness, such as sweating, tearing, and increased heart rate and blood pressure, can all be indicative of a light plane of anesthesia and should always be considered in conjunction with the BIS monitor. Although EEG monitoring provides valuable information, these monitoring devices do not guarantee that a patient will not experience awareness under anesthesia.

Neuromonitoring

While rarely monitored by the anesthesiologist directly, neurologic monitoring may be performed intraoperatively for procedures that can impact the brain or spinal cord. The anesthetics employed can impact the data gathered by these monitors. More specifically, somatosensory evoked potentials (SSEPs), motor evoked potentials (MEPs), brain–auditory evoked potentials (BAEPs), and lastly visual evoked potentials (VEPs) can all be utilized to monitor specific neurologic pathways. For example, procedures involving the spinal cord will include monitoring that is focused on MEPs via the corticospinal tract and on SSEPs via the spinothalamic tract. This monitoring is performed by sending electrical signals through these spinal cord pathways and measuring the potentials generated. A waveform is generated by a given electrical signal, and increases in latency or decreases in amplitude may indicate injury to the nerve tract. SSEPs and MEPs are very sensitive to volatile anesthetic agents. Therefore, when neuromonitoring is expected to be used, volatile agents should be avoided. Use of NMB agents would also abolish all forms of MEP due to the inability of muscle to respond to a stimulus. Total intravenous anesthesia without long-acting neuromuscular blockade is usually utilized for these cases. BAEPs and VEPs are rarely used. VEPs share a similar sensitivity to

SSEPs with regard to anesthetics. BAEPs are the most resistant to anesthetic agents but are limited as to what information they provide, given they are only an indicator that the brainstem and auditory neurological tracts are intact.

Review Questions

1. Which of the following monitors is not considered part of the standard of care during general anesthesia, as defined by the American Society of Anesthesiologists?

   (a) Blood pressure
   (b) Electrocardiography
   (c) Pulse oximetry
   (d) End-tidal carbon dioxide
   (e) Urine output

2. Which of the following is the best proxy measurement for left ventricular function during intraarterial blood pressure monitoring?

   (a) Dicrotic notch
   (b) Baseline value of a waveform
   (c) Systolic upstroke
   (d) Area under an individual waveform
   (e) Second peak of an arterial waveform

Answers

1 (e) While urine output is a valuable tool to measure renal perfusion, as a proxy for general perfusion and intravascular volume status, it is not considered a standard monitor during general anesthesia.

2 (c) The slope of the systolic upstroke is considered a surrogate for left ventricular contraction. If a patient has systolic heart failure, the slope of the systolic upstroke would be decreased, and thus slower to rise.

Further Reading

American Society of Anesthesiologists. Standards for basic anesthetic monitoring. 2015. Available from: www.asahq.org/standards-and-guidelines/standards-for-basic-anesthetic-monitoring.

Butterworth JF, Mackey DC, Wasnick JD. Chapter 5. Cardiovascular monitoring. In: JF Butterworth, DC Mackey, JD Wasnick, eds. *Morgan & Mikhail's Clinical Anesthesiology*, 5th ed. New York, NY: McGraw Hill; 2013. Available from: https://accessanesthesiology.mhmedical.com/content.aspx?sectionid=42800535&bookid=564.

Butterworth JF, Mackey DC, Wasnick JD. Chapter 6. Noncardiovascular monitoring. In: JF Butterworth, DC Mackey, JD Wasnick, eds. *Morgan & Mikhail's Clinical Anesthesiology*, 5th ed. New York, NY: McGraw Hill; 2013. Available from: https://accessanesthesiology.mhmedical.com/content.aspx?sectionid=42800536&bookid=564.

Gelb AW, Morriss WW, Johnson W, *et al.*; International Standards for a Safe Practice of Anesthesia Workgroup. World Health Organization-World Federation of Societies of Anaesthesiologists (WHO-WFSA) international standards for a safe practice of anesthesia. *Anesth Analg.* 2018;126(6):2047–55. Available from: https://journals.lww.com/anesthesia-analgesia/Fulltext/2018/06000/World_Health_Organization_World_Federation_of.39.aspx.

Mark JB. Direct arterial blood pressure monitoring: normal waveforms. In: JB Mark. *Atlas of Cardiovascular Monitoring.* New York, NY: Churchill Livingstone; 1998, pp. 91–8.

Wasnick JD, Hillel Z, Kramer D, Littwin S, Nicoara A. Chapter 3. Perioperative rhythm abnormalities. In: JD Wasnick, Z Hillel, D Kramer, S Littwin, A Nicoara, eds. *Cardiac Anesthesia and Transesophageal Echocardiography.* New York, NY: McGraw Hill; 2011. Available from: https://accessanesthesiology.mhmedical.com/content.aspx?sectionid=43896238&bookid=418.

Inhalational Anesthetics

Ricardo Diaz Milian

Introduction

Inhalational anesthetics (IAs) are a group of medications utilized, almost exclusively, for the induction and maintenance of anesthesia during surgery. The demonstration of ether anesthesia in 1846 marked the beginning of the use of IAs in clinical practice. Today, modern IAs are used widely, mainly due to their reliability, minimal interindividual variation of the desired pharmacological effect, and the ease of continuous monitoring during anesthesia. Interestingly, the exact mechanism of action of modern IAs is not completely understood. However, recent developments in basic neuropharmacology have elucidated a probable mechanism of action. IAs display unique pharmacokinetics due to the fact that they are gases and are delivered directly to the lungs via the anesthesia machine. Consequently, the interactions of IAs with the body (pharmacokinetics) are very different in comparison to other anesthetics that are administered intravenously. IAs have proven to be instrumental in the modern practice of anesthesia. However, they are not without unwanted adverse effects, some of which can be life-threatening. A deep understanding of these potent drugs and their effects on patients is indispensable for the practice of anesthesiology. This chapter will briefly review the history of IAs and describe the pharmacology of these drugs, including potential complications.

History

Diethyl ether has been known for centuries. However, in 1842, Crawford Williamson began experimenting with the administration of the drug as an anesthetic for small surgeries. This event initiated a course of events that paved the way to the use of volatile gases to provide anesthesia [1]. In October 16, 1846, William Thomas Green Morton demonstrated the use of inhaled ether to an audience at the Massachusetts General Hospital in Boston on what is now known as "ether day" [2]. Although he is not credited as the first person to utilize an IA, his demonstration received worldwide attention and revolutionized the practice of medicine. Nitrous oxide was discovered in 1772 by Joseph Priestley, and in 1844, the first demonstration of its medical use was performed during dental extractions [3]. This makes nitrous oxide the oldest IA currently in use.

Modern fluorinated hydrocarbon anesthetics are very simple chemical compounds with an interesting historical origin. Their development was facilitated by the ultrasecret Manhattan Project, which was commissioned to develop nuclear weapons during the Second World War. Prior to this effort, there was little interest in the chemistry of such compounds. However, during the late 1930s, a sudden and intense interest in fluorine chemistry emerged as fluorine was recognized as a valuable adjuvant in the process of uranium enrichment. Enriched uranium is a critical constituent of atomic weapons. Shortly after, it was recognized that fluorinated hydrocarbons had anesthetic properties [4]. However, it was not until 1956 that Raventos discovered halothane, the first fluorinated anesthetic of clinical utility. The development of the modern fluorinated hydrocarbon anesthetics currently in use (desflurane, isoflurane, and sevoflurane) was the result of extensive research and experimentation with the objective of improving the characteristics of earlier-generation anesthetics [5].

Pharmacology

All IAs are gases with different chemical structures, but similar clinical effects. Chemically, they comprise halogenated hydrocarbons, ethers, alkanes, noble gases, aromatic molecules, and alcohols [6]. Modern anesthetics in current use include the fluorinated hydrocarbons desflurane (CF_2 H-O-CFH-CF3), isoflurane (CF_2 H-O-CCIH-CF3), and sevoflurane (CFH2-O-CH[CF3]2) [7], and the inorganic gas nitrous oxide (N_2O). Other anesthetics such as halothane and enflurane are still used in some developing countries. Interestingly, a resurgence of ether has also been proposed [8]. However, the use of these older anesthetics is generally disfavored due to their side effect profile. This chapter will only discuss the modern halogenated anesthetics and nitrous oxide.

Pharmacodynamics

General anesthesia can be defined as a reversible state of drug-induced unconsciousness, amnesia, analgesia, and immobility in response to a surgical stimulus [9]. The exact mechanism by which IAs can induce and maintain general anesthesia has not yet been fully elucidated and remains one of the biggest mysteries of neuropharmacology. However, recent developments have given some insight into the likely pathways of unconsciousness caused by these drugs.

A unique property of IAs is that they exert the same biological effects in all living organisms, including animals, plants, and even prokaryotes [10]. This means that all organisms, complex or unicellular, can be reversibly anesthetized [6]. The extent to which these drugs affect the entirety of earth's biodiversity supports a target molecule or group of molecules that are fundamental to life, and therefore universally preserved throughout the evolution of species. These target molecules have remained elusive; however, it is known that anesthetics affect vital intracellular processes, including mitochondrial energy pathways, cytoskeletal structure, and ion channel function. An important clinical consequence of the homogeneity of effects of IAs is that there is very little interspecies difference in response among all different genotypes. This means that there is a strong and predictable correlation between IA concentration and observed effects in most humans. This property, combined with the ability to continuously monitor their end-tidal concentrations, is what makes them very reliable drugs for maintenance of anesthesia during surgery.

At the beginning of the twentieth century, Meyer and Overton independently discovered the correlation between lipid solubility and anesthetic potency. This led to the Meyer–Overton "lipoid" hypothesis [11], which formulates that IAs exert their effects by changing the lipid solubility of neuronal cellular membranes. This change in solubility leads to a nonspecific effect that alters the activity of molecules embedded in the membrane. Among those molecules are ion channels that can change the membrane potential, and thus the likelihood of neuronal depolarization. However, newer evidence has shown that IAs interact directly with protein targets [10], including direct inhibition of luciferase and other proteins that affect modulatory mechanisms linked to neurotransmitter receptors, neuronal ion channels, and the cytoskeleton. A group of potassium channels (TREK-1) were recently discovered that are strongly activated by IAs. The importance of these channels in the mechanisms of general anesthesia is evidenced by knockout TREK-1 animals that exhibit anesthetic resistance. Recently, a novel mechanism of TREK-1 activation via disruption of phospholipase D2 and disruption of lipid–protein domains, known as "lipid rafts" [12], has been demonstrated [13]. This would represent a direct effect of IAs on membrane lipids and membrane proteins that then exert effects on ion channels – perhaps explaining Meyer and Overton's results from the last century.

Pharmacokinetics

One of the most important pharmacokinetic characteristics of IAs is the blood/gas partition coefficient. This coefficient describes how the particles of each gas will distribute between the alveoli and the blood after equilibrium has been achieved. It affects the anesthetic uptake, and therefore its onset of action, as well as its clearance. Age, body mass index, gender, and hemoglobin do not appear to have any effect on the blood/gas coefficient [14]. The water/gas partition coefficient of isoflurane is 0.59, sevoflurane 0.37, and desflurane 0.27

[14]. The higher the partition coefficient, the higher the solubility and potency of the IA. Higher solubility correlates inversely with onset of anesthesia; therefore, the more soluble an IA is, the slower its onset [15]. The partition coefficients between the gas and blood, and blood and brain (the target organ) are known and shown in Table 5.1. Notice that isoflurane is the most soluble of the halogenated hydrocarbon anesthetics, and therefore the most potent. This correlates with its comparatively low minimum alveolar concentration (MAC). Inversely, it also has the slowest onset of action.

Clearance of IAs occurs almost exclusively via the lungs, since liver metabolism of available modern IAs is minimal [16]. Consequently, the most important factor in the clearance of IAs is ventilation, and there is a direct correlation between rate of clearance and ventilation. Theoretically, the lower the blood/gas partition coefficient of an anesthetic, the faster it should be cleared. However, this assumption is not supported by clinical evidence [17]. The duration of administration of an IA also correlates directly with the rate of clearance [18]. An increase in the alveolar concentration of an IA can occur when it is used concomitantly with a gas with a high uptake rate (nitrous oxide). This phenomenon is known as the second gas effect. Conversely, during emergence, nitrous oxide is quickly removed from the circulation and it increases the clearance of other gases [19]. Oxygen is one of such gases, and therefore, emergence of nitrous oxide anesthesia can be complicated by hypoxemia. Consequently, administration of 100% inhaled oxygen is recommended after the administration of nitrous oxide anesthesia.

Nitrous Oxide (N_2O)

Nitrous oxide is a natural gas with analgesic and anesthetic properties. It is the least potent of the IAs [20]. Owing to its low solubility, it has a rapid uptake and this property is utilized to facilitate the rapid uptake of other IAs. Another consequence of this property is the displacement of other gases in body

Table 5.1 Pharmacokinetic properties of inhalational anesthetics

Agent	Blood:gas PC	Brain:blood PC	MAC
Isoflurane	1.4	2.6	1.2
Desflurane	0.42	1.3	6.0
Sevoflurane	0.65	1.7	2.0

PC, partition coefficient; MAC, minimum alveolar coefficient. *Source:* Adapted from Sakai *et al.* [24].

compartments, including oxygen in the lungs; this is known as diffusion hypoxia. Nitrous oxide can cause hematopoietic adverse reactions and teratogenicity. However, the clinical significance in humans is debatable and seems to be neglibile [20].

Sevoflurane [CH2 F-O-CH(CF3)2]

Sevoflurane is a fluorinated methyl-isopropyl ether, liquid at room temperature, that lacks odor and is not pungent [21]. This characteristic makes it the ideal IA for inhalational induction of general anesthesia. Sevoflurane undergoes degradation into olefin compounds (hydrocarbons), named compounds A, B, C, and D [21]. Compound A is generated when sevoflurane is administered in a semi-closed circuit with high-alkali-containing carbon dioxide as a scavenger, especially when used at low fresh gas flows [22]. Compound A has been shown to cause renal damage in animals. However, this is likely of no clinical significance in humans [21, 22].

Isoflurane (CHF2-O-CHCl-CF3)

Isoflurane is a difluoromethyl ether that is pungent and associated with airway irritation [23]. Isoflurane is more soluble in tissues than desflurane [23], a property that increases the time of emergence from general anesthesia and is directly correlated with the length of time of administration.

Desflurane (CF2 H-O-CFH-CF3)

Desflurane is a fluorinated methyl-ethyl ether and the least soluble of potent IAs [21]. It is liquid at room temperature and exists as a combination of two isomers with similar biological activity [21]. It is the only widely used anesthetic that requires a special vaporizer with external heating for accurate dosing. This is because at room temperature its vapor pressure is similar to the atmospheric pressure. Therefore, a standard vaporizer would deliver inaccurate doses of the gas at that temperature [21]. Desflurane has the lowest lipid-to-blood solubility; this property has the hypothetical advantage of lessening fat absorption of the drug in obese patients [24]. This should equate to faster emergence of anesthesia after long surgeries (>2 hours). However, clinical studies have demonstrated only modest difference in emergence timing, compared to sevoflurane and isoflurane [24]. Due to its pungency, desflurane is not an appropriate anesthetic to use for induction of general anesthesia.

Adverse Reactions

Like all drugs, IAs have the potential to cause adverse reactions, including life-threatening complications. This underscores the importance of an in-depth understanding of the pharmacology of these drugs by anesthesiologists. Some adverse effects are common to all modern IAs. All IAs cause postoperative nausea and vomiting, albeit to a different extent. Similarly, all modern fluorinated hydrocarbon anesthetics cause hypotension by decreasing vascular tone. It is important to appreciate that although volatile anesthetics are associated with adverse reactions, they remain very important agents for maintenance of anesthesia. Perhaps the most important reason that IAs remain the most common drugs utilized for this objective is the ability to continuously monitor their exhaled concentration. Consequently, they are considered protective against the very important complication of intraoperative awareness. When total intravenous anesthesia is used as an alternative to IAs, patients are at a tenfold increase risk of this complication [25].

Postoperative Nausea and Vomiting

Both fluorinated hydrocarbons and nitrous oxide produce postoperative nausea and vomiting in an exposure time-dependent fashion [26]. Total intravenous anesthesia, in comparison, is associated with a lower risk of postoperative nausea and vomiting [26].

Nitrous Oxide and Effects on Cavities

The most important consideration for the use of nitrous oxide is its potential to expand physiologic and pathologic formed air-filled cavities. Therefore, nitrous oxide should be avoided, or used with caution, in patients with pneumothorax, pneumocephalus, pneumomediastinum, pulmonary blebs, and bowel obstruction with dilated bowel loops. The mechanism by which nitrous oxide causes this expansion is explained by the rate at which the gas can enter a cavity. Nitrous oxide is more soluble than air, and therefore, its uptake into the blood is reduced after it enters a cavity. The result is that the cavity expands in a time-dependent fashion [27]. Due to this time dependency, short administration of nitrous oxide is likely acceptable in some of these conditions.

Unwanted Physiological Effects of Fluorinated Hydrocarbons

Intracellular biological processes that are affected by anesthetics include mitochondrial energy production, cytoskeletal structural formation, and the function of ion channels [10]. Modern halogenated IAs can cause expected, but adverse, physiological effects, including hypotension, increase in heart rate, QT interval prolongation, decreased tidal volume and increased respiratory frequency, and airway irritation. Rarely, they can also cause increased intracranial pressure. Older IAs are linked to hepatotoxicity and nephrotoxicity. There are no reported cases of either complication with currently used IAs.

Malignant Hyperthermia

All volatile anesthetics, with the exception of nitrous oxide, are considered trigger agents for malignant hyperthermia (MH) [28]. MH is a rare, but potentially lethal, hypermetabolic reaction to anesthesia. It is characterized by hypercapnia that is refractory to aggressive ventilation, muscle rigidity, hyperthermia, metabolic acidosis, electrolyte imbalances, cardiac arrhythmias, and death. Patients with an MH episode and their families are at risk of developing an episode of MH. Therefore, IAs are not to be used in patients who are at risk (personal or family history of MH).

Nephrotoxicity and Hepatotoxicity

Older IAs are associated with rare, yet significant, adverse reactions caused by products of their liver metabolism. Methoxyflurane (discontinued) produces nephrotoxicity via the fluoride ion. Similarly, halothane is associated with fulminant hepatitis by trifluoroacyl chloride, a metabolite produced by the drug's liver metabolism [16]. For this reason, the metabolism of modern anesthetics has undergone exhaustive scrutiny. Modern anesthetics undergo minimal liver metabolism, via cytochrome p450 enzymes, to toxic metabolites. However, the concentrations produced clinically have failed to demonstrate any significant effect. Of initial concern, compound A does not seem to be linked to nephrotoxicity in humans.

Carbon Monoxide Toxicity

All modern anesthetics produce carbon monoxide when reacting with a desiccated carbon dioxide absorbent (scavenging system) [24]. The production of carbon monoxide is likely related to potency and is greater with desflurane than with isoflurane. Sevoflurane produces negligible amounts of the toxic gas [24]. Care should be taken to examine the state of the carbon dioxide absorbent to prevent this complication, particularly in the first case of the day. Accidental flow of gas through the anesthesia machine for prolonged periods of time (e.g., weekends) enables desiccation of carbon dioxide absorbents.

Protective Effects of Inhaled Anesthetics

Several decades of basic science research have supported the concept of anesthetic preconditioning of the myocardium, a process where short periods of ischemia provide protection against subsequent prolonged ischemia. This had also been suggested by several meta-analyses that included patients undergoing cardiac surgery. However, a recent randomized prospective controlled trial that compared the use of total intravenous anesthesia to IAs for maintenance of anesthesia in cardiac surgery failed to demonstrate a mortality benefit [29].

Monitoring of Depth of Anesthesia

The purpose of monitoring the depth of anesthesia is to prevent memory formation during procedures (intraoperative awareness). Intraoperative awareness is a dreaded complication of general anesthesia that has an incidence of 0.1–0.2% [30]. It can have devastating effects on quality of life and can lead to posttraumatic stress disorder. The gold standard for monitoring of depth of anesthesia is continuous measurement of end-tidal concentration of the anesthetic drug. This concentration can be utilized to determine the age-adjusted MAC. The MAC (or MACM) of an anesthetic is defined as the minimal end-tidal concentration at which 50% of a population will not move as a response to a surgical stimulus. Consequently, MAC values for the fluorinated hydrocarbon anesthetics are as follows: isoflurane 1.2, desflurane 6.0, sevoflurane 2.0, and nitrous oxide 104 [20, 24]. Importantly, MAC values are additive (e.g., 0.5 MAC of sevoflurane + 0.5 MAC of desflurane = 1 MAC). IAs prevent movement by acting on both the spinal cord and the brain [31] and they produce amnesia through their direct effects on the brain. Consequently, there is a MAC for movement (MACM), and a MAC for awareness (MACA). MACA is the end-tidal concentration of an anesthetic at which 50% of a population do not remember events during anesthesia. The necessary concentration to prevent awareness is significantly lower than the concentration needed to prevent movement and is generally accepted to be around 0.3 of MACM. At twice this concentration, or 0.6 MACM, 99% of the individuals will not form memories. A general recommendation is to keep anesthetized patients at 0.7 MAC, to prevent intraoperative awareness. It is important to consider the factors that affect the MAC of anesthetics. The most important factor that predictably affects MAC is age. Increased age decreases MAC by a factor of 7% per decade above 40 years of age. Conversely, MAC increases by the same factor of 7% each decade below 40 years of age, peaking at the age of 6 months [31]. Temperature, sodium concentration, and genetic makeup are other important variables that affect MAC [31]. Drugs that affect MAC include intravenous anesthetics, which decrease MAC. Opioids are known to reduce MAC; however, this needs to be carefully interpreted. Opioids can reduce MACM by inhibition of movement by acting on receptors in the spine. However, this mechanism lacks amnestic effects on the brain and it is known that they do not affect MACA. Consequently, they should not be relied on to prevent awareness. Central nervous system (CNS) stimulants, including cocaine and amphetamines, increase MAC during an acute intoxication; however, chronic use decreases MAC [31]. Acute ethanol intoxication, a CNS depressant, causes a decrease in MAC. Nevertheless, chronic use decreases MAC requirements. Chronic use of other CNS depressants, including benzodiazepines and antiepileptics, increases MAC requirements and is a risk factor for intraoperative awareness.

Brain activity monitors (BAIs) utilize raw electroencephalographic data to calculate a dimensionless number that indicates whether the patient is anesthetized or at risk of intraoperative awareness. Multiple trials have addressed the question of performance superiority between age-adjusted MAC and BAIs in preventing episodes of intraoperative awareness. The first randomized controlled trial suggested superiority of BAIs over MAC; however, the study design was limited by concerns of the Hawthorne effect in the BAI group [32]. Subsequent studies have addressed that concern and found no difference between MAC and BAI performance [33, 34]. Due to this limitation of BAIs, age-adjusted MAC remains the gold standard measurement to monitor anesthetic depth when using IAs for maintenance of anesthesia.

Conclusion

IAs currently in use include a naturally occurring gas and three fluorinated hydrocarbons. The exact mechanism of action of these drugs is yet to be elucidated. The most important pharmacokinetic property of these drugs is the blood/air partition coefficient, as it determines their anesthetic potency. Adverse reactions that are relatively common include postoperative nausea and vomiting and hypotension. Rare, life-threatening complications can also occur, the most important being MH. However, they remain to be the most commonly used drugs for maintenance of anesthesia due to their reliability and the ability to monitor their alveolar concentration.

References

1. Whalen FX, Bacon DR, Smith HM. Inhaled anesthetics: an historical overview. *Best Pract Res Clin Anaesthesiol*. 2005;19(3):323–30. DOI: 10.1016/j.bpa.2005.02.001.

2. Chaturvedi R, Gogna RL. Ether day: an intriguing history. *Med J Armed Forces India*. 2011;67(4):306–8. DOI: 10.1016/S0377-1237(11)60098-1.

3. Lew V, McKay E, Maze M. Past, present, and future of nitrous oxide. *Br Med Bull*. 2018;125(1):103–19. DOI: 10.1093/bmb/ldx050.

4. Holmes CMK. The Manhattan legacy. *Anaesth Intensive Care*. 2007;35(Suppl. 1):17–20. DOI: 10.1177/0310057x0703501s03.

5. Terrell RC. The invention and development of enflurane, isoflurane, sevoflurane, and desflurane. *Anesthesiology*. 2008;108(3):531–3. DOI: 10.1097/aln.0b013e31816499cc.

6. Lynch C. Meyer and Overton revisited. *Anesth Analg*. 2008;107(3):864–7. DOI: 10.1213/ane.0b013e3181706c7e.

7. Eger EI. New inhaled anesthetics. *Anesthesiology*. 1994;80(4):906–22.

8. Chang CY, Goldstein E, Agarwal N, Swan KG. Ether in the developing world: rethinking an abandoned agent. *BMC Anesthesiol*. 2015;15(1):1–5. DOI: 10.1186/s12871-015-0128-3.

9. Brown EN, Pavone KJ, Naranjo M. Multimodal general anesthesia: theory and practice. *Anesth Analg*. 2018;127(5):1246–58. DOI: 10.1213/ANE.0000000000003668.

10. Kelz MB, Mashour GA. The biology of general anesthesia from paramecium to primate. *Curr Biol*. 2019;29(22):R1199–210. DOI: 10.1016/j.cub.2019.09.071.

11. Krasowski M. Contradicting a unitary theory of general anesthetic action: a history of three compounds from 1901 to 2001. *Bull Anesth Hist*. 2003;21(3):1–7.

12. Sezgin E, Levental I, Mayor S, Eggeling C. The mystery of membrane organization: composition, regulation and roles of lipid rafts. *Nat Rev Mol Cell Biol*. 2017;18 (6):361–74. DOI: 10.1038/nrm.2017.16.

13. Pavel MA, Petersen EN, Wang H, Lerner RA, Hansen SB. Studies on the mechanism of general anesthesia. *Proc Natl Acad Sci U S A*. 2020;117(24):13757–66. DOI: 10.1073/pnas.2004259117.

14. Esper T, Wehner M, Meinecke CD, Rueffert H. Blood/gas partition coefficients for isoflurane, sevoflurane, and desflurane in a clinically relevant patient population. *Anesth Analg*. 2015;120(1):45–50. DOI: 10.1213/ANE.0000000000000516.

15. Vallejo MC, Zakowski MI. Pro–con debate: nitrous oxide for labor analgesia. *Biomed Res Int*. 2019;2019:4618798. DOI: 10.1155/2019/4618798.

16. Kharasch ED. Biotransformation of sevoflurane. *Anesth Analg*. 1995;81:27S–38S. DOI: 10.1097/00000539-199512001-00005.

17. Stevanovic A, Rossaint R, Fritz HG, *et al*. Airway reactions and emergence times in general laryngeal mask airway anaesthesia: a meta-analysis. *Eur J Anaesthesiol*. 2015;32(2):106–16. DOI: 10.1097/EJA.0000000000000183.

18. Carpenter RL, Eger RI, Johnson BH, Unadkat JD, Sheiner LB. Does the duration of anesthetic administration affect the pharmacokinetics or metabolism of inhaled anesthetics in humans? *Anesth Analg*. 1987;66(1):1–8. DOI: 10.1213/00000539-198701000-00001.

19. Peyton PJ, Chao I, Weinberg L, Robinson GJB, Thompson BR. Nitrous oxide diffusion and the second gas effect on emergence from anesthesia. *Anesthesiology*. 2011;114(3):596–602. DOI: 10.1097/ALN.0b013e318209367b.

20. Zafirova Z, Sheehan C, Hosseinian L. Update on nitrous oxide and its use in anesthesia practice. *Best Pract Res Clin Anaesthesiol*. 2018;32(2):113–23. DOI: 10.1016/j.bpa.2018.06.003.

21. Young J, Apfelbaum JL. Inhalational anesthetics: desflurane and sevoflurane. *Rev Lit Arts Am*. 1995;8180(95):564–77.

22. Sondekoppam RV, Narsingani KH, Schimmel TA, McConnell BM, Buro K, Özelsel TJP. The impact of sevoflurane anesthesia on postoperative renal function:

a systematic review and meta-analysis of randomized-controlled trials. *Can J Anesth*. 2020;67(11):1595–623. DOI: 10.1007/s12630-020-01791-5.

23. Eger EI. Characteristics of anesthetic agents used for induction and maintenance of general anesthesia. *Am J Heal Pharm*. 2004;61(Suppl. 4):S3–10. DOI: 10.1093/ajhp/61.suppl_4.s3.

24. Sakai EM, Connolly LA, Klauck JA. Inhalation anesthesiology and volatile liquid anesthetics: focus on isoflurane, desflurane, and sevoflurane. *Pharmacotherapy*. 2005;25(12I):1773–88. DOI: 10.1592/phco.2005.25.12.1773.

25. Zhang C, Xu L, Ma YQ, *et al*. Bispectral index monitoring prevent awareness during total intravenous anesthesia: a prospective, randomized, double-blinded, multi-center controlled trial. *Chin Med J (Engl)*. 2011;124(22):3664–9. DOI: 10.3760/cma.j.issn.0366-6999.2011.22.012.

26. Horn C, Wallisch W, Homanics G, Williams J. Pathophysiological and neuro-chemical mechanisms of postoperative nausea and vomiting. *Eur J Pharmacol*. 2014;5(722):55–66. DOI: 10.1016/j.ejphar.2013.10.037.Pathophysiological.

27. Eger EI, Saidman LJ. Hazards of nitrous oxide anesthesia in bowel abstruction and pneumothorax. *Anesthesiology*. 1965;26(1):61–6.

28. Rosenberg H, Pollock N, Schiemann A, Bulger T, Stowell K. Malignant hyperther-mia: a review. *Orphanet J Rare Dis*. 2015;10(1):1–19. DOI: 10.1186/s13023-015-0310-1.

29. Landoni G, Lomivorotov VV, Nigro Neto C, *et al*. Volatile anesthetics versus total intravenous anesthesia for cardiac surgery. *N Engl J Med*. 2019;380(13):1214–25. DOI: 10.1056/nejmoa1816476.

30. American Society of Anesthesiologists Task Force on Intraoperative Awareness. Practice advisory for intraoperative awareness and brain function monitoring: a report by the American Society of Anesthesiologists Task Force on Intraoperative Awareness. *Anesthesiology*. 2006;104(4):847–64. DOI: 10.1097/00000542-200604000-00031.

31. Aranake A, Mashour GA, Avidan MS. Minimum alveolar concentration: ongoing relevance and clinical utility. *Anaesthesia*. 2013;68(5):512–22. DOI: 10.1111/anae.12168.

32. Myles PS, Leslie K, McNeil J, Forbes A, Chan MTV. Bispectral index monitoring to prevent awareness during anaesthesia: the B-Aware randomised controlled trial. *Lancet*. 2004;363(9423):1757–63. DOI: 10.1016/S0140-6736(04)16300-9.

33. Avidan M, Zhang L, Burnside B, Finkel K, Searlman A. Anesthesia awareness and the bispectral index. *N Engl J Med*. 2008;358(11):1097–108.

34. Avidan M, Jacobsohn E, Glick D, Burnskide B. Prevention of intraoperative awareness in a high risk surgical population. *N Engl J Med*. 2011;365(7):591–600.

Chapter

6

Intravenous Anesthetics and Adjunctive Agents

Matthew M. Colontonio, Mitchell C. Fuller, Harish Bangalore Siddaiah, Shilpa Patil, and Alan David Kaye

Introduction

Intravenous (IV) anesthetics were first discovered for their clinical utility in 1656 by Sir Christopher Wren, an architect, physicist, and astronomer at the University of Oxford, while using a goosequill to inject opium into a dog to produce sleep [1]. In 1909, Ludwig Burkhardt became the first surgeon to deliberately use IV ether in a 5% solution to sedate patients for head and neck surgery, finding that a higher concentration caused thrombophlebitis and hemolysis, whereas a lower concentration proved too weak a sedative. The first barbiturate hexobarbital was used in 1932, soon being used for over 10 million cases by 1944. In 1989, the first propofol lipid emulsion formulation was launched in the United States, marking the beginning of the modern age of IV sedation pharmacology [2].

Inhaled anesthetics were commonplace in the operative theatre long before IV use, although IV propofol is used in nearly all operations today, which is estimated to be 300 million annually [3]. Propofol, along with volatile anesthetic agents, are the main components of present-day general anesthesia, accounting for a multitude of advantageous outcomes in clinical practice and perioperative medicine [4]. A current high-powered meta-analysis found that the three biggest benefits of propofol-based total IV anesthesia (TIVA) included decreased risk of postoperative nausea and vomiting (PONV), lower pain scores (i.e., high patient satisfaction), and decreased time in the postanesthesia care unit (PACU) [4]. Another meta-analysis of over 4000 subjects investigating the superior safety profile of TIVA found low-quality evidence that propofol-based TIVA decreases the likelihood of postoperative cognitive dysfunction (e.g., postoperative delirium) [5]. This finding was of particular interest to geriatric surgery, which boasts a higher risk of post-operative delirium and has an increasing incidence of surgery each year.

IV anesthetic repurposing is emerging for classic disease processes such as sedation for the coronary artery bypass graft (CABG) procedure and sedation with etomidate for endoscopic retrograde cholangiopancreatography (ERCP). For example, volatile anesthetics such as sevoflurane have long been the mainstay anesthetic agent for CABG procedures; yet emerging evidence suggests that propofol-based TIVA is noninferior [6]. On another note, ERCP has long been performed under propofol-based TIVA; yet use of etomidate is now validated as a safe alternative [7].

Additionally, a new frontier of IV anesthetic use is rapidly emerging for clinical entities such as depression and status epilepticus. Ketamine, an N-methyl-D-aspartate (NMDA) antagonist, is becoming a well-accepted alternative pharmacotherapy in treatment-resistant depression and nonsuicidal self-injurious behavior [8, 9]. This is a novel and impactful discovery in an age of increasing mental disease. And the list of IV agents for treatment of refractory status epilepticus now boasts midazolam, propofol, pentobarbital, thiopental, and ketamine [10].

As exciting new pharmacotherapies are decreasing perioperative morbidity, we review barbiturates, benzodiazepines, ketamine, etomidate, dexmedetomidine, and propofol in this article as mainstay anesthesia agents. In addition, the adjunctive use of perioperative multimodal therapy, including opioids, local anesthetics, midazolam, and dexmedetomidine, is discussed. Finally, we will review in detail the inclusion of TIVA and adjunctive agents in Enhanced Recovery After Surgery (ERAS) protocols, a niche of anesthesia that is becoming widely popular in the United States.

Intravenous Anesthetic Agents

The hunt continues for the ideal IV agent. There are currently several options that are in clinical practice that all serve their own purpose; however, not one single agent has been able to encompass all ideal effects. The ideal IV anesthetic would provide amnesia with ultrarapid action, causing little to no cardiorespiratory depression, with concurrent ultrarapid metabolism. In addition to the aforementioned characteristics, the IV agent would be highly potent, reversible, stable in formulation, void of irritants, affordable, and easy to administer [11].

IV agents also have innumerable techniques of use, including, but not limited to, premedication, induction of general anesthesia, sedation for procedures and monitored anesthesia care (MAC) cases, and treatments of ailments including seizures, pain, and PONV. Further specific indications and uses are described, categorized by medication, below.

As seen below in Table 6.1, the majority of IV anesthetics used today have targets of gamma-aminobutyric acid (GABA) receptor modulation. With a primary objective of increasing GABA's efficiency, this mechanism occurs via GABA potentiation, as well as via inhibition of counteracting and excitatory neurotransmission of glutamate [12, 13]. If large boluses of these types of medications with this action are administered, they can cause burst suppression on electroencephalography (EEG) and act as an anticonvulsant, with the exception of methohexital.

Table 6.1 Mechanisms of action/pharmacokinetics

	MOA	Absorption	Distribution	Biotransformation	Excretion
Barbiturates	GABAA	IV, IM, PO PR	Redistribution	Hepatic oxidation to water-soluble, N-dealkylation, desulfuration	Renal, bile (methohexital)
Ketamine	NMDA antagonist	IV, IM, IN, PO, SC, E	Redistribution	Hepatic, N-demethylation	Renal
Propofol	GABAA	IV	Redistribution	CYP P450, plasma esterases	Renal
Etomidate	GABAA	IV	Redistribution	Conjugation, extrahepatic metabolism	Renal
Benzodiazepines	GABAA	IV, IM, IN, PO, PR, SL, B	Redistribution	Glucuronidation to water-soluble	Renal
Dexmedetomidine	α2-agonism	IV, IN	Redistribution	Rapid hepatic conjugation, N-methylation, hydroxylation	Renal, bile

IV, intravenous; IM, intramuscular; PO, *per os*; PR, per rectal; IN, intranasal; SC, subcutaneous; E, epidural; SL, sublingual; B, buccal.

Source: Adapted from [11], [13], and [15].

Regarding pharmacokinetics, all IV anesthetics share very similar properties. Their distribution throughout the body is determined by blood flow to vessel-rich organs (brain, heart, kidneys, liver), before transitioning to muscles, with eventual deposition in vessel-poor tissues (fat, bone) [13]. Their metabolism is considerably hepatic, with renal excretion, though there are exceptions (see Table 6.1). The more lipid-soluble the anesthetic, the more readily it crosses the blood–brain barrier (BBB), which implies a faster onset of action. Dosing for IV anesthetics can range based on the desired effect, as shown in Table 6.2; the various organ effects are shown in Table 6.3.

Naturally, IV agents that contain irritants or stabilizing agents, such as propylene glycol or phenols, consequently cause pain on injection [14], notably thiopental, diazepam, lorazepam, propofol, and etomidate. All of the IV medications can be administered as a single bolus versus an infusion, which will alter immediate organ effects. If considering an infusion, it is important to understand the concept of context-sensitive half-life, which is discussed later in this chapter. Context-sensitive half-life, or context-sensitive half-time, is defined as the time taken for blood plasma concentration of a drug to decline by half after an infusion designed to maintain a steady state has been stopped [13]. As shown in Figure 6.1, the context-sensitive half-times of various IV agents are plotted against time. Context-sensitive half-time can help predict when a drug is cleared and the patient is no longer sedated by that respective agent.

Barbiturates include thiopental, thiamylal, methohexital, and phenobarbital. They work by depressing the reticular activating system (RAS), directly potentiating the gamma-aminobutyric acid-A (GABAA) receptor, prolonging the duration of chloride channel opening. Historically, these agents served well as induction agents for both pediatric and adult anesthetics; however, with the advent of propofol, their routine use has decreased. Barbiturates treat raised intracranial pressure (ICP) and may be beneficial as neuroprotective agents against ischemia during deep hypothermic circulatory arrest, stroke, and aneurysm surgery. It is worth noting that production of porphyrins is increased through stimulation of aminolevulinic acid synthetase and therefore should be avoided in patients with porphyria.

Benzodiazepines include short-acting (midazolam and triazolam), intermediate-acting (alprazolam, clonazepam, lorazepam, oxazepam, temazepam), and long-acting (chlordiazepoxide, diazepam, flurazepam) agents. They work similarly to barbiturates, with potentiation of the GABAA receptor, but differently by increasing the frequency of chloride channel opening. Benzodiazepines assist as an excellent preoperative medication for anxiolysis, sedation, and induction of anesthesia. As previously mentioned, they suppress seizure activity by inhibiting GABA. Midazolam is the most commonly used benzodiazepine in the operating room. Typically, 1–2 mg IV before induction

Table 6.2 Dosing of anesthetics

	Premedication	Sedation	Induction	Maintenance
Thiopental			2.5–5 mg kg^{-1}	
Methohexital 1%		0.2–0.4 mg kg^{-1} IV	1–2 mg kg^{-1} IV	50–150 µg/(kg min)
Ketamine		2.5–15 µg/(kg min)	1–2 mg kg^{-1} IV 3–5 mg kg^{-1} IM	0.1–0.5 mg min^{-1}
Propofol		25–100 µg/(kg min)	1–2.5 mg kg^{-1} IV	50–200 µg/(kg min)
Etomidate		0.1–0.2 mg kg^{-1} load, 0.05 mg kg^{-1} Q5 min PRN	0.2–0.5 mg kg^{-1} IV	
Midazolam	0.02–0.15 mg kg^{-1} IV/IM 0.1–0.2 mg kg^{-1} PO	0.01–0.1 mg kg^{-1}	0.1–0.4 mg kg^{-1}	0.25–1 µg/(kg min)[a]
Dexmedetomidine	0.5–1 µg kg^{-1} IN	0.5–1 µg kg^{-1} load[b], 0.3–0.7 µg/(kg hr)	N/A	

[a] As an adjunct to volatiles

[b] Over 15 minutes. *Source:* Adapted from [11], [13], and [15].

Table 6.3 Organ effects of anesthetics

Agents	Neuro (CBF/ICP/CMRO$_2$)	CV (BP/HR/CO)	Respiratory (TV/RR)	Renal (RBF/GFR)	Unique characteristics
Barbiturates	↓↓/↓↓↓/↓↓↓	↓/↑/N	↓↓/↓↓	↓/↓	Rate of administration can vary effects dramatically, can precipitate porphyria
Ketamine	↑↑/↑↑/↑	N	N	N	Closest to "ideal" IV agent as provides amnesia, analgesia, and unconsciousness
Propofol	↓↓↓/↓↓↓/↓↓↓	↓↓/V/↓^{a}	↓↓↓/↓↓	N	No tolerance; however, PRIS
Etomidate	↓↓↓/↓↓↓/↓↓↓	N	N	N	Transient inhibition of 11-β hydroxylase, myoclonic activity
Benzodiazepines	↓↓/↓↓/↓↓	↓/V/↓	(↓/↓)^a	N/N	Most effective anxiolytic
Dexmedetomidine	N/N/V	↓/VV/V	N/N	N/N	No GABA effect

^{a} Clinically insignificant.

CBF, cerebral blood flow; ICP, intracranial pressure; CMRO$_2$, cerebral metabolic rate of oxygen; BP, blood pressure; HR, heart rate; CO, cardiac output; TV, tidal volume; RR, respiratory rate; RBF, renal blood flow; GFR, glomerular filtration rate; IV, intravenous; N, no change, minimal, or offsetting effects; V, variable effect; PRIS, propofol infusion syndrome; GABA, gamma-aminobutyric acid.

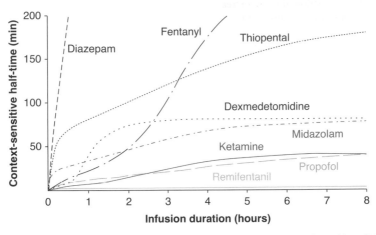

Figure 6.1 Context-sensitive half-time effects of anesthetics. *Source:* Adapted from [20].

provides substantial anxiolytic effects, and reduced dosage should be considered in the elderly. Benzodiazepines have dose-dependent respiratory depression and caution should be exercised when co-administering opioids, as hypotension can occur in hemodynamically unstable patients.

Ketamine is an analog of phencyclidine, causing dissociation of the thalamus from the limbic cortex. Ketamine works by noncompetitive inhibition of the NMDA receptor. It is also the only analgesic of IV agents discussed in this chapter that has weak opioid agonist activity ($\mu > \kappa > \delta$). Additionally, it has properties of a weak GABA agonist, adrenergic agonist ($\alpha 1$ and $\beta 2$), and muscarinic antagonist. Ketamine is a direct myocardial depressant, but an indirect sympathomimetic. Ketamine is the only IV anesthetic that has low protein binding [15].

Ketamine uses include induction of general anesthesia, intramuscular use for uncooperative patients, for adults and children without IV access, deep sedation, and newer ideas, including treatment of treatment-resistant depression and refractory status epilepticus. Ketamine can be helpful in difficult airway cases, as respiratory function appears to be preserved, though an antisialagogue should be considered. Ketamine is a helpful aid in trauma patients, and is commonly used for chest tube placement and bone reduction by orthopedic surgeons. It has also been beneficial as an adjunct to analgesia in the opioid-tolerant patient. Ketamine should be avoided in the critically ill who have exhausted their adrenergic capacity, in patients with severe right heart dysfunction due to increased pulmonary vascular resistance, and in those with severe hypovolemia.

Etomidate is another IV anesthetic, a carboxylated imidazole, that depresses the RAS, with GABAA receptor potentiation. Etomidate is notably dissolved in propylene glycol, which is known to cause pain on injection. Myoclonus is very common after administration, and there is dose-dependent inhibition of the adrenocortical system via 11β-hydroxylase; however, no studies have demonstrated an adverse effect on outcome [15]. Common applications for etomidate include deep sedation, as well as induction of general anesthesia, especially in those with compromised cardiac function.

Propofol is a lipid emulsion formulation, standardized to 1% propofol, 10% soybean oil, and 1.2% purified egg phospholipid as an emulsifier, with 2.25% glycerol as a tonicity-adjusting agent and sodium hydroxide to adjust the pH [16]. Bacterial retardants are added, as the above-mentioned formulation supports bacterial growth. Propofol should be used immediately or at least within 6 hours of vial opening [15].

It is the most commonly used IV anesthetic that currently exists in clinical practice [15]. It is also easily titratable and commonly used for maintenance of intraoperative and postoperative sedation. Children will typically require higher doses. Low-dose propofol can be used for central line placement, as well as as an alternative agent for PONV. If given in high-dose infusions for an extended period of time, propofol can cause propofol infusion syndrome (PRIS), which presents with metabolic acidosis, hypertension, hypertriglyceridemia, and renal failure.

Dexmedetomidine is a highly selective α2-adrenergic agonist, approximately eight times more specific than clonidine, with 1620:1 α2/α1 receptor favorability [17]. By stimulating α2 receptors in the locus ceruleus, there is a decrease in norepinephrine release. Action on the descending noradrenergic pathways inhibits norepinephrine release and inhibits pain transmission at the dorsal horn of the spinal cord [18, 19]. Dexmedetomidine has been used extensively as a nonopioid adjuvant for perioperative pain relief. Because of the central and peripheral receptors, dexmedetomidine can have a paradoxical effect on hemodynamics. Upon bolus administration, due to α1 activity, hypertension may result, which is avoided with a loading dose over 15 minutes. At peak effect of an infusion, hypotension and bradycardia are generally present. Dexmedetomidine has minimal to no respiratory depression, and therefore has been useful in sedation. Common applications include sedation for MAC and intensive care unit (ICU) patients, and preventing emergence delirium, as well as awakening from general anesthesia and ICU recovery [11].

Significant attenuation of stress response to tracheal intubation/extubation allows for assistance during awake fiberoptic techniques. Dexmedetomidine reduces minimal alveolar concentration, and therefore reduces opioid, muscle relaxant, and inhalational anesthetic requirements.

Novel Intravenous Agents

Attempts are being made for improvement in IV drug profile. More favorable characteristics would include less or no pain on injection, more predictable and consistent termination of action, and drug utility irrespective of, and unbound by, renal or liver failure. Shockingly, drug development approaches almost $3 billion dollars, with only roughly 12% approval rate for entering clinical development [21]. Although newer formulations are in the pipeline, drug development is not inexpensive.

Most current drugs in the development process share and emulate existing formulations with slight modifications to their structures. However, not all of these agents have been successful, and some have already been removed from the market. These agents include fospropofol, novel propofol formulations (and micro- to macro-emulsions), remimazolam, cyclopropyl-methoxycarbonyl metomidate, methoxycarbonyl etomidate, and AZD 3043.

Fospropofol is a prodrug of propofol appearing to allay microbial concerns, as well as causing decreased pain on injection as it is water-soluble. Fospropofol used in endoscopic procedures is approved for use of MAC sedation, not general anesthesia. However, fospropofol does have a longer onset of action, and therefore has less precision upon administration.

Remimazolam is an amnestic that has a similar onset time to midazolam and remifentanil. Because it is metabolized by tissue esterases, no concerns about accumulation of the products are warranted.

Cyclopropyl-methoxycarbonyl metomidate also appears to be demonstrating some early promise in animal studies [11]. The less potent brother of etomidate has a shorter duration of action and less adrenocortical suppression. It is metabolized by blood and tissue esterases, but the drug remains in early clinical trials.

Adjuvant Agents

Adjuvants are medications that can be administered in smaller doses when used in combination to achieve maximum benefits while minimizing side effects [22]. Multimodal general anesthesia utilizes the advantage of various drug combinations targeting different sites in the nociceptive pathway and arousal systems [22]. As previously discussed, the ideal IV agent would fulfill many characteristics, but adjuvants can supplement those gaps. Adjuvant agents include antiinflammatories, analgesics, and local anesthetics, which will be discussed heavily in their respective chapter, but also gabapentin and magnesium. This chapter will also discuss below adjuvant use in conjunction with regional anesthetics.

Ketorolac is a nonsteroidal antiinflammatory drug (NSAID) that acts by inhibiting cyclooxygenase-1 and 2 (COX-1 and COX-2), which decreases the production of prostaglandins. Prostaglandins are produced in response to tissue damage, leading to inflammation and pain. Ketorolac is a potent analgesic that is recommended for moderate to severe pain and a very useful IV adjuvant in attempts to spare the use of opioids. Ketorolac is typically used for a short period of time to avoid gastrointestinal bleeding and damage to the kidneys. Though the intramuscular route is an option, IV dosing includes 15–30 mg every 6 hours, but not exceeding 60–120 mg a day (dependent on kidney function).

Acetaminophen is produced in many formulations, and the mechanism of action remains unknown. It is suggested that it works similarly to ketorolac in that it decreases the production of prostaglandins, though likely a more central process than with NSAIDs, which work at the site of tissue damage. Acetaminophen is beneficial in treating mild to moderate pain and should be used as an adjuvant to analgesia in the anesthetic. Rectal and oral routes are commonly used successfully in pediatric analgesics. However, IV dosing includes 15 mg kg^{-1} (not to exceed 75 mg kg^{-1} per day in children <12 years old), given over 15–30 minutes every 6 hours, but not exceeding 4 g, with caution in those with liver disease.

Opioids act primarily at several receptors (μ, κ, δ) and prevent nociceptive transmission at the level of the spinal cord, brain, and peripheral nociceptors. Their action is mediated via the G protein-coupled receptor mechanism, causing hyperpolarization of afferent sensory neurons [22–24]. They are often used as adjuvants with local anesthetics to prolong the duration and quality of postoperative analgesia [23]. Table 6.4 provides dosing through different sites of administration for different opioids.

Advantages include effective analgesia, diminished hemodynamic stress response to noxious stimuli, facilitation of airway manipulation by blunting of cough and gag reflexes, and synergistic effects, and thereby dose reduction, when given along with other IV induction agents [25].

Adverse effects include respiratory depression, sedation, nausea, vomiting, muscle rigidity, constipation, ileus, pruritus, urinary retention, and addiction and dependence. Individual opioids are discussed more thoroughly in their respective chapter.

Lidocaine is a commonly used local anesthetic agent given IV for decreasing the sympathetic response to intubation and extubation. Local anesthetics decrease the minimum alveolar concentration, subsequently augmenting the effects of other agents. It is also commonly used as pretreatment to decrease pain on injection with propofol and etomidate. Lidocaine acts by blocking sodium channels and preventing conduction of action potentials in peripheral nerves. As an adjuvant, it can be used in the form of an infusion for perioperative pain relief. Infusions can start with or without a loading dose and range from 1 to 3 mg/(kg hr) [28]. When providing an infusion, close monitoring for cardio- and neurotoxicity is paramount. Toxicity may present in the intubated patient as cardiac arrhythmias, hypertension, and seizures.

Table 6.4 Opioids as adjuvants

Name of the drug	Intravenous	Intravenous patient-controlled analgesia (for opioid-naïve patients)	Intrathecal	Epidural	Peripheral nerve block	Comments
Morphine	0.03–0.15 mgkg^{-1}: for postoperative analgesia	Conc: 1 mg mL^{-1} Demand dose: 0.5–2 mg Maximum: 7.5 mg hr^{-1} Lockout: 5–10 min	100–200 µg	1–5 mg	No	Hydrophilic and more widespread analgesia
Fentanyl	0.5–1.5 µg kg^{-1}: for postoperative analgesia	Conc: 10 µg mL^{-1} Demand dose: 5–20 µg Maximum: 75 µg hr^{-1} Lockout: 4–10 min	10–25 µg		No	

Sufentanil	0.25–20 µg kg⁻¹: for intraoperative analgesia		1.5–5 µg	0.75–1 µg mL⁻¹	
Hydromorphone	0.01–0.02 mg kg⁻¹: for postoperative analgesia	Conc: 0.2 mg mL⁻¹ Demanc dose: 0.2–0.4 mg Maximum: 1.5 mg h⁻¹ Lockout interval: 6–10 min	100 µg	500–600 µg	
Buprenorphine (opioid agonist–µ-antagonist–κ)	0.3 mg	75–150 µg	150–300 µg	0.3 mg	Lipophilic, ceiling effect on respiratory depression due to partial agonist property
Tramadol		10–50 mg	1–2 mg kg⁻¹		

Source: Adapted from [23] and [25–27].

Magnesium is a less commonly nonopioid strategy used despite its analgesic and sedative effects. The proposed mechanism of action includes competitive and noncompetitive NMDA antagonism at the hippocampal presynaptic calcium channels, which regulate aspartate and glutamate [29]. Both pathways are thought to contribute to the prevention of central sensitization [29]. Though magnesium is making waves as a revival, there is substantial variability in dosing. Dosing generally includes a 30–50 mg kg^{-1} load, followed by an infusion of 6–25 mg/(kg hr). Fortunately, magnesium is forgiving due to its large therapeutic window, though toxicity risks remain and patients should be monitored closely for risks of hypermagnesemia [29].

Gabapentin is an anticonvulsant that is a structural analog of GABA but acts at the α–2δ subunit of presynaptic P/Q-type voltage-gated calcium channels [30]. Gabapentin is also less frequently used in the operating room but does play a small role in adjuvant therapy. Gabapentin dosing also varies due to lack of evidence over effective dosing. Gabapentin likely works by decreasing the analgesic requirements due to neuropathic pain relief. More studies need to be performed to demonstrate consistent responses and effective dosing for optimal analgesia.

IV anesthetics and adjuncts have also been trialed in the field of regional anesthesia. Regional techniques have proven benefits in alleviating postoperative pain and decreasing the amount of narcotics used in the perioperative period. By decreasing the amount of opioids used, there is decreased PONV and adverse effects. With pain being a common obstruction to discharge from PACU, regional techniques have drastically become a necessity. IV anesthetics have been combined with various peripheral nerve blocks and neuraxial techniques in anticipation of superior effects. This includes addition of opioids, benzodiazepines, dexmedetomidine, and other adjuvants to local anesthetics, including epinephrine and sodium bicarbonate. For example, dexmedetomidine prolongs the sensory/motor block duration and decreases the requirement for rescue analgesics when used as an adjuvant with local anesthetics in epidural and regional blocks.

Incorporation of Intravenous Anesthetics in ERAS Protocols

ERAS is an evidence-based multimodal perioperative protocol directed towards stress reduction, reduced morbidity, and promotion of return of function [31, 32]. The introduction of target-controlled infusion (TCI) regimes since 1989 has broadened the applicability of TIVA in clinical practice. Benefits of incorporation of ERAS protocols were investigated in a retrospective study in single-level lumbar microdiscectomy by Kılıç *et al.* They found that application of ERAS protocols was clinically, as well as economically, beneficial when compared to the subset of patients who belonged to the preERAS group. This study highlights the benefits of use of

ERAS protocols in terms of relatively shorter operation duration and lesser blood loss, and therefore reduced requirement of crystalloid and colloid administration. In addition, patients experienced improved pain relief, early mobilization, reduced incidence of nausea/vomiting, and overall reduced hospital stay [33]. In this review, TIVA using fentanyl and propofol describes ease of titration, minimum stress response, opioid-sparing effect, lower risk of airway issues, and facilitation of optimum surgical conditions [33].

Interestingly, prediction of emergence and early extubation have been attempted in patients undergoing video-assisted thoracotomy surgery (VATS) under TIVA. A response surface equation to evaluate the effect of combination of drugs not only for anesthesia induction and maintenance, but also for emergence, was utilized by Chiou *et al.* [34]. Fentanyl, propofol, and rocuronium were used for induction and maintenance for the duration of the procedure. The benefits of early extubation in patients undergoing thoracic surgery in reducing airway and pulmonary complications have been extensively studied [34, 35]. Wang *et al.* described that TIVA combined with thoracic epidural anesthesia (TEA) plays a role in better postoperative outcome, improved pulmonary function, better pain relief, and early mobilization [36].

Opioids have been implicated in inducing hyperalgesia, lowering pain threshold manifesting as tolerance to opioids and abnormal pain symptoms in the form of allodynia [37]. To this effect, IV ketamine has been incorporated in ERAS protocols because of its antihyperalgesia and antiinflammatory properties [38]. Ketamine is useful in patients with chronic pain or chronic opioid use. This is not only because of a reduction in central sensitization by NMDA antagonism and reduction in opiate tolerance, but also because of the balance between excitatory and inhibitory neurotransmitters [39, 40].

IV lidocaine infusion has been used widely for its analgesic, antiinflammatory, and antihyperalgesic effects [39]. Clonidine and dexmedetomidine are also useful adjuncts that have been used for analgesia in ERAS programs. Propofol is beneficial for patients at high risk of PONV.

ERAS protocols for colorectal surgeries have been extensively reviewed in several meta-analyses and randomized controlled trials. The practice of following this protocol has demonstrated 40–50% reduced morbidity and a reduction in length of hospital stay by 2–3 days [31, 41]. Parrish *et al.* conducted a retrospective review from 14 centers in Southern California and found that implementing ERAS protocols for ambulatory anorectal surgeries decreased postoperative pain and unplanned emergency room return visits [42].

Use of Total Intravenous Anesthetics

Propofol, midazolam, ketamine, remifentanil, and dexmedetomidine are commonly used for TIVA. TIVA involves use of medications IV for induction and maintenance of anesthesia. It is commonly used in both adult and pediatric populations, and those at risk of malignant hyperthermia. TIVA is also heavily favored in neurosurgical cases when various neuromonitoring techniques are the standard of care and where there is potential for nerve injury during surgical resection. Pediatric patients differ from adults in several aspects. They have an increased volume of distribution, a smaller size, higher fat metabolism and cardiac output, and higher clearance. Infusions can be controlled manually or as automated TCI. The availability of TCI pumps with data sets programmed for pediatric age groups has been highly valuable, but caution should be exercised in neonates, young infants, and obese and hemodynamically unstable pediatric patients [43]. IV tubing dead space has to be borne in mind while administering drugs IV. Propofol is better avoided in patients with mitochondrial disease because of an increased risk of PRIS and in those with medium-chain acyl-CoA dehydrogenase deficiency [44]. In addition to standard monitors and clinical judgment, processed EEG monitoring is useful in titrating TIVA for prolonged procedures [45].

Advantages

(See reference [45].)

1. Optimum surgical conditions and preferred when airway is shared, e.g., bronchoscopy or laryngoscopy.
2. Prevention of PONV, especially with propofol (2,6-diisopropylphenol).
3. Reduced airway responsiveness and prevention of stridor, bronchospasm, and laryngospasm at induction or emergence, more so in children with reactive airway disease.
4. Improved ciliary function and less airway irritation.
5. Smooth emergence, quicker recovery, and prevention of emergence delirium.
6. Reduced environmental pollution.
7. Absolute indication in patients with a history of/at risk of malignant hyperthermia.
8. Suitable for use in patients with neuromuscular disease and muscular dystrophy/myopathy, and reduces postoperative problems by avoiding the use of neuromuscular blocking agents.
9. Children with phobia about face mask.
10. Propofol and remifentanil combination is preferred while monitoring spinal cord function with sensory or motor evoked potential during corrective surgery for scoliosis [43].
11. Suitable for radiological investigations or procedures.

Disadvantages

1. Need for IV access and specialized equipment such as infusion pumps.
2. Need for special equipment for reliable depth of anesthesia.
3. Concern for PRIS with higher rates of infusion (>4 mg/(kg hr)) over prolonged periods (>48 hours). PRIS is characterized by acute refractory bradycardia culminating in asystole and associated with one or more of metabolic acidosis, rhabdomyolysis, myoglobinuria, lipemia, or fatty liver enlargement [43].
4. Bacterial contamination risk.

Conclusion

In summary, IV drugs are the mainstay of anesthesia practice. They work to produce pain relief, sedation, anxiolysis, and amnesia in highly dynamic and complex patients undergoing surgery. It is critical that IV anesthetics are considered as a single component of the multimodal perioperative anesthesia plan, along with inhaled and regional anesthetic approaches. ERAS protocols are increasingly involving IV anesthesia, as studies show improved patient outcomes, in addition to major economic benefit. Emerging IV drugs such as fospropofol, remimazolam, and cyclopropyl-methoxycarbonyl metomidate are optimizing the landscape of IV anesthesia practice by allowing the anesthesiologist to give quick on/off sedation and analgesia. The future of clinical anesthesia will continue to rely heavily on IV therapy and on the drugs covered in this review.

Review Questions

1. An example of a barbiturate anesthetic is:

    (a) Ketamine
    (b) Methohexital
    (c) Etomidate
    (d) Midazolam

2. An advantage of remimazolam is:

    (a) It is metabolized by tissue esterases and therefore, there is no concern over accumulation of metabolites
    (b) It is strongly renally eliminated
    (c) It is a prodrug of midazolam
    (d) It has a longer duration than alprazolam

3. Dexmedetomidine:
   (a) Is a highly selective α2-adrenergic agonist and is approximately eight times more specific than clonidine
   (b) Possesses both central and peripheral receptors
   (c) Can have a paradoxical effect on hemodynamics upon bolus administration
   (d) Has minimal to no respiratory depression and therefore has been useful in sedation
   (e) All of the above

Answers

1. (b)
2. (a)
3. (e)

References

1. Roberts M, Jagdish S. A history of intravenous anesthesia in war (1656–1988). *J Anesth Hist.* 2016;2(1):13–21.

2. Baker MT, Naguib M. Propofol: the challenges of formulation. *Anesthesiology.* 2005;103(4):860–76.

3. Weiser TG, Regenbogen SE, Thompson KD, *et al.* An estimation of the global volume of surgery: a modelling strategy based on available data. *Lancet.* 2008;372 (9633):139–44.

4. Schraag S, Pradelli L, Alsaleh AJO, *et al.* Propofol vs. inhalational agents to maintain general anaesthesia in ambulatory and in-patient surgery: a systematic review and meta-analysis. *BMC Anesthesiol.* 2018;18(1):162.

5. Miller D, Lewis SR, Pritchard MW, *et al.* Intravenous versus inhalational maintenance of anaesthesia for postoperative cognitive outcomes in elderly people undergoing non-cardiac surgery. *Cochrane Database Syst Rev.* 2018;8(8):CD012317.

6. Landoni G, Lomivorotov VV, Nigro Neto C, *et al.* Volatile anesthetics versus total intravenous anesthesia for cardiac surgery. *N Engl J Med.* 2019;380(13):1214–25.

7. Park CH, Park SW, Hyun B, *et al.* Efficacy and safety of etomidate-based sedation compared with propofol-based sedation during ERCP in low-risk patients: a double-blind, randomized, noninferiority trial. *Gastrointest Endosc.* 2018;87(1):174–84.

8. Tadler SC, Mickey BJ. Emerging evidence for antidepressant actions of anesthetic agents. *Curr Opin Anaesthesiol.* 2018;31(4):439–45.

9. Mathew SJ, Shah A, Lapidus K, *et al.* Ketamine for treatment-resistant unipolar depression: current evidence. *CNS Drugs.* 2012;26(3):189–204.

10. Reznik M, Berger K, Claassen J. Comparison of intravenous anesthetic agents for the treatment of refractory status epilepticus. *J Clin Med*. 2016;5(5):54.

11. Barash PG, Cullen BF, Stoelting RK, *et al*. Clinical anesthesia. In: PG Barash, BF Cullen, RK Stoelting, *et al*., eds. *Clinical Anesthesia*, 8th ed. Philadelphia, PA: Wolters Kluwer; 2017, pp. 486–504.

12. Brohan J, Goudra BG. The role of GABA receptor agonists in anesthesia and sedation. *CNS Drugs*. 2017;31(10):845–56.

13. Butterworth JF, Mackey DC, Wasnick JD. Clinical anesthesiology. In: JF Butterworth, DC Mackey, JD Wasnick, eds. *Morgan & Mikhail's Clinical Anesthesiology*, 5th ed. New York, NY: McGraw Hill; 2013, pp. 175–88.

14. Desousa KA. Pain on propofol injection: causes and remedies. *Indian J Pharmacol*. 2016;48(6):617–23.

15. Stoelting RK, Miller RD. Basics of anesthesia. In: RK Stoelting, RD Miller, eds. *Basics of Anesthesia*, 5th ed. Philadelphia, PA: Elsevier; 2007, pp. 97–111.

16. Feng AY, Kaye AD, Kaye RJ, Belani K, Urman RD. Novel propofol derivatives and implications for anesthesia practice. *J Anaesthesiol Clin Pharmacol*. 2017;33 (1):9–15.

17. Srivastava U, Sarkar ME, Kumar A, *et al*. Comparison of clonidine and dexmede-tomidine for short-term sedation of intensive care unit patients. *Indian J Crit Care Med*. 2014;18(7):431–6.

18. Tang C, Xia Z. Dexmedetomidine in perioperative acute pain management: a non-opioid adjuvant analgesic. *J Pain Res*. 2017;10:1899–904.

19. Grewal A. Dexmedetomidine: new avenues. *J Anaesthesiol Clin Pharmacol*. 2011;27 (3):297–302.

20. [No authors]. Context-sensitive half-time. *J Neurocrit Care*. Available from: www.e-xjnc .org/journal/Figure.php?xn=jnc-8-2-x53.xml&id=f1-jnc-8-2-53&number= 199&p_name=0516_199.

21. DiMasi JA, Grabowski HG, Hansen RW. Innovation in the pharmaceutical indus-try: new estimates of R&D costs. *J Health Econ*. 2016;47:20–33.

22. Brown EN, Pavone KJ, Naranjo M. Multimodal general anesthesia: theory and practice. *Anesth Analg*. 2018;127(5):1246–58.

23. Swain A, Nag DS, Sahu S, Samaddar DP. Adjuvants to local anesthetics: current understanding and future trends. *World J Clin Cases*. 2017;5(8):307–23.

24. Busch-Dienstfertig M, Stein C. Opioid receptors and opioid peptide-producing leukocytes in inflammatory pain: basic and therapeutic aspects. *Brain Behav Immun*. 2010;24(5):683–94.

25. Casserly E, Alexander JC. Perioperative uses of intravenous opioids in adults: general considerations. Waltham, MA: UpToDate; 2022. Available from: www

.uptodate.com/contents/perioperative-uses-of-intravenous-opioids-in-adults-general-considerations.

26. Butterworth JF, Mackey DC, Wasnick JD, eds. *Morgan & Mikhail's Clinical Anesthesiology*, 6th ed. New York, NY: McGraw Hill; 2018.

27. Jonan AB, Kaye AD, Urman RD. Buprenorphine formulations: clinical best practice strategies recommendations for perioperative management of patients undergoing surgical or interventional pain procedures. *Pain Physician*. 2018;21(1):E1–12.

28. Dunn LK, Durieux ME. Perioperative use of intravenous lidocaine. *Anesthesiology*. 2017;126(4):729–37.

29. George R, Condrey J, Wilson S. "Oh Mg!" Magnesium: a powerful tool in the perioperative setting. 2018. Available from: www.asra.com/guidelines-articles/ori ginal-articles/article-item/asra-news/2018/07/23/-oh-mg!-magnesium-a-powerful-tool-in-the-perioperative-setting.

30. Schmidt PC, Ruchelli G, Mackey SC, Carroll IR. Perioperative gabapentinoids. *Anesthesiology*. 2013;119(5):1215–21.

31. Pędziwiatr M, Mavrikis J, Witowski J, *et al.* Current status of enhanced recovery after surgery (ERAS) protocol in gastrointestinal surgery. *Med Oncol*. 2018;35(6):95.

32. Patel HRH, Cerantola Y, Valerio M, *et al.* Enhanced recovery after surgery: are we ready, and can we afford not to implement these pathways for patients undergoing radical cystectomy? *Eur Urol*. 2014;65(2):263–6.

33. Tarıkçı Kılıç E, Demirbilek T, Naderi S. Does an enhanced recovery after surgery protocol change costs and outcomes of single-level lumbar microdiscectomy? *Neurosurg Focus*. 2019;46(4):E10.

34. Chiou Y-W, Ting C-K, Wang H-Y, Tsou M-Y, Chang W-K. Enhanced recovery after surgery: prediction for early extubation in video-assisted thoracic surgery using a response surface model in anesthesia. *J Formos Med Assoc*. 2019;118 (10):1450–7.

35. Gao S, Barello S, Chen L, *et al.* Clinical guidelines on perioperative management strategies for enhanced recovery after lung surgery. *Transl Lung Cancer Res*. 2019;8 (6):1174–87.

36. Wang H-Y, Ting C-K, Liou J-Y, Chen K-H, Tsou M-Y, Chang W-K. A previously published propofol–remifentanil response surface model does not predict patient response well in video-assisted thoracic surgery. *Medicine (Baltimore)*. 2017;96(19): e6895.

37. Mitra S. Opioid-induced hyperalgesia: pathophysiology and clinical implications. *J Opioid Manag*. 2008;4(3):123–30.

38. Gao M, Rejaei D, Liu H. Ketamine use in current clinical practice. *Acta Pharmacol Sin*. 2016;37(7):865–72.

39. Dunkman WJ, Manning MW. Enhanced recovery after surgery and multimodal strategies for analgesia. *Surg Clin North Am.* 2018;98(6):1171–84.

40. Loftus RW, Yeager MP, Clark JA, *et al.* Intraoperative ketamine reduces perioperative opiate consumption in opiate-dependent patients with chronic back pain undergoing back surgery. *Anesthesiology.* 2010;113(3):639–46.

41. Greco M, Capretti G, Beretta L, Gemma M, Pecorelli N, Braga M. Enhanced recovery program in colorectal surgery: a meta-analysis of randomized controlled trials. *World J Surg.* 2014;38(6):1531–41.

42. Parrish AB, O'Neill SM, Crain SR, *et al.* An enhanced recovery after surgery (ERAS) protocol for ambulatory anorectal surgery reduced postoperative pain and unplanned returns to care after discharge. *World J Surg.* 2018;42(7):1929–38.

43. Cowie P, Baxter A, McCormack J. Total intravenous anaesthesia in children: a practical guide. *Anaesth Intensive Care Med.* 2019;20(6):348–52.

44. Anderson BJ, Bagshaw O. Practicalities of total intravenous anesthesia and target-controlled infusion in children. *Anesthesiology.* 2019;131(1):164–85.

45. Gaynor J, Ansermino JM. Paediatric total intravenous anaesthesia. *BJA Educ.* 2016;16(11):369–73.

Chapter 7

Pharmacology of Local Anesthetics

Chang H. Park and Garrett W. Burnett

Introduction

Cocaine, derived from the coca leaf indigenous to South America, was the first drug to be utilized as a topical local anesthetic by Dr. Carl Koller for glaucoma surgery in 1884. Dr. William Stewart Halstead and Dr. Richard John Hall were the first to demonstrate nerve blockade with cocaine for dental surgery later in that same year. Due to the undesirable effects of cocaine, novocaine and subsequent other local anesthetics were developed.

Local anesthetics function through nerve conduction blockade and provide surgical or perioperative analgesia. Local anesthetics may be administered in a variety of routes, including local subcutaneous infiltration, topical, neuraxial, or peripheral nerve blockade, or intravenously. Each delivery method should be chosen based on the clinical situation or the provider's skill set.

Basics of Local Anesthetics

Structure

The basic structure of local anesthetics includes a lipophilic aromatic ring and a hydrophilic tertiary amine linked by either an amide or an ester linkage (see Figure 7.1). Local anesthetic types are therefore divided into ester local anesthetics and amide local anesthetics, depending on their linkage. Ester local anesthetics are rapidly metabolized by pseudocholinesterase in plasma, whereas amide local anesthetics are metabolized by hepatic microsomal enzymes. Examples of ester and amide local anesthetics are shown in Table 7.1.

Mechanism of Action

In order to understand the mechanism of action of local anesthetics at the level of the nerves, it is important to understand the physiology of nerve signals. Signal conduction in the nervous system relies on propagation of an action potential via depolarization of neuronal cell membranes. Depolarization can occur with the opening of voltage-gated sodium channels in the neuronal membrane; these voltage-gated sodium channels can exist in one of three

Table 7.1 Common ester and amide local anesthetics with associated characteristics

	Speed of onset	Duration of action	Maximum dose (mg kg^{-1})	Maximum dose (with epinephrine) (mg kg^{-1})
Esters				
Cocaine	+++	+	1.5 (topical)	–
Benzocaine	+++	+	–	–
Procaine	+	+	7	10
Chloroprocaine	+++	+	11	14
Amides				
Prilocaine	++	+	6	8
Lidocaine	++	++	4.5	7
Mepivacaine	++	++	5	7
Bupivacaine	+	+++	3	–
Ropivacaine	+	+++	3	–

Maximum doses reported in the literature are shown, but it is important to consider the route and location of administration when calculating the maximum dosages of local anesthetics.
+, least; +++, most.

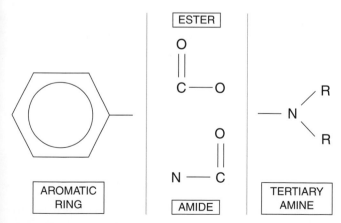

Figure 7.1 Structure of local anesthetics, including an aromatic ring group linked to a tertiary amine via an amide or ester linkage.

states: resting, open, or inactive. Voltage-gated sodium channels are in the resting state at the neuron's resting state (−70 mV). Initial depolarization occurs when sodium channels are in the open state, leading to an influx of sodium ions into the cell. Upon reaching a threshold potential (−55 mV), an action potential fires and a signal is propagated down the nerve's axon (see Figure 7.2). Following an action potential, the sodium channel repolarizes and the voltage-gated sodium channels temporarily revert to an inactive state. This inactive state is responsible for the refractory period in which a nerve signal cannot be sent until the sodium channels return to their resting state.

Local anesthetics reversibly inhibit voltage-gated sodium channels and prevent propagation of action potentials by preventing depolarization to the threshold potential. Binding of local anesthetics to voltage-gated sodium channels results in a sustained inactivated state. Voltage-gated sodium channels are most susceptible to inhibition by local anesthetics when in the open or inactivated state. Because of this preference for the open or inactivated state, nerves which fire more often are more susceptible to local anesthetic effects.

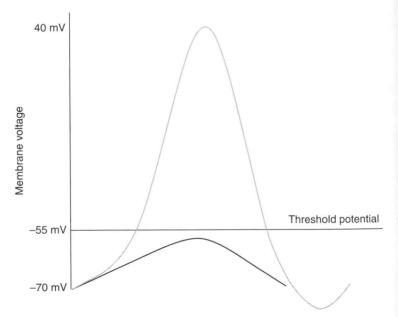

Figure 7.2 Depolarization of a nerve to the threshold potential leading to firing of an action potential (grey). Local anesthetic limits the nerve's ability to reach the threshold potential (black). Following a successful action potential, the refractory period leads to hyperpolarization of the nerve prior to returning to the resting potential of −90 mV.

Nerve Fiber Sensitivity and Differential Blockade

Local anesthetics do not affect all nerve fiber types identically. Differential blockade refers to varied susceptibility to local anesthetic effects among different nerve fibers and may be responsible for pain signal blockade without motor signal blockade. Typically, smaller nerves and myelinated nerves are more susceptible to blockade by local anesthetics. Myelinated fibers have small gaps along their axons called the nodes of Ranvier. Three consecutive nodes of Ranvier must be blocked to reliably block nerve signal conduction.

Autonomic nerves (C- and B-type fibers) are often the first to be blocked by local anesthetics, followed by sensory and motor nerves. Resolution of blockade follows the inverse of this pattern.

Pharmacodynamics

Onset of action for local anesthetics is dependent on the proportion of drug in the unionized form, as this form is able to cross the neuronal membrane to bind the cytoplasmic side of the target sodium channel (see Figure 7.3). This balance of unionized to ionized local anesthetic is dependent on the drug's pKa and the pH of the environment in which the drug is located. The pKa is defined as the pH at which 50% of the drug is in the unionized form and the remaining 50% in the ionized form. Most local anesthetics are weak bases with a pKa of 7.5–9.0, while physiologic pH is generally 7.35–7.45. The closer

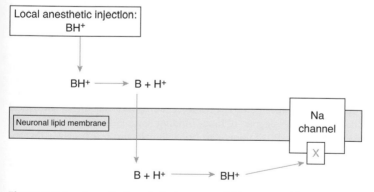

Figure 7.3 Local anesthetics exist in the water-soluble, unionized form when injected. Local anesthetics must be in the ionized form to cross the neuronal lipid membrane and bind to the effector site (X) on the cytoplasmic portion of the sodium (Na) channel. Local anesthetics with pKa values closest to the pH of physiologic tissue will have greater amounts of the ionized form. Local anesthetic binding to the Na channel prevents Na influx into the neuronal cell and subsequent action potential propagation.

a drug's pKa is to physiologic pH, the more the drug is in the unionized form, which leads to a faster onset of action. The exception to this is for drugs such as chloroprocaine, which has a higher pKa of 9.0 but is rapid-acting due to the concentration at which it is administered (3%).

Local anesthetic potency is related to lipid solubility, a property determined by the benzene ring of the drug. As lipid solubility of a drug goes up, the greater the potency of that local anesthetic. Additionally, molecular size impacts local anesthetic potency. This is due to larger, more lipophilic drugs being more apt to cross the lipid membrane of the cell to reach their target receptor. Common concentrations of clinically available local anesthetics range from 0.25% to 4%, with more potent local anesthetics being prepared at lower concentrations.

Duration of action of local anesthetics is a property of protein binding. Albumin and α1-acid-glycoprotein are the most common proteins bound to local anesthetics. The more protein binding, the longer the duration of action of the local anesthetic. Protein binding is directly related to the pH of the environment, with decreased protein binding in acidic environments. Additionally, more lipid-soluble drugs are more likely to be bound to protein in blood; therefore, lipid solubility and potency are associated with greater duration of action.

Additional considerations for duration of action of local anesthetics is the rate of clearance of the drug from target sites. Local anesthetics directly cause local vasodilation due to their effects on smooth muscle, which leads to decreased duration of action. To counter this, some practitioners add vasoconstrictors, such as epinephrine, to the local anesthetic to prolong the duration of action.

Pharmacokinetics

Systemic absorption of local anesthetics varies on the route of administration, as well as on the type of local anesthetic used. See Table 7.2, which illustrates various levels of systemic absorption of local anesthetics by route of administration. The local anesthetic itself affects systemic absorption, with local anesthetics with high degrees of tissue binding (e.g., etidocaine, bupivacaine) or larger volumes of distribution (e.g., prilocaine) having less systemic absorption. Additionally, with larger total doses of local anesthetic, there will be increased systemic absorption. The addition of vasoconstrictors limits systemic absorption. For the same reason, it increases the duration of action. Vasoconstrictors limit local blood flow.

Following systemic absorption, local anesthetics are distributed to organs with high levels of blood flow such as the brain, heart, kidney, or liver. Because of this distribution, toxic effects of local anesthetics will exert effects on these systems.

Table 7.2 Systemic absorption of local anesthetics by route of administration

Systemic absorption of local anesthetics
Intravenous
Tracheal
Intercostal
Caudal
Epidural
Brachial plexus
Sciatic
Subcutaneous

The intravenous route has the highest rate of systemic absorption, whereas the subcutaneous route has the lowest rate of systemic absorption.

Metabolism of local anesthetics is dependent on the type of local anesthetic. Ester local anesthetics are rapidly metabolized by pseudocholinesterase. Metabolism of the ester local anesthetics procaine and benzocaine results in the formation of para-aminobenzoic acid (PABA), which can result in anaphylaxis to both of these drugs. Amide local anesthetics are metabolized by cytochrome p450 hepatic microsomal enzymes and are therefore dependent on hepatic blood flow and hepatic function.

Following metabolism of local anesthetics, their metabolites are excreted via the kidneys.

Characteristics of Individual Local Anesthetic Agents

Cocaine

Cocaine was the first local anesthetic to be developed and has the unique property of being the only local anesthetic with an intrinsic vasoconstrictive effect. It is most commonly administered topically in head and neck surgery because of its unique combination of local anesthetic and vasoconstrictor properties. Cocaine is typically administered as a 4% solution. Toxic doses of cocaine must be avoided, as this can result in a hypertensive crisis or myocardial ischemia. Due to these inherent risks associated with cocaine toxicity, the clinical use of cocaine has become much less common, with practitioners opting to use safer local anesthetics, such as lidocaine, with vasoconstrictors such as phenylephrine.

Procaine

Procaine was the first synthetic local anesthetic to be developed in order to address problems associated with cocaine. Procaine use is limited due to its combination of short duration of action with limited tissue penetration. It may be administered subcutaneously or as a short-duration spinal anesthetic. Procaine is typically administered as a 5% solution. It cannot be administered topically and has unreliable results when administered via epidural or peripheral nerve injection. As previously mentioned, procaine is metabolized to PABA, which is responsible for procaine's associated allergic reactions.

2-Chloroprocaine

2-Chloroprocaine is a rapidly acting local anesthetic with a short duration of action of approximately 30–60 minutes. It is more reliable than procaine for nerve conduction blockade and can be used for spinal or epidural anesthesia, peripheral nerve blockade, and subcutaneous injection. 2-Chloroprocaine is typically administered as a 2–3% solution. Although the pKa of 2-chloroprocaine is high, the onset of action is fast because of the high concentration at which the drug is administered. Due to this rapid onset, it may be used for emergent cesarean sections in patients with an epidural catheter in place.

Benzocaine

Benzocaine is a local anesthetic available in the form of a topical spray. It is used as a topical local anesthetic for awake fiberoptic intubation or endoscopy procedures. Similar to procaine, benzocaine is metabolized to PABA and may lead to allergic reactions. Additionally, benzocaine is associated with the development of methemoglobinemia at high doses. Because of these risks, use of benzocaine is limited.

Lidocaine

Lidocaine is the most commonly used local anesthetic worldwide. It has reliable nerve conduction blockade, a relatively fast onset of action, intermediate duration, and minimal significant side effects. Lidocaine may be administered in a variety of routes, with good effect, including subcutaneous injection, epidural injection, peripheral nerve blockade, and topically. It is typically administered as a 1–4% solution. Although lidocaine can be administered as a spinal injection, its high association with transient neurologic syndrome limits this use.

Mepivacaine

Mepivacaine can be used in a method very similar to lidocaine. It has reliable nerve conduction blockade, a relatively fast onset of action, and a slightly longer duration of action than lidocaine. It may be administered as an epidural or spinal injection, peripheral nerve blockade, or a subcutaneous injection. It is typically administered as a 1–2% solution.

Bupivacaine

Bupivacaine is a long-acting local anesthetic with a slow onset of action. It can be administered in a variety of routes, including spinal and epidural injection, peripheral nerve blockade, and subcutaneous injection. Bupivacaine is typically administered as a 0.25–0.75% solution. It is also a local anesthetic that is the most likely to contribute to cardiotoxicity. Local anesthetic cardiotoxicity caused by bupivacaine is more likely to involve ventricular arrhythmias compared to toxicity caused by lidocaine. Cardiopulmonary resuscitation is also less effective in local anesthetic systemic toxicity caused by bupivacaine than that caused by other local anesthetics. Bupivacaine's pronounced effect on cardiac depression is thought to be caused by stronger sodium channel blockade that leads to a greater decrease in depolarization of Purkinje fibers and ventricular muscle, as well as a delayed recovery of sodium channels from local anesthetic blockade that makes fewer of them available between action potentials.

Ropivacaine

Ropivacaine is also a long-acting local anesthetic and was developed to address the concern about bupivacaine-related cardiotoxicity. In order to minimize cardiotoxicity, ropivacaine was developed as a single enantiomer with fewer cardiotoxic effects than bupivacaine. It is typically used for epidural injection or peripheral nerve blockade and is typically administered as 0.2–1% solutions. Animal studies have demonstrated that ropivacaine leads to less profound cardiovascular collapse and fewer severe arrhythmias, while providing comparable therapeutic benefit for regional anesthesia. Similarly, levobupivacaine is also a single (S)-stereoisomer of bupivacaine; it is also believed to be less cardiotoxic than bupivacaine.

EMLA Cream

Eutectic Mixture of Local Anesthetics (EMLA) cream is a topical local anesthetic consisting of lidocaine 2.5% and prilocaine 2.5%. It is commonly applied to intact skin and sometimes on genital mucous membranes for dermal procedures. It can also be used for intravenous catheter placement among pediatric patients. If applied properly on intact skin and covered with an occlusive dressing, EMLA cream should begin to take effect within about

45–60 minutes and reach peak effect within about 2–3 hours. Although adverse reactions associated with EMLA cream is not common, precautions should be taken among specific patient populations. Since it contains lidocaine and prilocaine, patients with an allergy to amide local anesthetics should avoid using EMLA cream. Patients should exercise caution when using EMLA cream while taking class I or III antiarrhythmic drugs, out of concern that the cardiotoxic effects could be potentially additive or synergistic. In addition, patients with congenital methemoglobinemia or glucose-6-phosphate dehydrogenase deficiency, infants under a year old who are undergoing treatment with methemoglobin-inducing agents, and other people at risk of methemoglobinemia should use EMLA cream with caution out of concern about an increased risk of inducing methemoglobinemia.

Complications Associated with Local Anesthetics

Cauda Equina Syndrome

Cauda equina syndrome (CES), a condition in which the nerve roots of the cauda equina are damaged, can be caused during anesthetic procedures involving local anesthetics. These causes include maldistribution of local anesthetics, intraneural injection of local anesthetics during spinal anesthesia, needle trauma, infection, and patient positioning. Lidocaine is classically associated with CES; however, case reports have also demonstrated that bupivacaine also can cause CES.

Symptoms of CES include severe back pain, saddle anesthesia, bladder dysfunction, bowel incontinence, sexual dysfunction, sensory loss and/or motor weakness of the lower extremities, and loss of reflexes. Any combination of these symptoms should prompt an urgent workup of CES. An immediate MRI should be considered for diagnosis. A suspicion of CES warrants a neurologic consult, as prompt surgical intervention offers the best chance of improvement of neurologic dysfunction and preventing further damage.

Transient Neurologic Symptoms

Transient neurologic symptoms (TNS) is a painful condition that can occur after undergoing spinal anesthesia. Symptoms of TNS often present as pain and dysesthesia in the buttocks, lower back, and lower extremities, typically within 12–24 hours after spinal anesthesia. Although most of the local anesthetics can cause TNS, lidocaine is considered the most common offending agent. Unlike CES, there are no neurologic deficits. MRI and electrophysiologic studies are normal in patients exhibiting TNS. Symptoms typically resolve within 2–3 days but rarely can last up to 10 days. Treatment during this duration consists of supportive care with nonsteroidal antiinflammatory drugs.

Methemoglobinemia

Methemoglobinemia, a condition in which elevated methemoglobin in the blood decreases oxygen delivery to tissues, can be caused by local anesthetics. The two most commonly described local anesthetics that cause methemoglobinemia are prilocaine and benzocaine. Prilocaine is metabolized into ortho-toluidine in the liver, which can then oxidize hemoglobin into methemoglobin. Benzocaine directly oxidizes hemoglobin into methemoglobin, but the underlying mechanism of this process is not well understood.

Signs and symptoms of methemoglobinemia include headache, dizziness, shortness of breath, cyanosis, and mental status changes. Methemoglobinemia can progressively lead to loss of consciousness, seizures, coma, dysrhythmia, and death when methemoglobin levels reach >50% of total hemoglobin levels. Patients with methemoglobinemia have an acceptable level of partial pressure of oxygen despite a low oxygen saturation level; methemoglobinemia requires co-oximetry for an accurate diagnosis. Patients' blood also exhibits a classically characteristic chocolate brown appearance. The mainstays of treatment of methemoglobinemia are oxygen and methylene blue. Methylene blue reduces methemoglobin back to hemoglobin to allow oxygen delivery.

Allergic Reactions

True allergic reactions to local anesthetics are rare and represent a very small percentage of adverse reactions associated with their use. Other reactions to local anesthetics that may present similarly to allergic reactions include responses to epinephrine added to local anesthetics, responses to preservatives, and systemic toxicity. Ester local anesthetics form PABA as a metabolite, which is known to trigger allergic reactions. Hence, allergic reactions to ester local anesthetics are sometimes reactions to PABA. Methylparaben, which is used in both amide and ester local anesthetic solutions, is also a known allergen.

A true allergic response to local anesthetics would manifest with any of the following symptoms: rash, itching, hives, swelling, and wheezing. Severe allergic reactions can result in bronchospasm, laryngeal edema, hypotension, hypoxia, and tachycardia, and can lead to anaphylactic shock. An allergic reaction to local anesthetics would likely be treated based on clinical suspicion and history, but the diagnosis can later be supported by measuring serum tryptase levels and performing intradermal allergy testing. Treatment of allergic reactions depends on the symptoms but may include administration of steroids, bronchodilators, epinephrine, fluids, and oxygen.

Local Anesthetic Systemic Toxicity

Local anesthetics are very safe when recommended dosages are used at the intended sites. However, when large doses of local anesthetics reach the bloodstream, local anesthetic systemic toxicity (LAST) may occur. LAST affects the central nervous system and cardiovascular system; symptoms tend to become more severe in a dose-dependent fashion. Initial symptoms for both the central nervous system and cardiovascular system tend to be more excitatory in nature, but as the plasma concentrations of local anesthetics increase, symptoms in both systems begin to exhibit signs of depression.

Symptoms of central nervous system toxicity include dizziness, agitation, tinnitus, metallic taste, and slurred speech. Severe symptoms include mental status changes, seizures, coma, and respiratory arrest. The cardiovascular system tends to be more resistant to toxicity. Cardiovascular toxicity can initially present with hypertension and tachycardia but later progresses to hypotension and bradycardia. Electrocardiographic changes manifest as prolongation of the PR interval and widening of the QRS complex. More malignant dysrhythmias can occur later, including complete heart block. Eventually, complete cardiovascular collapse and death can ensue. Although symptoms of LAST may present in any order, there is a common pattern of symptom progression, as shown in Table 7.3.

Given the severity of the adverse effects of LAST, it is important to try to prevent it from occurring in the first place. Since unintentional intravascular injection can lead to LAST, it is important to confirm that no blood is aspirated prior to every local anesthetic injection. Small incremental doses of

Table 7.3 Common order of symptom onset in local anesthetic systemic toxicity

Order of symptoms in local anesthetic systemic toxicity	
Late	Cardiovascular collapse
	Respiratory depression
	Coma
	Convulsions
	Altered mental status
Early	Paresthesia
	Tinnitus
	Agitation
	Metallic taste in mouth

Although this order is commonly seen, symptoms may present in any order.

local anesthetic should be injected each time, while monitoring for potential signs of toxicity. Exceeding the recommended maximum dose of local anesthetics is another cause of systemic toxicity; thus, a thorough knowledge of the maximum doses is vital.

Once LAST is suspected, practitioners must promptly begin aggressive supportive care and advanced cardiovascular life support (ACLS). The airway should be secured and the patient should be ventilated with 100% oxygen. Care must be taken to avoid hypoxia, hypercapnia, and acidosis, all of which could exacerbate the effects of LAST. If the patient is experiencing seizures, treatment should be initiated with benzodiazepines or barbiturates; propofol should be avoided as an antiepileptic agent if the patient is exhibiting cardiovascular instability.

Lipid emulsion therapy is the recommended treatment for LAST. The exact mechanism of action of lipid emulsion is not known, but it is believed that it decreases the plasma concentration of local anesthetics by increasing their clearance. Lipid emulsion is also thought to reverse cardiac depression caused by local anesthetics by reversing mitochondrial dysfunction. According to the American Society of Regional Anesthesia and Pain Medicine's (ASRA) LAST checklist, a 1.5 mL kg^{-1} bolus of 20% lipid emulsion (or 100 mL for patients weighing >70 kg) should be administered over 2–3 minutes, followed by repeat boluses as needed. An infusion of 0.25 mL/ (kg min) should also be started, and doubled if the patient remains unstable. Treatment with lipid emulsion should continue for 15 minutes, even after the patient becomes stable, or for an approximate maximum dose of 12 mL kg^{-1}.

ACLS in the setting of LAST differs from standard resuscitation in a few ways. It still involves chest compressions, defibrillation, and use of vasopressors. However, the dose of epinephrine should be reduced to <1 µg kg^{-1}. Medications that can potentially worsen cardiac depression, such as local anesthetics, beta-blockers, and calcium channel blockers, should be avoided. Vasopressin is best avoided due to evidence of adverse outcomes in animal models. Given the refractory nature of cardiovascular collapse due to LAST, early consideration for extracorporeal membrane oxygenation (ECMO) is warranted, and thus the nearest facility with cardiopulmonary bypass capability should be notified if such capability is not immediately available.

Conclusion

Local anesthetics provide excellent anesthesia and analgesia, and are vital to the practice of modern anesthesiology. Knowledge of the pharmacology of local anesthetics will guide anesthesiologists' ability to select an appropriate local anesthetic for every clinical scenario.

Further Reading

Clatayud J, Gonzalez A. History of the development and evolution of local anesthesia since the coca leaf. *Anesthesiology*. 2003;98(6):1503–8.

Taylor A, McLeod G. Basic pharmacology of local anaesthetics. *BJA Educ*. 2020;20 (4):34–41.

Chapter 8

Anesthesia Techniques: Mild, Moderate, and Deep Sedation in Clinical Practice

Mark R. Jones, Boris C. Anyama, Chikezie N. Okeagu, Meredith K. Shaw, Madelyn K. Craig, and Alan David Kaye

Background

Selection of the anesthetic technique to be employed during a procedure begins during the preoperative evaluation with consideration of factors such as the patient's comorbidities and preferences and the type of procedure to be performed. Oftentimes, general anesthesia is not necessary and the procedure can be performed under a lesser depth of sedation. Procedural sedation is a technique that allows the patient to tolerate the discomfort of a procedure while still maintaining cardiorespiratory function. In order to accomplish this, the anesthesia provider administers sedative, dissociative, and/or analgesic agents alone or in combination [1].

Although commonly regarded as one entity, procedural sedation is a heterogeneous anesthetic technique that encompasses a variety of levels of consciousness. The various depths of sedation are differentiated by the physiologic changes induced by the agents used and the patient's response to stimuli. The American Society of Anesthesiologists's (ASA) continuum of sedation divides sedation into three categories: minimal, moderate, and deep. Table 8.1 describes these categories of anesthetic depth. Minimal sedation is a drug-induced state defined by preserved response to verbal stimulation. While cognitive function and/or physical coordination may be impaired, a patient under minimal sedation maintains the ability to protect their own airway and ventilate spontaneously. Furthermore, cardiovascular function is unaffected when under minimal sedation. Under moderate sedation, patients retain the ability to respond purposefully to verbal or tactile stimuli. Patients maintain the ability to protect their own airway and perform adequate spontaneous ventilation without intervention from the anesthesia provider. Cardiovascular function also is usually maintained. This level of sedation is sometimes referred to colloquially as "conscious sedation." Deep sedation is the greatest depth of sedation before a patient is considered to be under general anesthesia. A patient under deep sedation is still able to respond purposefully to stimuli but only demonstrates this

Table 8.1 Depth of anesthesia

	Minimal sedation	Moderate sedation	Deep sedation	General anesthesia
Responsiveness	Normal response to verbal stimulation	Purposeful response to verbal or tactile stimulation	Purposeful response to repeated or painful stimulation	No response, even to painful stimulation
Airway	Unaffected	No intervention required	Intervention could be required	Intervention typically required
Spontaneous ventilation	Unaffected	Adequate	May be inadequate	Frequently inadequate
Cardiovascular function	Unaffected	Usually maintained	Usually maintained	May be impaired

ability following repeated or painful stimulation. Importantly, reflex withdrawal from painful stimuli is not considered purposeful. Patients under deep sedation may exhibit impairment of spontaneous ventilation and may require intervention to aid in protecting their airways. Just as in the lesser depths of sedation, cardiovascular function is usually maintained in patients under deep sedation. Since sedation is a continuum, it is difficult, and sometimes impossible, to predict how a particular patient will respond to the administered medications. As such, providers should always be prepared to "rescue" a patient from a level of sedation that is deeper than anticipated. Of note, the term monitored anesthesia care (MAC) is often used to describe situations in which patients are under a depth of sedation that is less than general anesthesia. It is important to note that MAC is not a particular depth of sedation, but rather a billing designation that indicates the involvement of an anesthesiologist [2].

Procedural sedation is appropriate for a wide array of procedures and can be performed in a variety of locations. In the hospital, procedural sedation is often required in the emergency department to facilitate procedures such as laceration repair and fracture reduction. Similarly, endoscopic procedures, such as colonoscopy, esophagogastroduodenoscopy (EGD), and transesophageal echocardiography, are often performed under sedation. Sedation is also utilized in the operating room for patients undergoing surgery. In these instances, it is often combined with other techniques such as regional or local anesthesia. Lastly, sedation can be performed out of the hospital in office-based settings to aid in the performance of procedures such dental or dermatologic procedures. Regardless of location or procedure, it is important for the provider in charge of administering sedation to possess the appropriate skill set and monitoring and resuscitation equipment to do so safely.

Provider Roles

A board-certified anesthesiologist is a physician who has completed medical school, was enrolled in, and completed, a certified anesthesiology residency program, and has passed all accreditation and licensing examinations, whether written or oral. The ASA believes that at least one physician anesthesiologist should be involved in the care of each patient receiving anesthetics [3]. This physician anesthesiologist may be directly providing care for the patient or often supervising another practitioner [4–6]. These practitioners can include a physician currently enrolled in training, either residency or fellowship, or a nonphysician anesthesia care provider. A nonphysician anesthesia care provider can include a certified registered nurse anesthetist (CRNA), a registered nurse who has completed an accredited program for nursing, has completed a set amount of time working in an intensive care unit environment, and has completed training and the accompanying licensing examinations as part of the nurse anesthetist accreditation [3–5]. Additionally, nursing providers in both the preoperative area and the postanesthesia care unit, as well as intraoperatively, are important in providing assistance to the anesthesia care team. They are often able to identify or anticipate issues that may arise, be an advocate for the patient, and provide additional assistance to the anesthesiologist if necessary [7]. Thus, there are a multitude of individuals in various healthcare professions and levels of training who make important contributions to the perioperative care team of the patient.

Drug Selection

This section will discuss the most commonly utilized pharmacologic agents in sedation anesthesia practice. Table 8.2 provides a summation of the below medications.

Benzodiazepines

Benzodiazepines act on type A gamma-aminobutyric acid (GABA) receptors in the brainstem, causing anxiolytic, amnesic, and sedative effects, without an analgesic effect [1]. Lorazepam, diazepam, and midazolam are commonly used benzodiazepines in anesthesia. These drugs have various ways of

Table 8.2 Commonly used anesthetic agents in sedation practice and their pharmacologic properties

Drug	Administration	Initial intravenous dosage	Infusion rate	Sedative effect
Benzodiazepine (midazolam)	Intravenous, oral, intramuscular	0.02–0.04 mg kg^{-1}	0.25–1.0 g/(kg min)	+++
Propofol	Intravenous	20–30 mg bolus	25–75 µg/(kg min)	+++
Opioids (fentanyl, remifentanil, alfentanil)	Intravenous, oral, intramuscular	Fentanyl: 2–50 µg kg^{-1} Remifentanil: 1 µg kg^{-1} Alfentanil: 8–100 µg kg^{-1}	Bolus in 5-min intervals to obtain titrated effect 0.1 µg/(kg min) 0.5–3 µg/(kg min)	Intensifies effects of other sedative anesthetics
Dexmedetomidine	Intravenous, oral	1 g kg^{-1} over 10 minutes	0.3–0.7 g/(kg hr)	++
Ketamine	Intravenous, oral, intramuscular	0.25–0.5 mg kg^{-1}	2.5–15 µg/(kg min)[a]	+++
Nitrous oxide	Inhaled	n/a	n/a	+/– Intensifies effects of other sedative anesthetics

[a] Usually administered with propofol.

+, weak effect; ++, moderate effect; +++, strong effect; –, no effect.

administration for sedation (e.g., intravenously, intramuscular, oral). Lorazepam and diazepam are insoluble (formulated with propylene glycol) and well absorbed in the gastrointestinal tract, making oral administration favorable [2]. Midazolam is water-soluble at low pH and commonly used as an anesthesia premedication in adults intravenously or intramuscularly (0.02–0.04 mg kg^{-1}) and orally in children (0.4–0.8 mg kg^{-1}) [1]. Minimal risk of cardiopulmonary depression exists when using midazolam in small dosages for procedural sedations. Midazolam is also preferred to maintain hypnosis and amnesia, with continuous infusion rates of 0.25–1.0 g/(kg min), while given with an inhalational agent or opioids. In addition, midazolam can enhance the effects of other opioids and sedatives when administered concomitantly [3]. Due to a prolonged emergence, administration of midazolam as an infusion for sedation should be reserved for short cases or patients who are expected to remain intubated [1]. Benzodiazepines can be pharmacologically reversed with flumazenil (0.5–1 mg intravenously), a competitive antagonist, making them favorable for sedation in the setting of a threatened airway [1]. Benzodiazepines are usually avoided during pregnancy because newborns can exhibit withdrawal symptoms from benzodiazepine administration to the mothers.

Propofol

Propofol is a rapid- and short-acting drug that acts on the type A GABA channel to provide sedative, amnesia, and antiemetic properties [2, 4]. Similar to benzodiazepines, propofol does not cause analgesia. Propofol is commonly used for moderate procedural sedation by intermittent boluses (20–30 mg) or titrated infusion (25–75 μg/(kg min)) intravenously [1]. Children will need a higher dose to overcome the accelerated clearance and larger volume of distribution to achieve an ideal sedative effect. Propofol has a narrow therapeutic index and can deepen the levels of sedation quickly. Consequently, close monitoring for adverse effects (e.g., myocardial depression) in patients receiving propofol is imperative. Because there is no reversal agent for propofol, oversedated patients should be managed with supportive therapy (e.g., airway support) until the agent is metabolized [1, 2]. Prolonged use of a high-dose propofol infusion in a critically ill population may cause propofol infusion syndrome (PRIS), which is characterized by rhabdomyolysis, cardiac failure, renal failure, metabolic acidosis, hepatomegaly, hyperkalemia, and hypertriglyceridemia [1]. If PRIS is suspected, propofol must be discontinued immediately and an alternative sedative should be used.

Opioids

Opioids bind to specific receptors (μ, κ, δ, and σ) throughout the central nervous system and peripheral nervous system to provide analgesia and supplemental sedation [1, 2]. Fentanyl, remifentanil, and alfentanil are common opioids used in anesthesia for sedation. Opioids alone mainly have analgesic properties, but when used with other agents (e.g., propofol and midazolam), they can intensify the effect of sedation. Fentanyl, short-acting, is administered intravenously in 2–50 µg kg^{-1} boluses at 5-minute intervals to obtain a titrated effect [2]. Remifentanil, ultrashort-acting, is administered as a typical bolus dose of 1 µg kg^{-1}, followed by an infusion of 0.5–20 µg/(kg min). Alfentanil, ultrashort-acting, is administered as a bolus dose of 8–100 µg kg^{-1}, followed by an infusion rate of 0.5–3 µg/(kg min). Keep in mind that opioid dose should be halved when midazolam is used, to decrease the risk of adverse effects from opioids (e.g., ventilatory depression, increased vagal tone, muscle rigidity) [1, 2]. Naloxone, an opioid receptor antagonist, may be administered (0.5–1 µg kg^{-1}) every 3–5 minutes until the clinical signs of opioids are reversed.

Dexmedetomidine

Dexmedetomidine, a centrally acting and selective α2-agonist, provides sedative, anxiolytic, and some analgesic effects without major respiratory depression [1, 5]. Administration can be intravenously (most common), orally, nasally, intramuscularly, or rectally. Dexmedetomidine given as an intravenous infusion is titrated (0.3–0.7 g/(kg hr)), based on the level of sedation and the stability of the patient's hemodynamics. An initial loading dose (1 g kg^{-1} over 10 minutes) can be given but warrants consideration due to an increased risk of hemodynamic instability. The onset of action is slower and sedation tends to be prolonged compared to other sedatives, making dexmedetomidine a less favorable sedation of choice for certain procedures [6].

Ketamine

Ketamine, a rapid-acting and short-duration N-methyl-D-aspartate (NMDA) receptor antagonist, provides analgesia, dissociative amnesia, and sedation, with minimal respiratory depression [1, 7]. In clinical practice, ketamine is administered intravenously and intramuscularly [2]. For sedation, ketamine is usually given in combination with propofol (2.5–15 µg/(kg min) intravenously) or alone with an initial bolus of 0.25–0.5 mg kg^{-1} [7]. Ketamine sedation may cause the patient's eyes to stay open, but remaining unresponsive to stimuli [1, 7]. Ketamine causes a release of catecholamines, resulting in increased heart rate, blood pressure, and cardiac output. Patients with catecholamine depletion can have myocardial depression [1, 2, 7]. Other adverse effects, such as laryngospasm from increased oral secretions and emergence reactions (vivid dreams and hallucinations), can be reduced by taking pharmacological agents concomitantly (e.g., glycopyrrolate and benzodiazepines).

Nitrous Oxide

Nitrous oxide, a rapid-onset and -offset inhalational anesthetic agent, provides analgesic, anxiolytic, and sedative effects, with minimal hemodynamic effects [1, 2]. Nitrous oxide is typically used as a supplemental agent for maintenance of general anesthesia to increase the depth of sedation, resulting in less dose requirements for the inhalational or intravenous anesthetic agent being used. Nitrous oxide when co-administered with other volatile inhalational agents can increase the speed of the anesthetic onset and offset, known as the "second gas" effect [1, 2, 9]. Prolonged use of nitrous oxide can cause anemia (by irreversibly inhibiting methionine synthetase) [1]. Because nitrous oxide is extremely soluble (35 times more soluble than nitrogen), some conditions are contraindicated for the usage of the inhalational agent (e.g., pneumothorax, air embolism, acute intestinal obstruction with bowl distension) [2].

Preprocedure

History and Physical

An essential component of every anesthesia practice is preoperative evaluation and risk assessment to screen patients prior to the delivery of anesthesia and to intervene, when necessary, to minimize perioperative morbidity and mortality. A key component of the preoperative evaluation is the history and physical examination. A patient's medical comorbidities and its therapies, surgical history, social history, physical examination, and functional capacity are needed to assess a patient's anesthetic risks, optimize chronic medical conditions, and develop an anesthetic plan [8, 9]. All patients undergoing anesthesia should be assessed for their risk of cardiac and pulmonary complications, PONV, delirium, and bleeding or clotting complications [10]. The physical examination should include at least an assessment of the patient's airway, heart, and lungs. Other systems examination should be based on the patient's comorbidities and the planned surgery. Inadequate evaluation or optimization of chronic medical conditions increases the risk of perioperative complications [9].

ASA Physical Status

The ASA physical status classification system is an assessment tool that allows clinicians to communicate an adult patient's medical comorbidities. When used in combination with other risk assessments tools, it aids in predicting perioperative outcomes. A healthy patient without chronic medical comorbidities who is having surgery for an acute problem is classified as ASA I. ASA II classification is for patients with systemic disease(s) that are mild or well controlled and do not cause functional limitations. Examples include well-controlled hypertension or diabetes, smoking, pregnancy, and obesity with a body mass index (BMI) <40. Patients with systemic disease that is severe or uncontrolled and limits functionality are assigned ASA III status. Poorly controlled hypertension or diabetes, BMI >40, end-stage renal disease with scheduled dialysis, systolic heart failure with moderately reduced ejection fraction, chronic obstructive pulmonary disease (COPD), and cerebrovascular accident are all examples of systemic disease listed under ASA III classification. If the systemic disease is a constant threat to the patient's life, then the patient is considered ASA IV. A patient not expected to survive without the operation is ASA V. ASA VI is reserved for patients who have been declared brain-dead and are having organ procurement surgery. An "E" is added for emergency surgeries of which a delay could result in an increased threat to the patient's life or limb [11].

Fasting Guidelines

The ASA published practice guidelines to aid in determining the timing of preoperative fasting for elective procedures. Categories include clear liquids, breast milk, infant formula, nonhuman milk, and solids. Every patient should remain nil *per os* (NPO) for at least 2 hours, and even longer, depending on the type of liquid or solid ingested. If only clear liquids were consumed, procedures requiring any type of sedation may be performed after 2 hours of fasting. Neonates and infants may ingest breast milk up to 4 hours prior to anesthesia. However, infant formula requires an additional 2 hours of fasting for a total of 6 hours NPO. A fasting period of at least 6 hours is recommended for a light meal or nonhuman milk. If fatty/fried foods or meats were ingested, a fasting time of 8 or more hours is appropriate. It is also important to consider the amount of food consumed and adjust the fasting time accordingly [12].

Preoperative Testing and Consultation

Routine preoperative testing, such as blood tests, CXR, and ECG, has low clinical utility and is generally not recommended. The majority of patients undergoing elective surgery require minimal, if any, testing [10]. A routine ECG is indicated for patients having high-risk surgery or patients with cardiovascular or respiratory disease who are not having low-risk surgery. Patients with a BMI >40 who have an additional risk factor for cardiovascular disease may also warrant a preoperative ECG. The 2014 American College of Cardiology/American Heart Association guidelines on perioperative cardiovascular evaluation for noncardiac surgery contain a simple algorithm to determine which patients should undergo a preoperative stress test. Transthoracic echocardiography (TTE) is recommended for patients with known valvular disease or heart failure who have new or worsening symptoms or who have not had TTE within a year. A new murmur found on physical examination is another indication for preoperative TTE. A routine CXR may be warranted for patients with known cardiovascular or pulmonary disease, including smokers, those aged >50 who have upper abdominal or thoracic surgery, those with a BMI >40, or patients who have had a recent upper respiratory infection (URI). Pulmonary function tests (PFTs) may be indicated for patients with symptomatic asthma or COPD, depending on the type of surgery being performed. Screening for obstructive sleep apnea (OSA) is recommended for most patients by using the STOP-Bang tool. Preoperative hemoglobin and hematocrit may be indicated in elderly patients and patients with a history of anemia or hematologic disorder, or for surgeries with severe blood loss. Patients with hematologic or hepatic disease should have a preoperative platelet count assessed. Patients taking warfarin should have prothrombin time measured. Other coagulation tests may be indicated for patients with bleeding disorders or kidney or liver disease, or those undergoing certain procedures. Serum chemistry may be indicated for elderly patients, patients with kidney disease, patients taking certain medications, or those requiring cardiac risk stratification. It is recommended that all females of childbearing age have a preoperative pregnancy test. As long as there are no significant changes in a patient's medical conditions, tests obtained within 6 months of an elective procedure are deemed acceptable. Testing should be guided by the presence of disease state or risk factors that will impact anesthetic management. Unnecessary preoperative tests may lead to harm, including increased costs and patient distress, especially when further testing is unlikely to change perioperative management [9, 10].

Monitoring and Equipment

The ASA has determined a standard of care for the administration of anesthetics that includes monitoring of ventilation, oxygenation, circulation, and body temperature of any patient under the care of an anesthesiologist [13]. These monitors provide information that assists the anesthesiologist in determining the amount of anesthetic medication to provide analgesia and amnesia, while simultaneously attempting to maintain the patient's normal cardiac and pulmonary homeostasis.

Monitoring ventilation is done through end-tidal carbon dioxide ($ETCO_2$) detection and continuous quantification, as well as through capnographic waveform monitoring. These allow the anesthesiologist to ensure the patient is maintaining adequate minute ventilation in order to provide their tissues, often in a hypermetabolic state, with oxygen [13–15]. Additionally, oxygenation of the patient is supervised through oxygen analyzers on the anesthesia machine, which are programmed to prevent delivery of a hypoxic mixture of gases, and a pulse oximeter, which is placed directly on the patient. These ensure that the anesthesiologist is providing an adequate amount of oxygen to the patient and that oxygen is being delivered to the patient's arterial system

[13, 15, 16]. Providing sedation *without* continuous quantitative $ETCO_2$ is below local, regional, and national standards of care, and can be a critical reason for morbidity and mortality in the delivery of sedation. In this regard, tubing that is connected to nasal cannulae or, when not available, a cut plastic intravenous cannula can be taped under the nose directly into the $ETCO_2$ tubing and can be employed to ensure real-time ventilation information for the clinical anesthesia provider. Prone patients are at even greater risk when being provided with moderate or deep sedation and these procedures are common in interventional pain sites, gastrointestinal procedure suites, and other procedure areas.

The patient's circulation is observed through ECG and either noninvasive or invasive blood pressure monitoring [13, 15, 16]. ECG monitoring, which should be at a minimum three-lead, allows the anesthesiologist to watch for abnormalities in response to the demands placed on the patient's body by the anesthetic medications and the surgeon's manipulation. Blood pressure monitoring, which should be recorded at a minimum of every 3– 5 minutes, ensures that the patient maintains adequate perfusion of their vital organs [13–15].

Finally, the patient's temperature should be monitored as redistribution from anesthetic medications can cause core heat loss. Additionally, it is a way by which, in addition to the other monitors listed previously, the anesthesiologist providing care to the patient can evaluate the patient for adverse reactions to medications given [13, 14, 17]. The most discussed is malignant hyperthermia, which presents with an acute increase in $ETCO_2$, muscle rigidity, and elevated temperature, in addition to severe metabolic abnormalities.

Thus, all the monitors required by the ASA allow the anesthesiologist to provide the highest quality of care to the patient, by allowing accurate administration of anesthetic medications to the patient, and to avert adverse consequences in response to those anesthetic administrations.

Conclusion

Various techniques and practices are available to the anesthetic provider when considering the utilization of sedation during interventions or surgeries. This chapter discussed the recognized categories of sedation depth, necessary patient and provider considerations prior to implementing sedation, pharmacologic agents available to achieve the desired depth, and requirements for safe maintenance of monitoring of the patient under sedation. As always, the utmost importance is placed on patient safety, and providers may refer to this chapter as a guide for appropriate conduction of sedation when practicing modern anesthesia, regardless of the clinical setting.

References

1. Whitlock EL, Pardo MC Jr. *Choice of Anesthetic Technique*, 7th ed. Philadelphia, PA: Elsevier; 2018.

2. American Society of Anesthesiologists. Continuum of depth of sedation: definition of general anesthesia and levels of sedation/analgesia. 2019. Available from: www .asahq.org/standards-and-guidelines/continuum-of-depth-of-sedation-definition-of-general-anesthesia-and-levels-of-sedationanalgesia.

3. American Society of Anesthesiologists. Statement on the anesthesia care team. 2019. Available from: www.asahq.org/-/media/sites/asahq/files/public/resources/st andards-guidelines/statement-on-the-anesthesia-care-team.pdf? la=en&hash=9674E540AB92E575C1FD8AB9B48159F7656B9AEB.

4. Abenstein JP, Warner MA. Anesthesia providers, patient outcomes, and costs. *Anesth Analg*. 1996;82(6):1273–83.

5. Jones TS, Fitzpatrick JJ. CRNA – physician collaboration in anesthesia. *AANA J*. 2009;77(6):431–6.

6. American Society of Anesthesiologists. Statement on the anesthesia care team. 2019. Available from: www.asahq.org/standards-and-guidelines/statement-on-the-anesthesia-care-team.

7. Sun EC, Miller TR, Moshfegh J, Baker LC. Anesthesia care team composition and surgical outcomes. *Anesthesiology*. 2018;129(4):700–9. DOI: 10.1097/ ALN.0000000000002275.

8. Committee on Standards and Practice Parameters; Apfelbaum JL, Connis RT, Nickinovich DG, American Society of Anesthesiologists Task Force on Preanesthesia Evaluation; Pasternak LR, Arens JF, Caplan RA, *et al*. Practice advisory for preanesthesia evaluation. *Anesthesiology*. 2012;116(3):522–38. DOI: 10.1097/aln.0b013e31823c1067.

9. Okocha O, Gerlach RM, Sweitzer BJ. Preoperative evaluation for ambulatory anesthesia: what, when, and how? *Anesthesiol Clin*. 2019;37(2):195–213. DOI: 10.1016/j.anclin.2019.01.014.

10. Bierle DM, Raslau D, Regan DW, Sundsted KK, Mauck KF. Preoperative evaluation before noncardiac surgery. *Mayo Clin Proc*. 2020;95(4):807–22. DOI: 10.1016/j. mayocp.2019.04.029.

11. American Society of Anesthesiologists. ASA physical status classification system. 2020. Available from: www.asahq.org/standards-and-guidelines/asa-physical-status-classification-system.

12. [No authors listed]. Practice guidelines for preoperative fasting and the use of pharmacologic agents to reduce the risk of pulmonary aspiration: application to healthy patients undergoing elective procedures. *Anesthesiology*. 2017;126(3):376–93. DOI: 10.1097/ALN.0000000000001452.

13. American Society of Anesthesiologists. Standards for basic anesthetic monitoring. 2020. Available from: www.asahq.org/standards-and-guidelines/standards-for-basic-anesthetic-monitoring.

14. Manohar M, Gupta B, Gupta L. Closed-loop monitoring by anesthesiologists: a comprehensive approach to patient monitoring during anesthesia. *Korean J Anesthesiol.* 2018;71(5):417–18. DOI: 10.4097/kja.d.18.00033.

15. Checketts MR, Alladi R, Ferguson K, *et al.* Recommendations for standards of monitoring during anaesthesia and recovery 2015: Association of Anaesthetists of Great Britain and Ireland. *Anaesthesia.* 2016;71(1):85–93. DOI: 10.1111/anae.13316.

16. Association of Anaesthetists. Checking anaesthetic equipment. 2012. Available from: https://anaesthetists.org/Home/Resources-publications/Guidelines/Checking-Anaesthetic-Equipment.

17. Sessler DI. Temperature monitoring and perioperative thermoregulation. *Anesthesiology.* 2008;109(2):318–38. DOI: 10.1097/ALN.0b013e31817f6d76.

Chapter
9

Anesthesia Techniques: General Anesthesia Techniques in Clinical Practice

Mark R. Jones, Edward S. Alpaugh, Boris C. Anyama, Chikezie N. Okeagu, Meredith K. Shaw, Madelyn K. Craig, and Alan David Kaye

Background

Preoperatively, the patient will transition from different depths of anesthesia, including the levels of sedation, to general anesthesia (GA). Sedation is a continuum of symptoms that range from minimal symptoms of anxiolysis to symptoms of moderate and deep sedation. Moderate sedation is defined by the patient remaining asleep but being easily arousable. Deep sedation is achieved when the patient is only arousable to painful stimulation. GA refers to medically induced loss of consciousness with concurrent loss of protective reflexes and skeletal muscle relaxation. GA is most commonly achieved via induction with intravenous sedatives and analgesics, followed by maintenance of volatile anesthetics [1]. Table 9.1 lists the depths of anesthesia and associated characteristics.

The stages of anesthesia can be based on Guedel's classification, which includes four stages:

- Stage I – analgesia or disorientation: The patient is not yet unconscious and may have just begun to feel the effects of anesthesia. Patients typically will remain conversational, and breathing will often be slow and regular.

- Stage II – excitement or delirium: There are many possible patient reactions while beginning this phase. Disinhibition, delirium, uncontrolled movements, hypertension, and tachycardia are commonly associated. The airway will remain intact and will have a higher sensitivity to stimulation. Airway manipulation must be avoided during this phase.

- Stage III – surgical anesthesia: Surgical anesthesia is achieved once the patient has reached the appropriate anesthetic level for procedures requiring GA. At this phase, it is safe to manipulate the airway. The patient will begin to show signs of respiratory depression, and eye movements will no longer be present.

- Stage IV – overdose: If the patient has received too much of an anesthetic agent, the patient is at higher risk of worsening brain function. The stage will begin with respiratory cessation and ends with potential death. The

Table 9.1 Definitions of different anesthetic depths and associated characteristics

	Minimal sedation/anxiolysis	Moderate sedation/analgesia ("conscious sedation")	Deep sedation/analgesia	General anesthesia
Responsiveness	Normal response to verbal stimulation	Purposeful response to verbal or tactile stimulation	Purposeful response following repeated or painful stimulation	Unarousable even with painful stimulus
Airway	Unaffected	No intervention required	Intervention may be required	Intervention often required
Spontaneous ventilation	Unaffected	Adequate	May be inadequate	Frequently inadequate
Cardiovascular function	Unaffected	Usually maintained	Usually maintained	May be impaired

patient can become hypotensive, with decreased cardiac output and peripheral vasodilation. The patient can also present with weak and thready pulses [2].

Preoperative Evaluation

The preoperative evaluation of the patient before surgery requires a detailed history and physical examination, ordering necessary laboratory workup, identifying the ASA physical status classification, and taking appropriate fasting precautions. The ASA physical status categorizes patients by their preanesthesia medical comorbidities. Classification is a clinical decision based on multiple factors, with the final assessment made on the day of anesthesia care. Table 9.2 describes the parameters of each ASA class.

The preanesthesia history will include all the components of the patient's current and past medical history, surgical history, family history, social history, allergies, current and recent medication regimen, and history of prior anesthetics. It is important to screen for any recent infections, specifically upper and lower respiratory tract infections. Screening for a family history of adverse reactions to anesthetics will help avoid adverse reactions due to hereditary metabolic syndromes. Prenatal and birth history should also be obtained in pediatric cases. A specific assessment of prematurity at birth, perinatal complications, and congenital chromosomal or anatomic abnormalities is also useful.

While obtaining the medication history, it is important to monitor for recent use of medications that may interfere with anesthetic agents. For example, monoamine oxidase inhibitors should be discontinued 2–3 weeks before surgery. Oral contraceptive therapies should also be discontinued at least 6 weeks before elective surgery due to the increased risk of venothromboembolism. Herbal supplements have been considered by the ASA and are recommended to be stopped 2 weeks before surgery.

The preanesthesia physical examination should focus on airway assessment, examination of the heart and lungs, and documentation of the patient's vital signs. It is important to identify comorbid diseases during history taking and physical examination that would necessitate further workup and consultations. The anesthesia provider should pay special attention to pulmonary, cardiac, renal, central nervous system (CNS), and bleeding disorders, and follow through with appropriate laboratory, study, or imaging [3]. Table 9.3 describes the indications for specific preoperative tests.

Before surgery, recommendations for fasting status of various foods and liquids are provided for GA, regional anesthesia, and procedural sedation and analgesia. The patient may ingest clear liquids for up to 2 hours, breast milk for up to 4 hours, infant formula for up to 6 hours, and solids and nonhuman milk for up to 6 hours. An additional fasting time of up to 8 hours or more is recommended in patients consuming fried foods, fatty foods, or

Table 9.2 Characteristics of American Society of Anesthesiologists' physical classification

ASA physical status classification	Definition	Adult examples (including, but not limited to)
ASA I	A normal healthy patient	Healthy, nonsmoker, no or minimal alcohol use
ASA II	A patient with mild systemic disease	Mild diseases without functional limitations, including current smoker, social alcohol drinker, pregnancy, obesity (30 < BMI < 40), well-controlled DM/HTN, mild lung disease
ASA III	A patient with severe systemic disease	Functional limitations with one or more moderate to severe diseases. Examples include poorly controlled DM or HTN, COPD, morbid obesity (BMI ≥40), active hepatitis, moderately reduced EF, ESRD regularly undergoing dialysis, premature infant, history of MI, CVA, TIA, or CAD/PCI
ASA IV	A patient with severe systemic disease that is a constant threat to life	Examples include recent MI, CVA, TIA, or CAD/PCI (<3 months), ongoing cardiac ischemia or severe valve dysfunction, severely reduced EF, sepsis, DIC, ARF or ESRD not regularly undergoing dialysis
ASA V	A moribund patient who is not expected to survive without the operation	Examples included ruptured abdominal/thoracic aneurysm, massive trauma, intracranial bleed with mass effect, ischemic bowel with threat to cardiac pathology or multiple organ/system dysfunction
ASA VI	A declared brain-dead patient whose organs are being removed for donor purposes	

BMI, body mass index; DM, diabetes mellitus; HTN, hypertension; COPD, chronic obstructive pulmonary disease; EF, ejection fraction; ESRD, end-stage renal disease; MI, myocardial infarction; CVA, cerebrovascular accident; TIA, transient ischemic attack; CAD, coronary artery disease; PCI, percutaneous coronary intervention; CVA, cerebrovascular accident; DIC, disseminated intravascular coagulopathy; ARF, acute renal failure.

Table 9.3 Indications for specific preoperative tests

Complete blood count

- Major surgery
- Chronic cardiovascular, pulmonary, renal, or hepatic disease, or malignancy
- Known or suspected anemia, bleeding diathesis, or myelosuppression

International normalized ratio (INR), activated partial thromboplastin time (aPTT)

- Anticoagulant therapy
- Bleeding diathesis
- Liver disease

Electrolytes and creatinine

- Hypertension
- Renal disease
- Diabetes
- Pituitary or adrenal disease
- Digoxin or diuretic therapy, or other drug therapies affecting electrolytes

Fasting glucose

- Diabetes (should be repeated on day of surgery)

Electrocardiography

- Heart disease, hypertension, diabetes
- Other risk factors for cardiac disease (may include age)
- Subarachnoid or intracranial hemorrhage, cerebrovascular accident, or head trauma

Chest radiograph

- Cardiac or pulmonary disease
- Malignancy

meat [4]. Table 9.4 describes the fasting and pharmacologic recommendations for induction of anesthesia.

Induction of Anesthesia

Inhalational Induction

Inhalation anesthesia began with the introduction of diethyl ether in 1846. Modern halothane was produced in 1956, leading to a new method of rapid and safe inhalational induction. Inhalational induction with halothane had been primarily utilized in pediatric populations and patients with difficult airways. Sevoflurane was later introduced in the 1990s and gained popularity

Table 9.4 Fasting and pharmacologic recommendations

Fasting recommendations	
Ingested material	**Minimum fasting period (hours)**
Clear liquids	2
Breast milk	4
Infant formula	6
Nonhuman milk	6
Light meal	6
Fried foods, fatty foods, or meat	8 or more
Pharmacologic recommendations	
Medication type and common examples	**Recommendation**
Gastrointestinal stimulants: • Metoclopramide	May be used/no routine use
Gastric acid secretion blockers: • Cimetidine • Famotidine • Ranitidine • Omeprazole • Lansoprazole	May be used/no routine use
Antacids: • Sodium citrate • Sodium bicarbonate • Magnesium trisilicate	May be used/no routine use
Antiemetics: • Ondansetron	May be used/no routine use
Anticholinergics: • Atropine • Scopolamine • Glycopyrrolate	No use

due to minimal airway irritation. Inhalational induction has been shown to have a perceived advantage over propofol through its avoidance of suppression of airway reflexes.

Sevoflurane can also provide relatively stable cardiac and hemodynamic conditions in patients at risk of hypotension, hypertension, and tachycardia. Studies have also shown similar outcomes when measuring cardiovascular stability during tracheal intubation in hypertensive patients compared to propofol. There are also documented case studies utilizing rapid sequence induction with sevoflurane in cesarean section without any reported adverse advents. Due to changes in the respiratory physiology in pregnant patients, induction is accelerated. It will have a decreased minimum alveolar concentration (MAC) due to increased ventilation with a reduced functional reserve capacity [1].

Intravenous Induction

Inhalational induction was initially the only practiced technique before the introduction of thiopental in 1934. Intravenous induction became a popular method, allowing the care provider more options to utilize safe induction agents. Compared to inhalation anesthesia, specific intravenous anesthetic medications decreased overall side effects. Intravenous induction agents include barbiturates, phenols, imidazoles, phencyclidines, and benzodiazepines [1].

Thiopental is a barbiturate, producing a smooth onset of hypnosis and rapid recovery. There have been reportedly low incidences of restlessness, nausea, and vomiting. The liver slowly metabolizes thiopental via first-order kinetics. Elimination will remain constant with increases in doses. It also acts as a negative inotrope depressing contractility of the heart. This will have a subsequent reduction in cardiac output and blood pressure. It is also common to have respiratory depression and can be seen following a bolus dose.

Propofol is a short-acting general anesthetic medication and the onset of action is approximately 30 seconds. Induction will typically be smooth, and patients generally experience a rapid recovery from anesthesia due to its short half-life of 2–4 minutes. Induction with propofol can be associated with drops in blood pressure, secondary to systemic vasodilation, and can have associated reflex tachycardia.

Etomidate is an imidazole ester and is associated with the least amount of cardiovascular side effects of intravenous anesthetics. It can, however, have cardiovascular effects and can cause a mild reduction in cardiac output and blood pressure. It is rapidly metabolized by the liver, yielding inactive metabolites, and is eliminated via the urine, with a half-life of 1–5 hours. Standard recovery is rapid due to redistribution to muscle and fat. Etomidate was used in shocked, elderly, and cardiovascular-compromised patients but has recently become less commonly used.

Ketamine is a derivative of phencyclidine, which was a formerly used anesthetic agent. It is metabolized in the liver and excreted in the urine. Common associations on induction include tachycardia, hypertension, and increased cardiac output. Due to these effects, it is also chosen as induction agent in shocked and unwell patients. Airway reflexes remain intact and it produces minimal effects on the respiratory drive.

Benzodiazepines, including midazolam and diazepam, are the most commonly used agents for anxiolysis, and α2 inhibitors and melatonin are also used, albeit much less often. Controlling anxiety has demonstrated decreased complications in perioperative care. More specifically, it has decreased hemodynamic instability, decreased anesthetic consumption during anesthesia, and improved postoperative pain, recovery time, and hospital stay [5].

Airway Management

Mask Ventilation

Mask ventilation is fundamental to the practice of anesthesia. This basic skill is one of the most important tools in airway management. It is performed before endotracheal intubation and used as a rescue maneuver if intubation is difficult or fails. Obtaining a tight seal with the face mask is an important aspect of successful mask ventilation. The face mask should fit over the bridge of the nose and enclose the mouth, with the bottom positioned between the lower lip and the chin. Leaks may develop if the mask is not the correct size, the cushion is improperly inflated, or the patient has a beard or an abnormal anatomy. Risk factors for difficult mask ventilation include a beard, increased BMI, edentulousness, limited mandibular protrusion, Mallampati III or IV, history of snoring or obstructive sleep apnea (OSA), airway masses or tumors, history of neck radiation, male gender, and age >55. The triple maneuver (jaw thrust, head extension, and chin lift) should be used to maximize pharyngeal patency. Once the triple maneuver is performed, the left hand holds this position, with the mask sealed tightly to the face, while the right hand squeezes the reservoir bag. If maintaining the triple maneuver position or an adequate seal with one hand proves difficult, the two-handed mask ventilation technique should be utilized and a second provider assists ventilation with the bag. An oral or nasal airway may be required to overcome obstruction, resulting from the tongue falling back to the posterior pharyngeal wall. It is important to note that using an oral airway may elicit a gag reflex or cause laryngospasm if the depth of anesthesia is inadequate. A nasal airway is better tolerated in these situations. Ventilating pressure should not exceed 20 cmH_2O to avoid gastric distension, regurgitation, and aspiration. If mask ventilation proves difficult or impossible, alternative strategies to ventilate the patient must be attempted such as intubation or placement of a supraglottic airway (SGA) [1, 5].

Supraglottic Airways

SGA devices are an alternative method to mask ventilation and endotracheal intubation. They have made their way into the difficult airway algorithm with their ease of use and rescue ventilation ability. Quick placement, less sympathetic stimulation, avoidance of neuromuscular blockers, and maintenance of spontaneous ventilation are a few advantages of SGAs over endotracheal tubes (ETTs). SGAs may be used as primary airway devices for selected patients and surgeries, in emergencies in and out of the hospital, to facilitate endotracheal intubation, and most importantly for airway rescue in the unable-to-ventilate-or-intubate situation. Nonfasting status, morbid obesity, and pregnancy are contraindications for laryngeal mask airway (LMA) use as the primary airway. OSA, gastro-esophageal reflux disease (GERD), gastroparesis, and position other than supine are factors that increase the risk of complications when using SGAs [2].

The LMA Classic, one of the first SGAs, is a reusable device made of silicone. A disposable, single-use version of the LMA Classic is the LMA Unique. Designed for intraoral procedures, the LMA Flexible has a wire-reinforced shaft to allow flexible positioning away from the surgical site. The LMA Fastrach, an intubating LMA, has a rigid, curved shaft and handle that facilitate placement of an ETT through its ventilating tube with or without the assistance of a fiberoptic scope. The reusable LMA ProSeal was the first LMA designed with a drainage tube to reduce the risk of aspiration. This drainage tube also facilitates placement of an orogastric tube. The LMA ProSeal's design creates an improved airway seal without adding pressure to the oropharyngeal tissue. A disposable alternative to the LMA ProSeal is the LMA Supreme. In addition to the gastric drainage tube like the LMA ProSeal, the LMA Supreme has a curved shaft like the LMA Fastrach. The LMA Classic Excel is an intubating version of the LMA Classic. The AirQ (disposable) and Intubating Laryngeal Airway (reusable) were designed with unique features to assist endotracheal intubation but may also be used as a primary airway. The Cobra Perilaryngeal Airway (PLA) differs from the previously discussed SGAs with its high-volume, low-pressure pharyngeal cuff that sits just proximal to the cuffless mask. It also allows passage of an ETT. The Esophageal-Tracheal Combitube and the King Laryngeal Tube were designed to achieve ventilation after blind insertion, making them useful for prehospital use or by unskilled operators. Their double cuff design allows ventilation via the larynx by inflating the esophagus's distal cuff and the hypopharynx's proximal cuff. The uniquely designed I-GEL device uses a cuffless mask made of a gel material that conforms to the larynx. It has a gastric drainage tube that allows passage of an orogastric tube [3].

Endotracheal Intubation

Endotracheal intubation is achieved with an ETT via an orotracheal or naso-tracheal approach. There are several types of ETTs used to achieve endotra-cheal intubation. The standard cuffed ETT is single lumen and comes in various sizes, based on the internal diameter of the tube. Specialty single-lumen tubes include oral and nasal Ring–Adair–Elwyn (RAE) tubes, wire-reinforced tubes, laser-resistant tubes, and electromyogram (EMG) tubes. Oral and nasal RAE tubes have a preformed bend to allow positioning of the tube and circuit away from the surgical field for facial, oral, or dental surgeries, or neurosurgery. Wire-reinforced tubes contain a metal wire spiraled along their length to minimize kinking or allow positioning away from the surgical field. Laser-resistant tubes are used during laser surgery of the upper airway to decrease the risk of airway fire. EMG monitoring tubes, such as the neural integrity monitor (NIM) tube, allow monitoring of the recurrent laryngeal nerve during thyroid and other neck surgeries [4, 6].

Several techniques are available for endotracheal intubation. Orotracheal intubation is most commonly performed via direct laryngoscopy using a Macintosh (curved) or Miller (straight) blade to visualize the glottic opening and insert the ETT. Indirect visualization using a video laryngoscope may be chosen for patients with suspected difficult airway or immobilization of the cervical spine. Video laryngoscopes are categorized as either channeled or nonchanneled. Nonchanneled videoscopes include the more commonly used Glidescope, C-MAC, and McGrath. While these devices provide improved glottic visualization, there can still be difficulty directing the ETT into the glottis. Channeled videoscopes have a guide channel into which the ETT is preloaded and directs the tube towards the glottic opening. Airtraq and King Vision Video Laryngoscope are types of channeled devices. A disadvantage of these devices is that the thicker blades require a greater interincisor distance. Fiberoptic intuba-tion is another option for management of a known or suspected difficult airway. It allows intubation in an awake patient; however, this technique requires airway anesthesia. Nasotracheal intubation is typically chosen for intraoral and man-dibular surgeries. It can be performed blindly, with the assistance of direct or video laryngoscopy or a fiberoptic scope [7, 8]. Table 9.5 describes the currently available techniques for endotracheal intubation.

Maintenance of Anesthesia

After induction of GA and management of the airway, it is necessary to maintain the patient at an appropriate depth of anesthesia to allow for the surgery's completion. This is almost exclusively achieved with

Table 9.5 Intubation techniques

Technique	Indications	Contraindications	Equipment
Oral route	Airway protection Prolonged mechanical ventilation General anesthesia for surgery	Penetrating trauma of upper airway	Laryngoscope/fiberoptic Stylet Bougie/Eschmann Airway exchange catheter Intubation introducer/catheter
Nasal route	Intraoral surgery Mandibular surgery Poor mouth opening	Basilar skull fracture Nasal fractures Epistaxis Nasal polyps Coagulopathy	Laryngoscope/fiberoptic McGills Red rubber
Direct laryngoscopy	Airway protection Prolonged mechanical ventilation General anesthesia for surgery	Poor mouth opening Documented difficult airway Airway mass/tumor	Light handle Blade
Video laryngoscopy	History of difficult intubation Suspected difficult intubation Inability to extend the neck Cervical instability	Severe bleeding of upper airway	Videoscope handle and screen
Flexible fiberoptic intubation	History of difficult intubation Suspected difficult intubation Compromised airway Inability to extend the neck Cervical instability Trauma to upper airway	High-grade stenosis of airway Severe bleeding of upper airway Pharyngeal abscess	Fiberoptic scope

See references [7] and [9].

intravenous or inhalational agents, although it is theoretically possible to accomplish maintenance of anesthesia with repeated intramuscular injections of an agent such as ketamine. Selection of the most appropriate method requires considering the patient history, surgical requirements, availability of equipment, and patient preferences [10]. While it is possible to maintain anesthesia through the sole use of a single modality (i.e., intravenous or inhalational), maintenance of anesthesia is more commonly carried out by utilizing a balanced approach that involves the administration of multiple agents of different classes. This allows less of each agent to be used, thereby increasing the likelihood of observing the intended effect without undesired side effects [11]. A thorough understanding of the approaches to maintenance of anesthesia is essential to making informed decisions regarding which is most appropriate for an individual patient.

Inhalational Anesthetics

Upwards of 90% of general anesthetics utilize inhalational agents in the maintenance phase [10]. Their use began in the 1800s when it was discovered that agents such as nitrous oxide, diethyl ether, and chloroform could be used to produce analgesia and hypnosis during painful procedures. These discoveries developed other inhalational anesthetics such as halothane, enflurane, methoxyflurane, isoflurane, desflurane, and sevoflurane. Due to largely unfavorable properties (i.e., high flammability of ether) and side effects (i.e., high rates of hepatotoxicity seen with chloroform and halothane use, nephrotoxicity with methoxyflurane use, and seizure activity with enflurane), many of these agents fell out of favor. In addition to the gaseous nitrous oxide, the volatile anesthetics isoflurane, sevoflurane, and desflurane are commonly used in modern anesthesia [12]. Table 9.6 describes inhalational anesthetic agents and their properties.

Despite decades of use in the maintenance of anesthesia, the mechanisms by which inhalational anesthetics produce their effects are still unclear and there is no consensus regarding what constitutes the anesthetized state. Immobility is easier to assess than other parameters such as analgesia or awareness and, as such, is often used as a surrogate to measure the depth of GA. The MAC measures the anesthetic required to suppress movement in response to a surgical incision in 50% of patients. At 1.2 MAC, 95% of patients should not move in response to a surgical incision, and 99% of patients should not move in response to an incision at 1.3 MAC of an inhaled anesthetic. Approximately 0.7 MAC is the concentration required to prevent awareness and recall. The MAC is inversely proportional to the potency – the higher the MAC of an agent, the less potent it is. Of the commonly used inhalational agents, isoflurane is the most potent with a MAC of 1.2, followed by sevoflurane with a MAC of 1.8 and desflurane with a MAC of 6.6. The MAC of nitrous oxide is 103 (>100%); therefore, it cannot be used by itself to achieve GA. The residual effects of induction

Table 9.6 Inhalational anesthetic agents and their properties

	Minimum alveolar concentration (MAC)	Blood/gas partition coefficient	Oil/gas partition coefficient
Chloroform	0.77	8	400
Desflurane	6.6	0.42	18.7
Diethyl ether	1.92	12	65
Enflurane	1.68	1.9	98
Halothane	0.75	2.4	220
Isoflurane	1.2	1.4	97
Methoxyflurane	0.2	11.0	950
Nitrous oxide	103	0.47	1.4
Sevoflurane	1.8	0.6	53

agents decrease the MAC, resulting in lower concentrations of gas necessary to achieve the desired level of anesthesia. Several other factors also affect the MAC. Factors such as hyperthermia, young age, hyperthyroidism, chronic alcohol use, anxiety, and stimulant use increase the MAC. In contrast, increased age, hypothyroidism, hypothermia, acute alcohol use, pregnancy, hypercarbia, and drugs such as opioids, benzodiazepines, and α2-adrenergic agonists decrease the MAC [10, 12, 13].

The MAC of an inhalational anesthetic relates to its potency, which, in turn, correlates with its solubility in oil [12, 13]. This is important as it highlights the importance of interactions with predominantly hydrophobic targets within the body (CNS) [13]. The more lipophilic an agent, the more easily it will cross the blood–brain barrier to exert its effect. This is measured by the oil:gas coefficient of the agent. Conversely, the blood:gas coefficient measures the solubility of an agent in blood and reflects how fast the agent is taken up into the blood from the alveoli. Agents with high oil:gas coefficients have low blood:gas coefficients and will have a relatively slow uptake, but they are highly potent.

Total Intravenous Anesthesia

It is possible to conduct GA through the exclusive use of intravenous agents, referred to as total intravenous anesthesia (TIVA). The choice of TIVA over inhalational agents is based on individual patient factors. TIVA has several advantages, including reduced postoperative nausea and vomiting (PONV), lower rates of postoperative delirium (especially in the elderly), the ability to rapidly titrate medications, independence from ventilation, reduced atmospheric pollution, and ease of inter-/intrahospital transfer. Importantly, TIVA eliminates the risk of triggering malignant hyperthermia (MH) and is therefore compulsory in patients with a history of, or strong risk factors for, MH. Disadvantages include increased costs, compared to inhalational anesthesia, and difficulty in evaluating the drug effects. Unlike inhalational agents, with end-tidal concentration measured to assess the depth of anesthesia, there is no way of measuring effect site concentrations of intravenous agents, thus presenting the potential for awareness [10].

Various agents are available for use in TIVA, including propofol, the N-methyl-D-aspartate (NMDA) receptor antagonist ketamine, α2-agonists such as dexmedetomidine, opioids, benzodiazepines, and barbiturates. A common approach employs infusion of propofol combined with boluses or an infusion of short-acting opioids (e.g., alfentanil, sufentanil, remifentanil). These agents are lipophilic and distribute into lipid-rich tissues after prolonged infusion. This results in prolonged context-sensitive half-times, the time it takes for blood or plasma drug concentrations to decrease by 50% after discontinuation of drug administration, and delayed emergence may be observed if this phenomenon is not accounted for. Of note, due to its rapid metabolism by nonspecific plasma and tissue esterases, remifentanil is exempt from this lengthening of context-sensitive half-time.

Neuromuscular Blockers

Neuromuscular blocking drugs (NMBDs), particularly nondepolarizing NMBDs, are used frequently in the maintenance phase of anesthesia. These agents interrupt transmission of nerve impulses at the neuromuscular junction, resulting in paralysis or paresis. This provides immobility during surgical procedures to help optimize working conditions. Commonly used nondepolarizing NMBDs include pancuronium, vecuronium, rocuronium, atracurium, cisatracurium, and mivacurium. The choice of NMBD is made considering the patient history and the drugs' characteristics. Of note, use of NMBDs has been shown to increase the risk of awareness during surgery, and care must be taken to ensure that patients are adequately anesthetized. Reversal of NMBDs is necessary at the end of the procedure. This has been achieved traditionally through the administration of an acetylcholinesterase inhibitor (i.e., neostigmine), coupled with an anticholinergic agent (i.e., glycopyrrolate) to prevent undesirable cholinergic side effects (i.e., bradycardia, bronchorrhea, bronchospasm, emesis, and diarrhea). More recently, a γcyclodextrin agent called sugammadex has been used to reverse certain non-depolarizing NMBDs. This drug works by encapsulating and inactivating the NMBDs and transporting them away from the neuromuscular junction. Sugammadex works rapidly and can reverse even profound neuromuscular blockade without untoward side effects [14].

Monitors

Monitors allow the physician to obtain data and interpret the physiologic conditions patients are undergoing and the responses to interventions performed by anesthesiology or surgical team members. The American Society of Anesthesiologists (ASA) has adopted a standard for basic monitors, mandating the use of monitors for ventilation, oxygenation, circulation, and body temperature [15]. These standards have been determined to provide the minimum amount of information about the patient while undergoing anesthesia care.

Oxygenation

The ASA requires that oxygenation of the patient is monitored by pulse oximetry and that oxygen analyzers with low oxygen concentration limit alarms are used throughout anesthetic administration. Pulse oximetry involves light to determine the amount of oxygen in the patient's blood. Monitors can be placed on parts of the body that allow the light to pass easily, such as the finger, nose, or ear. Using the Beer–Lambert law, which relates solute concentration to absorbance, two wavelengths of light can be measured – red correlating with oxyhemoglobin at 660 nm, and infrared correlating with deoxyhemoglobin at 940 nm. However, various conditions can alter the accuracy of pulse oximetry, including patient movement, low blood flow conditions, dysfunctional hemoglobin such as methemoglobin and carboxyhemoglobin, and intravascular dye administration [15–18].

Ventilation

Capnographic waveform monitoring and end-tidal carbon dioxide monitoring confirm that patients undergoing anesthesia are ventilating sufficiently. In addition to oxygenation monitors, these aim to ensure that patients are not receiving hypoxic mixtures of gases and receiving adequate ventilation to prevent severe hypercarbia [15–18].

Circulation

ECG monitoring in the operating room allows the anesthesia provider to monitor the patient's cardiac rhythm for abnormalities in response to surgical manipulation, and to monitor for episodes of ischemia. ECGs in the operating room at a minimum should be three lead. However, most providers opt for a five-lead ECG, as monitoring precordial leads greatly enhances the detection of ischemia. The addition of leads II, V4, and V5 increases the sensitivity from 75% with lead V5 alone to nearly 96% in detecting ischemia [15–18].

Blood pressure monitoring, whether noninvasive or invasive, is required at least every 3–5 minutes. In cases where wide variations in blood pressures are expected or rigorous control of blood pressures is required, direct arterial pressure monitoring can provide closer monitoring of blood pressures at every beat of the patient's heart. The anesthesiology provider should attempt to maintain the patient's mean arterial pressure within 20% of the patient's preoperative baseline [15–18].

Temperature

Temperature can be monitored by an exterior probe such as axillary, or an interior probe such as oropharyngeal or nasal. Anesthetics cause a decline in thermoregulatory function, as redistribution effects cause core heat loss. Core temperatures can decrease from 1 to 1.5°C in the first hour after induction. Although body temperature is not the first visible signal detecting MH in response to anesthetics, monitoring a patient's temperature is a way to avert adverse consequences in anesthetic administration [15–19].

Emergence

For patients to emerge from anesthesia and achieve successful extubation, they must return to their baseline state of physiologic function. They must regain their basic neurologic function to protect their airway, demonstrate spontaneous, independent ventilation, and often follow commands [20–22].

Before independent ventilation can be established, the patient must have a patent and protected airway. This is established through suctioning, head positioning, and often with placement of airway adjunct tools, such as an oral airway, to clear the airway from obstruction. The patient can demonstrate airway reflexes through swallowing secretions, coughing, and gagging, indicating their basic reflexes have been reestablished. To demonstrate intact airway reflexes, the patient requires reversal of the paralytic and often discontinued inhaled gases or intravenous anesthetic medications. Through these measures, the patient will be able to regain function of their ventilation and oxygenation, and thereby produce adequate spontaneous minute ventilation [20–23].

In some cases, deep extubation may be performed when coughing and straining must be avoided during emergence. In that case, while the patient is still under enough anesthetics to tolerate surgical stimuli, but can demonstrate adequate spontaneous minute ventilation, the ETT can be removed. The anesthesia provider in that case will apply oxygen via a face mask as the patient gradually emerges.

Options to reverse neuromuscular blockade include anticholinesterase inhibitors such as neostigmine, edrophonium, or pyridostigmine. These medications inhibit acetylcholinesterase and thus prolong the existence of acetylcholine at the motor end plate, thereby reversing the motor blockade. These medications are paired with glycopyrrolate or atropine to prevent the adverse side effects of these drugs secondary to their muscarinic effects. In addition, for rocuronium and vecuronium, an alternative option exists. Sugammadex, a novel cyclodextrin, reverses neuromuscular blockade with two nondepolarizing muscle relaxants by binding the molecules of the neuromuscular blocker, allowing for rapid removal of these molecules from the plasma [23–25].

Peripheral nerve stimulation or train-of-four (TOF) monitoring should be used to determine dosing for neuromuscular blockade reversal. This involves a small electrical current delivered to the patient to evaluate peripheral nerve activity to attempt to quantify the amount of paralytic medication still in effect by a subjective quantitative method. Stimulation of the ulnar nerve and monitoring of the adductor pollicis muscle are the preferred site, as the nerve activity cannot be confounded by direct muscle stimulation; however, in certain situations, access to the patient's arms is not available during surgical procedures secondary to surgical sites or positioning. In such a situation, the facial nerve is often used for monitoring. TOF measurements are not entirely accurate, as direct muscle stimulation can occur and measurements are subjective to the examiner as to the height of the twitch. Some newer methodology is available to quantify the twitches in response to peripheral nerve stimulation; however, they are not widely used [23, 26, 27].

Conclusion

This chapter may guide the clinician providing GA to patients in various scenarios. GA, defined as medically induced loss of consciousness with concurrent loss of protective reflexes and skeletal muscle relaxation, is essential to the safe and successful performance of many interventional and surgical therapies. This chapter discussed the necessary methods behind GA, including preoperative evaluation, specific preoperative tests, fasting and pharmacologic recommendations, and induction of anesthesia (inhalational versus intravenous), as well as airway management to include mask ventilation, SGAs, and endotracheal intubation. Maintenance of the desired anesthetic depth and available pharmacologic agents involved in inhalation anesthesia versus TIVA were reviewed, in addition to properly monitoring the patient's circulation, oxygenation and ventilation, and temperature. Lastly, emergence from anesthesia and safe, appropriate conditions were discussed.

References

1. El-Orbany M, Woehlck HJ. Difficult mask ventilation. *Anesth Analg.* 2009;109 (6):1870–80. DOI: 10.1213/ANE.0b013e3181b5881c.

2. Gordon J, Cooper RM, Parotto M. Supraglottic airway devices: indications, contraindications and management. *Minerva Anestesiol.* 2018;84(3):389–97. DOI: 10.23736/S0375-9393.17.12112-7.

3. Hernandez MR, Klock PA, Ovassapian A. Evolution of the extraglottic airway: a review of its history, applications, and practical tips for success. *Anesth Analg.* 2012;114(2):349–68. DOI: 10.1213/ANE.0b013e31823b6748.

4. Haas CF, Eakin RM, Konkle MA, Blank R. Endotracheal tubes: old and new. *Respir Care.* 2014;59(6):933–55. DOI: 10.4187/respcare.02868.

5. Malhotra SK. Practice guidelines for management of the difficult airway. In: SK Malhotra, VP Kumra, B Radhakrishnan, SM Basu, eds. *Practice Guidelines in Anesthesia.* New Delhi: Jaypee Brothers Medical Publishers; 2016, pp. 127–31. DOI: 10.5005/jp/books/12644_18.

6. Gray AW. Endotracheal tubes. *Clin Chest Med.* 2003;24(3):379–87. DOI: 10.1016/S0272-5231(03)00052-2.

7. Hurford WE. Techniques for endotracheal intubation. *Int Anesthesiol Clin.* 2000;38 (3):1–28. DOI: 10.1097/00004311-200007000-00003.

8. Cooper RM. Strengths and limitations of airway techniques. *Anesthesiol Clin.* 2015;33(2):241–55. DOI: 10.1016/j.anclin.2015.02.006.

9. Koerner IP, Brambrink AM. Fiberoptic techniques. *Best Pract Res Clin Anaesthesiol.* 2005;19(4):611–21. DOI: 10.1016/j.bpa.2005.07.006.

10. Walton TEF, Palmer J. Maintenance of anaesthesia. *Anaesth Intensive Care Med.* 2020;21(3):121–6. DOI: 10.1016/j.mpaic.2019.12.007.

11. Brown EN, Pavone KJ, Naranjo M. Multimodal general anesthesia: theory and practice. *Anesth Analg.* 2018;127(5):1246–58. DOI: 10.1213/ANE.0000000000003668.

12. McKay RE. Inhaled anesthetics. In: MC Pardo, Jr, RD Miller, eds. *Basics of Anesthesia*, 7th ed. Philadelphia, PA: Elsevier; 2018, pp. 83–103. DOI: 10.1016/B978-0-323-40115-9.00007-4.

13. Perouansky M, Pearce RA, Hemmings HC, Franks NP. Inhaled anesthetics: Mechanisms of action. In: MA Gropper, ed. *Miller's Anesthesia*, 9th ed.

Philadelphia, PA: Elsevier; 2020, pp. 487–508. DOI: 10.1016/B978-0-323-59604-6.00019-5.

14. Naguib M, Lien C, Meistelman C. Pharmacology of neuromuscular blocking drugs. In: RD Miller, LI Eriksson, LA Fleisher, JP Wiener-Kronish, NH Cohen, WL Young, eds. *Miller's Anesthesia*, 8th ed. Philadelphia, PA: Elsevier Saunders; 2014, pp. 958–94. DOI: 10.1016/B978-0-323-40115-9.00011-6.

15. American Society of Anesthesiologists. Standards for basic anesthetic monitoring. 2020. Available from: www.asahq.org/standards-and-guidelines/standards-for-basic-anesthetic-monitoring.

16. Manohar M, Gupta B, Gupta L. Closed-loop monitoring by anesthesiologists – a comprehensive approach to patient monitoring during anesthesia. *Korean J Anesthesiol*. 2018;71(5):417–18. DOI: 10.4097/kja.d.18.00033.

17. Checketts MR, Alladi R, Ferguson K, *et al*. Recommendations for standards of monitoring during anaesthesia and recovery 2015: Association of Anaesthetists of Great Britain and Ireland. *Anaesthesia*. 2016;71(1):85–93. DOI: 10.1111/anae.13316.

18. Association of Anaesthetists. Checking anaesthetic equipment. 2012. Available from: https://anaesthetists.org/Home/Resources-publications/Guidelines/Checking-Anaesthetic-Equipment.

19. Sessler DI. Temperature monitoring and perioperative thermoregulation. *Anesthesiology*. 2008;109(2):318–38. DOI: 10.1097/ALN.0b013e31817f6d76.

20. Difficult Airway Society Extubation Guidelines Group; Popat M, Mitchell V, Dravid R, *et al*. Guidelines Difficult Airway Society guidelines for the management of tracheal extubation. *Anaesthesia*. 2012;67(3):318–40. DOI: 10.1111/j.1365-2044.2012.07075.x.

21. Bala Bhaskar S. Emergence from anaesthesia: have we got it all smoothened out? *Indian J Anaesth*. 2013;57(1):1–3. DOI: 10.4103/0019-5049.108549.

22. Miller KA, Harkin CP, Bailey PL. Postoperative tracheal extubation. *Anesth Analg*. 1995;80(1):149–72. DOI: 10.1097/00000539-199501000-00025.

23. Murphy GS, Szokol JW, Marymont JH, Franklin M, Avram MJ, Vender JS. Residual paralysis at the time of tracheal extubation. *Anesth Analg*. 2005;100(6):1840–5. DOI: 10.1213/01.ANE.0000151159.55655.CB.

24. Krause M, McWilliams SK, Bullard KJ, *et al*. Neostigmine versus sugammadex for reversal of neuromuscular blockade and effects on reintubation for respiratory failure or newly initiated noninvasive ventilation: an interrupted time series design. *Anesth Analg*. 2020;131(1):141–51. DOI: 10.1213/ANE.0000000000004505.

25. Naguib M. Sugammadex: another milestone in clinical neuromuscular pharmacology. *Anesth Analg*. 2007;104(3):575–81. DOI: 10.1213/01.ane.0000244594.63318.fc.

26. Ali HH, Savarese JJ, Lebowitz PW, Ramsey FM. Twitch, tetanus and train-of-four as indices of recovery from nondepolarizing neuromuscular blockade. *Anesthesiology*. 1981;54(4):294–7. DOI: 10.1097/00000542-198104000-00007.

27. Kopman AF, Yee PS, Neuman GG. Relationship of the train-of-four fade ratio to clinical signs and symptoms of residual paralysis in awake volunteers. *Anesthesiology*. 1997;86(4):765–71. DOI: 10.1097/00000542-199704000-00005.

Postanesthesia Care Unit

Iliana Ramirez-Saldana

Introduction

The postanesthesia care unit (PACU) or recovery unit is the place where patients go to after leaving the operating room (OR) and before being discharged home or to the wards. Monitoring the patients for common complications is of utmost importance in the immediate postoperative period. This requires the presence of trained personnel and staff that can quickly identify common problems and treat the patient. Patients must have a return to baseline before getting discharged home. Emergency equipment and drugs should be readily available at all times.

Phases of Postoperative Care

The PACU, recovery room, or postoperative care unit are staffed by nurses specifically trained in the care of patients who have just received general, neuraxial, or peripheral blocks or monitored anesthesia care types of anesthesia. They should have expertise in recognizing and handling the most common complications after surgery. Nurses in the PACU are trained in airway management skills and must be certified in advanced cardiac life support. Usually patients in the PACU are under the medical direction of an anesthesiologist [1, 2].

- *Phase 1*: Marks the beginning of the immediate postoperative period. Typically, nursing care is one nurse to two patients. It is the position of the American Society of PeriAnesthesia Nurses (ASPN) that the number of patients assigned to a nurse in phase 1 should depend on multiple factors, including acuity level, complexity of care, comorbidities, and the American Society of Anesthesiologists (ASA) status, among other factors [2]. Vital signs are recorded every 15 minutes or more often if the patient condition warrants. In some institutions, critical care patients go directly from the OR back to the intensive care unit (ICU), bypassing the PACU.

- *Phase 2*: Typical staffing consists of one nurse to three patients. Some monitored anesthesia care (MAC) cases performed on ASA I or II patients can be fast-tracked into phase 2 directly from the OR. During this phase, the patient and caregivers are educated for care at home or prepared for extended observation.

- *Phase 3*: It is an extended care phase staffed by one nurse to 3–5 patients. Patients are ready to leave the recovery unit but might wait here until a bed is available.

ASA Standards for Postoperative Care

1. Postanesthesia management should be provided to any patient receiving MAC or regional or general anesthesia. An anesthesiologist should be responsible for the supervision and care of PACU patients.

2. The patient should be transported by a member of the anesthesia care team who can continually monitor, evaluate, and treat any condition that might arise until handing off to the PACU nurse.

3. A verbal report should be provided to the nurse receiving the patient that includes the patient's past medical history, allergies, relevant home medications, surgery undergone, any airway issues, intraoperative course and medications or infusions, pertinent laboratory results or radiological film reports, fluid balance, blood products administered, lines and intravenous cannulae or intravenous catheters, whether peripheral or central, regional or neuraxial procedures, complications, concerns, and pending tasks for the immediate postoperative period. This is the moment when the nurse is alerted about any particular concerns.

4. The patient will be continually evaluated in this setting by the nurse for any signs of deterioration. Vital signs are recorded at set intervals, including arterial saturation, blood pressure, respiratory rate, cardiac rhythm, temperature, and mental status. Assessment of pain, nausea, and vomiting should be routine during emergence and recovery.

5. A physician is responsible for discharging the patient from the PACU, and the name should be noted on the record [3].

Transport and Delivery to the Postanesthesia Care Unit

Patients should receive supplemental oxygen during transport to delay the hypoxemia that can ensue from residual effects of anesthetics, opioids, and neuromuscular blocking agents administered. Depending on the stability of the patient, a pulse oximeter, ECG, and blood pressure monitors may suffice for transport. Vigilance is always required. Upon arrival to the PACU, a report is provided to the nurse as described previously. The anesthesia provider places orders for any patient's needs that might arise such as pain and antiemetic medications. Also, orders for supplemental oxygen and neuraxial anesthesia when applicable should be available. Monitoring of vital signs at regular intervals, usually every 5 minutes and then every 15 minutes, continues. The patient's breathing patterns, airway patency, respiratory rate, saturations, blood pressure, temperature, pain, and level of consciousness are routinely assessed.

Most Common Problems Encountered in the PACU

Surgery can trigger inflammation due to tissue damage, and anesthesia can cause alterations in hemodynamics that can further compromise organs. Whether patients are healthy or not, many systems are affected by these alterations, giving rise to potential problems (see Table 10.1).

1. *Hypertension*: The goal is to identify the most probable cause and treat accordingly. The patient might be asymptomatic or complain of visual changes or headaches, or can feel short of breath and restless. Some blood pressure medications are held prior to surgery. If this is the case, consider restarting. Always review the patient's chart to look at the baseline pressure to target your goal. Also, consider the context and note any other associated signs and symptoms that might point you to a different source. For instance, examine the pupils and alertness level, which can help you rule out a developing intracranial pathology. Ask the patient if they are having pain and use a number scale, for instance, to quantify. If so, titrate pain medication to effect. By looking at the history, you can verify if the patient has a history of alcohol or drug abuse contributing to withdrawal signs. Consider fluid overload or transfusion-associated cardiac overload. Examine the suprapubic area if the patient has had no urine output after neuraxial anesthesia. A bladder ultrasound can be helpful. Revise the drugs given to the patient recently, and make sure that vasopressor infusions are held or checked for correct concentration and dosing.

2. *Hypotension*: Keep in mind that cardiac output will depend on heart rate and stroke volume. Blood pressure is the product of cardiac output and systemic vascular resistance. One way to approach this is by considering whether the patient is volume-depleted, there is a delivery problem, the vessels are dilated, or the pump is failing. This can give you a start on how to navigate and find the culprit. Check the intraoperative record for fluid balance and estimated blood loss. Review the urine output and recent laboratory results, including hemoglobin. Look at the drains and surgical incisions for swelling or frank bleeding. If the lungs sound clear, consider a fluid bolus and observe the response. Consider whether your patient can tolerate the Trendelenberg position while you continue to troubleshoot. Be mindful of patients who are known to have poor cardiac and/or valvular dysfunction, as deterioration can rapidly ensue after a fluid challenge or changes in position. Consider recently dialyzed patients who are volume-depleted. Look at the ECG for conduction abnormalities; ask the

Table 10.1 Problems encountered in the PACU, with a summary of the potential reasons for each problem

System	Problem	Possible reasons
Cardiac	Hypertension Hypotension Arrhythmias	Preexisting hypertension, pain, hypercarbia, bladder distension, drugs – methergine, fluid overload, withdrawal, increased ICP
		Volume depletion, ongoing bleeding, sepsis, arrhythmias, heart failure, allergic reaction, myocardial infarction, neuraxial anesthesia, tamponade, pneumothorax, pulmonary embolism
		Electrolyte imbalances, pacemaker/defibrillator issue, toxicity, acidosis, hypoxemia
Renal	Oliguria Anuria Polyuria	Volume depletion
		Residual neuraxial anesthesia effects, obstruction
		Diabetes insipidus
Neurological	Delirium Stroke Somnolence	Secondary to drugs received, preexisting dementia
		Intracranial bleed due to HTN, surgery, or blood thinners
		Hypoglycemia, residual anesthetic effects, hypermagnesemia, hypercarbia
Respiratory	Hypoxia and hypercarbia	Residual NMBDs, atelectasis, opioid overdose, benzodiazepine overdose, pneumothorax, asthma exacerbation, airway obstruction, edema, allergic reactions, pulmonary edema, neck hematomas, subcutaneous emphysema
Other		
Drug-related		Allergic reactions, PONV, shivering, Parkinson-like
Injuries		Teeth, nerve, lip, cornea, nose
Pain		Infiltrated IV, failed block, high tolerance, inadequate dose
Recall		Light anesthesia, cardiac surgery, NMBDs, substance abuse, young age, emergency surgery

ICP, intracranial pressure; HTN, hypertension; NMBD, neuromuscular blocking drug; PONV, postoperative nausea and vomiting.

patient if they have chest pain, and look for other signs that can suggest a cardiac event. Also, consider allergic/anaphylactic reactions and examine the skin; listen for stridor, and look for signs of angioedema. If the patient had neuraxial anesthesia, review the details on record. In the case of a patient who received a blood transfusion, consider a transfusion reaction. In patients who had a procedure at the electrophysiology laboratory or trauma patients, consider tamponade. Consider pneumothorax, and examine those patients who had regional blocks, central lines, laparoscopic surgery, and trauma to the chest, for example. For those on a ventilator, check the positive end-expiratory pressure (PEEP) settings. Sepsis can already be present in many patients who come to the OR, including those with obstructive kidney stones, and also in patients with burns and necrotizing fasciitis, among others. Look for a transesophageal echocardiogram in the chart, if available, and consider a cardiac consult for cardioversion if deemed appropriate. Consider antiarrhythmics and inotropic agents, and consider placement of invasive monitors such as an arterial line for continuous monitoring and for frequent laboratory draws when appropriate. When persistent hypotension ensues despite treatment, consider adrenal causes and hypothyroidism and plan for possible transfer to the ICU.

3. *Arrhythmias*: Some benign arrhythmias might be a consequence of electrolyte imbalances. This can be easily ruled out by sending a venous gas sample or, if an arterial line is already in place, by sending an arterial sample. Preexisting cardiac conditions, sympathetic discharge from surgical procedures, and acidosis can also affect electrical conduction through the heart. For bradycardias, consider the residual effects of beta-blockers, reversal agents, and opioids. Sinus bradycardia with a sustained blood pressure usually does not require treatment. Always assess your patient's mental status and look for other signs or symptoms. Look at the medical record for administered medications. Always verify infusion concentrations, dosages, and pump settings. Also consider the patient's history, as athletes tend to have normal sinus bradycardia. Irregular bradycardia with long pauses, missed beats, and low blood pressure might be the first sign of a third-degree atrioventricular block. These patients should be placed on a transcutaneous pacing monitor, and cardiology should be immediately consulted for further workup. For those patients who had a pacer or defibrillator setting changes before going to surgery, make sure to restore back to the presurgical settings before discharge home, and ensure that it is working. In the case of tachycardia, rule out pain, fever, low preload state, reversal agents, bleeding, and malignant hyperthermia, among many others.

4. *Oliguria/anuria/polyuria*: Oliguria is defined as the state in which a patient makes <0.5 mL/(kg hr) of urine. Consider if the patient is not making urine because of intravascular fluid depletion, tubular necrosis at the level of the

nephron unit, or obstruction to drainage. The most common cause will be fluid restriction techniques used where the intravascular space remains depleted. Consider administering a fluid challenge of 250–500 mL of crystalloid, and assess. Special precaution and slow infusion are recommended for patients known to have poor cardiac function or renal failure. A physical examination and chart review for laboratory results and context should take place. Administration of diuretics might not be indicated in every case and the effects will be temporary if the injury is at the level of the nephron. In this last scenario, further investigation by a specialist might be indicated. Renal hypoperfusion, toxins, and trauma might be responsible for intraparenchymal damage to the kidneys. Lastly, it is important to check that if a foley catheter is in place, it is not obstructed or dislodged. After prostate surgery, for example, large amounts of clots might obstruct drainage. Anuria is more commonly seen in known advanced stages of renal failure in patients undergoing dialysis. Sometimes it can also be seen as a result of a spinal anesthetic. In this case, straight catheterization is recommended until the spinal anesthetic wears off and the bladder regains normal function. Polyuria is seen after large volumes of fluid administration, diuresis with furosemide or osmotic diuretics, diabetes insipidus, and nonoliguric renal failure. It is important to monitor these patients for hemodynamic instability and electrolyte imbalances.

5. *Delirium*: Most commonly seen in the elderly population, those with preexisting dementia and psychiatric disorders, and drug-dependent patients. These patients present very agitated as they emerge, often requiring multiple persons to keep them from harming themselves. They can also be lethargic and disoriented. A number of drugs have been cited as a contributing factor, such as benzodiazepines, anticholinergics, opioids, large doses of metoclopramide, and ketamine, among others. It is important to rule out hypoxemia as the cause of agitation, bladder distension, electrolyte derangements, preexisting encephalopathies, preexisting delirium, and brain injuries, among others.

6. *Stroke*: Certain surgeries have a higher incidence of stroke. Cardiac, carotid, and intracranial surgeries, as well as polytrauma patients, have the highest risk. Vigilance and good clinical judgment are critical to recognizing some of the signs and symptoms of a stroke. When suspected, the stroke/neuro team should be immediately contacted as the outcomes are directly related to the time to intervention. The patient can present with slurred speech, facial asymmetry, visual disturbances, confusion, and paralysis. Blood pressure and airway control is warranted in some instances. Look for any recent administration of anticoagulants and the presence of dysrhythmias.

7. *Somnolence*: Hypoglycemia, hypothermia, and hypermagnesemia can lead to somnolence. Do a finger stick to check glucose. Check the temperature and provide the patient with warm blankets. Check magnesium levels to

avoid toxicity in those receiving an infusion (preeclampsia). A patient who is hypoventilating, with high carbon dioxide levels, can also become somnolent. Check saturations and draw an arterial blood gas if there is a suspicion of hypercarbia. Always know where your reintubation equipment is, in case you need it.

8. *Hypoxia*: The pulse oximeter should be one of the first monitors to be connected to the patient upon arrival to the PACU. Mild hypoxemia on room air is common in patients recovering from anesthesia. Sometimes airway obstruction by the tongue can be resolved by gentle jaw thrust or a nasal/oral airway. If the neck was a site of surgery, examine the patient for an enlarging neck hematoma and note the output on the drain when present. The attending physician and surgeon should be notified immediately of this, as it might warrant a return to the operating suite. When hypoxia is present, sit the patient up to increase the functional residual capacity if the type of surgery allows for it, and provide supplemental oxygen via nasal cannulae or other device. Titrate the oxygen level to achieve saturations near preoperative levels. Decreases in functional residual capacity and atelectasis are the most common cause of hypoxemia postoperatively. Encourage the patient to take deep breaths and provide suction if needed. Patients with chronic lung conditions might require oxygen supplementation for longer duration. If the patient's condition does not improve after maximal supplementation via a nonrebreather mask, for instance, and an arterial blood gas sample indicates continuous hypoxemia, consider reintubating the patient. For patients with obstructive sleep apnea, a trial of continuous positive airway pressure (CPAP) or bilevel positive airway pressure (BiPAP) first might make a difference. Make sure that you have reversed respiratory depressant drugs such as opioids, benzodiazepines, and neuromuscular blocking drugs. Think of the type of surgery the patient just underwent and consider atelectasis, mucus plugs, or gauze left behind in the airway during ear, nose, and throat procedures. Consider a CXR that can rule out the presence of aspiration, pneumothorax, or excess fluid in the lungs. Consider drawing blood to make sure hemoglobin is not at critical levels.

9. *Hypercarbia*: Hypoventilation leads to hypercarbia, and so does splinting. A patient who becomes hypercarbic ($PaCO_2$ >60 mmHg) becomes obtunded over time if not treated, which might be the reason why you are called in the first place. Examine the patient; assess their alertness level and listen to the breath sounds. Take note of the breathing pattern and frequency, and note the abdominal and thoracic movements. Revise the medications and the quantities that the patient has received over a period of time. Palpate the patient's chest in long laparoscopic cases and assess for subcutaneous emphysema. When appropriate and suspected, use reversal agents for opioids, benzodiazepines, and neuromuscular blocking drugs.

However, titrate these agents in small increments to avoid increases in sympathetic tone that can lead to hypertension and myocardial ischemia. Patients with obstructive sleep apnea might require assisted ventilation via a mask for a period of time. Assess for hypoventilation due to splinting and pain, and consider regional anesthesia if applicable. Use one of many methods for the patient to score pain. If hypoxia or hypercarbia are left untreated, they might quickly progress to cardiovascular and respiratory collapse requiring a higher level of management.

10. *Postoperative nausea and vomiting (PONV)*: This is a commonly encountered experience, which is multifactorial in nature. Some of the patient factors include young age, female gender, history of motion sickness, or prior history of PONV. Anesthetic factors, such as general anesthesia with volatile agents, nitrous oxide, and use of opioids, are also risk factors. In the case of a spinal anesthetic with sudden hypotension, this can trigger the chemoreceptor trigger zone in the area postrema of the brain, causing nausea. In this latter case, administering drugs that can increase blood pressure, such as phenylephrine, can resolve the symptoms. Some of the surgical procedures that present as a higher risk factor for PONV are strabismus, breast, and laparoscopic surgeries. In general, patients with multiple risk factors should receive prophylaxis as their risk is higher [4]. Use of multiple agents that act on different receptors is more effective than use of multiple doses of the same class of drug [4, 5]. Some examples of the drugs used are dexamethasone, ondansetron, and scopolamine patch. Consider the individual patient and the side effect profile before choosing a drug.

11. *Pain*: The patient with pain will be anxious and clearly uncomfortable, and will manifest high blood pressure and often tachycardia. Multiple scoring systems for pain exist that can be used to help the patient communicate the severity of their pain. This could be due to a failed nerve block, a high tolerance of narcotics due to drug use, or insufficient quantities of opioids given intraoperatively for the type of surgery. Use a combination of nonnarcotics and narcotics to treat pain. Consider a patient's renal and liver function during your selection, and be aware of whether the patient uses agonist/antagonist medications at home as part of their treatment plan. Consider an intravenous bolus of ketamine on a case-by-case basis or a postoperative regional block if applicable. Sickle cell patients who suffer an acute attack after surgery best respond to Dilaudid.

12. *Shivering and hypothermia*: Heat gets redistributed from the core to the peripheral compartments, causing hypothermia. Added to this are the vasodilatory effects of anesthetics, the cool ambient temperature, and the large exposure of body parts that can all contribute to significant hypothermia. Shivering is the body's response to increase its temperature.

Use of forced air warming devices has been effective at increasing body temperature. Be aware that shivering increases cardiac output, oxygen consumption, and carbon dioxide production, which might not be well tolerated by patients with fragile cardiac and pulmonary systems. Small doses of meperidine can reduce or stop shivering [5].

Discharge Criteria

Before a patient is discharged home, it is important that they meet certain criteria and each case be considered individually [5]. The patient must be awake and alert. Some patients with baseline dementia or neurologic pathologies will not be oriented. The patient's vital signs must be within preoperative values for at least 30 minutes. If they came from home on room air, they must be able to sustain their baseline saturations on room air for at least 15 minutes. Be very vigilant with patients with obstructive sleep apnea, and make sure you follow your institutional protocol for discharge of these patients. Make sure that pain is under control and nausea has been addressed. For patients who received regional or neuraxial anesthesia, it is important to document regression of their sensory and motor blockade. Patients should be educated about fall prevention when a block has been performed, with or without continuous catheters in place, and given a knee brace when indicated. They should also be alerted about the prolongation of a neuraxial block that might indicate the presence of a hematoma in the subdural or epidural space. According to the ASA practice guidelines for postanesthetic care, it is agreed that having an adult accompany the patient home should be mandatory as it increases patient comfort and satisfaction, as well as reduces adverse outcomes. Urination before discharge should only be mandatory for selected day-surgery patients. ASA members were equivocal on whether drinking fluids before discharge should be mandatory and it should be done rather on a case-by-case basis. Lastly, patients should remain in the recovery unit until cardiac and respiratory issues have resolved and are sustained before discharge home. Minimum stays are not required if the patient is in a stable condition. A physician should be in charge of the discharge home order [5].

References

1. American Association of Nurse Anesthesiology. Postanesthesia care practice considerations. 2019. Available from: www.aana.com/search?keyword=postanesthesia%20care

2. American Society of PeriAnesthesia Nurses. *2017–2018 Perianesthesia Nursing Standards, Practice Recommendations and Interpretive Statements*. Cherry Hill, NJ: American Society of PeriAnesthesia Nurses; 2016.

3. American Society of Anesthesiologists. Standards for postanesthesia care. 2019. Available from: www.asahq.org/standards-and-guidelines/standards-for-postanesthesia-care.

4. Gan TJ, Meyer TA, Apfel CC, *et al.* Society for Ambulatory Anesthesia guidelines for the management of postoperative nausea and vomiting. *Anesth Analg.* 2007;105:1615–28.

5. Apfelbaum JL, Silverstein JH, Chung FF, *et al.* Practice guidelines for postanesthetic care: an updated report by the American Society of Anesthesiologists Task Force on Postanesthetic Care. *Anesthesiology.* 2013:118:291–307.

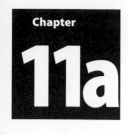

Chapter

11a

Regional Anesthesia: Blocks of the Upper and Lower Extremities

Peter Amato, Brittany Deiling, Erik Helander, Jinlei Li, Chikezie N. Okeagu, Michael McManus, Annemarie Senekal, Christopher M. Sharrow, Ashley Shilling, Alan David Kaye, and Michael P. Webb

Introduction

A regional block, also known as a localized block, is a type of anesthetic that blocks nerve transmission to prevent or alleviate pain. Regional anesthesia is the process of injecting an anesthetic substance into a peripheral nerve and inhibiting transmission to avoid or treat pain. It is distinct from general anesthesia in that it does not alter the patient's level of awareness to alleviate pain. There are numerous advantages of regional anesthesia over general anesthesia, including avoidance of airway manipulation, lower dosages, fewer systemic medication adverse effects, shorter recovery period, and considerably less discomfort following surgery.

Postoperative recovery time has been demonstrated to be significantly shortened because of significantly lowered pain levels and early involvement in physical therapy. Regional anesthesia can be used in combination with general anesthesia, postoperatively, and often for treatment of a variety of acute and chronic pain problems.

Upper Extremity/Brachial Plexus Blocks

Interscalene

The interscalene block (ISB) targets the brachial plexus at the level of the roots and trunks. This block traditionally could be done with a landmark approach and/or nerve stimulator but is now routinely accomplished with the use of ultrasound (US) guidance. ISBs are often performed for analgesia in surgeries involving the shoulder such as total shoulder arthroplasties and rotator cuff repairs, proximal humerus fractures, or surgeries of the distal clavicle. This approach reliably blocks the superior and middle trunks of the brachial plexus but will often result in sparing of the inferior trunk (C8–T1), commonly termed "ulnar sparing."

To perform the ISB, the patient is placed in either a semi-sitting or a lateral position. If the patient is placed in the semi-sitting position, the head is turned towards the contralateral side. Identification of the target anatomy is done using a high-frequency US probe beginning at either the supraclavicular fossa or the cricoid cartilage. If starting at the supraclavicular fossa, first the sub-clavian artery is identified, with the brachial plexus sitting superior and lateral to the artery. Then the probe is slid cranially, tracking the brachial plexus. Another starting point is to place the probe on the lateral neck at the level of the cricoid cartilage (C6). The brachial plexus can be identified between the anterior and middle scalene muscles as a rounded, stacked structure resembling a "snowman" or "stop light." Injections of 10–20 mL of local anesthetic are often used.

This block is performed in the neck and in proximity to the cervical sympathetic chain, recurrent laryngeal nerve, and phrenic nerve. Thus, it can result in Horner syndrome or hoarseness, and has a near 100% incidence of blocking the ipsilateral phrenic nerve. The resulting hemidiaphragm paralysis often goes unnoticed in healthy patients but can make it potentially unsuitable for patients with underlying respiratory disease. Other complications include vertebral artery injection, which may result in immediate seizures with injection of local anesthetic, and intrathecal injection resulting in total spinal anesthesia, pneumothorax, and permanent nerve injury.

Supraclavicular

The supraclavicular block (SB) is a block of the brachial plexus at the supra-clavicular fossa that provides surgical anesthesia and analgesia to the upper extremity. The block requires deposition of local anesthetic around the brachial plexus as it courses through the neck in close association with the subclavian artery. This block is often referred to as the "spinal of the arm" due to its reliability and provision of excellent anesthesia for the entire length of the arm.

Prior to the advent of US-guided regional anesthesia, this block was rarely performed, owing to the proximity of the brachial plexus to the dome of the pleura. US reinvigorated clinicians to use this block routinely, as direct visualization of the plexus, pleura, and the first rib provided a wide margin of safety. The relative superficial depth of the brachial plexus at this location also provided for good imaging of the needle, further enhancing the safety of the SB.

The plexus can be readily seen in close proximity to the subclavian artery as the latter courses over the first rib and between the anterior and middle scalene muscles. The first rib is seen beneath the artery and plexus as a hyperechoic structure superficial to the mobile, "sliding," and hyperechoic pleura. The upper, middle, and lower trunks of the brachial plexus coalesce into multiple round, hyperechoic structures within an investing fascia that sits lateral to the artery. The SB targets the brachial plexus at the level of the trunks and divisions. The practitioner needs to be aware of the path of the dorsal scapular artery, which often lies close to the plexus and can sometimes lie in the path of the needle trajectory.

This block is most commonly performed under US guidance with an in-plane approach. The block can be performed in a supine or semi-recumbent position, with the patient's head turned to the contralateral side. A high-frequency, linear probe (10–12 MHz) is commonly employed and placed in the midpoint of the supraclavicular fossa and angled caudally to best visualize a cross-section of the subclavian artery. Color Doppler scanning can be used here to visualize any vessels that may lie in the anticipated needle trajectory, including the dorsal scapular artery, which can sometimes be seen arching over the brachial plexus. The needle is brought in plane to the deepest aspect of the brachial plexus and is associated with a palpable "pop" as the investing fascia of the plexus is pierced. A volume of approximately 20 mL of local anesthetic is required to achieve surgical anesthesia of the arm. Traditionally, local anesthetic is deposited close to the subclavian artery just above the first rib to ensure that there is spread of the drug in the deepest part of the plexus to avoid "ulnar sparing." This is often referred to as "the corner pocket" and provides a characteristic appearance of the artery peeling off the first rib and spreading around the plexus. To ensure complete spread of the anesthetic, injections at multiple sites around the plexus may be necessary. Complications of the SB include intravascular injection, nerve injury, Horner syndrome, hemidiaphragm paralysis (phrenic nerve blockade), and pneumothorax.

Axillary

The axillary brachial plexus block is used for surgery of the elbow, forearm, and hand. This block derives its name from the approach used to perform it, as the nerves branched from the brachial plexus are accessed through the axilla. The axillary block is relatively easy to perform and mitigates some of the risks associated with comparable blocks such as the ISB (spinal cord or vertebral artery puncture) and SB (pneumothorax). The risk of phrenic nerve palsy is also considerably less than with brachial plexus blocks performed above the level of the clavicle. There are several techniques by which the block can be performed; these include transarterial approach, via nerve stimulation, and via US-guided techniques. US guidance is often favored as it allows for direct visualization of the nerves to be targeted, the needle tip, and the distribution of local anesthetic. To perform the block under US guidance, the arm is abducted 90°; then the insertion of the pectoralis major onto the humerus is palpated, and the transducer is placed distal to this point, perpendicular to the axis of the arm. The axillary artery, the conjoint tendon, and the terminal branches of the brachial plexus can be brought into view by sliding the transducer proximally. Three of the nerves to be blocked are located directly adjacent to the axillary artery – the median nerve superiorly, the ulnar nerve inferiorly, and the radial nerve posteriorly/laterally. Local anesthetic should be distributed between the nerves and the artery to ensure distribution within the neurovascular bundle. The musculocutaneous nerve is located either between the coracobrachialis and biceps muscles or within the coracobrachialis muscle itself. For this reason, vigilance on the part of the operator is required to avoid an incomplete block. It can be identified by its characteristic medial to lateral course in the axilla, as well as by its characteristic change in shape as it courses through the axilla (round adjacent to the artery, flat within the coracobrachialis muscle, and triangular after exiting the muscle).

Intercostobrachial

The intercostobrachial nerve (ICBN) block is commonly performed as a supplemental block in conjunction with blocks of the brachial plexus to obtain total upper arm analgesia. The ICBN supplies cutaneous sensation to the upper half of the medial/posterior arm and a portion of the anterior axilla. The nerve primarily originates from the second thoracic nerve but can have contributions from T1 and T3. As it is not part of the brachial plexus, it is not anesthetized when blocks of the brachial plexus are performed. Blocking of the ICBN may help to alleviate pain caused by tourniquet application to the upper arm, a common practice during surgeries of the arm, forearm, and hand. It is also useful in procedures involving the medial/posterior upper arm and/or for anterior arthroscopic port placement. The block is typically performed by subcutaneously injecting 2–5 mL of local anesthetic superiorly and inferiorly along the axillary crease with a fine-bore needle. Alternatively, the block can be performed under US guidance. One method of achieving this involves externally rotating and abducting the shoulder 90°, placing the probe over the posteromedial axilla, and visualizing the ICBN just posterior to the axillary artery and vein, and just deep to the superficial fascia. Placing the probe too anteriorly may result in inadvertent visualization of the medial cutaneous nerve of the arm, median nerve, or ulnar nerve.

Lower Limbs

Femoral Nerve Block and Adductor Canal Block

The femoral nerve is one of the largest nerves from the lumbar plexus. This nerve supplies a large portion of the lower extremity. It travels along the anteromedial thigh, traversing the femoral triangle and adductor canal, and terminates as the saphenous nerve – a pure sensory branch. The femoral nerve and its branches innervate the anterior thigh above the knee joint and the medial side of the lower leg and ankle. The extent of the saphenous distribution in the ankle is variable, potentially including the entire medial malleolus, and this must be considered in the regional anesthetic approaches to foot and ankle surgery. Indications for femoral nerve block (FNB) and adductor canal block (ACB) include partial or complete pain control for the anterior thigh and the medial side of the lower leg, such as partial or total knee arthroplasty (TKA), knee ligamentous procedures such as anterior cruciate ligament repair (ACLR), patella tendon repair, and tibial plateau fracture repair. Typical volumes used in FNB and ACB are around 20–40 mL, with lower concentrations (0.2% ropivacaine, 0.25% bupivacaine) for motor-sparing block or higher concentrations (0.5% ropivacaine, 0.5% bupivacaine) of local anesthetics for a more complete sensory and motor block. The FNB can be performed at the level of the inguinal crease level with a linear transducer. At this level, the neurovascular contents of the femoral triangle can be visualized. Under US guidance, the femoral nerve sits lateral to the femoral artery and vein, below the fascia lata and iliaca, and superficial to the iliopsoas muscle. The ACB targets the saphenous nerve and, dependent on the level at which it is performed, the nerve to the vastus medialis. Local anesthetic is deposited into the adductor canal between the sartorius and the adductor longus muscle in the middle third of the thigh under direct US guidance with a linear transducer. The ACB has increasingly replaced the FNB in procedures around or below the knee such as TKA, ACLR, and ankle surgeries, largely due to its ability to preserve quadriceps muscle strength and facilitate early ambulation, while maintaining similar level of analgesia as the FNB. The FNB has retained its indication for pain control in procedures or pathology more proximal to the adductor canal, such as procedures around the hip and proximal femur.

Obturator Nerve Block

The obturator nerve is a major branch from the lumbar plexus that provides motor and sensory innervation to the adductor muscles in the thigh, and sensory innervation to the skin over the medial surface of the thigh up to the posterior–medial knee. The sensory distribution of this nerve makes its blockade valuable in hip and knee analgesia. The obturator nerve block (ONB) has been used in acute pain management after several types of procedures around the knee, such as total knee replacement and ACLR, where it has been shown to improve postoperative analgesia. In addition, the ONB has been shown to be effective in acute pain management after hip fracture surgery in conjunction with the lateral femoral cutaneous nerve (LFCN) block, likely due to the blockade effect of the articular branch of the obturator nerve that innervates the anteromedial hip joint capsule. Several approaches of US-guided ONB have been proposed. Ergonomically, the patient is positioned supine, with a linear transducer employed. In the distal ONB, a volume of 10–15 mL of local anesthetic is injected into the interfascial space between the pectineus/adductor longus and the adductor brevis muscles to block the anterior branch, and between the adductor brevis and adductor magnus muscles to block the posterior branch. Alternatively, a single injection of local anesthetic in a volume of 5–10 mL can be injected into the interfascial plane between the pectineus and obturator externus muscles to block the obturator nerve at its confluence before it divides into two branches.

It is worth mentioning specific block complications germane to the ONB, owing to the particular location of these branches and the potential for unfamiliarity with the landmarks and sonoanatomy. These include penetration of the pelvic cavity and subsequent perforation of the bladder or rectum, as well as perforation of other surrounding structures, such as the obturator vessels, resulting in visceral organ injury or hematoma formation. Corona mortis, a retropubic anastomosis between the external iliac and obturator arteries, is present in 10% of individuals and, if perforated, can cause extensive hemorrhage that is difficult to control. The medial circumflex femoral vessels that travel along the obturator branches between the pectineus, obturator externus, adductor brevis, and adductor magnus must be carefully avoided, as they may lie in the needle path.

Sciatic Nerve Block

The sciatic nerve is the largest peripheral nerve in the body. It originates from the lumbosacral plexus (L4–5 and S1–3) and provides sensory and motor innervation to the lower extremity. The sciatic nerve exits the pelvis through the greater sciatic foramen, inferior to the piriformis, and descends between the greater trochanter of the femur and the ischial tuberosity. The nerve lies deep to the gluteus maximus and courses down the midline of the posterior thigh towards the popliteal fossa. Upon reaching the popliteal fossa, the sciatic nerve branches into the common peroneal nerve (CPN) and tibial nerve (TN). The bifurcation typically occurs 5–12 cm from the popliteal crease, although it may occur more proximally. The smaller CPN branches laterally and descends along the head and neck of the fibula. It gives off articular branches to the knee joint and branches to the sural nerve before dividing into its terminal components: the superficial and deep peroneal nerves. The larger tibial component descends vertically through the fossa, giving off many collateral branches, before splitting into its terminal branches, the medial and lateral plantar nerves.

The sciatic nerve and its branches innervate the posterior aspect of the knee, the hamstring muscles, and the entire lower limb below the knee, with the exception of the cutaneous innervation of the medial leg and foot (supplied by the saphenous nerve). It also has numerous articular branches to the hip and knee. The skin of the posterior thigh is supplied by the posterior femoral cutaneous nerve (PFCN) and will be variably spared (up to 35%) by subgluteal approaches to sciatic nerve blockade. Indications for sciatic nerve block include foot and ankle surgery, lower leg surgery, below-knee amputation, and analgesia following knee surgery involving the posterior compartment.

Given the long course of the sciatic nerve through the posterior compartment, it can be targeted at any point along its course. The most common approaches are the subgluteal and popliteal. The subgluteal approach targets the sciatic nerve as it traverses the subgluteal space between the ischial tuberosity and the greater trochanter, taking advantage of the reliable bony landmarks to aid identification. This location is amenable to catheter techniques, and reliable blockade can be achieved with moderate volumes of local anesthetic. Its main drawbacks are that several vascular structures are present in this space, including the inferior gluteal vessels, and the aforementioned potential for sparing the PFCN. The popliteal approach targets the sciatic nerve as it divides into the CPN and the TN. At this level, the sciatic nerve lies more superficial and is superficial to the popliteal vein and artery. These vascular structures provide reliable anatomical landmarks to assist identification of the nerve. Care must be taken to ensure blocking proximally to the division of the CPN and TN, such that both nerves can be anesthetized within their common investing fascia. Local anesthetic volumes of 10–20 mL are typically sufficient for adequate sciatic nerve blockade (see Figure 11a.1).

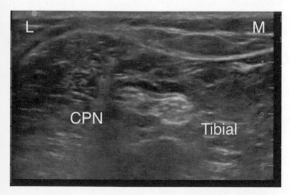

Figure 11a.1 The sciatic nerve in the popliteal fossa. CPN, common peroneal nerve.

iPACK

The infiltration between the popliteal artery and the capsule of the knee (iPACK) block was first introduced in 2012 as a motor-sparing, US-guided technique for providing analgesia to the posterior capsule of the knee in patients undergoing TKA. Subsequently, indications have spread to arthroscopic approaches to the knee, and it is commonly used with a femoral or saphenous nerve block. The traditional sciatic nerve block can provide excellent analgesia to the posterior knee; however, it also results in motor blockade of the foot and ankle, which can delay early rehabilitation and prevent recognition of a surgical injury to the CPN. These features make a sciatic nerve block an undesirable option for most patients undergoing knee surgery. The concept of the iPACK is to provide posterior knee analgesia while preserving motor function of the leg and foot by performing the block at the level of the sensory articular branches innervating the posterior capsule of the knee.

Anatomically, these articular branches originate from the tibial, common peroneal, and posterior division of the obturator nerve and traverse the space between the popliteal artery and the distal femur to provide sensation to the posterior knee.

The iPACK block is typically performed utilizing a high-frequency linear US transducer placed transversely in the popliteal crease or medially over the distal thigh, to image the distal femur/femoral condyles and the popliteal artery. Using an in-plane technique, the block needle is then advanced in a medial to lateral or anterior–medial to posterior–lateral direction, respectively, through the space between the popliteal artery and the femoral condyles until the needle tip is positioned approximately 2 cm past the popliteal artery. A judicious dose of local anesthetic (15–20 mL) can be deposited here to reliably block the nerves.

Specific potential complications of the iPACK block include needle injury to the CPN or TN and possible motor blockade secondary to local anesthetic spread to the TN and CPN within the popliteal space.

Lateral Femoral Cutaneous Nerve Block

The lateral cutaneous nerve of the thigh can be blocked individually or as part of a lumbar plexus technique. This block has gained considerable popularity for postoperative analgesia in hip surgery, meralgia paresthetica, and muscle biopsy of the proximal lateral thigh.

The anatomy of this nerve is highly variable. It branches off the L2 and L3 dorsal divisions of the lumbar plexus and courses on, or within, the iliacus muscle in the pelvis between two fascial layers. It then runs 1–2 cm medial to the anterior superior iliac spine and can be found above, below, or inside the inguinal ligament. Below the inguinal ligament, the nerve moves laterally, and in the proximal thigh, it can be identified in the groove between the sartorius and the tensor fascia lata. Owing to this variable course, landmark techniques are challenging and use of US to localize the nerve is recommended.

In performing the block, the patient should be positioned supine. Using a high-frequency probe (10–15 Hz), the femoral nerve is identified in the inguinal skin crease. The probe is slid laterally to identify the sartorius muscles and tensor fascia lata. The LCFN can be recognized as a single hyperechoic oval. A small dose of local anesthetic (approximately 5 mL) is sufficient for blockade of the nerve.

Pericapsular Nerve Group Block

The pericapsular nerve group (PENG) block is a novel analgesic block for surgery or pathology of the hip. The PENG block provides an alternative approach to treatment of hip pain that is desirable for its simplicity to perform and its sensory-specific qualities. More traditional nerve blocks for hip analgesia include the FNBs fascia iliaca plane block and "3-in-1" FNB. Blocks around the femoral nerve have been shown to improve pain following hip surgeries; however, these patients are at significantly higher risk of having motor weakness and subsequently falls. This is especially relevant to the outpatient setting where patients are not monitored and contend with household hazards.

The anterior portion of the hip capsule, which is the most highly innervated portion of the joint, is supplied by three nerves: the obturator nerve (posterior rami L2–4), the accessory obturator nerve (L3–4), and the femoral nerve (anterior rami L2–4). The PENG block was developed to selectively block the articular branches of these three nerves. Indications for a PENG block include hip arthroscopy, hip fractures, and anterior hip arthroplasty for analgesia of the hip joint. Initially, this technique was used in a small case series, with promising analgesic results, and demonstrated little motor sequelae.

Key landmark structures for this block are the anterior inferior iliac spine (AIIS) and the iliopubic eminence (IPE) (see Figure 11a.2). The articular branches from the femoral nerve and the accessory obturator nerve course between these two structures. The articular branches of the obturator nerve are found close to the inferomedial acetabulum. The common area for these nerves lies along the ilium deep to the psoas, between the IPE and the AIIS. The PENG block is performed with the patient in the supine position, using either a low-frequency curvilinear probe or a linear US probe. The probe is positioned in the inguinal crease and requires identification of the AIIS and the IPE. The local anesthetic is injected deep to the psoas tendon with an in-plane needle approach from lateral to medial. Successful performance of the block is demonstrated by "peeling" of the psoas off the ilium with instillation of the local anesthetic. A typical volume injected is 20 mL of either 0.5%

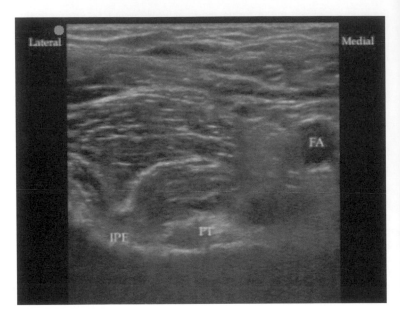

Figure 11a.2 PENG block. FA, femoral artery; PT, psoas tendon; IPE, iliopubic eminence.

ropivacaine or bupivacaine. The remoteness of the femoral nerve to this location makes motor blockade unlikely despite the relatively high volume of local anesthetic used.

Further Reading

Baker JF, *et al.* Post-operative opiate requirements after hip arthroscopy. *Knee Surg Sports Traumatol Arthrosc.* 2011;19:1399–402.

Birnbaum K, Prescher A, Hessler S, Heller KD. The sensory innervation of the hip joint – an anatomical study. *Surg Radiol Anat.* 1997;19:371–5.

Bruhn J, van Geffen GJ, Gielen MJ, Scheffer GJ. Visualization of the course of the sciatic nerve in adult volunteers by ultrasonography. *Acta Anaesthesiol Scand.* 2008;52:1298–302.

Burckett-St Laurant D, *et al.* The nerves of the adductor canal and the innervation of the knee: an anatomic study. *Reg Anesth Pain Med.* 2016;41(3):321–7.

Chan VW, Nova H, Abbas S, McCartney CJ, Perlas A, Xu DQ. Ultrasound examination and localization of the sciatic nerve: a volunteer study. *Anesthesiology.* 2006;104:309e14.

Feigl GC, Schmid M, Zahn PK, Gonzalez CA, Litz RJ. The posterior femoral cutaneous nerve contributes significantly to the sensory innervation of the lower leg: an anatomical investigation. *Br J Anaesth*. 2020;124:308e13.

Gerhardt M, *et al.* Characterization and classification of the neural anatomy in the human hip joint. *Hip Int*. 2012;22:75–81.

Giron-Arango L, *et al.* Pericapsular nerve group (PENG) block for hip fracture. *Reg Anesth Pain Med*. 2018;43:859–63.

Haslam L, *et al.* Survey of current practices: peripheral nerve block utilization by ED physicians for treatment of pain in the hip fracture patient population. *Can Geriatr J*. 2013;16(1):16–21.

Horner G, Dellon AL. Innervation of the human knee joint and implications for surgery. *Clin Orthop Relat Res*. 1994;301:221–6.

Johnson CS, Johnston RL, Niessen AD, Stoike DE, Pawlina W. Ultrasound-guided posterior femoral cutaneous nerve block: a cadaveric study. *J Ultrasound Med*. 2018;37:897–903.

Karmakar MK, Kwok WH, Ho AM, Tsang K, Chui PT, Gin T. Ultrasound-guided sciatic nerve block: description of a new approach at the subgluteal space. *Br J Anaesth*. 2007;98:390e5.

Kaye AD, Urman RD, Vadivelu N, eds. *Essentials of Regional Anesthesia*, 2nd ed. Cham: Springer; 2018.

Kuang MJ, *et al.* Is adductor canal block better than femoral nerve block in primary total knee arthroplasty? A GRADE analysis of the evidence through a systematic review and meta-analysis. *J Arthroplasty*. 2017;32(10):3238–48.e3.

Lenz K, *et al.* Comparing low volume saphenous-obturator block with placebo and femoral-obturator block for anterior cruciate ligament reconstruction. *Minerva Anestesiol*. 2018;84(2):168–77.

Li J, *et al.* Novel regional anesthesia for outpatient surgery. *Curr Pain Headache Rep*. 2019;23:69.

Mansour NY. Re-evaluating the sciatic nerve blocks: another landmark for consideration. *Reg Anesth*. 1993;18:322e3.

Runge C, *et al.* The analgesic effect of obturator nerve block added to a femoral triangle block after total knee arthroplasty: a randomized controlled trial. *Reg Anesth Pain Med*. 2016;41(4):445–51.

Sharma S, *et al.* Complications of femoral nerve block for total knee arthroplasty. *Clin Orthop Relat Res*. 2010;486:135–40.

Shelvin S, Johnston D, Turbitt L. The sciatic nerve block. *Br J Anaesth*. 2020;20(9):312–20.

Short AJ, *et al.* Anatomic study of innervation of the anterior hip capsule: implications for image-guided intervention. *Reg Anesth Pain Med*. 2018;43:186–92.

Sinha SK, *et al.* Ultrasound-guided obturator nerve block: an interfascial injection approach without nerve stimulation. *Reg Anesth Pain Med.* 2009;34(3):261–4.

Sinha SK, *et al.* Use of ultrasound guided popliteal fossa infiltration to control pain after total knee arthroplasty: a prospective, randomized, observer-blinded study. American Society of Regional Anesthesia and Pain Medicine, Spring Meeting. San Diego, CA; 2012, Poster A51.

Sinha SK, *et al.* Infiltration between the popliteal artery and capsule of the knee (iPACK): essential anatomy, technique, and literature review. *Curr Anesthesiol Rep.* 2019;9:474–8.

Sinha SK. How I do it: infiltration between popliteal artery and capsule of knee (iPACK). ASRA News. 2020. Available from: www.asra.com/news-publications/asra-newsletter /newsletter-item/asra-news/2020/05/03/how-i-do-it-infiltration-between-popliteal-artery-and-capsule-of-knee-(ipack).

Smith JH, *et al.* Adductor canal versus femoral nerve block after anterior cruciate ligament reconstruction: a systematic review of level I randomized controlled trials comparing early postoperative pain, opioid requirements, and quadriceps strength. *Arthroscopy.* 2020;36(7):1973–80.

Taha AM. Brief reports: Ultrasound-guided obturator nerve block: a proximal inter-fascial technique. *Anesth Analg.* 2012;114(1):236–9.

Vloka JD, Hadzic A, April E, Thys DM. The division of the sciatic nerve in the popliteal fossa: anatomical implications for popliteal nerve blockade. *Anesth Analg.* 2001;92:215e7.

Wertheimer LG. The sensory nerves of hip joint. *J Bone Joint Surg Am.* 1952;34:477–87.

Xing JG, *et al.* Preoperative femoral nerve block for hip arthroscopy: a randomized, triple-masked controlled trial. *Am J Sports Med.* 2015;43:2680–7.

Regional Anesthesia: Chest and Abdominal Plane Blocks

Jinlei Li, Annemarie Senekal, Michael P. Webb, Alan David Kaye, and Erik Helander

Thoracic Plane Blocks

Intercostal Nerve Block

The intercostal nerves are the continuations of the ventral ramus of the thoracic spinal nerves. To perform an effective ICB, the block should be performed proximal to the mid-axillary line, where the lateral cutaneous branch takes off. ICBs can be performed using landmarks, a nerve stimulator, or under ultrasound guidance. Evidence supports the effectiveness of ICBs for chest tube placement, rib fractures, and procedures of the breast and chest wall. Limitations of ICBs include the need to perform blocks at multiple levels (each level of fractured rib) and their association with a shorter duration of action, compared to other chest wall fascial plane blocks such as pectoralis (PECS) II block and serratus anterior plane block (SAP). This is mainly related to a high rate of absorption of local anesthetic within the intercostal space. These considerations make ICBs a less favorable option, as with each injection, there is a potential risk of complications, such as neurovascular injury and pneumothorax. The risk of local anesthetic systemic toxicity (LAST) may also be increased with multiple intercostal injections related to the highly vascularized bundle located underneath each rib, resulting in a high rate of absorption.

Pectoralis and Serratus Anterior Plane Blocks

PECS and SAP blocks belong to the group of newly developed chest wall fascial plane blocks. A PECS I block refers to the injection of 10–20 mL of dilute local anesthetics between the pectoralis major and the pectoralis minor muscles. This interpectoral injection targets the medial (C8–T1) and lateral pectoral nerves (C5–C7), which, respectively, originate from the medial and lateral cords of the brachial plexus. The PECS II block consists of the same interpectoral injection (PECS I), with an additional injection between the pectoralis minor and the serratus anterior muscle (SAM). The deeper subpectoral injection blocks the intercostal nerves, long thoracic nerve, and thoracodorsal nerve. The PECS II injection is traditionally performed at the level of the fourth rib on the anterior axillary line. Indications for PECS I and II blocks include breast surgery such as lumpectomy, mastectomy, breast expander insertion, and radical mastectomy with axillary lymph node dissection. In addition, PECS II can also be used to provide analgesia on the medial side of the arm for upper extremity procedures such as elbow surgery or arterial–venous fistula placement.

At the axillary fossa, the intercostobrachial nerve, lateral cutaneous branches of the intercostal nerves (T3–T9), long thoracic nerve, and thoracodorsal nerve are located in a compartment between the serratus anterior and the latissimus dorsi muscles, and between the posterior and mid-axillary lines. The SAP block is therefore performed at around the fourth to fifth rib, with local anesthetics injected either superficial to the SAM (see Figure 11b.1, right arrow) and deep to the latissimus dorsi muscle or deep to the SAM and superficial to the rib (see Figure 11b.1, left arrow), though the former technique might be associated with more effective analgesia.

Advantages of PECS blocks are that they can be used as alternatives to classic postoperative pain control modalities in the chest, such as thoracic epidural and thoracic paravertebral blocks (TPVBs), by providing somatic

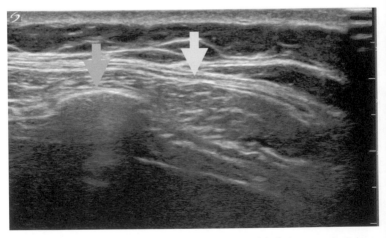

Figure 11b.1 Ultrasound-guided serratus anterior plane block. Arrow on the right pointing at the injection site between the latissimus dorsi muscle and the serratus anterior plane muscle, and arrow on the left pointing at the injection site between the serratus anterior plane muscle and the fifth rib.

pain control and with the potential for fewer complications such as hypotension and urinary retention. The analgesic effects of PECS and SAP blocks are well supported by the literature, though it may be limited to the anterior two-thirds of the chest wall.

These blocks can be done with the patient supine and therefore can be performed in patients with polytrauma and those on total spine precautions or in pelvic traction who cannot be turned lateral or sat up, such as when needed for placement of thoracic epidurals or paravertebrals. In addition, these blocks are relatively superficial in location and easy and safe to perform under ultrasound guidance with a linear ultrasound transducer, and have fewer stringent restrictions on the coagulation status. Potential risks of PECS and SAP blocks include injury to the thoracodorsal and long thoracic nerves, vascular injuries, LAST, and pneumothorax. The novel chest wall blocks share similar analgesic benefits of thoracic epidural and TPVBs and can be used in unilateral or bilateral surgery for upper thoracic procedures in the format of a single injection or a continuous catheter.

Thoracic Paravertebral Block

The TPVB is a truncal plane block with a goal of analgesia/anesthesia of the left or right hemithorax. The technique requires the deposition of local anesthesia in the paravertebral space – immediately adjacent to the path of spinal nerves emerging from the intervertebral foramina. The block can be performed for surgical anesthesia but is most often relied upon as a source of postsurgical or trauma analgesia. This block can be performed with a variety of techniques, but ultrasound-guided techniques have led to a resurgence of this block.

The thoracic paravertebral space is an anatomical wedge-shaped region that lies immediately adjacent to the sides of the vertebral column. This space is bounded medially by the intervertebral disc and the intervertebral neuro-vascular foramen, the base by the body of the vertebrae, and anteriorly by the pleura. The posterior wall is formed by the costotransverse ligament, a fenestrated ligament complex that provides a window to access the space. The apex of the space is formed by the lower border of the transverse process and the confluence of fascia from surrounding structures in the region. The contents of the space are loose fatty connective tissue and the spinal nerve, dorsal ramus, sympathetic chain, rami communicantes, and intercostal vessels.

TPVBs are most commonly performed under ultrasound guidance with an in-plane approach. The ultrasonographic landmarking relies primarily on the image acquisition of the transverse process of the desired dermatomal level. A linear high-frequency probe (10–12 MHz) is placed over the transverse process in the axial plane. An image of the "squared-off" hyperechoic transverse process, costotransverse ligament complex, and moving pleura is acquired. The target space lies deep to the ligament complex and superficial to the pleura. The needle is advanced adjacent to the transverse process, through the ligament complex, and adjacent to the pleura. Local anesthetic deposition in the paravertebral space results in visible caudal and cephalad spread, and the anterior bulging of the parietal pleura. The cephalad and caudal spread of local anesthesia provides multilevel dermatomal spread.

Erector Spinae Plane Block

The thoracic erector spinae plane block (ESPB) is a relatively new truncal plane block that also provides analgesia to the left or right hemithorax. In a fashion distinct from, but not dissimilar to, the TPVB, this block anesthetizes the spinal nerve roots as they traverse the interverterbral foramina. The exact mechanism of this block is unclear and is likely to require ingress of local anesthesia across the costotransverse ligament complex. It is an ultrasound-guided technique that provides analgesia for procedures or pain involving the hemithorax.

The erector spinae muscle complex is formed from a trio of long, vertical cephalocaudal muscles: the spinalis, longissimus thoracis, and iliocostalis muscles. There is a space deep to these muscles, and superficial to the transverse process and costotransverse ligament complex. It is believed that the effect of ESPBs is through the movement of local anesthetic from this plane into the deeper paravertebral and epidural spaces, and laterally into the intercostal spaces. The costotransverse ligament complex is fenestrated, and thus may allow the spread of local anesthetic into these deeper spaces, resulting in anesthesia of the sympathetic nerve roots, as well as the dorsal and ventral rami. Diffusion laterally allows anesthesia of the somatic (intercostal) nerve. However, spread of local anesthetic has not been consistently seen in cavaderic studies, leaving some question as to the exact mechanism of action.

Similar to the TPVB, the ESPB is performed most commonly with ultrasound guidance and an in-plane approach. A linear high-frequency (10–12 MHz) ultrasound probe in the axial plane is frequently used. The probe is placed over the transverse process that corresponds to the desired level of blockade. The transverse process image is acquired approximately 3 cm lateral to the midline spinous processes, and is distinguished from the rounded ribs and flat, faint lines of the thoracic laminae (which are further lateral and medial, respectively) by its "squared-off" appearance. Deep to these structures is the hyperechoic and moving parietal pleura. A needle is advanced in plane directly at the transverse process. The needle is stopped just short of the transverse process (and many practitioners will strike the transverse process before withdrawing slightly). Local anesthesia deposition at this location results in an expansion of the plane deep to the fascia, lifting it off the transverse process and costotransverse ligament. Local anesthesia is seen to spread cephalad and caudal from this deposition, and much like the TPVB, spread in the plane is variable, resulting in a variable dermatomal distribution.

Abdominal Plane Blocks

Rectus Sheath Block

The rectus sheath block is useful for midline incisions from the xiphoid to the pubis. Unlike an epidural, the rectus sheath block only affects somatic pain (no visceral coverage). A major benefit of the rectus sheath block is access to the posterior portion of the rectus abdominis.

The innervation of the anterolateral abdominal wall arises from the anterior rami of the spinal nerves of T7–11, the subcostal nerve (T12), and the iliohypogastric/ilioinguinal nerves (L1). The T7–11 nerves provide sensory innervation to the rectus muscle and the overlying skin. In obese patients, adipose tissue can sometimes be mistaken with the rectus abdominis. Scanning medially and laterally from the midline can help identify the tapering edges of the rectus abdominis on either side.

The amount of adipose tissue can influence the type of probe used, but ideally the linear probe is used with a starting estimated depth of around 3 cm. A practical place to begin is with the ultrasound probe placed midline in a transverse orientation. A hyperechoic layer of fascia can be identified deep to rectus abdominis muscle. Rectus sheath blocks should be performed bilaterally and not all dermatomes may be covered with a single injection. The needle can be advanced in plane from lateral to medial, with the optimal injection point just superficial to the posterior fascia. Once the needle is in position, a total of 10–20 mL of local anesthetic is injected. Complications are uncommon but can include inadvertent intraperitoneal injection, bowel perforation, intravascular injection, and block failure.

Transversus Abdominis Plane Block

The traditional transversus abdominis plane (TAP) block provides analgesia to the abdominal wall beneath the umbilicus (T10–12). It involves the injection of local anesthetic in between the internal oblique and the transversus abdominis muscles. With the use of ultrasound, the muscle layers are easily identifiable, which has also cultivated new variations of the TAP block. Subcostal, lateral, posterior, and ilioinguinal TAP blocks have been developed and provide analgesia to slightly different regions of the abdominal wall up to the level of T6. Due to their safety, efficacy, and ease, TAP blocks have become a valuable part in multimodal analgesia. One advantage of TAP blocks is that they can be performed after surgery while the patient is still anesthetized or in the postanesthesia care unit.

As previously mentioned, the innervation of the anterior abdominal wall arises from the anterior rami of spinal nerves T6–L1. The spinal nerves travel in between the muscle layers of the abdominal wall, coursing anteriorly on the superficial part of the transversus abdominis muscle. The nerves that travel on the superficial surface of the transversus abdominis muscle have lateral perforator branches, which are important for anesthetizing the anterolateral part of the abdominal wall. There is marked individual variation where these nerves enter and exit the transversus abdominis plane, which can lead to incomplete analgesia from TAP blocks, especially if they are performed too anteriorly. Thus, TAP blocks should be performed as laterally as possible to increase the likelihood of local anesthetic spread to these nerve branches before they exit the fascial plane.

When performing the TAP block, the patient can be in the supine or lateral position and usually 20–30 mL of dilute local anesthesia is prepared for each side to allow ample spread within the fascial plane. A linear high-frequency probe (10–15 MHz) is ideal, but in obese patients, a curvilinear low-frequency probe may be necessary. The probe is first positioned in a transverse plane, with the medial end of the probe over the umbilicus, to obtain an image of the rectus abdominis muscle. Next, the probe is slid laterally across the abdominal wall, generally to the anterior axillary line halfway between the costal margin and the iliac crest. As the probe is moved laterally, the typical view of the three muscle layers will become visible. The internal oblique is identifiable as the middle and thickest muscle layer, and the transversus abdominis muscle will be visible deep to that. Ideally the best site for injection is where all three muscle layers are present on the lateral abdominal wall. Needle insertion is in plane from the anteromedial side, traversing first the adipose tissue and then both the external and internal oblique muscles. The tip of the needle should be placed in the superficial part of the transversus abdominis muscle. To improve spread within the TAP, the needle is advanced while injecting the local anesthetic under direct vision and "unzipping" the fascial layers. To optimize needle visibility, the needle insertion point should be 3–5 cm away from the probe to provide for a more shallow approach that is perpendicular to the line of the ultrasound beam. Complications are infrequent but can occur, and include abdominal perforation, liver hematoma, block failure, pneumothorax, hematoma, and local anesthetic toxicity.

Quadratus Lumborum Blocks

Quadratus lumborum blocks (QLBs) are relatively new and emerging blocks, with limited, but growing, published data regarding their efficacy. There is interest in QLBs because they may provide analgesia with motor-sparing effects, while also avoiding the potential complications of epidurals and limitations of TAP blocks. Thus, this block may be effective in assisting in early mobilization in the postoperative period. The QLB is performed under ultrasound guidance and has been described to be effective in a multitude of surgeries, including open abdominal surgery, laparoscopic surgeries, and hip and femur surgeries.

The quadratus lumborum (QL) muscle resides in the lower back and forms part of the posterior wall of the abdominal cavity. It originates from the iliac crest and inserts onto the transverse processes of L1–4 and medial half of the twelfth rib. Anteromedial to the QL is the psoas major muscle. Posteromedially to the QL muscle lies the sacrospinalis muscle. Posterolaterally, the QL lies next to the latissimus dorsi, and lateral to the QL are the major muscles of the abdominal wall (external oblique, internal oblique, and transversus abdominis). The thoracolumbar fascia (TLF) sheathes the muscles of the lumbar and thoracic spine, and is formed by the aponeurosis of the internal oblique and transversus abdominis muscles. The TLF separates into three layers, with the posterior portion behind the erector spinae muscle, the middle portion between the QL and erector spinae muscles, and the anterior portion anterior to the QL.

Three different QLBs have been described: lateral, posterior QL2, and anterior QL3. These blocks can be performed with the patient in the supine or lateral position; however, posterior and anterior QLBs may be better performed with the patient in the lateral position. The mechanism of analgesia for QLBs is still debated and one theory is it may be due to spread of local anesthetic along the TLF and into the paravertebral space. Furthermore, the mechanism of action may be different for each approach to the QLB. The lateral QLB can be considered as a posterior TAP block whereby local anesthetic is deposited between the anterolateral border of the QL muscles and the TLF adjacent to the three muscles of the abdominal wall. This is generally used for surgeries below the umbilicus and covers the L1 dermatome. The posterior QLB involves injecting local anesthetic along the posterolateral border of the QL and may block dermatomes from T4 to L1. The anterior QLB can be the most challenging of the QLBs to perform and targets similar dermatomes to the posterior QLB. This is also the most posterior approach of the QLBs and involves injecting local anesthetic between the QL and the psoas muscle.

Lower extremity weakness can occur with QLBs but has the greatest potential with the QL3 block. Potential complications involve possible injury to intraabdominal organs, including the liver, spleen, and kidney.

Review Questions

1. Which of the following is an ultrasound-guided indication of appropriate deposition of local anesthetic in a thoracic paravertebral block?

(a) Aspiration of air prior to deposition

(b) Anterior bulging of the parietal pleura

(c) Local anesthetic spread deep to the erector spinae muscle complex and superficial to the transverse process

(d) Rapid onset of a dense bilateral sensory block of both hemithoraces

2. When performing an erector spinae plane block, what is the characteristic appearance of the thoracic transverse processes?

(a) Rounded appearance, 5 cm lateral to the midline

(b) Hypoechoic, "squared off"

(c) Hyperechoic, "squared off"

(d) Hyperechoic, moving with respiration

Answers

1 (b) The parietal pleura is anterior to the thoracic paravertebral space and will be depressed anteriorly, with deposition of local anesthetic causing it to bulge.

2 (c) The transverse processes of the thoracic spine give a characteristic square appearance, relative to the rib ends, which are rounded. Bone has a characteristic hyperechoic appearance on ultrasound.

Further Reading

Baldinelli F, Capozzoli G, Pedrazzoli R, Feil B, Pipitone M, Zaraca F. Are thoracic wall blocks efficient after video-assisted thoracoscopy surgery-lobectomy pain? A comparison between serratus anterior plane block and intercostal nerve block. *J Cardiothorac Vasc Anesth*. 2021;35(8):2297–302.

Carney J, Finnerty O, Rauf J, Bergin D, Laffey JG, Mc Donnell JG. Studies on the spread of local anesthetic solution in transversus abdominis plane blocks. *Anesthesia*. 2011;66(11):1023–30.

Forero M, Adhikary SD, Lopez H, Tsui C, Chin KJ. The erector spinae plane block: a novel analgesic technique in thoracic neuropathic pain. *Reg Anesth Pain Med*. 2016;41(5):621–7.

Karmakar MK. Thoracic paravertebral block. *Anesthesiology*. 2001;95(3):771.

Kaushal B, Chauhan S, Saini K, *et al*. Comparison of the efficacy of ultrasound-guided serratus anterior plane block, pectoral nerves II block, and intercostal nerve block for the management of postoperative thoracotomy pain after pediatric cardiac surgery. *J Cardiothorac Vasc Anesth*. 2019;33(2):418–25.

Kaye AD, Urman RD, Vadivelu N. *Essentials of Regional Anesthesia*, 2nd ed. Cham: Springer;2018.

Kim S, Bae CM, Do YW, Moon S, Baek SI, Lee DH. Serratus anterior plane block and intercostal nerve block after thoracoscopic surgery. *Thorac Cardiovasc Surg*. 2021;69 (6):564–9.

Kot P, Rodriguez P, Granell M, *et al*. The erector spinae plane block: a narrative review. *Korean J Anesthesiol*. 2019;72(3):209–20.

Wang W, Song W, Yang C, *et al*. Ultrasound-guided pectoral nerve block I and serratus-intercostal plane block alleviate postoperative pain in patients undergoing modified radical mastectomy. *Pain Physician*. 2019;22(4):E315–23.

Yang H, Dong Q, Liang L, *et al*. The comparison of ultrasound-guided thoracic para-vertebral blockade and internal intercostal nerve block for non-intubated video-assisted thoracic surgery. *J Thorac Dis*. 2019;11(8):3476–81.

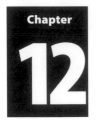

Chapter 12

Fluid and Electrolyte Balance

Ryan J. Kline, John A. Helmstetter, and Bethany L. Menard

Introduction

Maintaining fluid and electrolyte balance is one of the mainstays of anesthesia. Often patients present to the operating room with intravascular volume depletion secondary to nil *per os* (NPO) status, acute bleeding, and recent bowel preparation, as well as with electrolyte abnormalities due to coexisting disease. Physical examination is useful in determining volume status, coupled with static and dynamic hemodynamic monitoring.

Evaluation of Intravascular Volume

Determining the intravascular volume status can be difficult for the clinician. However, it is very important to be able to assess intravascular volume derangements in order to improve perfusion to vital organs. Patient history is the first step in evaluating volume status by assessing the NPO status and for the presence of persistent diarrhea and vomiting, intravenous fluid administration, recent blood administration, nasogastric suctioning, and hemodialysis. Physical examination further assists in assessing the volume status by assessing capillary refill time, skin turgor, heart rate, blood pressure, and intake and output and for the presence of jugular distension, as well as the presence of peripheral edema. Laboratory analysis can also provide some insight with serum lactate levels, as well as arterial blood gases, both of which will assess end-organ perfusion, which can be used as a surrogate for volume status.

Physical Examination and Laboratory Markers for Fluid Status

Hypovolemic patients may present with lethargy, hypotension, decreased skin turgor, and reduced jugular venous pressure. Laboratory values also display elevated blood urea nitrogen and serum creatinine levels, hyperkalemia or hypokalemia, hypernatremia or hyponatremia, and metabolic alkalosis as well as acidosis.

Hypovolemia is one of the most important volume derangements and can lead to perioperative complications, including acute kidney injury, acute cerebrovascular accidents, and decreased global tissue perfusion. This loss of intravascular volume may be due to "third spacing," as well as loss of sodium-containing fluids through the skin, gastrointestinal (GI) tract, or urine. The decreased intravascular volume can have many causes, including excessive preoperative fasting, mechanical bowel preparation, acute and chronic GI bleeding, sympathetic blockade secondary to neuraxial anesthesia, and myocardial depression and vasodilatation secondary to inhaled anesthetics.

Hypervolemic patients may present with elevated jugular venous pressure, edema of the lower extremities, S3 heart sound, and orthopnea. Laboratory findings include elevated B-type natriuretic peptide (BNP) and N-terminal pro-BNP (NT-proBNP) levels, in addition to radiographic findings of Kerlyy "B" lines due to increased pulmonary vascular and interstitial markings.

Hemodynamic Measurements

Static hemodynamic parameters that can be used to monitor intravascular fluid status include noninvasive blood pressure, heart rate, urine output, mixed venous oxygen saturation, and central venous pressure. These parameters are best used based on their trends to determine volume status. These parameters have many limitations, including in a hypovolemic patient unable to increase their heart rate secondary to beta-blocker use, as well as surgical stress and anesthetic gases leading to decreased urine output in a euvolemic patient.

Dynamic hemodynamic parameters are typically used as a guide for goal-directed fluid therapy, and compared to static parameters, they provide improved assessment of fluid challenge responsiveness. These parameters include arterial pressure waveform variations (stroke volume variation, pulse pressure variation, systolic blood pressure variation), transesophageal echocardiography (TEE), and serum lactate levels, as well as noninvasive devices (Vigileo FloTrac).

Intravenous Fluids

The two types of intravenous fluids include crystalloids and colloids. Crystalloid solutions consist of ions in water that are able to freely cross capillary membranes. Colloids consist of high-molecular-weight substances that cannot cross capillary membranes. Colloid solutions are beneficial in maintaining plasma oncotic pressure, whereas crystalloid solutions are able to equilibrate rapidly with the extravascular fluid space. There is no ideal resuscitation fluid; however, the choice of fluid, as well as the dose, may affect patient-centered outcomes. Unfortunately, systematic reviews, as well as randomized controlled trials, have not been able to prove increased safety or effectiveness of any one resuscitation fluid or shown a decrease in mortality.

Crystalloids

These solutions are widely available and low cost, and are typically the first-line resuscitation fluid for septic shock, hemorrhagic shock, burn injury, cardiac arrest, and brain trauma. Isotonic crystalloids can be separated into two types: balanced (lactated Ringer's, Plasma-Lyte) and saline (0.9% sodium chloride). Balanced solutions have a composition that more closely resembles that of extracellular fluid. This is achieved by including buffers that are excreted, as well as metabolized. They also contain sodium, chloride, and possibly potassium, as well as have a more similar composition of acids and bases to extracellular fluid, as shown in Table 12.1.

Normal saline contains solely sodium and chloride, with a chloride concentration of 154 mEq L^{-1} that is 50% more than is contained in extracellular fluid. This can lead to dilutional hyperchloremic acidosis after large volume administration due to its increased sodium and chloride content. As chloride concentration increases, a decrease in plasma bicarbonate concentration is also observed.

Balanced crystalloid solutions include lactated Ringer's, Plasma-Lyte, Normosol, and Isolyte. These solutions also contain sodium and chloride, but also have varying mixtures of added electrolytes (potassium, magnesium, and calcium) and buffers (lactate and gluconate). The addition of these electrolytes and buffers allows these fluids to have a more similar acid–base composition to extracellular fluid. There is long-standing debate regarding the effectiveness of balanced crystalloids versus saline for fluid replacement. Recent studies have indicated that balanced crystalloids can decrease the

Table 12.1 Crystalloid solutions and their composition

Electrolyte	Plasma (mEq L^{-1})	ICF (mEq L^{-1})	ECF (mEq L^{-1})
Sodium	142	10	140
Potassium	4	150	4.5
Magnesium	2	40	2
Calcium	5	1	5
Chloride	103	103	117
Bicarbonate	25	7	28

ICF, intracellular fluid; ECF, extracellular fluid.
Source: Table adapted from Miller RD, Pardo MC. *Basics of Anesthesia*. Philadelphia, Elsevier, 2001. Rhoades RA, Tanner GA. *Medical Physiology*. Boston, Little, Brown, 1995.

incidence of death, persistent renal dysfunction, and new renal replacement therapy.

Colloids

These solutions are higher cost and contain higher-molecular-weight molecules in a carrier fluid that are typically unable to pass through the semipermeable capillary membrane. This allows colloids to maintain and expand intravascular volume as they are less able to leave the intravascular space and instead maintain colloid oncotic pressure. This leads to a decreased volume required for resuscitation, also known as the volume-sparing effect. When resuscitating with colloids versus crystalloids, three times the amount of crystalloids are needed versus colloids to replace the lost intravascular volume. The two main types of colloids include human derived (albumin) and semisynthetic (starches).

Albumin consists of human protein removed from blood and added to saline. It is then heated in order to decrease the risk of viral transmission. Administration increases the intravascular oncotic pressure, which then leads to movement of fluid from the extravascular compartments into the intravascular compartments. In severe sepsis and critically ill patients, crystalloid solutions should be used for initial management, with albumin infusions considered if solely crystalloids are ineffectual, as per the Surviving Sepsis Campaign guidelines.

Semisynthetic colloids include hydroxyethyl starch solutions and dextran solutions, as well as others. These solutions are currently not in use in the United States but have found use in Europe, and as a first-line resuscitation fluid in military theaters. Current evidence is poor regarding clinical benefit, and risks of use include possible nephrotoxicity and changes in coagulation.

Perioperative Fluid Replacement

Preexisting fluid deficits, fluid and blood losses during surgery, and patient comorbidities can all increase the complexity of proper fluid replacement in the perioperative patient. Historically, a more liberal approach to intravenous fluid therapy was employed in order to replace fluid lost to "third spacing." Loss of fluid into the third space leads to fluid accumulation in the extravascular extracellular space. More recently, consensus has shifted towards a more goal-directed approach to fluid replacement therapy due to patients receiving excessive amounts of fluids in the perioperative period. The objective is to avoid underresuscitation, as well as overresuscitation, in the perioperative period. This is important as underresuscitaiton can lead to hypotension and impaired tissue oxygenation, as well as impaired perfusion. Overresuscitation may lead to anastomotic compromise and impaired GI function, as well as cardiac and pulmonary complications. Ultimately, fluid replacement should be based on the individual patient, their comorbidities, and surgical considerations.

Conventional Management

This management style consisted of replacing fluid with crystalloid by using the maintenance fluid rate multiplied by the duration of NPO, with the addition of insensible losses (6 mL/(kg hr) for small incisions), as well as replacement of three times the amount of blood loss with crystalloid. The addition of maintenance fluid is also based on the 4–2–1 rule (4 mL kg^{-1} for the first 10 kg body weight, 2 mL kg^{-1} for the second 10 kg body weight, and 1 mL kg^{-1} for the remaining body weight). This method of fluid replacement can lead to a large volume of fluids administered in the perioperative period, and has started to lose favor for more goal-directed fluid management strategies.

Goal-Directed Fluid Therapy

This management style consists of administering intravenous fluid to achieve a specific target. These targets include maintaining stroke volume, cardiac index, urine output, blood pressure, and heart rate. This is achieved by delivering small boluses of colloid (250 mL) in an effort to maintain cardiac output or stroke volume, rather than relying on a maintenance rate of fluid replacement. Use of goal-directed fluid therapy in high-risk patient populations and major surgeries was found to result in improved time to recovery of GI function and decreased length of stay, as well as decreased rates of pneumonia.

Perioperative Fluid Loss

One of the difficult tasks encountered during surgery is estimation of surgical blood loss. This can be complicated by hidden blood loss in the drapes, surgical flush use, and occult bleeding into the surgical wound. Visual estimation is used to determine the amount of blood in the surgical suction canister, as well as assessing the laparotomy pads and surgical sponges. Completely saturated laparotomy pads can contain 100 mL of blood, and surgical sponges can carry as much as 10 mL of blood.

Other fluid losses also occur during surgical procedures. Based on the size of the incision, evaporative losses can be calculated to further track fluid loss. Small incisions, such as hernia repairs, may lead to 0–2 mL kg^{-1} of volume loss per hour, moderate incisions up to 2–4 mL/(kg hr), and large incisions, such as open abdominal procedures, up to 4–8 mL/(kg hr).

Electrolyte Balance Management

Table 12.2 shows the normal electrolyte composition in body compartments.

Table 12.2 Normal electrolyte composition in body compartments

Electrolyte	Plasma (mEq L^{-1})	ICF (mEq L^{-1})	ECF (mEq L^{-1})
Sodium	142	10	140
Potassium	4	150	4.5
Magnesium	2	40	2
Calcium	5	1	5
Chloride	103	103	117
Bicarbonate	25	7	28

ICF, intracellular fluid; ECF, extracellular fluid.

Source: Table adapted from Miller RD, Pardo MC. *Basics of Anesthesia.* Philadelphia, Elsevier, 2001. Rhoades RA, Tanner GA. *Medical Physiology.* Boston, Little, Brown, 1995.

Sodium Homeostasis

Sodium homeostasis and plasma sodium concentration are generally reflective of total body osmolality. Table 12.2 above demonstrates the normal electrolyte composition in body compartments. Total body osmolality is the sum of extracellular and intracellular solutes divided by total body water. Plasma osmolality is regulated by thirst and secretion of antidiuretic hormone (ADH) from the posterior pituitary. When an increase in extracellular osmolality is sensed by cells in the hypothalamus, ADH is released and increases water reabsorption in the kidney to restore normal plasma osmolality. Normal plasma osmolality is typically in the range of 280–290 mOsm L^{-1}. On the other hand, when the extracellular fluid has a decreased osmolality, ADH secretion is reduced; the kidneys excrete more water, and plasma osmolality shifts back to normal. Thirst sensors in the hypothalamus also sense increases or decreases in extracellular fluid osmolality and stimulate or suppress thirst. One must evaluate plasma osmolality when assessing a patient with sodium level derangements.

Hyponatremia

Hyponatremia is defined as sodium concentration <135 mEq L^{-1} and occurs either due to an increase in total body water or through the body's excess sodium loss relative to water loss. Hyponatremia causes are often determined by evaluation of plasma osmolality. In a hyponatremic patient with a normal plasma osmolality, causes include marked hyperlipidemia or hyperproteinemia which are asymptomatic. It can also be due to glycine absorption during transurethral surgery that presents with symptoms. In those with an elevated plasma osmolality, causes of hyponatremia are attributed to either mannitol administration or hyperglycemia. Hyperglycemia causes what is known as pseudohyponatremia. Calculations can be made to determine the actual sodium level in the presence of severely elevated plasma glucose levels. Patients with both low sodium and low plasma osmolality are categorized as having decreased, normal, or increased total sodium content. In those with a decreased total sodium content, sodium losses can be renal or extrarenal. Renal losses are most commonly attributed to thiazide diuretics but can also be due to salt-losing nephropathies, mineralocorticoid deficiency, or renal tubular acidosis. Extrarenal sodium losses are the result of excessive diarrhea or vomiting, sweating, burns, or "third spacing." In patients with a normal total sodium content, causes include primary polydipsia, syndrome of inappropriate ADH secretion (SIADH), hypothyroidism, drug-induced, and glucocorticoid deficiency. Finally, in those with an increased total sodium content and hyponatremia, causes typically include congestive heart failure, cirrhosis of the liver, and nephrotic syndromes.

Symptoms and manifestations of hyponatremia are due to an increase in intracellular water. With this effect, symptoms are typically neurological and nonspecific. Some symptoms include malaise, weakness, and anorexia; however, they can progress to life-threatening situations such as seizures or coma and leading up to death. Serious symptoms typically occur when sodium levels are <120 mEq L^{-1}. Chronicity of sodium level derangements also factors into the severity of symptomatology. Those with chronic hyponatremia typically have mild symptoms or none at all.

When correcting for hyponatremia, one must first aim to identify the underlying cause of the metabolic derangement. This is often done through plasma and urine osmolality measurements, along with evaluation of the patient's volume status. Urine sodium levels are measured to evaluate whether sodium losses are extrarenal or renal in nature. The treatment of choice of hyponatremic patients with a decreased total body sodium content is typically isotonic saline. By contrast, in patients with normal or increased total body sodium content, treatment for hyponatremia is water restriction. Evaluation of a patient's underlying cause of hyponatremia is particularly important because treatment may be more specific to their disease process such as hormone replacement in a patient with, for example, a glucocorticoid or thyroid hormone deficiency. Since acute hyponatremia presents with the most serious of symptoms, it is generally recommended to treat patients to a sodium level of >120 mEq L^{-1}. Correction of sodium levels must be performed first by calculating the patient's total sodium deficit by use of the following formula: sodium deficit = total body water $\times$ (desired sodium − current sodium). Once this calculation has been determined, the sodium level should not be rapidly corrected due to the possibility of causing central pontine myelinolysis and permanent neurological damage. Acute hyponatremia, typically described as <48 hours, often presents with seizures and/or coma and must be addressed urgently. Several published cases suggest a correction of 4–6 mEq L^{-1} should be sufficient to suppress seizures secondary to hyponatremia. Fluid boluses of 3% saline are typically used to treat acute hyponatremia. One method for correcting sodium levels is to use an approximation formula of 1 mL kg^{-1} of 3% sodium chloride, which is expected to raise serum sodium levels by 1 mEq L^{-1}. One must always remember to address the underlying cause to evaluate if it is reversible. It is also recommended to monitor serum sodium levels approximately every 6–8 hours during correction periods. Typically, sodium levels of >130 are acceptable for a patient who will undergo general anesthesia. Those with symptoms should have the sodium levels corrected prior to anesthetic administration, especially those undergoing transurethral procedures and at risk of massive fluid absorption.

Hypernatremia

Hypernatremia occurs when there is an increase in sodium solutes in comparison to total body water. Hypernatremia is defined as sodium levels >145 mEq L^{-1}. It occurs either due to a relative loss of water more than sodium loss or as a result of sodium retention. Those in a hypernatremic state may have normal, low, or high total body sodium content. Patients with hypernatremia and low total body sodium content have lost sodium and water, but the water loss is greater than the relative sodium loss. This is often the result of osmotic diuresis, sweating, or diarrhea, and patients often appear hypovolemic on presentation. By contrast, hypernatremia, in the presence of normal total body sodium content, often is the result of central or nephrogenic diabetes insipidus. Lastly, patients with high total body sodium content and hypernatremia are often seen following infusions of hypertonic saline. Other instances of hypernatremia can be seen in patients with Cushing's syndrome or primary aldosteronism.

Manifestations of hypernatremia occur as a result of cellular dehydration. Chronic hypernatremia is typically better tolerated. Symptoms can range from hyperreflexia to lethargy. More acute developments of hypernatremia can lead to decreases in brain volume that can ultimately cause shearing of the cerebral veins and subsequent brain hemorrhage. Other common manifestations of acute hypernatremia include seizures, coma, neurological damage, and even death.

To manage hypernatremia, one must first identify if the issue is acute or chronic, and what the underlying cause is. One must calculate the patient's total body water deficit and aim to correct that deficit in a 48-hour span with a hypotonic solution, such as 5% dextrose in water. Patients with a low total body sodium content should first be treated with an isotonic solution prior to hypotonic solution treatment. If a hypernatremic patient has a high total body sodium content, they should also be given a loop diuretic to enhance sodium loss, along with hypotonic solution administration. The most important issue with hypernatremia correction is the rate at which it is corrected. One should not correct hypernatremia at a rate faster than 0.5 mEq/(L hr) in order to avoid cerebral edema and the risk of permanent neurological damage. Addressing hypernatremia is extremely important in the perioperative period because it has been shown in many studies to be an independent predictor of increased risk of 30-day morbidity and mortality. Increased rates of major coronary events, pneumonia, wound or surgical site infections, and venous thromboembolism are seen in patients with hypernatremia in the perioperative period. In many instances, patients with hypernatremia present for emergent surgery and correction of sodium levels prior to surgery may not be feasible.

Potassium Homeostasis

Potassium homeostasis is an important regulator and a determining factor in the resting cell membrane potential. As seen in the normal electrolyte range displayed in Table 12.2, the intracellular level of potassium is much higher (approximately 140 mEq L^{-1}) compared to the extracellular level (approximately 4 mEq L^{-1}). Maintenance of this gradient is important for normal cellular functions. Derangements can occur due to lower or higher total body potassium levels, along with redistribution between extracellular and intracellular components without an actual change in total body potassium levels. Shifts of potassium ions between intracellular and extracellular compartments occur with acid/base shifts and plasma pH alterations, catecholamine activity, insulin administration or circulation, and changes in plasma osmolality. Acidosis promotes the intracellular shift of hydrogen ions into the cell, with concomitant shift of potassium ions into the extracellular compartment, and hence an increase in plasma potassium levels. The opposite effect is seen with an alkalotic state, with an end-result of low plasma potassium levels.

Hypokalemia

Hypokalemia is defined when plasma potassium levels fall below 3.5 mEq L^{-1}. Hypokalemia can be attributed to any situation that leads to either a decreased potassium intake or excessive potassium losses, or shifts between the intracellular and extracellular compartments. Signs or manifestations of hypokalemia are broad and can significantly affect a patient undergoing anesthesia in the perioperative period.

One of the most serious effects is on the cardiovascular system, which is a result of cell membrane excitability. Hypokalemia can manifest as ECG changes, which can include ST segment depression, decreased T wave amplitude, and the presence of a U wave. Arrhythmias are also seen, with premature ventricular contractions (PVCs) being the most common; however, premature atrial contractions (PACs) are also seen in this state. Neuromuscular symptoms can also be manifested in the presence of hypokalemia. Muscle fatigue and restlessness, myalgias, and weakness can be seen in mild cases. When potassium levels are critically low, such as <2 mEq L^{-1}, extremity paralysis may occur and even potentially involve muscles of the trunk and muscles involved in respiratory mechanics. Other body systems can be affected by hypokalemia. In the renal system, polyuria, increased ammonia production, and increased bicarbonate reabsorption can occur. Hypokalemia can lead to decreased insulin and aldosterone secretion in the endocrine system. Patients with liver disease can develop encephalopathy and hypokalemia can also lead to an overall decreased nitrogen balance.

When addressing hypokalemia in the perioperative period, one must take into consideration the rate at which it is developing and what the underlying cause may be. Mild hypokalemia in the range of 3.0–3.5 mEq L^{-1} in the absence of ECG changes often is not associated with an increased anesthetic risk; however, more critically low potassium levels must be addressed to mitigate the above-mentioned risks. When potassium repletion is necessary, one should assess the necessary amount of potassium that must be administered to reach a safe threshold. Potassium supplementation should be done under close ECG monitoring. If more rapid potassium replacement is deemed necessary, it should be done via a central venous catheter. Intravenous fluids should not contain dextrose, as the risk of hyperglycemia could worsen hypokalemia. When intravenous potassium replacement is used, it is recommended this does not exceed 240 mEq per day. Another important anesthetic consideration in the setting of hypokalemia is the use of neuromuscular blocking drugs. There is increased sensitivity to these drugs in a hypokalemic patient; therefore, a provider should consider a reduction in the dose, along with close neuromonitoring with a nerve stimulator.

Hyperkalemia

Hyperkalemia is defined as serum potassium levels of >5.5 mEq L^{-1}. The differential diagnosis for hyperkalemia is extensive and can be multifactorial. The differential list can be broken down into a few categories, including pseudohyperkalemia, redistribution or extracellular movement of potassium, decreased renal excretion of potassium, and increased potassium uptake. Pseudohyperkalemia can be the result of using a tourniquet and/or a small-bore needle for blood collection. It can also be seen in the presence of marked thrombocytosis or leukocytosis. Because potassium is predominantly intracellular, potassium shifting out of the cell can obviously lead to an increase in plasma potassium levels. A number of medications can cause extracellular movement of potassium, including, but not limited to, beta-2 blockers, digoxin, and succinylcholine. It is predicted that succinylcholine causes approximately 0.5 mEq increase in the potassium level; however, this can be much higher in cases such as burns and massive tissue trauma. Insulin deficiency can cause hyperkalemia. Other causes of hyperkalemia due to redistribution include rhabdomyolysis and hemolysis due to any cause, as well as metabolic acidosis. Impaired renal excretion is another large category of patients with hyperkalemia, with the most obvious causes being renal failure and impaired glomerular filtration rates. Decreased mineralocorticoid activity can lead to hyperkalemia. Medications are also a very common cause of hyperkalemia. Some medications include potassium-sparing diuretics such as spironolactone and amiloride, angiotensin-converting enzyme (ACE) inhibitors, nonsteroidal antiinflammatory drugs (NSAIDs), trimethoprim, and pentamide. Increased potassium intake is unlikely to cause a problem in normal individuals, unless inadvertent large doses are given or if repletion is given too rapidly. One must remember that potassium levels can be increased when multiple blood transfusions are administered. After 21 days of storage, one unit of whole blood can potentially contain up to 30 mEq L^{-1} of potassium.

Hyperkalemia manifests with signs and symptoms mainly through effects on cardiac and skeletal muscle. Cardiac signs of hyperkalemia can be seen on ECG changes initially with peaked T waves and shortened QT interval, but can progress to widening of the QRS complex, PR interval prolongation, loss of the P wave, and ST segment depression. These changes can ultimately lead to a sine wave pattern before the most feared transition to ventricular fibrillation or even asystole. Hyperkalemia can be worsened in the presence of acidosis, hyponatremia, and hypocalcemia. Skeletal muscle manifestations are not usually present until potassium levels exceed 8 mEq L^{-1}, resulting in muscle weakness.

Because cardiac and skeletal muscle manifestations of hyperkalemia can lead to severe morbidity and mortality, potassium levels >6 mEq L^{-1} must be treated. Treatment of hyperkalemia is aimed at stabilizing the cardiac muscle cell membrane, shifting potassium into the intracellular space, and eliminating potassium from the body. Stabilizing the cardiac membrane is done through administration of intravenous calcium gluconate or calcium chloride. If a patient has metabolic acidosis, one should administer sodium bicarbonate to promote the intracellular movement of potassium. Other methods to shift the potassium intracellularly include inhaled beta agonists and intravenous insulin and glucose. To excrete potassium from the body in a patient with improved renal function, furosemide can be administered, with an onset of 5–15 minutes. A much slower method of excretion is through administration of sodium polystyrene sulfonate (Kayexalate); however, this can have an onset time of 2–24 hours. Finally, in cases of very severe or refractory hyperkalemia, dialysis can be done to remove potassium. Hemodialysis can remove approximately 50 mEq hr^{-1}, and peritoneal dialysis can remove about 10–15 mEq hr^{-1}.

As mentioned earlier, because of the lethal nature of this electrolyte abnormality, an anesthesia provider must be extremely careful in not proceeding with elective cases in the setting of significant hyperkalemia. Many institutions have their own "cutoffs" for potassium levels before proceeding with surgery. Often for elective surgery, a potassium level of >6.5 signifies a definitive cancellation and necessitates treatment. There are no specific levels or guidelines for other potassium levels; however, one must evaluate the acuity of not only the electrolyte imbalance, but also the patient's underlying disease process and situation, as well as the urgency of the surgery.

Calcium Homeostasis

Calcium homeostasis is particularly important because calcium ions participate in nearly every biological function and disruption in its balance can lead to profound effects on nearly all body systems. Over 98% of the body's calcium is in bone. Calcium is normally absorbed through the GI system and is mostly excreted by the kidneys. Disorders along any of this passage, as well as many other factors, can lead to hypocalcemia or hypercalcemia. Calcium exists in the body as either a free ionized form (50%) or bound to a protein (40%). Albumin is the major calcium-binding protein; therefore, alterations in albumin levels will alter total calcium levels. The remaining 10% of calcium is bound to other anions such as amino acids or citrate. Alterations in plasma pH can affect protein binding and hence alter ionized calcium levels. In other words, a decrease in plasma pH will decrease protein binding and lead to higher levels of the free ionized calcium.

Normal calcium homeostasis is maintained by three main substances – parathyroid hormone (PTH), vitamin D, and calcitonin. PTH is the most important regulator of plasma calcium levels. Decreased levels of calcium lead to secretion of PTH, which, in turn, mobilizes calcium from bone and enhances its absorption in the renal tubules. PTH also indirectly increases intestinal absorption of calcium. Vitamin D augments calcium absorption in the intestines and also helps facilitate the actions of PTH. Calcitonin is a hormone released by the thyroid gland when calcium levels are elevated. Calcitonin lowers calcium levels through increased urinary excretion and inhibition of bone resorption.

Hypocalcemia

Hypocalcemia is confirmed by total calcium levels. It must be corrected for in the presence of hypoalbuminemia. Other causes of hypocalcemia include hypoparathyroidism or pseudohypoparathyroidism. Vitamin D deficiency is a major cause of hypocalcemia and can be seen in a number of conditions such as malnutrition, malabsorption either secondary to postsurgical changes or inflammatory bowel disease, and altered vitamin D metabolism. Hyperphosphatemia, pancreatitis, rhabdomyolysis, fat embolism, and loop diuretics are other potential etiologies of low calcium levels. One must recall that stored blood products contain citrate as preservative. Following multiple transfusions, citrate can chelate calcium and lead to a decrease in calcium levels. A similar effect can also be seen after large albumin boluses.

Hypocalcemia can manifest with paresthesias, weakness, and muscle spasms in the carpopedal area and masseter known as the Trousseau's sign and Chvostek's sign, respectively. Seizures can also be seen in profound hypocalcemia. Important considerations for anesthesia include the risk of laryngospasm and bronchospasm. Cardiac manifestations are commonly seen as ECG changes and decreased cardiac contractility leading to hypotension or heart failure. The QT interval is prolonged and ST inversions can occur; however, it can also be normal in the setting of life-threatening hypocalcemia.

Significant hypocalcemia should be addressed and treated prior to someone being anesthetized. Hypocalcemia that is severe enough to cause symptoms should be promptly treated with intravenous calcium gluconate or chloride. Serial calcium levels should be checked regularly during the replacement period. Other anesthetic considerations of hypocalcemia include avoidance of alkalosis, as this can worsen hypocalcemia. Hypocalcemia can lead to unpredictable responses of neuromuscular blocking drugs, as well as potentiate the negative inotropic effects of volatile anesthetics.

Hypercalcemia

The most common cause of hypercalcemia is primary hyperparathyroidism. An increase in PTH secretion leads to increased blood calcium levels. Another common cause of increased calcium levels is malignancy. Bone metastasis can lead to bone destruction or secretion of mediators of hypercalcemia such as PTH-like substances, prostaglandins, and cytokines. Increased bone turnover in diseases such as Paget's disease can lead to increased calcium levels. Other causes include granulomatous disorders such as tuberculosis and sarcoidosis, chronic immobilization, milk-alkali syndrome, adrenal insufficiency, and drug-induced with medications such as thiazide diuretics and lithium.

Clinical signs and symptoms of hypercalcemia include nausea and vomiting, anorexia, weakness, and polyuria. Lethargy and confusion can lead to coma. As with most other electrolyte abnormalities, ECG changes can be seen. With hypercalcemia, the QT interval is shortened, as well as the ST segment. When hypercalcemia is symptomatic, it must be treated. Treatment includes first addressing the underlying cause of hypercalcemia. Initial therapies to lower calcium levels include normal saline administration, often at a rate of 2.5–3.0 mL/(kg hr). This is particularly important in the surgical patient and saline diuresis should be continued in the intraoperative period. Bisphosphonates, such as pamidronate, are the first-line drug of treatment in hypercalcemia. Other treatment modalities include administration of phosphate intravenous infusion or intravenous doses of calcitonin. Anesthesia providers in the perioperative period should monitor calcium levels serially, along with other electrolytes such as potassium and magnesium. During the perioperative period, in a patient with acidosis, one should consider controlled ventilation to avoid acidosis that could worsen hypercalcemia.

Magnesium Homeostasis

Magnesium balance plays an important role in many enzymatic pathways in the body, often serving as a cofactor. Majority of magnesium is located within the bone with only approximately 1–2% present in the extracellular compartment. Derangements of magnesium levels can have several anesthetic implications. Magnesium also serves as a therapy for some conditions and disease processes. Magnesium is absorbed in the small bowel and is excreted renally, where it can also be reabsorbed. Normal magnesium levels in the blood are between 1.7 and 2.1 mEq L^{-1}.

Hypomagnesemia

Hypomagnesemia is defined as plasma levels of <1.7 mEq L^{-1}. A number of different factors can lead to this condition. Decreased nutritional intake is a potential cause, along with malabsorption in the GI tract. Decreased absorption can be seen in syndromes of malabsorption, laxative use, prolonged nasogastric suctioning, or severe diarrhea or vomiting. Another potential etiology of hypomagnesemia is increased renal loss that can be seen with diuretic use, hyperaldosteronism, nephrotoxic drug use, hypophosphatemia, and diabetic ketoacidosis. Hypomagnesemia is commonly seen in chronic alcoholics, patients with pancreatitis, hyperthyroid patients, and burn victims.

As with nearly all other electrolyte abnormalities, low magnesium levels can present with ECG changes and cardiac muscle cell irritability. The most common changes seen are PR and QT interval prolongation. It is also associated with an increased risk of atrial fibrillation. Hypomagnesemia is commonly asymptomatic but can present with weakness, paresthesias, ataxia, confusion, and even seizures. Hypomagnesemia is often seen in patients with concomitant hypokalemia and hypocalcemia; therefore, it is often imperative to address these abnormalities in the perioperative period.

Treatment can be given either orally or intramuscularly; however; more serious presentations, such as seizures, should warrant intravenous treatment, which is often given in doses of 1–2 g over a 15- to 60-minute period. Since hypomagnesemia is associated with a risk of arrhythmias, anesthesia providers should treat low levels of magnesium and monitor ECG waveforms closely.

Hypermagnesemia

Elevated levels of magnesium are most commonly seen following exogenous administration; however, impaired renal excretion can also lead to elevated levels. Intravenous magnesium is sometimes used in the treatment of pre-eclampsia and eclampsia, and can lead to elevations in both mother and fetus. Magnesium functions in the body as a calcium blocker; therefore, one can expect hemodynamic compromise with critically high levels of magnesium. If a patient also has hyperkalemia, there is an increased risk of cardiac arrhythmias and cardiac arrest. Neuromuscular symptoms occur as a result of magnesium inhibiting acetylcholine release from the neuromuscular junction. The kidneys are typically able to maintain magnesium homeostasis until the glomerular filtration rate drops below 30 mL min^{-1}.

Hypermagnesemia often does not show signs or symptoms until magnesium levels reach >4 mg dL^{-1}. Some milder symptoms include weakness, nausea, dizziness, and confusion. As magnesium levels reach between 7 and 12 mg dL^{-1}, diminished deep tendon reflexes (DTRs) can be seen. This physical examination finding is often assessed for in preeclamptic patients receiving magnesium therapy. At these magnesium levels, patients can often experience worsening confusion, flushing, headaches, blurred vision, bladder paralysis, and/or constipation. Hypotension and bradycardia may also be apparent with these magnesium levels. As magnesium levels increase to >12 mg dL^{-1}, flaccid paralysis, decreased respiratory drive, and more pronounced hypotension and bradycardia can be seen. ECG changes often demonstrate a prolonged PR interval or atrioventricular blocks. With magnesium levels of >15 mg dL^{-1}, coma and cardiorespiratory arrest are often the unfortunate presentation.

Hypermagnesemia is an important consideration for the anesthesia provider. Because of the associated risk of cardiac instability and hemodynamic compromise, magnesium levels should be addressed prior to elective surgery. ECG waveforms should always be closely monitored in those receiving magnesium therapy, as well as in those with known elevated plasma levels of magnesium. Elevated levels of magnesium can inhibit acetylcholine release from the neuromuscular junction; thus, neuromuscular blocking drugs should be used with extreme caution, as these patients may have exaggerated responses. Close monitoring with a nerve stimulator is necessary and one should consider dosage reductions. Volatile and intravenous anesthetics may have a more pronounced negative inotropic effect in a patient with elevated magnesium levels. It has been suggested that magnesium can decrease overall anesthesia requirements and blunt cardiovascular effects from laryngoscopy and intubation, along with its muscle relaxation effect. Although magnesium can be used in a multitude of conditions, such as asthma, torsades de pointes, and preeclampsia and eclampsia in pregnancy, exogenous magnesium administration or inadvertent overdose can lead to serious consequences. In severe cases of elevated magnesium levels, intravenous calcium gluconate or calcium chloride should be administered to antagonize the effect of magnesium at the neuromuscular junction or in cardiac muscle. Normal saline administration is also recommended as a treatment modality in severe cases. If increased renal excretion is warranted, loop diuretics, such as furosemide, can be given. If kidney function is profoundly impaired and magnesium levels are critical or symptomatic, hemodialysis can be performed to effectively remove magnesium from the blood; however, this can also increase excretion of calcium and, in turn, worsen the symptoms of hypermagnesemia. If patients have severe respiratory or cardiopulmonary complications, ventilation and vasopressor administration may be warranted to stabilize the patient while treatment can ensue. Providers should always closely monitor ECG waveforms, along with serial measurements of plasma magnesium, as well as calcium, levels.

Review Questions

1. Goal-directed fluid therapy has been found to have improved outcomes, *except* which of the following?

   (a) Decreased rates of pneumonia
   (b) Decreased length of stay
   (c) Increased patient satisfaction
   (d) Improved time to recovery of gastrointestinal function

2. Which of the following medications *does not* cause hyperkalemia?

   (a) Furosemide
   (b) Spironolactone
   (c) Trimethoprim
   (d) Angiotensin-converting enzyme (ACE) inhibitors

Answers

1 (c) Goal-directed fluid therapy has been found to decrease rates of pneumonia, decrease length of stay, and improve time to recovery of gastrointestinal function.

2 (a) Spironolactone, trimethoprim, and ACE inhibitors can cause hyperkalemia. Other medications include amiloride, nonsteroidal antiinflammatory drugs, and pentamidine. Furosemide is one medication that can cause hypokalemia due to increased potassium loss in the kidneys.

Further Reading

Aguilera IM, Vaughan RS. Calcium and the anaesthetist. *Anaesthesia*. 2000;55:779–90. DOI: 10.1046/j.1365-2044.2000.01540.x.

Bajwa SJ, Sehgal V. Anesthetic management of primary hyperparathyroidism: a role rarely noticed and appreciated so far. *Indian J Endocrinol Metab.* 2013;17(2):235–9. DOI: 10.4103/2230-8210.109679.

Bunn F, Trivedi D. Colloid solutions for fluid resuscitation. *Cochrane Database Syst Rev.* 2012;7:CD001319.

Butterworth J, Mackey D, Wasnick J, Morgan G, Mikhail M, Morgan G. *Morgan & Mikhail's Clinical Anesthesiology*, 5th ed. New York, NY: McGraw Hill;2013.

Cascella M, Vaqar S. Hypermagnesemia. In: *StatPearls.* Treasure Island, FL: StatPearls Publishing; 2020. Available from: www.ncbi.nlm.nih.gov/books/NBK549811/.

Casey J, Brown R, Semler M. Resuscitation fluids. *Curr Opin Crit Care.* 2018;24(6):512–18. DOI: 10.1097/MCC.0000000000000551.

Corcoran T, Rhodes JE, Clarke S, Myles PS, Ho KM. Perioperative fluid management strategies in major surgery: a stratified meta-analysis. *Anesth Analg.* 2012;114(3):640–51. DOI: 10.1213/ANE.0b013e318240d6eb.

Gurjar M. *Textbook of Ventilation, Fluids, Electrolytes, and Blood Gases*. New Delhi: Jaypee Brothers Medical Publishers Ltd; 2020.

Herroeder S, Schönherr ME, De Hert SG, Hollmann MW. Magnesium – essentials for anesthesiologists. *Anesthesiology.* 2011;114:971–93. DOI: 10.1097/ALN.0b013e318210483d.

Huang L, Yarl W, Liu H. Patient with hyperkalemia for surgery: proceed or postpone? *Transl Perioper Pain Med.* 2019;6(1):17–19.

Leung AA, McAlister FA, Finlayson SR, Bates DW. Preoperative hypernatremia predicts increased perioperative morbidity and mortality. *Am J Med.* 2013;126(10):877–86. DOI: 10.1016/j.amjmed.2013.02.039.

Miller R, Pardo M, Stoelting R, eds. *Basics of Anesthesia*, 6th ed. Philadelphia, PA: Elsevier/Saunders;2011.

Myburgh JA, Mythen MG. Resuscitation fluids. *N Engl J Med.* 2013;369:1243–51.

Myles PS, Andrews S, Nicholson J, Lobo DN, Mythen M. Contemporary approaches to perioperative IV fluid therapy. *World J Surg.* 2017;41(10):2457–63. DOI: 10.1007/s00268-017-4055-y.

Perel P, Roberts I. Colloids versus crystalloids for fluid resuscitation in critically ill patients. *Cochrane Database Syst Rev.* 2012;6:CD000567.

Sahay M, Sahay R. Hyponatremia: a practical approach. *Indian J Endocrinol Metab.* 2014;18(6):760–71. DOI: 10.4103/2230-8210.141320.

Semler MW, Self WH, Wanderer JP, *et al.* Balanced crystalloids versus saline in critically ill adults. *N Engl J Med.* 2018; 378:829–39.

Simmons JW, Dobyns JB, Paiste J. Enhanced recovery after surgery: intraoperative fluid management strategies. *Surg Clin North Am.* 2018;98(6):1185–200. DOI: 10.1016/j.suc.2018.07.006.

Sterns RH, Nigwekar SU, Hix JK. The treatment of hyponatremia. *Semin Nephrol.* 2009;29:282–99.

Vincent JL, De Backer D, Wiedermann CJ. Fluid management in sepsis: the potential beneficial effects of albumin. *J Crit Care.* 2016;35:161–7. DOI: 10.1016/j.jcrc.2016.04.019.

Vitez TS, Soper LE, Wong KC, Soper P. Chronic hypokalemia and intraoperative dysrhythmias. *Anesthesiology.* 1985;63(2):130–3. DOI: 10.1097/00000542-198508000-00002.

Wong KC, Schafer PG, Schultz JR. Hypokalemia and anesthetic implications. *Anesth Analg.* 1993;77(6):1238–60. DOI: 10.1213/00000539-199312000-00027. Erratum in: *Anesth Analg.* 1994;78(5):1035.

Zhu Q, Li X, Tan F, *et al.* Prevalence and risk factors for hypokalemia in patients scheduled for laparoscopic colorectal resection and its association with post-operative recovery. *BMC Gastroenterol.* 2018;18(1):152. DOI: 10.1186/s12876-018-0876-x.

Chapter

13

Blood Transfusion Components and Complications in Anesthesiology

Christine T. Vo and Pamela R. Roberts

Packed Red Blood Cells

Processing, Storage, and ABO Compatibility

Donation of one unit of whole blood or apheresis can be used to obtain red blood cell (RBC) units. For apheresis RBCs, a donor is connected to an apheresis machine and RBCs are separated from other constituents, which are returned to the donor; this process may yield 2 units of RBCs or a single unit of RBCs, along with a unit of platelets and/or plasma. RBC units are stored in polyvinyl chloride bags with the plasticizer di-2-ethylhexylphthalate (DEHP) to maintain RBC membrane integrity during storage. Preservation includes an anticoagulant-preservative (A-P) solution, and the current additive solutions maintain pH and other parameters needed to allow RBC storage shelf life of 42 days [1]. ABO typing and matching are required to avoid reactions due to mismatch (see Table 13.1).

Components

One unit of RBCs has approximately 2–5 billion leukocytes, which convey risks of adverse reactions, including transmission of cytomegalovirus (CMV), intracellular organisms, and inflammatory or immunologically mediated reactions. Leukocyte reduction or depletion is the process of blood filtration to remove leukocytes. Leukoreduction done prestorage is preferred over depletion as it removes more leukocytes, has better quality control, and is a standardized process. Universal leukoreduction strategies decrease the leukocyte load by about 99.9%. Benefits of leukoreduction include reducing the incidence of febrile nonhemolytic transfusion reactions, transfusion-related acute lung injury (TRALI), and transmission of CMV and prions [2].

Clinical Application

Informed consent should be obtained prior to transfusion, except in emergencies. In the United States, average storage of RBCs is 15–19 days; numerous

Table 13.1 ABO and rhesus compatibility of the various blood components

Recipient blood type	Donor RBCs	Donor platelets	Donor FFP	Donor cryopreci-pitate
Rh compat-ibility	Indicated	Indicated	Not indicated	Not indicated
O	O	O, AB, A, B	O, A, B, AB	O, A, B, AB
A	A, O	A, AB, [a]B, [a]O	A, AB	A, AB
B	B, O	B, AB, [a]A, [a]O	B, AB	B, AB
AB	AB, A, B, O	AB, [a]A, [a]B, [a]O	AB	AB

[a] Consider other donors if known from apheresis process and resuspended in additive solutions.
RBC, red blood cell; FFP, fresh frozen plasma; Rh, rhesus.

randomized clinical trials demonstrated similar outcomes with fresh, standard issue, or long storage duration RBCs. RBC units require storage at 1–6°C to prevent bacterial growth and preserve viability. During any transport, RBCs must be kept between 1 and 10°C.

Indications for Transfusion

Symptomatic anemia and acute blood loss are indications for transfusion of RBCs. Physiologic triggers include orthostatic hypotension, shock with marginal hemoglobin levels, and evidence of end-organ damage due to inadequate tissue oxygenation. Clinical concerns of risks of transfusions led to studies revealing noninferiority of restrictive transfusion strategies aimed at hemoglobin levels of 7–8 g dL^{-1}. Single-unit transfusions with reassessment prior to further transfusion and treatment of iron deficiency with iron are both recommended by the Choosing Wisely Campaign, which is promoted by clinical groups from over 20 countries on five continents [3]. Recommendations for most hospitalized patients include a restrictive threshold of 7–8 g dL^{-1}, and for patients with preexisting cardiovascular disease, data support a threshold of 8 g dL^{-1}. Current recommendations are to assess for symptoms, as well as hemoglobin level, prior to deciding to transfuse. Anesthesia-related studies, such as a meta-analysis by Chong *et al.* [4], also support restrictive strategies in critically ill and surgical patients with improved outcomes, including reduced risk of stroke, transfusion reactions, hospital length of stay, and significantly reduced 30-day mortality in critically ill patients. Further studies are necessary to determine specific goals for perioperative stages and for varied surgical populations.

Potential Complications

Transfusion reactions are covered later in this chapter. Mistransfusion, iron overload, alloimmunization, and metabolic derangements can also occur. Some of these complications can be decreased by avoiding unnecessary transfusions or using electronic systems to ensure patient identification and blood matching for each patient.

Fresh Frozen Plasma

Processing, Storage, and ABO Compatibility

Plasma is centrifuged out from citrate-containing whole blood or apheresis donations. Plasma rises to the top. It is then collected and frozen to −18°C within 8 hours of collection. It should be noted that there are instances where collected plasma is frozen >8 hours, but <24 hours, from collection. This is termed PF24 for plasma frozen within 24 hours. The clinical difference is negligible, but there is a decrease in factor VIII and protein C levels during the thawing process [5]. FFP can be stored frozen for up to 1 year. ABO compatibility must be followed.

Components

FFP contains factors II, V, VII, VIII, IX, X, and XI. It also contains fibrinogen (400–900 mg per unit), albumin, protein C, protein S, antithrombin, tissue factor pathway inhibitor, and von Willebrand factor (vWF) [6].

Clinical Application

Once thawed, FFP must be used within 5 days for major hemorrhagic cases; otherwise it is recommended to transfuse FFP within 24 hours of thawing [7]. One unit of FFP is contained in approximately 250 mL of solution. Usual dose of 15–20 mL kg^{-1} is enough to raise clotting factors by approximately 20–30%. In general, raising clotting factors by 10% is enough for clinically significant hemostasis [8].

Indications for Transfusion

Plasma is mainly used to correct for clotting factor deficiencies in actively bleeding patients, especially when specific clotting factor concentrates are not readily available. Patients with significant liver disease have deficiencies in multiple clotting factors. When they are actively bleeding or there is concern for clinically significant bleeding with upcoming invasive procedures, and the international normalized ratio (INR) is >1.5, transfusion of FFP is generally indicated. Other acquired deficiencies in clotting factors are expected in patients taking vitamin K antagonists, those with acute disseminated intravascular coagulation (DIC), and those undergoing massive transfusion protocol. The significance of active bleeding weighed against the unavailability of specific clotting factor concentrates would make FFP a reasonable option for transfusion. FFP has also been indicated with thrombotic microangiopathies as a replacement fluid [9].

Potential Complications

FFP has been implicated in TRALI at a rate of approximately 1 in 2000 plasma transfusions, although the incidence may be higher due to limitations in passive reporting of adverse events. It is the second leading cause of transfusion-associated mortality in the United States, with FFP being the most common cause for this complication [10]. Caution should be taken to avoid FFP in patients with a congenital deficiency in immunoglobulin A in the presence of anti-IgA antibodies. These patients can develop severe anaphylactic reactions. FFP from IgA-deficient donors are advised for this specific patient population. Less than 1% may develop significant anaphylactic allergic or febrile reactions. Approximately 1% may have mild allergic reactions manifested as urticaria. Other complications include transfusion-associated circulatory overload (TACO), transmission of viral infections, hemolytic transfusion reaction (HTR), and citrate toxicity [9].

Platelets

Processing, Storage, and ABO Compatibility

Platelets are obtained either from whole blood or through an apheresis donation. The clinical efficacy is similar, with the only difference being that the recipient of the transfusion is exposed to more donors with platelets obtained from whole blood [9]. The platelets are then stored at room temperature of approximately 22°C, with continuous agitation, for no more than 5 days. ABO compatibility is not required, but recommended if derived from whole blood. Rhesus (Rh) compatibility is necessary.

Components

In general, platelets obtained from whole blood produces approximately $0.45–0.85 \times 10^{11}$ platelets. Therefore, multiple units are pooled together to produce a platelet concentrate of about 2.5×10^{11}, whereas platelets obtained from an apheresis donation produces a concentrate of about 3×10^{11}.

Clinical Application

One unit of pooled platelets from whole blood or one unit of platelets from apheresis will raise the platelet count by approximately 30,000–50,000 per microliter in an average adult. Once processed, platelets should be transfused within 4 hours of release.

Indications for Transfusion

Platelet transfusion is used for prophylactic and therapeutic treatment of significant bleeding in patients with severe thrombocytopenia or disorders of dysfunctional platelets [9]. For anesthesiologists, the suggested threshold for transfusion varies, but the general recommendation is to transfuse to a platelet count of above 50,000 per microliter for invasive procedures or major surgery. For surgeries where even microbleeds are devastating, such as ocular surgery or neurosurgery, it is recommended to transfuse to a platelet count of above 100,000 per microliter. During massive transfusions, it is recommended to transfuse to a threshold of 75,000 per microliter. Specific perioperative situations where platelet transfusions would be indicated include acute DIC with significant hemorrhage, disorders of platelet function with active bleeding, or during massive transfusions with active bleeding.

Potential Complications

Sepsis is a concern due to the storage of platelets at room temperature favoring an environment for bacterial growth. Therefore, the risk of bacterial infection is higher than viral transmission, with a rate of contamination of about 1 in 2000 transfusions. Mild allergic reactions can occur, as well as febrile non-hemolytic reactions, TRALI, TACO, alloimmunization to human leukocyte antigens (HLA) and human platelet antigens (HPAs), and posttransfusion purpura. Transfusion of platelets should be avoided in patients with thrombotic thrombocytopenic purpura and heparin-induced thrombocytopenia due to the risk of worsening thrombosis.

Cryoprecipitate

Processing, Storage, and ABO Compatibility

When FFP is thawed to 1–6°C, cryoprecipitate precipitates out from the solution. These cryoproteins are then suspended in a small volume of plasma and refrozen. It can be stored at −18°C for up to 1 year. To preserve the integrity of clotting factors, it takes approximately 20–30 minutes to thaw cryoprecipitate. ABO compatibility must be followed. Rh compatibility is not required.

Components

Cryoprecipitate contains fibrinogen, factors VIII and XIII, vWF, and fibronectin. The average fibrinogen content is 300 mg per unit. The average factor VIII content is 120 IU per unit, with the shortest half-life of 12 hours. The average factor XIII content is 60 IU per unit. The average vWF content is 125 IU per unit. Most facilities will pool multiple units together when distributing for transfusion [11].

Clinical Application

Cryoprecitipate must be transfused within 4–6 hours of thawing. Cryoprecipitate is typically given as 5–10 pooled units. For correcting fibrinogen deficits, one unit of cryoprecipitate generally raises the plasma fibrinogen concentration by about 7–10 mg dL^{-1} in an average 70-kg adult. The target fibrinogen level is above 100 mg dL^{-1}; thus 10 units of cryoprecipitate should be adequate to reach this target. It should be noted that there are insufficient data to recommend an optimal dose [7].

Indications for Transfusion

Cryoprecipitate is mainly used for clinically significant bleeding in patients with hematologic disorders consisting of deficiencies in clotting factors specific to components found in cryoprecipitate. These include patients with von Willebrand disease, DIC, liver disease, uremia with significant bleeding, and with low or dysfunctional fibrinogen. Cryoprecipitate is considered an alternative if first-line therapy is not available. Standard of care involves the use of specific recombinant or plasma-derived factor concentrates.

Potential Complications

There is a risk of viral transmission that is similar to packed RBC (PRBC) transfusion, but with the added effect of exposure to multiple donors due to pooled units typically being infused. Other risks are similar to that of FFP, but lower overall due to smaller total volumes of plasma transfused. These include TRALI, TACO, HTR, allergic reaction, and citrate toxicity.

Complications

Any suspected transfusion reaction should be reported to the local blood bank. With reactions being a rare event, their expertise is a valuable resource to help guide management, as well as provide details for further workup necessary to appropriately diagnose complications from a transfusion. Reporting is important to prevent future reactions to the patient, as well as for quality control measures. Table 13.2 summarizes and compares key elements of complications commonly associated with blood product transfusions.

Table 13.2 Complications commonly associated with transfusion of blood products

Complication	Timeline	Risk factors	Major signs and symptoms	Treatment and further workup
TRALI	Within 6 hours of transfusion	• Incompatibility to donor HLA/HNA antibodies • Direct or indirect lung injury	• Dyspnea • Pulmonary edema with copious frothy sputum • Diffuse bilateral infiltrates on CXR • Hypotension • Fever • Leukopenia • Exudative pleural fluid	• Stop the transfusion • CXR • Oxygen therapy • Ventilatory support • Volume administration and/or vasoactive therapy
TACO	Within 12 hours of transfusion	• Preexisting cardiac, pulmonary, or renal dysfunction • Age >70 • Increased number of units transfused • Increased rate of transfusion • Delayed diuresis [12]	• Tachypnea • Dyspnea • Pulmonary edema • Desaturations • Orthopnea • Tachycardia • Increased blood pressure • Increased JVP • Widened pulse pressure	• Stop the transfusion • Oxygen support • Ventilatory support • Diuresis • BNP or NT-proBNP • Fluid balance and/or serial weights • CXR • Possibly echocardiography

	Timing	Cause	Signs and symptoms	Diagnosis/Management
			• Enlarged cardiac silhouette and diffuse bilateral infiltrates on CXR	
Hemolysis	Immediately with ABO-incompatible blood transfusion 3–10 days after transfusion of ABO-compatible blood products	• Transfusion of ABO-incompatible blood products	• Flushing • Urticaria • Dyspnea • Anxiety • Bronchospasm • Chills/rigors • Abdominal pain • Tachycardia • Fever • Hypotension • Jaundice	• Low free hemoglobin levels • Low haptoglobin levels • High bilirubin levels • Positive direct Coombs' test • Hematuria • Supportive care • Maintain adequate urinary output
Febrile reactions	Within 1–6 hours of transfusion	• Transfusion of platelets or PRBCs	• Rise in temperature >1°C from baseline during transfusion • Chills • Rigors	• Rule out life-threatening etiologies • Supportive care
Allergic reactions	Within minutes of transfusion	• IgA deficiency • Peanut allergy	• Urticaria and pruritus • Flushing • Dyspnea • Desaturations • Possibly wheezing or stridor	• Epinephrine • Diphenhydramine • Airway patency support • IV fluids

Table 13.2 (cont.)

Complication	Timeline	Risk factors	Major signs and symptoms	Treatment and further workup
			• Hypotension • Angioedema	
Sepsis	Within 30 minutes to 5 hours of transfusion	• Platelet transfusion • Longer storage time • Pooled sources for blood products	• Fever • Chills • Dyspnea • Malaise • Organ dysfunction • Shock	• Supportive care • Rule out hemolytic transfusion reaction • Send blood component to microbiology for Gram staining and culture

TRALI, ; TACO, ; BNP, B-type natriuretic peptide; NT-proBNP, N-terminal pro-BNP.

Transfusion-Associated Circulatory Overload

TACO has been associated with the most common cause of death from transfusion since 2016 [13]. Aside from preexisting cardiac, pulmonary, and/or renal disease, the risk of developing TACO increases proportionally to the number of units transfused. It is important to avoid unnecessary and excessive transfusions.

Signs and Symptoms

Cardiopulmonary distress is a cardinal feature of TACO. This includes tachypnea, dyspnea, decreased oxygen saturations, tachycardia, and hypertension. Pulmonary edema will be present. At least three of the following criteria should be met to consider TACO as the etiology of respiratory compromise: acute or worsening respiratory status; acute or worsening pulmonary edema; signs of congestive heart failure not explained by preexisting cardiac history; signs of fluid overload; and/or increased B-type natriuretic peptide (BNP) or N-terminal pro-BNP (NT-proBNP) levels [14].

Treatment

Cessation of any ongoing transfusions should be immediately done for suspected TACO reactions. The focus should be on supportive care and balancing the overloaded fluid status. Patients will typically respond to diuretic therapy, with rapid improvement in their clinical status. Oxygen supplementation is indicated for patients with saturations <90%. Consideration for ventilatory support should be made for significant respiratory deterioration. This may include noninvasive positive pressure techniques versus endotracheal intubation. Since TACO is the result of a fluid-overloaded state, resumption of transfusion may be considered once the patient has reached a stable hemodynamic state.

Further Workup

Immediate referral to the blood bank/hospital transfusion medicine service is highly recommended for consultation on how to proceed with future transfusions and workup, as well as helping in distinguishing between TACO and TRALI. It is also crucial to notify these services to prevent future reactions on the affected patient. Ordering CXR, BNP or NT-proBNP, echocardiography, and following fluid balance, arterial blood gases (ABGs), and pulse oximetry may help guide diagnosis and responsiveness to therapy.

Transfusion-Related Acute Lung Injury

This complication of transfusion is defined as a new acute lung injury (ALI)/acute respiratory distress syndrome (ARDS) with hypoxemia (i.e., room air oxygen saturation of ≤90% or PaO_2/FiO_2 ratio of <300 mmHg) and bilateral infiltrates on

CXR occurring during or within 6 hours of blood product administration. If a temporally related alternative etiology or risk factor of ALI/ARDS, such as aspiration, toxic inhalation, sepsis, pneumonia, trauma, burn injury, or pancreatitis, coincided, then the term "possible TRALI" is commonly used. TRALI is a clinical diagnosis which does not require detection of antibodies [15]. The true incidence of TRALI is unclear but is thought to range between 1 in 5000 and 12,000, and is believed to vary among patient populations, with a higher incidence in critically ill patients than in general populations [16]. Recent TRALI mitigation strategies for platelet and plasma components appear to have contributed to decreases in its incidence. Prior to 2016, TRALI was the leading cause of transfusion-related mortality, but TACO has overtaken this. TRALI occurs in any patient, all age groups, and both sexes equally. Recipient risk factors vary in published studies but commonly include: shock prior to transfusion, chronic alcohol abuse, smoking, positive fluid balance prior to transfusion, sepsis, mechanical ventilation, and liver disease or transplantation. All blood components have been implicated in TRALI. The most prominent blood component risk factors are high plasma volume components which include plasma, apheresis platelet concentrates, and whole blood, as well as female gender and increased parity of the donor. Currently, the majority of TRALI cases occur after RBC transfusions and age of storage does not seem related to incidence. The risk of TRALI is likely mediated by incompatibility to donor HLA/HNA antibodies, instead of proportionally to the number of units transfused. To decrease TRALI, many countries use a strategy of supplying transfusable plasma products exclusively from male donors, female donors without a prior pregnancy, or donors who test negative for HLA antibodies. TRALI pathogenesis is proposed to be mediated by neutrophil sequestration and priming followed by neutrophil activation; further mechanistic details are beyond the scope of this chapter.

Signs and Symptoms

Symptoms of hypoxemic respiratory insufficiency often begin within 1–2 hours of beginning the transfusion but may be delayed as long as 6 hours. Pulmonary infiltrates with a classically normal cardiac silhouette are seen on CXR. If the patient is intubated, pink, frothy secretions may be seen. Other symptoms may include fever, hypotension, tachypnea, tachycardia, and cyanosis.

Treatment

If TRALI is suspected during a transfusion, it should be discontinued immediately. Clinical treatment of TRALI is supportive, with oxygen supplementation being the fundamental intervention. Noninvasive respiratory therapies, such as high-flow oxygen, continuous airway positive pressure (CPAP), or bilevel positive airway pressure (BIPAP), may be sufficient, but endotracheal intubation and mechanical ventilation may be necessary. ARDS treatment strategies should be used for these patients. Hemodynamic support should be aimed at ensuring end-organ perfusion and may require volume administration and/or vasoactive therapy. Early diuresis should be avoided as it may exacerbate hypotension. Differentiating TRALI from TACO or, in some patients, determining a coexistence of a combination of these entities is needed prior to considering diuretic therapy. As in other causes of ARDS, routine use of steroids is not recommended. An extensive review of perioperative transfusion-related lung injuries relevant to anesthesiologists is provided by McVey and colleagues [17].

Further Workup

Immediate referral to the blood bank/hospital transfusion medicine service will lead to a transfusion reaction workup with appropriate laboratory blood tests for the recipient. The blood bank will assemble a list of all products administered in the previous 6 hours and alert the supplier, who will recall donors and initiate HLA, and possibly HLN, antibody testing. Results of this testing will not change treatment of the patient but may lead to declining further donation from a donor.

Febrile Reactions

The presence of fever without other systemic complications leads one to consider a febrile nonhemolytic reaction. This is considered after other etiologies for fever have been ruled out. It is thought that this reaction occurs due to the release of donor cytokines from white blood cells of a blood product that had not been leukoreduced. These include interleukin (IL)-1, IL-6, IL-8, and tumor necrosis factor alpha (TNFα). Although febrile nonhemolytic reactions may occur with any blood product, it is more commonly associated with platelet or RBC transfusions. It is one of the most common types of transfusion reactions, occurring at a rate of 0.1–1% of all transfusions [18].

Signs and Symptoms

These include fever (defined as temperature rising 1–2°C above the baseline) within 1–6 hours of transfusion and potentially chills and rigors. This is a diagnosis of exclusion after ruling out other etiologies for fever, including sepsis, TRALI, and HTR.

Treatment

The transfusion should be terminated immediately. Inpatient admission should be considered for workup of more serious complications of fever. Once ruled out, treatment involves primarily supportive care. Antipyretics may be useful for treatment of fever, but evidence for routine prophylactic use is limited and has not conclusively shown benefit in reducing the incidence of a febrile reaction. Meperidine may be administered for significant chills with associated shivering.

Further Workup

The transfusion medicine service should be notified for reaction workup. No further workup for febrile nonhemolytic reaction is necessary as this is a benign self-limiting reaction, although workup for severe life-threatening complications should be initiated.

Hemolytic Transfusion Reaction

HTRs can range from clinically insignificant hemolysis to life-threatening accelerated destruction of RBCs causing massive hemolysis, acute renal failure, DIC, and potentially death [19]. HTRs most commonly occur with transfusion of ABO-incompatible RBCs where recipient native antibodies form complexes with donor cellular antigens, leading to complement activation and extravascular and/or intravascular hemolysis. Rarely do HTRs occur with other blood products, but they may contain antibodies that react with recipient RBCs [20]. Acute-onset HTRs typically involve IgM-mediated antibody–antigen complexes that result in complement activation and subsequent hemolysis. Bradykinin and histamine release leads to their corresponding signs and symptoms. Kidd, Kell, Duffy, and Rh RBC antigens have been implicated in patients with a history of transfusion and alloimmunization, more often causing delayed HTRs that occur about 3–30 days after transfusion. Delayed HTRs typically occur when the recipient has IgG alloantibodies to specific antigens (from prior exposure to allogeneic blood such as from a prior blood transfusion, pregnancy, or sharing intravenous needles) that are present in donor blood products and result in a clinically insignificant extravascular hemolytic response.

Signs and Symptoms

Acute HTRs are associated with fever, chills, back pain, hypotension, urticaria, bronchospasm, dyspnea, flushing, and anxiety that occur within minutes of transfusion of ABO-incompatible blood products. Under general anesthesia, these signs may not be apparent until significant hemolysis has occurred. Signs of DIC or hemoglobinuria may be seen under general anesthesia. Delayed HTRs generally result in mild fever, hyperbilirubinemia, and sometimes anemia.

Treatment

Acute HTRs are a medical emergency. Immediate termination of the transfusion and notifying the blood bank are critical. Hemodynamic support with vasoactive agents and intravenous hydration with 0.9% sodium chloride should not be delayed for further laboratory workup. Goals are to maintain hemodynamic stability and adequate urine output to prevent further renal injury.

Further Workup

Lab draws should be obtained from a different site from where the transfusion took place, ideally on a different extremity; otherwise a separate site on the same extremity will suffice. For acute HTRs, lab work should include the following: ABO compatibility, direct and indirect Coombs' tests, urine sample, free hemoglobin level, haptoglobin, lactate dehydrogenase, bilirubin, DIC workup, electrolytes (for hyperkalemia), and serial hemoglobin levels (for anemia) [20]. HTRs are isolated incidences, but the patient should be made aware to notify their provider/blood bank about the HTR for any future transfusions, so that proper crossmatching can occur. Laboratory workup for delayed HTRs should include general testing for hemolysis, as well as an antibody screen to identify the triggering RBC antigen.

Allergic Reactions

These reactions may range from mild urticaria and pruritus to significant life-threatening anaphylactic reactions. These reactions can occur with any blood component. Seemingly mild allergic reactions can quickly escalate to a significant anaphylactic reaction, as the early signs and symptoms may be similar for all allergic reactions. Anaphylactic reactions are usually IgE- or IgG-mediated immune responses with acute severe systemic release of histamine and tryptase by mast cell and basophil degranulation. The most common allergic reactions occur in patients with an IgA deficiency who have circulating IgG anti-IgA antibodies that respond to donor IgA antigens.

Signs and Symptoms

It may manifest as mild urticaria and pruritus that are a mere annoyance to significant dyspnea, wheezing, angioedema, and hypotension. Urticaria can occur at any point of the transfusion, whereas anaphylactic reactions generally manifest within minutes of transfusion initiation.

Treatment

The transfusion should be terminated immediately, and the blood bank notified. If an anaphylactic reaction is suspected, low-dose epinephrine should be administered (0.3 mg IM of a 1 mg mL^{-1} solution or 50–100 μg IV), confirming the diagnosis of anaphylaxis based on the immediate response to epinephrine. IV fluid resuscitation for hypotension and an epinephrine infusion may be necessary for hypotensive patients refractory to initial epinephrine administration. Oxygen and bronchodilators and/or maintenance of a patent airway may be indicated if clinically significant respiratory distress occurs from bronchospasm or angioedema, respectively. If a mild urticarial reaction is suspected, after terminating the transfusion and finding no evidence for an evolving anaphylactic reaction, the patient can be given 25–50 mg diphenhydramine PO or IV to assess for the resolution of hives. If there is improvement, with no signs of hemodynamic deterioration, the transfusion may be resumed.

Further Workup

Notifying the blood bank will help prevent further anaphylactic reactions by ensuring future IgA-deficient blood products are released for the patient; tryptase levels may be helpful to confirm a true anaphylactic reaction. Workup to rule out other transfusion reactions, such as TRALI, TACO, and sepsis, should be investigated since clinical manifestation can be similar with hypotension and dyspnea.

Sepsis

Bacterial contamination represents a significant source for transfusion-related fatalities. The source of contamination can occur at any point, from the donor's skin during the initial venepuncture to the water bath used to thaw blood products. Many organisms are reported as causative of transfusion-transmitted bacterial infections, including *Staphylococcus*, *Streptococcus*, *Bacillus*, *Clostridium*, *Escherichia coli*, *Klebsiella*, *Enterobacter*, and *Pseudomonas*. Platelets are associated with the highest risk of bacterial contamination secondary to their storage in warmer conditions. The incidence and magnitude of bacterial contamination increase with the duration of storage, with >4 days being associated with an almost sixfold increase in bacterial contamination [21]. It is standard practice to divert the initial 20–40 mL of donor blood into a separate chamber to minimize the risk of contaminating the entire donation [19].

Signs and Symptoms

Sepsis is associated with fever or an increase of >2°C from baseline, tachycardia, change in systolic blood pressure of >30 mmHg, chills, and rigors. Onset of signs and symptoms varies from within 30 minutes to 5 hours of transfusion. Gram-negative organisms are associated with a more severe presentation, a quicker onset, and a higher mortality risk [21].

Treatment

The transfusion should be terminated immediately, and the blood bank and microbiology laboratory notified. Supportive care should be initiated, with treatment aimed at potential septic shock. This may include fluid resuscitation and ventilatory and vasopressor support. Septic shock may lead to multiorgan dysfunction, with an elevated risk of death. If there is a high suspicion for sepsis, treatment with broad-spectrum antibiotics should be initiated, with the intention to tailor to more specific antibiotic therapy or discontinuation of antibiotics after results of blood cultures are obtained.

Further Workup

The offending blood component should be isolated, sealed, and sent to microbiology for Gram staining and culture. Workup should be initiated to rule out an HTR since clinical manifestation can be similar.

References

1. Vo C, Roberts PR. Blood component therapy. In: CS Scher, AD Kaye, H Liu, S Perelman, S Leavitt, eds. *Essentials of Blood Product Management in Anesthesia Practice*. Cham: Springer; 2020, pp. 21–8.

2. Kleinman S. Practical aspects of red blood cell transfusion in adults: storage, processing, modifications, and infusion. Waltham, MA: UpToDate; 2022. Available from: www.uptodate.com/contents/practical-aspects-of-red-blood-cell-transfusion -in-adults-storage-processing-modifications-and-infusion.

3. American Association of Blood Banks. Five things physicians and patients should question. 2014 (updated 2022). Available from: www.choosingwisely.org/wp-content/uploads/2015/02/AABB-5things-List_2022.pdf.

4. Chong MA, Krishnan R, Cheng D, Martin J. Should transfusion trigger thresholds differ for critical care versus perioperative patients? A meta-analysis of randomized trials. *Crit Care Med*. 2018;46(2):252–63.

5. Scott E, Puca K, Heraly J, Gottschall J, Friedman K. Evaluation and comparison of coagulation factor activity in fresh-frozen plasma and 24-hour plasma at thaw and after 120 hours of 1 to 6 degrees C storage. *Transfusion*. 2009;49(8):1584–91.

6. Khawar H, Kelley W, Stevens JB, Guzman N. Fresh frozen plasma (FFP). In: *StatPearls*. Treasure Island, FL: StatPearls Publishing; 2022. Available from: www .ncbi.nlm.nih.gov/books/NBK513347/.

7. Green L, Bolton-Maggs P, Beattie C, *et al*. British Society of Haematology Guidelines on the spectrum of fresh frozen plasma and cryoprecipitate products: their handling and use in various patient groups in the absence of major bleeding. *Br J Haematol*. 2018;181(1):54–67.

8. Hunt BJ. Bleeding and coagulopathies in critical care. *N Engl J Med*. 2014;370(9):847–59.

9. Liumbruno G, Bennardello F, Lattanzio A, Piccoli P, Rossetti G. Recommendations for the transfusion of plasma and platelets. *Blood Transfus*. 2009;7(2):132–50.

10. Pandey S, Vyas GN. Adverse effects of plasma transfusion. *Transfusion*. 2012;52 (Suppl 1):65S–79S.

11. Tobian A. Clinical use of cryoprecipitate. Waltham, MA: UpToDate; 2022. Available from: www.uptodate.com/contents/clinical-use-of-cryoprecipitate.

12. Lieberman L, Maskens C, Cserti-Gazdewich C, *et al*. A retrospective review of patient factors, transfusion practices, and outcomes in patients with transfusion-associated circulatory overload. *Transfus Med Rev*. 2013;27(4):206–12.

13. US Food and Drug Administration. Fatalities reported to FDA following blood collection and transfusion: annual summary for fiscal year 2018. 2018. Available from: https://www.fda.gov/media/136907/download.

14. Wiersum-Osselton JC, Whitaker B, Grey S, *et al*. Revised international surveillance case definition of transfusion-associated circulatory overload: a classification agreement validation study. *Lancet Haematol*. 2019;6(7):e350–8.

15. Kleinman S, Vlaar APJ, Toy P, *et al*. A consensus redefinition of transfusion-related acute lung injury. *Transfusion*. 2019;59(7):2465–76.

16. Kleinman S, Kor D. Transfusion-related acute lung injury (TRALI). Waltham, MA: UpToDate; 2022. Available from: www.uptodate.com/contents/transfusion-related-acute-lung-injury-trali.

17. McVey M, Kapur R, Cserti-Gazdewich C, Semple J, Karkouti K, Kuebler W. Transfusion-related acute lung injury in the perioperative patient. *Anesthesiology*. 2019;131(3):693–715.

18. Silvergleid AJ. Approach to the patient with a suspected acute transfusion reaction. Waltham, MA: UpToDate; 2022. Available from: www.uptodate.com/contents/approach-to-the-patient-with-a-suspected-acute-transfusion-reaction?topicRef=7947&source=see_link.

19. Barash PG, Cullen BF, Stoelting RK, Cahalan MK, Stock MC, Ortega R. *Clinical Anesthesia*, 7th ed. Philadelphia, PA: Lippincott Williams & Wilkins; 2013.

20. Silvergleid AJ. Hemolytic transfusion reactions. Waltham, MA: UpToDate; 2022. Available from: www.uptodate.com/contents/hemolytic-transfusion-reactions?topicRef=7947&source=see_link.

21. Spelman D, MacLaren G. Transfusion-transmitted bacterial infection. Waltham, MA: UpToDate; 2022. Available from: www.uptodate.com/contents/transfusion-transmitted-bacterial-infection.

Chapter 14

Cardiac Anesthesiology

Alan M. Smeltz, Logan Gray, Austin Erney,
Julia Kendrick, and Matthew Graves

Introduction

The anesthetic management of patients undergoing cardiac surgery involves
meticulous preparation and persistent vigilance. In this chapter, we will discuss the general anesthetic principles that apply to all cardiac surgical procedures in the preoperative, intraoperative, and early postoperative phases. By
doing so, we aim to provide a standard approach and rationale for monitoring
and managing complex cardiac surgical patients. We will then conclude by
highlighting anesthetic considerations that are unique to specific types of
cardiac procedures.

Preoperative Evaluation

Patients requiring cardiac surgery should undergo a thorough preoperative
evaluation. The results of this assessment impact preoperative optimization,
intraoperative anesthetic management, and postoperative planning.
Recommended preoperative tests and objectives are provided in Table 14.1
[1]. A sample of a standard cardiac anesthesia setup is listed in Table 14.2.

Maintaining adequate tissue oxygen delivery and hemostasis for patients
undergoing cardiac surgery can be challenging. Adequate blood products should
be prepared, as transfusion of blood products is often necessary, though the
associated risks may complicate the decision to transfuse. The Transfusion
Requirements in Cardiac Surgery III trial concluded a restrictive transfusion
threshold of 7.5 g dL^{-1} had noninferior outcomes to a more liberal transfusion
threshold and can be used to guide the administration of red blood cells [2]. Other
factors indicating inadequate oxygen delivery, such as low mixed venous oxygen
saturation and lactic acidosis, may also support the decision to either transfuse or
hemoconcentrate blood to raise the hemoglobin level and oxygen-carrying capacity. The use of plasma, platelets, cryoprecipitate, or other factors should be guided
by laboratory testing and clinical bleeding. For patients who refuse blood transfusions, a thorough discussion identifying acceptable alternative strategies in the
preoperative period is essential. These alternatives may include the preoperative
use of erythropoietin, iron, and vitamin B12 and folate supplementation, as well as
intraoperative acute normovolemic hemodilution, cell salvage, and recombinant

Table 14.1 Recommended tests before cardiac surgery

Test	Objective
Complete blood count	To detect anemia, thrombocytopenia, and infection
Basic metabolic panel	To detect renal disease, electrolyte abnormalities, and poor glycemic control
Hemoglobin A1c	To diagnose and determine the severity of diabetes mellitus
Liver function tests	To detect unknown liver disease
Coagulation profile	To detect unknown coagulation disorders
Pulmonary function tests	To aid in differentiating between restrictive and obstructive pathology, and in ventilator weaning
Brain natriuretic peptide	When elevated, there is increased risk of atrial arrhythmias and prolonged postoperative stay
Thyroid function tests	To detect thyroid dysfunction
Blood type and crossmatch	To allow for rapid blood preparation and transfusion, if needed
Echocardiography	To detect undiagnosed pathology that may determine hemodynamic goals, selection of appropriate monitors, and need for circulatory support
Cardiac catheterization	To evaluate coronary disease, patency of previous grafts, gather information about coronary anatomy and potential targets for grafting, and confirm chamber pressure and severity of pulmonary hypertension
Carotid Doppler[a]	To detect carotid stenosis and determine perioperative stroke risk
Chest radiograph	To evaluate lung fields, detect aortic calcification and pleural effusions, and help identify sternal wires that are a sign of prior sternotomy and implanted medical devices

[a] Recommended in patients with a history of transient ischaemic attack or stroke or patients >65 years old with carotid bruits or peripheral vascular disease.

Table 14.2 Cardiac anesthesia setup

Standard items:

- Airway equipment necessary to facilitate masking and endotracheal intubation
- Induction medications, emergency resuscitative medications, heparin, and protamine
- Rack of pumps, with infusions on a carrier
- Infusions (either available in the room or "on pump") may include vasopressors, vasodilators, inotropes, propofol, antibiotics, insulin, antifibrinolytics, etc.
- Equipment to place arterial and venous lines, including triple transducer setup and ultrasound machine
- Transesophageal echocardiography machine and probe, lubrication, bite block, and patient's information programmed
- Cooler with blood products, checked
- Miscellaneous: pacer box, patient sticker with barcode, defibrillator pads, and machine

Items to consider in special circumstances:

- Pulmonary artery catheter, continuous cardiac output monitor
- Lung isolation equipment
- Inhaled pulmonary vasodilator device
- Cerebral oximetry
- Bags of ice

clotting factors [3]. Of note, normovolemic hemodilution is contraindicated in severe aortic stenosis, left main coronary artery disease, and preoperative hemoglobin concentration <11 g dL^{-1}. Contraindications to using cell salvage include infection, malignancy, and use of topical hemostatic agents. Of note, platelets and coagulation factors are removed during the washing process, promoting dilutional thrombocytopenia and reduction in clotting factors. Additionally, attempts should be made to prevent fibrinolysis through the use of either tranexamic acid or aminocaproic acid.

Patients undergoing repeat cardiac surgery have adhesive scar encasement of cardiovascular structures and are at risk of sudden massive hemorrhage with repeat sternotomy and mediastinal dissection. CT of the chest should be performed to ascertain the retrosternal position of these structures [4]. In high-risk patients, it may be necessary to preemptively expose the femoral vessels or even establish peripheral cardiopulmonary bypass prior to sternotomy. Additional units of blood should be readily available and external defibrillator pads should be considered also for these cases.

Any implanted cardiac electronic device should be evaluated prior to cardiac surgery. Important variables to assess include the type of device (e.g.,

Table 14.3 Recommendations for holding medications prior to cardiac surgery

Medication	Recommendation
Adenosine diphosphate inhibitors	Stop at least 5 days prior to surgery
Coumadin	Stop 3–5 days prior to surgery
Direct thrombin inhibitor	Stop 2–4 days prior to surgery
Direct factor Xa inhibitor	Stop 2 days prior to surgery
Glycoprotein IIb/IIIa inhibitors	Do not take on the day of surgery
Angiotensin-converting enzyme inhibitors	Do not take on the day of surgery
Angiotensin receptor blockers	Do not take on the day of surgery

single- or dual-lead pacemaker, biventricular resynchronization pacemaker, implantable cardiac defibrillator), pacemaker dependency, device functionality, and the patient's underlying rhythm. Pacemakers usually require reprogramming to pace in asynchronous mode, with any tachytherapies disabled to avoid device activation or inhibition by electrical artifacts. In particular, the use of surgical electrocautery in close proximity to the device leads to extensive electromagnetic interference. Patients with disabled tachytherapies should always have external defibrillator pads in place.

Chronically taken cardiac-specific medications that should be continued throughout the perioperative period include statins, aspirin, and beta-blockers. Those that may need to be held prior to cardiac surgery are listed in Table 14.3. Additional medications to consider in the preoperative setting include a benzodiazepine for anxiolysis and fentanyl for analgesia during preinduction arterial catheter placement. Benzodiazepines and fentanyl should be used judiciously, however, to avoid excessive sedation, hypoventilation, hypercarbia, hypoxemia, and increased pulmonary arterial pressure. This is especially concerning in patients with preexisting pulmonary hypertension and/or right ventricular dysfunction.

Intraoperative Management

Monitoring

In addition to standard American Society of Anesthesiologists monitors, patients receiving cardiac surgery also require monitoring of continuous five-lead ECG with automated ST-segment analysis, processed EEG to minimize the risk of intraoperative awareness, nerve stimulation of motor activity to ensure immobility, arterial and central venous pressure monitoring to detect sudden changes in hemodynamics, both nasal and bladder temperature monitoring to trend changes induced by cardiopulmonary bypass (CPB), urinary output for assessing end-organ perfusion, and possibly also pulmonary artery pressure, mixed venous oxygen saturation, and cerebral oximetry. Prevailing evidence does not support routine pulmonary artery catheterization. Reasons to place a pulmonary artery catheter include significantly reduced left or right ventricular function, severe diastolic dysfunction, recent myocardial infarction, significant pulmonary hypertension, or high surgical complexity [5]. Transesophageal echocardiography (TEE) is an invaluable tool that is also utilized in cardiac anesthesia. Tables 14.4, 14.5, and 14.6 describe some of the many applications of TEE in cardiac anesthesia, as well as indications and contraindications to use [6].

Frequent perioperative laboratory tests include activated clotting time (ACT) to ensure adequacy of anticoagulation, and "loaded" arterial blood gas analysis to evaluate dynamic changes in glucose levels, hemoglobin, electrolytes, and acid–base status. It may also be necessary to assess intraoperative coagulation parameters such as platelet count, international normalized ratio, fibrinogen level, and viscoelastic tests, to identify specific mechanisms that contribute to nonsurgical bleeding.

Induction of General Anesthesia

To prevent an insurmountable spiral of circulatory collapse, efforts should be made to minimize hemodynamic fluctuations throughout the induction of general anesthesia. Strategies to achieve this might include an opioid and benzodiazepine combination, etomidate, ketamine, an inhalational agent, or small titrated boluses of agents such as propofol, with concurrent monitoring of hemodynamics and vasopressor or inotrope administration. In addition, other peri-induction agents given to facilitate orotracheal intubation include intravenous lidocaine and neuromuscular blockade. There are specific situations where preservation of spontaneous ventilation should be attempted, such as severe pulmonary hypertension, right ventricular failure, or cardiac tamponade. Patients with these disease processes are especially sensitive to effects of positive pressure ventilation, leading to increases in right ventricular afterload and right ventricular failure. Some additional indications to further tailor the technique of anesthetic induction are described below in corresponding sections under "Surgery-Specific Considerations."

Access

An intraarterial catheter is typically placed prior to the induction of anesthesia. A second arterial line can also be placed for continuous monitoring of blood pressure, while obtaining blood samples and monitoring blood pressure on either side of a vascular repair. Large-bore peripheral and central venous access is

Table 14.4 Role of transesophageal echocardiography in cardiac surgery

Evaluation	Impact
LV and RV systolic function	Aids in determining appropriate monitors, fluid resuscitation, pharmacologic agents, and perioperative mechanical circulatory support
LV diastolic function	Aids in determining optimum heart rate to allow for maximum cardiac output
Regional wall motion abnormalities	Aids in early detection of ischemia and is predictive of long-term adverse cardiac events
Ventricular dimensions	Aids in determining failure of the left or right ventricle. Ventricles that undergo chamber dilatation are less sensitive to preload and extremely sensitive to increased afterload
Valvular function	Evaluating the severity of valvular lesions aids in determining hemodynamic goals and may prompt surgical intervention
Aortic atheroma	The presence of large or mobile atheromas have been associated with a higher incidence of postoperative stroke
Pericardial diseases and effusion	Large pericardial effusions could indicate tamponade pathology. Patients with pericarditis or pericardial constriction typically have significant blood loss
Anatomic defects	Previously undiagnosed anatomic defects may alter the surgical plan. Septal defects can result in RV volume overload and pulmonary hypertension. It is important to look for additional associated congenital cardiac anomalies (i.e., coronary sinus defects, partial anomalous venous connection, or cleft anterior mitral valve leaflet)
Arterial or mural thrombus	Thrombus in the left atrial appendage or apex of the left ventricle may prompt thrombectomy or ligation of the left atrial appendage. The presence of the thrombus should be confirmed with TEE both during and after surgery
Guide line/cannula placement	Direct visualization can aid in placement of lines and cannulae
De-airing procedures	Direct visualization of the ventricle can aid in this procedure to avoid air embolism
Surgical feedback	Immediate feedback with the surgical team regarding the adequacy of surgical repairs and possible collateral injury can prompt additional intervention prior to leaving the operating room

LV, left ventricular; RV, right ventricular; TEE, transesophageal echocardiography.

Table 14.5 Indications for transesophageal echocardiography

Valvular procedures
Thoracic aortic surgical procedures
Transcatheter intracardiac procedures (undergoing general anesthesia)
Congenital heart surgery with cardiopulmonary bypass
Hypertrophic cardiomyopathy surgery
Resection of cardiac mass
Ventricular remodeling surgery
Heart transplantation
Pericardiectomy
Ventricular assist device insertion
Cannula positioning
Septal defect closures
Atrial appendage obliteration
CABG[a]
Unexplained hemodynamic instability during any surgical procedure

[a] Should be considered for CABG and off-pump CABG. Generally recommended for patients with abnormal ventricular function, though may play an important role in all cases.
CABG, coronary artery bypass graft.

routinely obtained to monitor pressures and enable rapid administration of intravenous fluids, blood products, and vasoactive and inotropic medications. Ultrasound guidance should be used to guide placement of central catheters to assess for venous patency and minimize the risk of iatrogenic puncture of neighboring neural, vascular, or pleural structures. An introducer can be used to place a pulmonary artery catheter, a catheter with additional lumens, temporary transvenous pacing wires, or a retrograde cardioplegia catheter.

General Precardiopulmonary Bypass Management

General anesthesia can be maintained with volatile and/or intravenous agents, with special attention paid to both the hemodynamics, as well as the depth of anesthesia, given the high incidence of intraoperative awareness associated

Table 14.6 Contraindications to transesophageal echocardiography

Absolute contraindications	Relative contraindications
Esophageal stricture	Esophageal varices
Esophageal trauma	Acute esophagitis
Esophageal tumor	Barrett's esophagus
Postesophageal surgery	Restriction of neck mobility (severe cervical arthritis/atlantoaxial joint disease)
Tracheoesophageal fistula	History of radiation of the neck and mediastinum
Acute upper GI bleed	Coagulopathy History of GI surgery Recent upper GI bleed Acute peptic ulcer disease

GI, gastrointestinal.

with cardiac surgery. Long-acting neuromuscular blockade and adequate analgesia should be maintained throughout the procedure to achieve immobility and blunt the autonomic pain response, respectively. Mean arterial pressure should be maintained within 20% of each patient's baseline, with systolic blood pressure reduced to 100 mmHg prior to arterial cannulation to minimize the risk of aortic dissection. Once the arterial cannula is in place, blood pressure should again be raised to ensure blood pressure is adequate to tolerate retrograde autologous priming ("RAP") of the CPB circuit where blood is withdrawn from the patient. In anticipation of the expected hemodilution that occurs with the initiation of CPB, it may be necessary to prime the bypass circuit with packed red blood cells for patients starting off with extreme anemia. Lung-protective ventilation, such as tidal volumes of 6 mL kg^{-1} of ideal body weight, positive end-expiratory pressure of 5 mmHg, and maintaining peak airway pressure <40 mmHg, should generally be employed. Notable exceptions to this include use of smaller tidal volumes to minimize lung expansion during internal mammary artery dissection and redo sternotomy. Ventilation is usually held altogether for first-time sternotomy. Many factors contribute to both surgical and nonsurgical bleeding in cardiac surgical patients. Preemptive preparation of blood products and blood conservation techniques are covered in "Preoperative Evaluation."

Anticoagulation

Exposure of blood to the synthetic surfaces of the CPB circuit triggers inflammatory cascades, platelet dysfunction, and activation of both the intrinsic and extrinsic coagulation pathways. Thankfully, widespread thrombosis can generally be prevented altogether by using high doses of anticoagulation prior to the initiation of CPB. Due to the availability of a direct reversal agent, the primary anticoagulant used is unfractionated heparin. Heparin binds antithrombin III (AT-III) to decrease the activity of thrombin and factor Xa. For patients with ongoing platelet factor 4 (PF4) antibodies predisposing them to heparin-induced thrombocytopenia (HIT) or a known hypersensitivity reaction to heparin, alternatives include bivalirudin, argatroban, and removal of PF4 antibodies by plasmapheresis. The short half-life of bivalirudin makes it a more favorable second choice, though argatroban may be preferable in patients with reduced kidney function [7].

Initial dosing of heparin is 300–400 units kg^{-1}, with additional doses titrated to achieve an ACT of 400–480 seconds [8]. An alternative measure of anticoagulation involves the use of ex vivo heparin dose–response testing, which, despite failure to demonstrate a reduction in bleeding or blood transfusions, has been used with increasing popularity. Heparin "resistance" can occur in patients with hereditary or acquired AT-III deficiency and may be seen in patients with sepsis, platelet dysfunction, or heparin-binding proteins, or in those on long-term heparin therapy [9]. This deficiency can be overcome through the administration of fresh frozen plasma or recombinant AT-III. Once heparinized, ACT should be monitored at least every 30 minutes.

Management on Cardiopulmonary Bypass

Both initiation and separation from CPB are critical events during cardiac surgery that require careful coordination among the surgeon, anesthesiologist, and perfusionist. Sample checklists outlining the necessary items that must occur prior to each of these events are provided in Table 14.7. Following the initiation of CPB, there is an expected drop in blood pressure as systemic viscosity rapidly declines, and vasopressor support may be necessary if blood pressure does not recover within 1 minute. As CPB flows are increased to "full flow" (2.2–2.4 L/(min m^2)), the heart and lungs become fully bypassed, pulsatility is lost on the arterial waveform and pulse oximeter, the ventilator can be turned off, as necessary, to minimize movement of the operative field, and anesthesia machine alarms and pulse oximetry volume should be temporarily suspended. Unless a total intravenous anesthetic is being used, the delivery of volatile agent will need to transition from the ventilator to the CPB circuit. Vasopressors and dilators should be used to achieve a mean arterial pressure ≥65 mmHg and a mixed venous oxygen saturation ≥75%. Given a shared responsibility of all members to maintain adequate hemodynamics when on CPB, and the myriad of situations where flow might be low (whether intentionally or not), close communication with the perfusionist is essential to

Table 14.7 Checklist for initiating and separating from cardiopulmonary bypass

	Initiating CPB	Separation from CPB
Laboratory values	ACT at least 400–480 seconds Hct adequate to tolerate hemodilution	Ensure normal Hct and electrolytes (lower K^+ and give Ca^{2+})
Anesthetic	Decide: anesthesiologist versus perfusionist (volatile versus TIVA)	Transition from perfusionist to anesthesiologist, as appropriate
Machine	Ventilator may be turned off when on full bypass Alarms suspended to bypass mode Pulse oximetry muted MAP BP only	Recruit lungs, resume ventilation Alarms turned back on Normal settings
Monitors	Ensure functional monitoring of arterial pressure, CVP, PCWP, and TEE	Normothermia and other vital signs normal Transducers rezeroed and leveled TEE turned back on
Patient/field	Cannulae in place, no kinks or air, no SVC drainage obstruction Empty urinary catheter	TEE: rule out intracardiac air; evaluate volume, contractility, surgical repair, etc. Evaluate SVR and rhythm; consider pacing wires
Support	As necessary	As necessary (pharmacologic ± mechanical)

ACT, activated clotting time; K^+, potassium; Ca^{2+}, calcium; TIVA, total intravenous anesthesia; MAP, mean arterial pressure; CVP, central venous pressure; PCWP, pulmonary capillary wedge pressure; TEE, transesophageal echocardiography; SVC, superior vena caval; SVR, systemic vascular resistance.

manage hemodynamics. Electrolytes should be maintained normal and glucose should be kept <180 mg dL^{-1}. Core temperature might be lowered to decrease tissue oxygen demand and injury during periods of ischemia.

Common Problems Immediately Postcardiopulmonary Bypass

Numerous complications can manifest following CPB, among which the more common include myocardial dysfunction, vasoplegia, disorders in hemostasis, and incomplete surgical repair or new collateral injury. These might result from inadequate myocardial protection during periods of ischemia, reperfusion injury, coronary spasm, kinked graft or embolism of debris or air, heightened inflammatory responses, endocrine dysfunction, labile volume status and decreased myocardial tolerance of chamber distension, electrolyte imbalances, and accumulation of pericardial material (e.g., hematoma) following chest closure. Given the expansive differential diagnosis of hypotension and inadequate perfusion following cardiac surgery, comprehensive echocardiographic, laboratory, and hemodynamic pressure monitoring is necessary to guide the administration of fluids, blood products, vasoactive agents, inhaled pulmonary vasodilators, inotropes, and clotting factors. Depending on how refractory complications are to management, it may be appropriate to discuss with the surgical team whether it would be appropriate to initiate some form of mechanical circulatory support, including an intraaortic balloon pump (IABP), ventricular assist device (VAD), or extracorporeal membrane oxygenation (ECMO). Once it has been determined that the patient will not need to return to CPB for further intervention, heparin is reversed with protamine (1 mg per 100 units heparin) to achieve normalization of ACT. Careful administration of protamine is vital as it can cause profound hypotension, for example if it is administered too quickly.

Postoperative Management

Transport

Transport of critically ill cardiac surgical patients carries significant risk. Depending on the condition of the patient, patient transport may include a surgeon, an anesthesiologist, a perfusionist, and a respiratory therapist. Roles during transport include moving the bed, tending to the vital sign monitor, medication infusion settings, and rack of pumps and lines, providing ventilation for the patient manually or via a transport ventilator, and transport of a cooler of blood products, extracorporeal circuit(s), VAD monitor, and inhaled pulmonary vasodilator device. Additional items to bring include a full tank of supplemental oxygen, a pacemaker box, suction devices for chest tube drains, emergency medications, airway equipment, and devices capable of delivering rescue electrical shocks, as necessary. Clear communication and thorough handoff of care are paramount to mitigate lapses in attention given to important issues.

Extubation

Previous Enhanced Recovery After Surgery pathways for cardiac surgery have promoted the use of short-acting hypnotic drugs, ultrashort-acting opioids, and reduced total opioid doses [10]. This has resulted in earlier time to extubation (within 6 hours of surgery) and shorter intensive care unit (ICU) stay, with no increased need for reintubation, and no difference in morbidity and mortality or overall hospital stay. Prolonged mechanical ventilation after cardiac surgery, on the other hand, is associated with longer hospitalization, higher morbidity and mortality, increased cost, and increased incidence of ventilator-associated pneumonia and dysphagia. Finally, patients should be free of myocardial ischemia, infarction, or heart failure, and be hemodynamically stable, with limited inotropic support and adequate blood gas values while on minimal ventilator settings prior to extubation.

Historically, parenteral opioids were the mainstay of postoperative pain management after cardiac surgery. However, cardiac anesthesia has recently shifted from a high-dose narcotic technique to a more multimodal approach using moderate-dose narcotics, shorter-acting muscle relaxants, and volatile anesthetic agents, facilitating earlier tracheal extubation. Some nonnarcotic modalities include regional nerve blocks, supplementary nonsteroidal antiinflammatory drugs (NSAIDs), and acetaminophen.

Surgery-Specific Considerations

In addition to the involved setup and proceedings common to the majority of cardiac surgical procedures, there are many specific situations that further complicate anesthetic management. Selected types of cases and their unique challenges to the anesthesiology team are detailed below.

Valve Replacement/Repair

Specific hemodynamic goals for patients with valvular disease are given in Table 14.8. A thorough TEE evaluation is essential both before and after valve replacement/repair to aid in surgical planning and then to identify/grade the severity of residual disease. In particular, there are several potential complications that can result from anatomical distortion and placement of circumferential sutures around the valvular annulus. In particular, defects to the electrical conduction system, neighboring valve injury, compromised coronary blood flow, and new dynamic left ventricular outflow tract obstruction should be ruled out.

"Off-Pump" Cases

The use of CPB enables adequate perfusion and gas exchange, despite heart and lung manipulation, as well as rapid blood temperature control.

Table 14.8 Induction and maintenance strategies for various valvular pathology

Valvular disease	Induction	Maintenance
Aortic stenosis	Avoid hypotension (treat aggressively with fluids and α-agonists), avoid tachycardia, caution with dilators (NTG), preload-dependent	Increase LV preload, normal to slow HR, NSR, maintain contractility, modest increase in SVR, maintain PVR
Aortic regurgitation	High normal HR with afterload reduction	Normal to increased LV preload, modest increase in HR, NSR, maintain contractility and PVR, decrease SVR
Mitral stenosis	Avoid hypotension/hypovolemia, careful with pulmonary edema, maintain SVR, avoid tachycardia	Normal to increased LV preload, decreased HR, NSR, maintain contractility, normal SVR, avoid increased PVR
Mitral regurgitation	Maintain preload and contractility, reduce afterload, avoid increased PVR	Normal to increased LV preload, increased HR, NSR, maintain contractility, decrease SVR, avoid increased PVR
Tricuspid regurgitation	Maintain preload and contractility, avoid increased PVR	Adequate preload, normal to increased HR, normal contractility, avoid increased PVR

NTG, nitroglycerin; LV, left ventricular; HR, heart rate; NSR, normal sinus rhythm; SVR, systemic vascular resistance; PVR, pulmonary vascular resistance.

However, many procedures can be performed "off pump." For these cases, it may be difficult to maintain stable hemodynamics and close communication with the surgical team is paramount. In particular, myocardial stabilizers, surgical retractors that minimize cardiac movement, and manipulation of cardiovascular structures may compromise chamber filling and ejection. Also, though full aortic cross-clamps are not used, partial "side-biting" clamps might be used, restricting blood flow. It is also important to maintain ambient room temperature and utilize external conductive and/or convective warming systems to minimize the effects of evaporative cooling. Minimizing ventilatory tidal volumes is often necessary to decrease the movement of cardiac structures. A perfusionist is always present during these cases, should the patient become too unstable and require CPB.

Minimally Invasive Procedures

For minimally invasive procedures, surgeons perform either a partial sternotomy or a thoracotomy, instead of a full sternotomy, for access and exposure. For these cases, lung isolation and/or smaller tidal volumes are often necessary. Less surgical exposure might lead to lengthier procedures, the need for intravascularly placed lines or devices (e.g., retrograde cardioplegia catheter insertion through an introducer or a balloon-tipped catheter to occlude flow in the ascending aorta, in lieu of an external cross-clamp), and difficult repair of surgical mishaps. Further, in the event of cardiac arrest, direct cardiac massage or delivery of an electric shock might not be possible and therefore, peripheral cannulation access for CPB and external defibrillator pads are important considerations.

Aortic Arch Repairs

For repairs of the distal ascending aorta and aortic arch, the presence of aortic disease and need for surgical exposure may preclude aortic cannulation and cross-clamping for CPB. In lieu of these techniques, alternative strategies of cerebral protection are required. Depending on the extent of vascular disease, vessels such as either the innominate or the right axillary artery, can be cannulated to initiate CPB and full body induction of deep hypothermia. To facilitate cerebral cooling, bags of ice can be applied externally to the patient's head. Once metabolic demand is sufficiently reduced, either temporary whole-body circulatory arrest or selective cerebral perfusion may be performed while the surgeon completes the final anastomoses. Afterward, full CPB flows are restored to the body and rewarming begins.

For these procedures, bilateral invasive blood pressure monitoring is usually required. This can be especially useful to monitor the pressure of anterograde cerebral perfusion (i.e., using a right upper extremity arterial line) and detect discrepancies in flow on either side of the final repair. Coagulopathy and platelet dysfunction can be especially difficult to manage following deep hypothermia.

Septal Myectomy

Patients undergoing septal myectomy (also known as "debulking") are at especially high risk of hemodynamic collapse with the induction of anesthesia, resulting from dynamic left ventricular outflow tract obstruction and diastolic dysfunction. Efforts should therefore be made to avoid tachycardia and maintain adequate systemic vascular resistance and left ventricular preload, especially prior to the repair. Hypotension should be preferentially managed with phenylephrine and volume resuscitation over inotropic agents, and normal sinus rhythm should be maintained. Following the repair, care should be maintained to rule out any new iatrogenic defects of the electrical conduction system and/or interventricular septum.

Left Ventricular Assist Devices

Patients with advanced heart failure may require implantation of a left ventricular assist device (LVAD) to function as either destination therapy or as a bridge to heart transplantation. Factors that might complicate or contraindicate LVAD placement include greater than mild right ventricular dysfunction, mural thrombus at the LVAD inflow cannulation site, extensive ascending aortic disease at the LVAD outflow cannulation site, and small left ventricular internal chamber size. Cardiac pathology requiring concurrent repair to enable proper LVAD function includes intracardiac shunting, including a patent foramen ovale, greater than mild aortic insufficiency, greater than mild mitral stenosis, and severe tricuspid regurgitation. LVADs are generally placed on CPB, but without aortic cross-clamping and cardiac arrest – that is, assuming no other concurrent repairs are necessary. TEE is invaluable in assisting the surgical team with proper cannula positioning and titration of optimal pump flow. Excessive LVAD flows can lead to left ventricular chamber collapse (also known as "suck-down"), a condition that leads to an abrupt cessation of blood flow. Maintenance of adequate function of the right ventricle is especially critical, as a properly functioning LVAD increases right ventricular preload, which can lead to progressive chamber dilatation and failure.

Heart Transplantation

Multidisciplinary coordination of when anesthesia and surgical preparation of a heart transplant recipient should commence is challenging, yet very important. Additional preparation unique to this procedure may include the need for aspiration precautions, initiation of perioperative immunosuppression, reversal of prophylactic anticoagulation (e.g., for patients on warfarin for an LVAD), and additional hemostatic agents/blood products. Posttransplantation, TEE should be used to evaluate for early graft dysfunction and stenoses at anastomotic sites. Additional pharmacologic or mechanical support may be necessary to manage right ventricular failure, decreased systemic vascular resistance, and bleeding following CPB separation.

Pericardial Window or Resection of Anterior Mediastinal Mass

Whether due to pericardial fluid or an anterior mediastinal mass, external compression on central cardiovascular structures can lead to cardiac tamponade pathophysiology. In this setting, some or all chambers of the heart are restricted in their ability to fully expand and fill between contractions, compromising cardiac output. In general, the thinner-walled right-sided chambers tend to be the most affected. These patients benefit from maintenance of adequate heart rate, preload, contractility, and systemic vascular resistance. Of utmost importance, efforts should be made to minimize any further increases in intrathoracic pressure and pulmonary vascular resistance. This often involves the maintenance of spontaneous ventilation throughout the induction of anesthesia, via either inhalational agents or ketamine, or small titrated doses of agents such as etomidate or propofol. In addition to predisposing to the collapse of cardiovascular structures with positive pressure ventilation, the presence of mediastinal masses also predisposes to airway collapse. Induction strategies include awake fiberoptic intubation to place the tip of a reinforced endotracheal tube beyond the point of obstruction. It is recommended that rigid bronchoscopy be readily available, as needed, in these patients. Due to the heightened risk in these patients, it is advisable to have the surgical team in the room, with the patient prepped and draped for surgery prior to the induction of anesthesia.

Catheter-Based Cardiac Procedures

Catheter-based cardiac procedures serve as an alternative to surgery for many types of cardiac diseases. On the one hand, avoidance of large surgical incisions and CPB has been associated with improved outcomes and decreased hospital length of stay. On the other hand, procedures performed outside of a standard operating room setting in the absence of surgical access pose unique challenges. For many of these procedures, a cardiothoracic surgery team and CPB machine should be in the room in case they are needed to repair an iatrogenic injury in the event of a mishap. Possible inadvertent damage can include an aortic or ventricular wall perforation, cardiac tamponade, valve leaflet or subvalvular apparatus tear, acute coronary ostial obstruction, and electrical conduction defect. Whether or not the patient is under sedation or intubated for general anesthesia can determine whether or not transthoracic echocardiography or TEE is used to monitor and diagnose periprocedural success and complications.

Lead Extraction

Reasons pacemaker leads might require LASER-assisted extraction include infection, venous occlusion, device recall/failure, and device upgrade. Perioperatively, the device should be evaluated and reprogrammed, and a temporary transvenous pacemaker and/or transcutaneous pads may be placed. Avulsion injury to cardiac structures can occur with lead extraction, leading to complications similar to those that may be seen with transcatheter procedures (see "Catheter-Based Cardiac Procedures"), as well as pneumothorax.

References

1. Szelkowski LA, Puri NK, Singh R, *et al.* Current trends in preoperative, intraoperative, and postoperative care of the adult cardiac surgery patient. *Curr Probl Surg.* 2015;52:531–69.

2. Shehata N, Whitlock R, Fergusson DA, *et al.* Transfusion Requirements in Cardiac Surgery III (TRICS III): study design of a randomized controlled trial. *J Cardiothorac Vasc Anesth.* 2018;32:121–9.

3. Hughes DB, Ullery BW, Barie PS. The contemporary approach to the care of Jehovah's Witnesses. *J Trauma.* 2008;65:237–47.

4. Roselli EE. Reoperative cardiac surgery: challenges and outcomes. *Tex Heart Inst J.* 2011;38:669–71.

5. Sandham JD, Hull RD, Brant RF, *et al.* A randomized, controlled trial of the use of pulmonary-artery catheters in high-risk surgical patients. *N Engl J Med.* 2003;348:5–14.

6. Nicoara A, Swaminathan M. Diastolic dysfunction, diagnostic and perioperative management in cardiac surgery. *Curr Opin Anaesthesiol.* 2015;28:60–6.

7. Agarwal S, Ullom B, Al-Baghdadi Y, *et al.* Challenges encountered with argatroban anticoagulation during cardiopulmonary bypass. *J Anaesthesiol Clin Pharmacol.* 2012;28:106–10.

8. Shore-Lesserson L, Baker RA, Ferraris VA, *et al.* The Society of Thoracic Surgeons, The Society of Cardiovascular Anesthesiologists, and The American Society of ExtraCorporeal Technology: clinical practice guidelines – anticoagulation during cardiopulmonary bypass. *Ann Thorac Surg.* 2018;105:650–62.

9. Avidan MS, Levy JH, van Aken H, *et al.* Recombinant human antithrombin III restores heparin responsiveness and decreases activation of coagulation in heparin-resistant patients during cardiopulmonary bypass. *J Thorac Cardiovasc Surg.* 2005;130:107–13.

10. Myles PS, Daly DJ, Djaiani G, *et al.* A systematic review of the safety and effectiveness of fast-track cardiac anesthesia. *Anesthesiology.* 2003;99:982–7.

Chapter 15

Vascular Anesthesia
Jeffrey Park

Introduction

Anesthetic management of vascular surgery is highly demanding, due to physiologic perturbations caused by major vascular procedures, as well as the high burden of existing atherosclerotic disease or disease equivalents that are often poorly controlled in this patient population. The perioperative care of the vascular patient is often complex, requiring a thorough preoperative evaluation, sophisticated intraoperative management, and attentive postoperative care. Of paramount importance to the anesthesiologist is the likelihood of major adverse cardiac events (MACEs), the incidence of which may be mitigated by appropriate risk stratification and a detailed understanding of specific major vascular surgical procedures.

Preoperative Assessment and Risk Stratification

Among noncardiac surgical procedures, the risk of MACEs has remained highest in vascular surgery, accounting for 7.7% of cases between 2004 and 2013 [1]. Prior myocardial infarction (MI) or stroke are both important independent risk factors for MACE, so appropriate screening, evaluation, and testing of these and other high-risk patients who present for elective vascular surgery may reduce their overall risk.

Preoperative testing for nonemergent vascular surgery varies widely; it is important to note that there are no Class I recommendations for testing supported by the American College of Cardiology (ACC) and American Heart Association (AHA). The following table outlines the recommendations of the ACC/AHA for supplemental tests that may be of use in specific clinical scenarios and patient populations (see Table 15.1). The decision for testing should be made with consensus agreement among the surgeon, anesthesiologist, and cardiologist, if applicable.

There is more substantial evidence regarding coronary revascularization and management of such patients. Routine coronary revascularization is not recommended, but patients who meet cardiac indications for undergoing percutaneous coronary intervention should delay noncardiac surgery, depending on the intervention (14 days after percutaneous old balloon

Table 15.1 Common preoperative tests and recommendations in noncardiac surgery

12-lead ECG	• Class IIa recommendation – should be considered for a history of coronary artery disease, significant arrhythmia, peripheral artery disease, and stroke • Class IIb recommendation – may be considered in asymptomatic patients without a history of the above
Transthoracic echocardiography	• Class IIa recommendation – should be considered in patients with a history of HF and a change in clinical status, and dyspnea without known origin • Class IIb recommendation – may be considered in clinically stable HF patients without a recent (<1 year) echocardiogram • Class III recommendation – there is no evidence of benefit in performing routine echocardiography in asymptomatic patients
Exercise or pharmacologic stress testing	• Class IIa recommendation – patients with excellent functional capacity (>10 METs) require no further testing • Class IIb recommendation – a stress test can be performed for patients with poor or unknown functional capacity if the test result will change management
Coronary angiography	• Class III recommendation – routine preoperative coronary angiography is not recommended

HF, heart failure; MET, metabolic equivalent.
Source: Adapted from 2014 ACC/AHA recommendations.

angioplasty (POBA), 30 days after bare metal stent (BMS), and 365 days after drug-eluting stent (DES)) [2].

Special circumstances and pathologies may warrant additional investigation. The presence of valvular lesions, pulmonary hypertension and/or right ventricular (RV) dysfunction, and indwelling pacemakers or an automatic implantable–cardioverter defibrillator (AICD) should prompt further evaluation and involve expert consultation, if possible, as these factors tend to be independently associated with a greater incidence of MACEs [3].

The anesthesiologist should also consider, in addition to the risk of MACEs, the impact of major vascular surgery on postoperative renal function. The balance of oxygen supply and demand is often disrupted during intraoperative fluid shifts and the physiologic demands of anesthesia; maintenance of mean arterial pressure within strict parameters can help to preserve baseline renal perfusion. Renal comorbidities (chronic kidney disease, hypertension, insulin-dependent diabetes, peripheral vascular disease) and intraoperative risk factors (intraabdominal surgery, aortic reconstruction and/or cross-clamping, use of intraoperative bypass) all contribute to the incidence of postoperative acute kidney injury (AKI) [4]. Measurement of serum creatinine concentration and urine output may be helpful in managing suspected AKI; however, options for pharmacologic management are limited, with some evidence supporting the use of dexmedetomidine infusion in cardiac surgery [5]. Diuretic therapy and previously touted renal protective agents, such as dopamine and fenoldopam, have not been proven to reduce postoperative AKI. Severe injury may progress to acute renal failure, and in these cases, the decision of whether or not to initiate renal replacement therapy (RRT) should be considered within the larger clinical context; there are some data to suggest that there may be a trend towards decreased mortality in intensive care unit (ICU) patients who are started on RRT early versus late [6].

Carotid Endarterectomy

Atherosclerotic plaques of the carotid arteries contribute to embolic and ischemic cerebrovascular disease, with significant, high-grade lesions (symptomatic patients with >70% luminal stenosis) clearly benefiting from surgical intervention over medical management [7]. Data for carotid endarterectomy (CEA) are equivocal in those with symptomatic stenosis ranging from 30% to 69%, and suggest that in those with minimally stenotic lesions (<30% luminal narrowing), surgery may be harmful [8].

Minimally invasive techniques have also gained traction in treating carotid artery stenosis. Stenting and angioplasty may be beneficial in patients with comorbidities that prevent safe execution of traditional CEA; the Carotid Revascularization Endarterectomy Versus Stenting (CREST) trial demonstrated no difference in composite primary outcome (4-year perioperative stroke, MI, or death); however, stenting was associated with a higher risk of perioperative stroke versus CEA, which carried a higher risk of MI [9].

Anesthetic techniques for CEA should be tailored for individual patients and their comorbidities, but the overall goals are to maintain hemodynamic stability in the perioperative period and to facilitate a prompt postoperative neurologic examination. The General anaesthesia versus local anaesthesia for carotid surgery (GALA) trial is the largest study to compare general anesthesia versus local anesthesia for CEA; a similar composite outcome to the CREST trial was used, which included stroke, MI, and death up to 30 days after surgery. No difference was seen between the two groups for the primary composite outcome [10]. As with the surgical technique for treating carotid

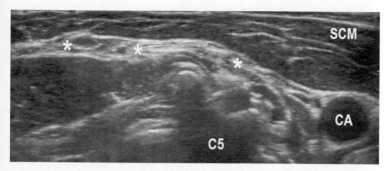

Figure 15.1 Ultrasound anatomy highlighting placement of local anesthetic for superficial cervical plexus block. * denotes the superficial cervical plexus. SCM, sterno-cleidomastoid muscle; CA, carotid artery; C5, C5 vertebral body.

artery stenosis, provider expertise and patient characteristics should determine the appropriate anesthetic technique.

Whichever modality of anesthetic is selected, the anesthesiologist has a large armamentarium of monitoring options for patients presenting for intervention. An awake patient undergoing CEA under local and regional anesthesia (via superficial cervical plexus blockade) (see Figure 15.1) provides the surgeon and anesthesiologist with the most reliable method of neurologic assessment, given appropriate patient selection; cortical function and motor and sensory pathways can be easily assessed during critical portions of the surgery. EEG may also be used and is considered the most sensitive modality when general anesthesia is used, effectively detecting regional or global ischemic events intraoperatively [8]. Somatosensory evoked potentials (SSEPs) and transcranial Doppler (TCD) are additional methods that may be used at institutions to assess global or regional cerebral blood flow during critical portions of the revascularization procedure.

Arterial line placement is mandatory for all cases, as stringent control over hemodynamics will allow for maintenance of adequate cerebral perfusion pressures. Surgeon preference and institutional practices will largely determine the use of selective hypertension during carotid artery cross-clamping, stump pressure measurements, shunt placement to promote collateral flow, or a combination of the three, along with the aforementioned monitoring modalities [7]. The anesthesiologist must judiciously use fluids and vasopressors to ensure adequate cerebral blood flow whether an awake or general anesthetic technique is used. Special attention should be given to the carotid cross-clamping period, and ongoing communication between the surgeon and the anesthesiologist is crucial to the success of the case.

Postoperative care of the patient undergoing CEA is as instrumental in preventing morbidity and mortality as intraoperative management. Immediate assessment of neurologic function is paramount, as embolization of air or plaque (especially if a carotid shunt was placed intraoperatively) is a major contributing factor to postoperative stroke. Maintenance of adequate cerebral perfusion (by avoidance of hypo- or hypertension) mitigates the risk of postoperative cerebral ischemia and hyperperfusion injury. Additional postoperative assessments include close monitoring for neck hematoma, potential airway compromise, and myocardial ischemia.

Abdominal Aortic Aneurysm

Defined as an enlargement of the aorta of >3.0 cm in diameter, abdominal aortic aneurysm (AAA) has known associations with advanced age, male gender, and a history of smoking at any point. The risk of rupture is associated with increasing AAA diameter, advanced age, female gender, and poorly controlled blood pressure [11]. The US Preventive Services Task Force has recommended one-time ultrasound screening for AAA in men aged 65–75 years who have ever smoked, but found little benefit in routine screening in all groups [12].

Patients presenting for elective repair of AAA may opt for open aneurysm repair (OAR) versus an endovascular aneurysm repair (EVAR). Selection often occurs based on patient frailty, the complexity of the repair to be performed, and surgeon and institutional experience. Two early European trials (EVAR-1 and DREAM) demonstrated that EVAR conferred a 30-day perioperative mortality benefit over OAR; however, the incidence of reintervention and "catch-up" deaths in the EVAR arm of both trials over years of follow-up data has put this benefit into question, even suggesting that patients undergoing EVAR may experience higher long-term mortality [13, 14]. A more recent study from the United States, the OVER trial, showed similar long-term mortality in its endovascular and open aortic repair arms [15].

From the perspective of intraoperative management, EVAR has a number of advantages over OAR for the anesthesiologist. Hemodynamic perturbations are minimal, as volume loss and fluid shifts are significantly less when using an endovascular technique [11]. Arterial blood pressure monitoring is still mandatory, given patient comorbidities, the potential for conversion to open repair, and frequent sampling for arterial blood gas and activated clotting time (ACT) monitoring. Central venous cannulation can be considered in case large-bore intravenous access is not easily obtainable. The specific anesthetic technique should be determined by the length of the procedure, patient comorbidities, and other special considerations (e.g., presence or absence of a lumbar drain, specialized lower or upper extremity vascular access by surgeon, patient comfort, etc.). Local, regional, and general anesthesia have all been used successfully in the patient undergoing EVAR, although data on outcomes comparing anesthetic techniques are conflicting and lag significantly behind advances in surgical technique and approach [16].

While the intraoperative physiologic changes of EVAR may not be as dramatic as a traditional OAR, unique anesthetic challenges remain. Patient positioning and location are often remote; principles of out-of-OR procedures often apply, with the anesthesiologist having limited access to the patient due to the geography of angiography or hybrid OR suites. Heparinization is commonly employed throughout, with use of ACT to guide therapy until procedure end and protamine reversal. Maintenance of normothermia may prove challenging, as patient exposure for angiographic evaluation can be extensive and prolonged, based on the complexity of the graft and length of procedure. Spinal cord ischemia is perhaps the most feared complication related to EVAR, and the anesthesiologist and surgeon must communicate and employ multiple strategies to mitigate the risk of partial or complete occlusion of collateral vessels that supply the anterior spinal artery. Permissive hypertension and/or drainage of the cerebrospinal fluid (CSF) are the two mainstays of increasing spinal cord perfusion in patients at high risk of spinal cord ischemia. Risk increases with longer procedures, complex fenestrated grafts, and reduced preoperative renal function [17].

Postoperative endoleak from EVAR may occur after endovascular repair and, depending on the pressure gradient created by the leak, may place the patient at continued risk of aneurysmal rupture despite graft deployment. The type of leak will be determined by examination and angiographic evaluation, and may necessitate re-repair (see Figure 15.2).

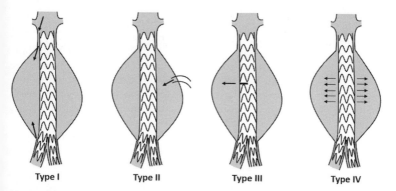

Figure 15.2 Endoleaks seen with EVAR. Type I results from a poor seal at the proximal (type IA) or distal (type IB) end of the aortic graft. Type II results from filling of the aneurysmal sac by collateral vessels. Type III can result from a defect or failure of the graft. Type IV is due to graft porosity.

Anesthetic principles of OAR are similar to those of EVAR – maintenance of hemodynamic stability and avoidance of hypotension to reduce the risk of decreased spinal cord perfusion. The physiologic changes with OAR can be dramatic, especially with large-volume shifts and aortic cross-clamping, and often necessitate additional invasive monitoring and vascular access.

Much like in EVAR, OAR requires a great deal of preparation for successful management. General endotracheal anesthesia is most commonly employed for OAR, given the nature of the procedure and the multitude of invasive lines and monitors commonly placed intraoperatively. Arterial cannulation and large-bore intravenous access should be obtained prior to, or immediately after, induction of anesthesia. A central venous catheter should be considered if peripheral access is inadequate or intra- and postoperative infusions are anticipated. Pulmonary arterial catheterization was once commonly employed in OAR but has since fallen out of favor as an intraoperative monitoring tool [18]. Transesophageal echocardiography can be considered for intraoperative assessment of volume status and may provide valuable information regarding global and regional cardiac function during demanding portions of the case. Lumbar drains placed preoperatively can be used both during and after OAR to slowly drain the CSF (10 mL hr^{-1}) to increase spinal cord perfusion pressure [19]. Blood products (a minimum of 4 units of packed red blood cells and 4 units of fresh frozen plasma) should be crossmatched to the patient presenting for elective OAR.

The physiology of aortic cross-clamping is complex and deserves special attention when discussing the management of OAR. Cardiac output and end-organ perfusion depend on the position of the aortic cross-clamp, the existence or absence of collateral blood flow, and anesthetic management. Systemic vascular resistance and mean arterial pressure increase dramatically with aortic cross-clamping, often resulting in a decrease in overall cardiac output. The level of the clamp, with respect to the renal and splanchnic arteries, most often determines the physiologic response [11]. Supraceliac aortic clamps often shift blood volume to the proximal organs and tissues, resulting in increased venous return and preload. Infraceliac aortic clamps will often shift blood volume to the splanchnic vasculature, with variable changes in venous return, depending on the underlying splanchnic venous smooth muscle tone [20]. Regardless of where the clamp is placed, the anesthesiologist must be prepared to monitor and appropriately manage a potentially massive increase in mean arterial pressure and myocardial oxygen demands. Short-acting, easily titratable vasodilating agents may be used as an intermediary, while the body adapts to the mechanical and humoral changes caused by aortic cross-clamping. Judicious use of these agents is recommended, as distal organ and tissue perfusion (spinal cord) must be maintained throughout the cross-clamping period.

Unclamping during OAR is equally fraught with risk, as it is strongly associated with reactive hyperemia and often profound hypotension if not treated appropriately. The cause for this unique physiology is thought to occur due to hypoxia, vasodilating substances, and myogenic mechanisms [20]. Aggressive treatment with fluids, vasopressors, inotropes, and calcium has been used successfully to counteract hypotension; slow release of the aortic cross-clamp after prolonged cross-clamping time is recommended to avoid a sudden surge of ischemic "washout" products from distal organs and tissues.

Consideration should be given to the placement of a preoperative thoracic epidural, if there are no contraindications. In a large retrospective analysis of elective OAR, a combined general anesthetic with a thoracic epidural was associated with improved survival, compared to general anesthetic alone, over a 9-year study period [21]. The study authors determined that the comparative decrease in mortality was likely due to the reduction in postoperative complications; the traditional benefits of an epidural conferred in elective OAR included improved analgesia, reduced postoperative pulmonary complications, and reduced incidence of bowel ischemia [2, 21].

Hemodialysis Access

Dialysis dependence has significantly increased due to rising rates of cardiovascular disease and disease equivalents, most commonly poorly controlled hypertension and diabetes. Vascular access is critical in patients with end-stage renal failure in order to maintain fluid and electrolyte homeostasis. And while the creation of an arteriovenous shunt is uncomplicated, patients who present for fistula or graft placement are among the most medically complex cared for by the anesthesiologist. A thorough preoperative assessment should be conducted to rule out active or decompensated cardiopulmonary disease, assess for appropriate volume status and the need to correct metabolic imbalances, and optimize preoperative blood pressure to avoid intraoperative hyper- or hypotension.

There are unique challenges associated with patients presenting for permanent hemodialysis access. Intravenous access is challenging due to long-standing vasculopathy and often requires ultrasound assistance. The aforementioned medical complexity of these patients necessitates careful planning for anesthetic management. Regional anesthesia is often preferred, as multiple studies have pointed towards an association with improved long-term shunt patency, and possibly fewer perioperative complications, as compared to general anesthesia [22, 23]. The brachial plexus at the supraclavicular level is often the preferred route of delivery for surgical anesthesia; however, the anesthesiologist must make a tailored decision, with consideration for where the shunt will be placed, as well as patient comorbidities (severe obstructive or restrictive lung disease, contralateral phrenic nerve injury or palsy) that may preclude more proximal brachial plexus blockade.

Surgery for Critical Limb Ischemia: Limb Salvage and Amputation

Lower extremity limb ischemia as a result of peripheral arterial disease (PAD) necessitates a wide array of treatment strategies to improve ischemic pain, promote vascular blood flow to poorly healing wounds, and preserve limb function by preventing amputation. Progressive disease despite revascularization is not uncommon, however, and limb amputation is often an inevitable outcome for many patients with severe PAD.

Open lower extremity bypass (LEB) has remained the cornerstone for surgical revascularization, facilitated most commonly by the use of saphenous vein grafts. Although the 5-year patency for LEB is high, complications can abound, including graft thrombosis, surgical site infection, and MACEs [24]. Endovascular techniques also have gained traction, though no significant difference is seen in amputation-free survival at 3 years [25].

The anesthetic technique for LEB, like most vascular surgery, should be individually tailored; general anesthesia is more commonly employed, but regional and neuraxial anesthesia may be useful in patients who are at risk of postoperative pulmonary complications and have no contraindications (e.g., inherited or acquired coagulopathy). Regional anesthetics may be beneficial in certain circumstances but have not demonstrated improved overall outcomes [26].

Despite optimal medical and surgical therapies, limb amputations are often an inevitable result for patients with PAD. Regional anesthetic techniques are preferred, with indwelling peripheral nerve catheters significantly reducing the need for postoperative opioid analgesia, though data on prevention of chronic phantom limb pain are mixed [27, 28].

Review Questions

1. After removal of the cross-clamp for a complex repair of an infrarenal aortic aneurysm, a patient develops refractory hypotension. What is the next best step in the management of this patient?

   (a) 100 μg bolus of phenylephrine
   (b) Immediate transfusion of packed red blood cells
   (c) Initiate advanced cardiovascular life support (ACLS)
   (d) Reclamping of the aorta by the surgeon
   (e) Administer 500 mL of crystalloid bolus

2. A 68-year-old male with peripheral arterial disease, hypertension, insulin-dependent diabetes mellitus, and stage 2 chronic kidney disease presents for lower extremity bypass. He cannot generate >4 METs due to lower extremity claudication but denies chest pain at rest or orthopnea. His vitals are: heart

rate 48 bpm, blood pressure 155/105 mmHg, respiratory rate 16 breaths/min, and SpO$_2$ 98%. Which of the following preoperative tests is indicated?

(a) Pulmonary function testing
(b) Dobutamine stress test
(c) Left heart catheterization
(d) 24-hour urine vanillylmandelic acid

Answers

1 (d) This patient has undergone a complex aortic repair, with what is presumed to be prolonged aortic cross-clamp time. The use of vasopressors and fluids may be useful when preparing for cross-clamp release, in anticipation of hypotension that results from the release of ischemic and vasoactive substances distal to the clamp. In the case of refractory hypotension, however, the next best step would be to have the surgeon partially or totally reclamp the aorta.

2 (b) For a patient whose exercise tolerance is unclear and who presents for planned major vascular surgery, in the setting of multiple risk factors for coronary artery disease, it would be reasonable to proceed with pharmacologic stress testing if it will change anesthetic management. Coronary angiography is not recommended as a routine test, even if the patient has risk factors, in the absence of symptoms. It would be especially risky for this patient, given his underlying chronic kidney disease.

References

1. Smilowitz NR, Gupta N, *et al*. Trends in perioperative major adverse cardiovascular and cerebrovascular events associated with non-cardiac surgery. *JAMA Cardiol.* 2017;2(2):181–7.

2. Fleisher L, Fleischmann K, *et al*. 2014 ACC/AHA guideline on perioperative cardiovascular evaluation and management of patients undergoing noncardiac surgery: a report of the American College of Cardiology/American Heart Association task force on practice guideline. *Circulation.* 2014;130(24):e278–333.

3. Chou J, Gylys M, *et al*. Preexisting right ventricular dysfunction is associated with higher postoperative cardiac complications and longer hospital stay in high-risk patients undergoing nonemergent major vascular surgery. *J Cardiothorac Vasc Anesth.* 2019;33(5):1279–86.

4. Meersch M, Schmidt S, *et al*. Perioperative acute kidney injury: an under-recognized problem. *Anesth Analg.* 2017;125(4):1223–32.

5. Ji F, Li Z, *et al*. Post-bypass dexmedetomidine use and postoperative acute kidney injury in patients undergoing cardiac surgery with cardiopulmonary bypass. *PLoS One.* 2013;8(10):e77446.

6. Nadim MK, Forni LG, *et al.* Cardiac and vascular surgery-associated acute kidney injury: the 20th International Consensus Conference of the ADQI (Acute Disease Quality Initiative) Group. *J Am Heart Assoc.* 2018;7(11):e08834.

7. Howell SJ. Carotid endarterectomy. *Br J Anaesth.* 2007;99(1):119–31.

8. Ferguson GG, Eliasziw M, *et al.* The North American Symptomatic Carotid Endarterectomy Trial: surgical results in 1415 patients. *Stroke.* 1999;30 (9):1751–8.

9. Brott TG, Hobson RW, *et al.* Stenting versus endarterectomy for treatment of carotid-artery stenosis. *N Engl J Med.* 2010;363:11–23.

10. GALA Trial Collaborative Group. General anaesthesia versus local anaesthesia for carotid surgery (GALA): a multicenter, randomised controlled trial. *Lancet.* 2008;372:2132–42.

11. Smaka TJ, Miller TE, *et al.* Anesthesia for vascular surgery. In: PG Barash, BF Cullen, *et al.*, eds. *Clinical Anesthesia*, 7th ed. Philadelphia, PA: Lippincott Williams & Wilkins; 2013, pp. 1128–39.

12. US Preventive Services Task Force. Screening for abdominal aortic aneurysm: US Preventive Services Task Force Recommendation Statement. *JAMA.* 2019;322 (22):2211–18.

13. The UK EVAR Trial Investigators.Endovascular versus open repair of abdominal aortic aneurysm. *N Engl J Med.* 2010;362:1868–71.

14. De Bruin JL, Baas AF, *et al.* Long-term outcome of open or endovascular repair of abdominal aortic aneurysm. *N Engl J Med.* 2010;362:1881–9.

15. Lederle FA, Kyriakides TC, *et al.* Open versus endovascular repair of abdominal aortic aneurysm. *N Engl J Med.* 2019;380:2126–35.

16. Baril DT, Kahn RA, *et al.* Endovascular abdominal aortic aneurysm repair: emerging developments and anesthetic considerations. *J Cardiothorac Vasc Anesth.* 2007;21(5):730–42.

17. Spanos K, Kolbel T, *et al.* Risk of spinal cord ischemia after fenestrated or branched endovascular repair of complex aortic aneurysms. *J Vasc Surg.* 2019;69(2):357–66.

18. Valentine RJ, Duke ML, *et al.* Effectiveness of pulmonary artery catheters in aortic surgery: a randomized trial. *J Vasc Surg.* 1998;27(2):203–12.

19. Estrera AL, Sheinbaum R, *et al.* Cerebral fluid drainage during thoracic aortic repair: safety and current management. *Ann Thorac Surg.* 2009;88:9–15.

20. Gelman S. The pathophysiology of aortic cross-clamping and unclamping. *Anesthesiology.* 1995;82:1026–57.

21. Bardia A, Sood A, *et al.* Combined epidural-general anesthesia vs general anesthesia alone for elective abdominal aortic aneurysm repair. *JAMA Surg.* 2016;151 (12):1116–23.

22. Levin SR, Farber A, *et al.* Association of anesthesia type with outcomes after out-patient brachiocephalic arteriovenous fistula creation. *Ann Vasc Surg.* 2020;68:67–75.

23. Marsh C, Holloway J, *et al.* Outcomes of local and regional anesthesia for super-ficialization of brachiobasilic arteriovenous fistulas. *Ann Vasc Surg.* 2020;65:40–4.

24. Farber A, Eberhardt T. The current state of critical limb ischemia: a systematic review. *JAMA Surg.* 2016;151(11):1070–7.

25. Adam DJ, Beard JD, *et al.*; BASIL trial participants. Bypass versus angioplasty in severe ischaemia of the leg (BASIL): multicentre, randomised controlled trial. *Lancet.* 2005;366:1925–34.

26. Sgroi MD, McFarland G. Utilization of regional versus general anesthesia and its impact on lower extremity bypass outcomes. *J Vasc Surg.* 2019;69(6):1874–9.

27. Madabhushi L, Reuben SS, *et al.* The efficacy of postoperative perineural infusion of bupivacaine and clonidine after lower extremity amputation in preventing phantom limb and stump pain. *J Clin Anesth.* 2007;19(3):226–9.

28. Ayling OGS, Montbriand J, *et al.* Continuous regional anaesthesia provides effective pain management and reduces opioid requirement following major lower limb amputation. *Eur J Vasc Endovasc Surg.* 2014;48(5):559–64.

Thoracic Anesthesia

Kimberley C. Brondeel, Frederick R. Ditmars, and Alan David Kaye

Preoperative Evaluation and Optimization

Cardiac Risk Stratification

This is by far the most important aspect of preoperative assessment. Any patient with a score >2 should be referred to cardiology for additional testing. The Revised Cardiac Risk Index is shown in Table 16.1.

The Thoracic Revised Cardiac Risk Index has four components, each of which is weighted. Patients with a score ≥2 should be referred to a cardiologist for risk stratification and additional testing if needed [1].

Assessment of Lung Resectability

The initial step in assessing lung resectability is a cardiopulmonary examination using the Thoracic Revised Cardiac Risk Index. Once cleared from a cardiac standpoint, the patient's pulmonary function must be examined to generate predictive postoperative values (ppoFEV$_1$ and ppoDLCO), calculated based on the maximum proposed number of segments removed:

$$\text{ppoFEV}_1 \% = \text{preoperative FEV}_1 \% \times (1 - \% \text{ functional lung tissue removed}/100)$$

$$\text{ppoDLCO} \% = \text{preoperative DLCO} \% \times (1 - \% \text{ functional lung tissue removed}/100)$$

Reductions in ppoFEV$_1$ and ppoDLCO are both associated with an increased risk of postoperative pulmonary complications (PPCs), including increased 30-day readmission, prolonged length of stay, and decreased overall survival. According to the American College of Chest Physicians (ACCP), patients with ppoFEV$_1$ and ppoDLCO >60% are considered low risk for PPCs and do not require additional cardiopulmonary testing. Those with ppoFEV$_1$ or ppoDLCO <60% and >30% are recommended to undergo informal evaluation of their cardiopulmonary reserve. This could include the stair climbing test, shuttle walk test, 6-minute walk test, or exercise oxygen desaturation test. Conversely, those with a high risk

Table 16.1 Thoracic Revised Cardiac Risk Index

Risk factors	Points
History of cerebrovascular disease	1.5
History of coronary artery disease	1.5
Pneumonectomy	1.5
Serum creatinine >177 µmol L^{-1} or 2 mg dL^{-1}	1

Risk of major cardiovascular event	
Points	Risk (%)
0	0.9
1–1.5	4.2
2–2.5	8
>2.5	18

cardiac evaluation, poor results on informal exercise testing, or a ppoFEV$_1$ or ppoDLCO <30% are recommended to undergo formal laboratory exercise testing or cardiopulmonary exercise testing. Those with low VO$_2$ max <10 mL/(kg min) or <35% predicted are considered to be at high risk. These patients should be counseled on sublobar resections, less invasive surgical options, nonoperative treatments, and palliative care. A flowchart summarizing the recommendations of the American College of Chest Physicians (ACCP) for preoperative evaluation is shown in Figure 16.1.

Remember, these equations and procedures reflect the typical relationship between the extent of resection and postoperative complications. Values such as ppoDLCO decrease as more functional lung tissue is removed; thus, there is an increase in morbidity and mortality. Notable exceptions include disease processes that reduce lung compliance and/or functional capacity. For example, in patients with chronic obstructive pulmonary disease (COPD), the removal of emphysematous lung may actually improve the degree of ventilation/perfusion mismatch postoperatively. Therefore, in these patients, regional lung studies may provide a more accurate prediction of postoperative pulmonary function.

Finally, many thoracic procedures are related to previous cancer diagnosis. Therefore, it is important for anesthesiologists to understand the

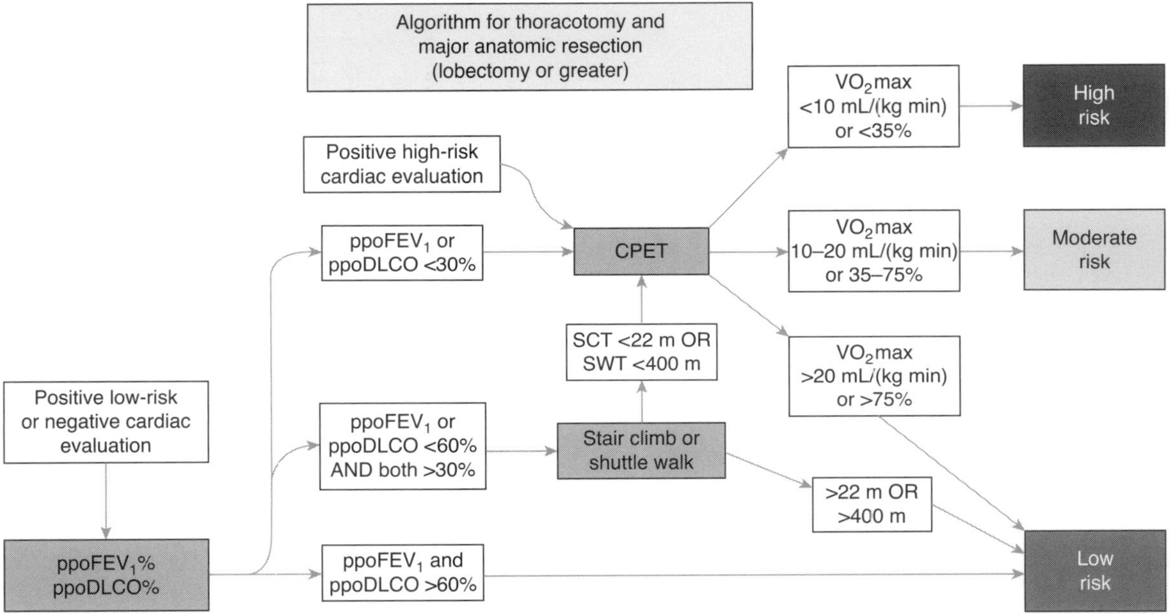
Algorithm for thoracotomy and major anatomic resection (lobectomy or greater)
Positive high-risk cardiac evaluation
Positive low-risk or negative cardiac evaluation
ppoFEV1% ppoDLCO%
ppoFEV1 or ppoDLCO <30%
ppoFEV1 or ppoDLCO <60% AND both >30%
ppoFEV1 and ppoDLCO >60%
CPET
SCT <22 m OR SWT <400 m
Stair climb or shuttle walk
>22 m OR >400 m
VO2max <10 mL/(kg min) or <35%
VO2max 10–20 mL/(kg min) or 35–75%
VO2max >20 mL/(kg min) or >75%
High risk
Moderate risk
Low risk

Figure 16.1 The American College of Chest Physicians (ACCP) algorithm for cardiopulmonary preoperative assessment of patients requiring lung resection. According to the ACCP, low risk indicates a mortality rate below 1%. In patients deemed moderate risk, morbidity and mortalityrates vary, based on pulmonary function, exercise tolerance, and the extent of resection. High-risk patients may have perioperative mortality rates in excess of 10%. CPET, cardiopulmonary exercise test; DLCO, diffusing capacity of the lungs for carbon monoxide; FEV_1, forced expiratory volume in first second; ppo, predicted postoperative; SCT, stair climbing test; SWT, shuttle walk test; VO_2 max, maximal oxygen consumption. *Source:* Reprinted with permission from Brunelli A, Kim A, Burger KI, Addrizzo-Harris, DJ. Physiologic evaluation of the patient with lung cancer being considered for resectional surgery: diagnosis and management of lung cancer, 3rd ed: American College of Chest Physicians evidence-based clinical practice guidelines. *Chest*. 2013;143(5 Suppl):e166S–90S.

anesthetic implications of various malignancies. Broadly, nonsmall-cell cancers have better outcomes with surgical treatment than small-cell cancers. However, metabolic activity, size, and location can play a large role in airway and intraoperative management. Therefore, it is critical to perform a focused evaluation on the "4 Ms" in all patients with pulmonary masses:

- Mass effects – obstructive pneumonia, lung abscess, superior vena cava syndrome, tracheobronchial distortion, Pancoast syndrome, nerve palsy, chest wall or mediastinal extension
- Metabolic – Lambert–Eaton syndrome, hypercalcemia, hyponatremia, Cushing's syndrome
- Metastases – particularly to the brain, bone, liver, and adrenals
- Medications – chemotherapy agents: pulmonary, cardiac, and renal toxicity.

Preoperative Optimization

Smoking cessation, in particular, is important for thoracic surgeries. Smoking is the most common cause of lung disease and is associated with an increased postoperative 30-day mortality rate, as well as an increased risk of postoperative pulmonary complications. Furthermore, these outcomes are directly correlated with the number of pack-years smoked. While the required duration of smoking cessation preoperatively to mitigate these risks is unknown, recent studies have suggested that smoking cessation of <8 weeks is still beneficial.

Lung Isolation Techniques

Lung isolation, or one-lung ventilation (OLV), is desired in surgery to optimize surgical access and exposure and prevent puncturing of the lung, and can prevent contamination of healthy lung tissue by a diseased lung in cases of severe infection or bleeding [2]. Tables 16.2 and 16.3 show indications for OLV, two methods of OLV, and relevant information.

Double-lumen tubes (DLTs) are the main method of anatomic and physiologic isolation in most thoracic surgery cases. Selective ventilation of an individual lung can also be achieved using a bronchial blocker, with an open-tipped model applying continuous positive pressure and suction in the airway therefore being a more useful choice to use, rather than a closed-tip. Single-lumen endotracheal tubes are preferred for patients younger than 6 months [2].

Physiology of One-Lung Ventilation

In order to improve gas exchange and ventilation efficiency during OLV, recruitment maneuvers should be employed. Peak airway pressure for recruitment in healthy lung should remain <40 cmH$_2$O, with a PEEP slowly

Table 16.2 Indications for lung isolation

Surgical indications	Absolute (nonsurgical) indications	Relative contraindications
• Mediastinal surgery • Esophageal surgery • Thoracic spine surgery • Minimally invasive cardiac valve surgery • Pulmonary resection (including pneumonectomy, lobectomy, and wedge resection) *Relative strong:* • Thoracic vascular surgery • Pneumonectomy • Upper lobectomy *Relative weak:* • Esophageal surgery • Video-assisted thoracoscopic surgery (including wedge resection, biopsy, and pleurodesis) • Middle and lower lobectomy	*Protective isolation of one lung from pathologic processes occurring in the contralateral lung, such as:* • Pulmonary hemorrhage • Infection or purulent secretions *Control of ventilation in circumstances, such as:* • Tracheobronchial trauma • Bronchopleural or bronchocutaneous fistula • Giant cyst or bullae due to risk of rupture with PPV • Unilateral lung lavage	• Patient unable to tolerate OLV/dependence on bilateral ventilation • Intraluminal airway masses (making DLT placement difficult) • Hemodynamic instability • Severe hypoxia • Severe COPD • Severe pulmonary hypertension • Known or suspected difficult intubation

PPV, positive pressure ventilation; OLV, one-lung ventilation; DLT, double-lumen tube; COPD, chronic obstructive pulmonary disease.

Source: Modified from Mehrotra M, Jain A. *Single Lung Ventilation.* In: StatPearls [Internet]. Treasure Island (FL): StatPearls Publishing; 2021. Available from: www.ncbi.nlm.nih.gov/books/NBK538314/

Table 16.3 Methods of one-lung ventilation

Double-lumen tubes	Bronchial blockers
• Main method of anatomic and physiologic lung isolation in most thoracic surgery cases • Most commonly used DLT is left-sided (irrespective of which side requires isolation) due to left-sided being easier and minimized risk of dislodgement or impaired ventilation of the right upper bronchus	• Open-tipped BB is a more useful alternative to closed-tipped due to the ability to apply continuous positive pressure and suction to the airway
Advantages: • Best device for absolute lung separation • Large luminae facilitating suctioning • Allows for easy transition between one- and two-lung ventilation	*Advantages:* • Utility in airway trauma • Best device for patients with difficult airways • No cuff damage during intubation • Ability to be placed through an existing endotracheal tube → no need to replace a tube if mechanical ventilation is needed • Ability to selectively block a lung lobe • Easy recognition of the anatomy if the tip of a single tube is above the carina
Disadvantages: • Placement difficult due to larger size and design • Damage to tracheal cuff	*Disadvantages:* • Especially difficult to place, particularly in the RUL • More likely to get dislodged

Table 16.3 (cont.)

Double-lumen tubes	Bronchial blockers
• Difficulties in selecting proper sizes • Difficult to place during laryngoscopy • Major tracheobronchial injuries • Contraindications: difficult airway, limited jaw mobility, tracheal constriction, preexisting trachea or stoma, inability to perform direct laryngoscopy	• May cause local trauma to tracheal mucosa during placement • Overinflation of balloon that is too large can damage the mucosa of the airway • Inflation within the trachea blocks ventilation of both lungs • Small channel for suctioning • Conversion from one- to two-lung ventilation, then to one-lung ventilation (problematic for novice) • High-maintenance device (dislodgement or lost seal during surgery)

DLT, double-lumen tube; BB, bronchial blocker. RUL, right upper lobe.

Source: Mehrotra M, Jain A. *Single Lung Ventilation.* In: StatPearls [Internet]. Treasure Island (FL): StatPearls Publishing; 2021. Available from: www.ncbi.nlm.nih.gov/books/NBK538314/. Purohit A, Bhargava S, Mangal V, Parashar VK. Lung isolation, one-lung ventilation and hypoxaemia during lung isolation. *Indian J Anaesth.* 2015 Sep;59(9):606–17.

increasing up to 20 cmH$_2$O, and lower in a diseased lung [3, 4]. Final recruitment maneuvers with two-lung ventilation should be performed at lower pressure levels to prevent disrupting surgical staples. The end result of these techniques improves oxygenation, increases compliance, and decreases dead space, while also potentially reducing inflammatory cytokine release [5]. Thoracic surgical procedures should use all of the American Society of Anesthesiologists standard basic anesthetic monitoring. Summarized below are the most important vitals to monitor during OLV:

- FiO$_2$: lowest to maintain SpO$_2$ >90%
- TV: 4–6 mL kg^{-1} based on ideal body weight
- PEEP: 5–10 cmH$_2$O to dependent lung
- CPAP: 2–5 cmH$_2$O (disrupt when visibility impaired) to nondependent lung
- PaCO$_2$: <60–70 mmHg.

Addressing Hypoxemia

Hypoxemia is defined as an oxygen saturation below 85–90% PaO$_2$ while inspired FiO$_2$ is 1.0 [6]. This occurs in approximately 5–10% of patients. In this scenario, nonurgent procedures should be stopped, and dual-lung ventilation should be restored until oxygenation improves. If hypoxia persists or recurs, check placement of the DLT or bronchial blocker, as they are the most common cause. Table 16.4 summarizes the management of hypoxemia during OLV [5].

Goal-Directed Fluid Management

Hypovolemia results in insufficient oxygen delivery and flow-dependent organ dysfunction, as opposed to hypervolemia, which leads to pulmonary interstitial edema with impaired oxygen diffusion and poor collagen regeneration. Table 16.5 shows the parameters that need to be monitored to maximize cardiac output and oxygen delivery while minimizing perioperative complications [8–10].

Nonintubating Technique for Thoracic Surgical Procedures

Although the mainstay of all thoracic surgery patients has been intubation with endotracheal tube/DLT after induction of general anesthesia, nonintubating techniques have been gaining popularity over recent years.

Benefits include reduced postoperative morbidity, faster discharge, decreased hospital costs, and a globally reduced perturbation of the patient's well-being. Important results from a meta-analysis suggests that nonintubating general anesthesia for thoracic procedures can reduce

Table 16.4 One-lung ventilation hypoxemia management

Increase FiO$_2$	Increasing FiO$_2$ can often improve oxygenation, but 100% FiO$_2$ may lead to absorption atelectasis
PEEP	PEEP is a catch-22: (1) it can recruit more alveoli to participate in oxygenation on the nonoperative side; but (2) it may also increase shunting from the nonoperative side to the operative side
Increase I:E ratio	Oxygenation occurs during inspiration; increased I:E ratio will potentially help oxygenation
Suction of DLT	If secretion, blood, mucus, etc. in the airway or DLT → suction is very effective
DLT positioning	If DLT shifts position → ventilation and/or lung isolation will be affected
Operative-side CPAP	Applying low-flow CPAP to the operative side often improves oxygenation but may affect surgical field exposure
Intermittent two-lung ventilation	If previously described measures do not improve oxygenation adequately → intermittent two-lung ventilation is the last resort

PEEP, positive end-expiratory pressure; I:E ratio, inspiratory-to-expiratory ratio; DLT, double-lumen tube; CPAP, continuous positive airway pressure.
Source: Table 16.4 is modified from *Thoracic Anesthesia Procedures* by Dr. Alan Kaye and Dr. Richard Urman, p. 104. [7].

Table 16.5 Volume- and goal-directed therapy hemodynamic parameters

SV	SV decreases due to hypovolemia, based on the Starling curve; HR increases as a compensatory response
CO	CO decrease in hypovolemia if no contractility and HR increased
EDLV/EDLVP	EDLV – best indicator of volume status; EDLVP – used as parameter of left ventricular volume status instead
U/O	The oldest indicator of volume status but can still be useful
SVV	The most used parameter for goal-directed fluid therapy
PPV	Often used also in goal-directed fluid therapy

SV, stroke volume; HR, heart rate; CO, cardiac output; EDLV, end-diastolic left ventricular volume; EDLVP, end-diastolic left ventricular pressure; U/O, urine output; SVV, stroke volume variation; PPV, pulse pressure variation.
Source: Table 16.5 is modified from *Thoracic Anesthesia Procedures* by Dr. Alan Kaye and Dr. Richard Urman, p.105. [7].

Table 16.6 Thoracic procedures – sedation indications

Surgery in the pleural space	• Drainage of pleural effusion • Pleurodesis under TEA; thoracic, paravertebral, and local anesthesia • Pleurostomy or decortication under TEA • Paravertebral block • Pneumothorax treatment under TEA (i.e., pleurectomy) • Empyema drainage under epidural or paravertebral block [9] • Bleb resection
Surgery on the lung	• Pneumonectomy under TEA • Lobectomy with thoracotomy and thoracoscopy under TEA • Bilobectomy under TEA • Wedge resection under TEA/LA • Thoracoscopic lobectomy and segmentectomy under TEA • Lung metastasis resection under TEA • Lung volume reduction surgery and bullectomy under TEA
Biopsies	• Anterior mediastinal mass biopsy • Pleural/lung biopsy under TEA
Surgery in the mediastinum	• Pericardial window • Tracheal resection with cervical epidural from C7 to T1 (use local anesthetic to minimize cough response)

TEA, thoracic epidural analgesia; LA, local anesthesia.
Source: Modified from source: Kiss G, Catillo M. Nonintubated anesthesia in thoracic surgery: general issues. *Ann Transl Med.* 2015;3(8):110 [12].

operative morbidity and hospital stay when compared to equipollent procedures performed under general anesthesia [11]. See Table 16.6 for indications of sedation for thoracic procedures [12].

Regional Techniques

The types of blocks used in thoracic techniques can be complicated. Table 16.7 summarizes the different types of anesthetic blocks, and their complications are described in Table 16.8.

Table 16.7 Sedation indications and techniques for thoracic procedures

Block type	Regional coverage	Indications	Technical degree	Allow use of catheter	Ultrasound required	Requires holding anticoagulation
Thoracic epidural	Anterior, lateral, and posterior thoracic wall	Breast, cardiac, chest wall, esophageal, and thoracic wall surgery; multiple rib fractures	High	Yes	No (could be used to identify landmarks)	Yes
Thoracic paravertebral	Anterior, lateral, and posterior thoracic wall	Breast, cardiac, chest wall, esophageal, thoracic wall surgery, multiple rib fractures	High	Yes	No (could be used to identify landmarks and perform block)	Yes
Intercostal nerve block	Anterolateral, lateral, and posterolateral thoracic wall	Breast, chest, and thoracic wall surgery; chest tube placement; rib fracture(s)	Intermediate	Yes	No (could be used to identify landmarks and perform block)	No

Block	Coverage	Indications				
PECS I and II blocks	Anterolateral and lateral thoracic wall	Breast surgery, including axillary dissection; chest wall and thoracic wall surgery	Intermediate	No	Required	No
Serratus anterior plane block	Anterolateral and lateral thoracic wall	Breast surgery, including axillary dissection; chest wall and thoracic wall surgery	Low	No	Required	No
Erector spinae plane block	Anterolateral, lateral, and posterolateral thoracic wall	Breast, chest wall, and thoracic wall surgery	Low	Yes	Required	No
Transversus thoracis muscle plane block	Anterior thoracic wall	Anterior thoracic wall and breast surgery, ICD placement	Intermediate	No	Required	No

ICD, implantable cardioverter-defibrillator.

Source: Table 16.7 is modified from *Thoracic Anesthesia Procedures* by Dr. Alan Kaye and Dr. Richard Urman, pp. 273–4 [7].

Table 16.8 Sedation complications for thoracic procedures

Block type	Complications
Thoracic epidural	• Accidental intrathecal injection • Epidural abscess • Epidural hematoma • Intravascular injection • Local anesthetic systemic toxicity • Nerve root or spinal cord injury • Pneumothorax
Thoracic paravertebral	• Accidental epidural or intrathecal injection • Hematoma • Horner syndrome (transient) • Intravascular injection via intercostal artery or vein • Local anesthetic toxicity • Pneumothorax • Spinal or intercostal nerve injury
Intercostal nerve block	• Intercostal nerve injury • Intravascular injection via intercostal artery or vein • Local anesthetic toxicity • Pneumothorax

PECS I and II blocks	• Intravascular injection via pectoral branch of the thoracoacromial artery • Local anesthetic toxicity • Neuraxial spread • Pneumothorax
Serratus anterior plane block	• Intercostal nerve injury • Intravascular injection via intercostal artery or vein • Local anesthetic toxicity • Pneumothorax
Erector spinae plane block	• Local anesthetic toxicity • Pneumothorax
Transversus thoracis muscle plane block	• Intravascular injection via the internal thoracic artery or vein • Local anesthetic toxicity • Pericardial puncture • Pneumothorax

Source: Table 16.8 is modified from *Thoracic Anesthesia Procedures* by Dr. Alan Kaye and Dr. Richard Urman, p. 274.

Special Considerations in Surgical Procedures

Anterior Mediastinal Masses

Preoperative

All patients should undergo X-ray and chest CT before surgery. X-ray is useful for determining a mediastinal:thoracic ratio or the ratio between the widest diameter of the mediastinal mass, with the width of the thorax at T5–T6. Importantly, a ratio >0.5 is associated with a higher incidence of postrespiratory complications. CT is useful for assessing involvement of the tracheobronchial tree. A tracheal narrowing of >50% in cross-section is associated with increased airway obstruction during anesthesia. Furthermore, these patients should be assessed with echocardiography to evaluate cardiac, systemic, or pulmonary compromise [13].

These risks were best summarized by Blank and de Souza [13]:

- *Low risk*: Asymptomatic or minimally symptomatic, with no postural complaints or indication of substantial compression of tissues on radiographic examination.
- *Intermediate risk*: Postural symptoms ranging from mild to moderate and <50% compression of the trachea.
- *High risk*: Severe postural symptoms, stridor, cyanosis, tracheal compression of >50%, or tracheal compression in conjunction with bronchial compression, pericardial effusion, or superior vena cava (SVC) syndrome.

Even with these precautions, total airway obstruction can occur unexpectedly during induction of anesthesia in mediastinal mass patients. The reasons for this are multifactoral, including decreased lung volume (as low as 500 mL), increased mass effect due to relaxing of bronchial smooth muscle, and loss of normal transpleural pressure gradient on diaphragmatic paralysis, which further enhances the effect of extrinsic compression. Moreover, the supine position can cause an increase in central blood volume, which may increase the tumor's blood mass. On the other hand, positive pressure ventilation during induction is dangerous as the increased gas flow across the stenosis increases intraluminal pressure, thus increasing the likelihood of collapse. **Overall, when general anesthesia is required, spontaneous respiration and avoiding paralysis can preserve normal transpulmonary pressure and maintain airway patency** [14, 15].

Intubation, Sedation, and Positioning

Distal tracheal compression allows for placement of a reinforced endotracheal tube beyond the site of obstruction. However, if the carina or mainstem bronchi are compressed, awake fiberoptic intubation is useful.

Possible Complications: Cardiovascular Collapse

If the mediastinal mass is able to compress the most vital components of circulation (SVC, heart, pulmonary artery, and aorta), it can result in fatal cardiovascular collapse. Intraoperative monitoring with transesophageal echocardiography can be useful in these cases. Vasopressors can be used to preserve coronary flow in ventricular outflow obstruction. Occasionally, circulatory compromise can be due to reduced preload. This can be treated with fluid, although it should be done conservatively, as fluid can exacerbate right ventricular dysfunction. Similar techniques can be used in SVC syndrome [16].

Pneumonectomy

Preoperative

Pneumonectomy has the highest morbidity of all pulmonary resections, with a mortality rate of 3.7–7.8%. Before the procedure, patients must undergo an extensive risk assessment of cardiac health, respiratory mechanics, and lung parenchymal function. This testing is extensive, and risk profiles are summarized in Figure 16.2 [17].

Anesthesia management of this procedure is summarized best in "Physiology of One-Lung Ventilation."

Considerations
Extrapleural Pneumonectomy

This is associated with significant blood loss due to involvement of chest wall vessels.

- Venous return to the heart can be compromised by blood loss, compression of the SVC by the tumor, or surgical causes.
- Cardiac herniation with hemodynamic instability can occur when the patient is moved from the lateral decubitus to supine position.
- Patients typically remain intubated due to the extended duration of surgery and large fluid shifts.
- If using a DLT, it is typically exchanged to a single-lumen endotracheal tube at the end of the procedure.
- The perioperative morbidity rate is 0–82.6%, and mortality rate 0–11.8%.
- The 5-year survival rate is 0–78%.
- Complications include acute respiratory distress syndrome, pericardial tamponade, cardiac herniation, pulmonary embolism, respiratory infections, respiratory failure, atrial arrhythmia, and myocardial infarction [17, 18].

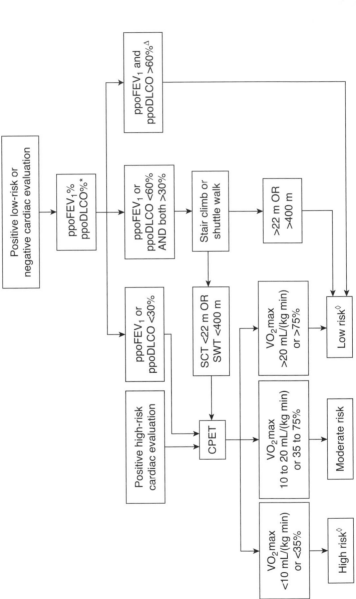

Figure 16.2 Risk stratification for cardiac evaluation.

Tracheal Sleeve Pneumonectomy/Carinal Pneumonectomy

- Ventilation during tracheobronchial resection and anastomosis can be achieved with:

    ○ Cross-field ventilation – a long, single-lumen, sterile endobronchial tube is advanced through the surgical field and into the left mainstem bronchus, or

    ○ High-frequency jet ventilation.

- Intermittent apnea is used during placement of anastomotic sutures.
- Occasionally performed with cardiopulmonary bypass (CPB) or extracorporeal membrane oxygenation (ECMO).
- Flexible bronchoscopy is performed prior to extubation, to check anastomosis and clear endobronchial secretions.
- Morbidity (11–50%) and mortality rates (3–20%) are higher, and 5-year survival rate (20%) is lower than with other pulmonary resections.
- Postpneumonectomy pulmonary edema is a common complication after right sleeve pneumonectomy.
- Acute respiratory distress syndrome occurs in up to 20% of patients and has a mortality rate of 50–100% [17, 18].

Hemodynamic Management

Pulmonary artery and veins are isolated and ligated during standard pneumonectomy. During isolation and clamping, it is crucial that the anesthesiologist and surgeon communicate to maintain a stable cardiac output, as the entire pulmonary circulating volume begins to pass through one lung. Significant increases in central venous pressure (CVP) or hemodynamic perturbations indicate insufficient compliance of the right ventricle and can lead to lung collapse, with a significantly higher risk of cardiac complications and mortality. Furthermore, resulting increases in peripheral venous return (PVR) can rapidly start a chain reaction causing left- and right-sided heart failure [19].

Pain Management

Pain management is especially important in pneumonectomy, as patients need the ability to cough and clear secretions. Thoracic epidural catheters should be placed for intra- and postoperative pain control, unless contraindicated [19].

Esophagectomy

Preoperative Assessment

Patients presenting for esophagectomy often have many comorbidities, such as COPD, cardiovascular disease, and gastro-esophageal reflux disease

(GERD), as well as alcohol and tobacco use. The American College of Cardiology/American Heart Association guidelines should be used for preoperative evaluation.

Monitoring

Pay careful attention to ECG placements of leads II and V5, as cardiac arrhythmias and ischemia are possible during mediastinal manipulation. Furthermore, standard OLV monitoring of blood gas and venous return should be conducted.

Induction

Minimizing aspiration risk is of particular importance during esophagectomy. Given this risk, rapid sequence induction or awake endotracheal intubation should be performed with the head of the bed elevated. Airways should be secured with a cuffed single-lumen or double-lumen endotracheal tube, depending on the approach. After the airway is secured, a nasogastric tube should be placed for gastric decompression [19].

Pain Management

Thoracic epidural analgesia is the gold standard for pain management in open surgical approaches. Truncal blocks may also be considered for esophagectomy approaches requiring laparotomy in patients where neuraxial analgesia is contraindicated or technically challenging [19].

Intraoperative Complications

Hypotension is a major intraoperative concern of esophagectomy surgery and can result from compression and manipulation of the heart and major vascular structures during dissection, hypovolemia, neuraxial analgesia, or cardiac arrhythmias. Tracheal injury is quite rare and is typically detected through the smell of the anesthetic gas. In the event of a tracheal injury, the endotracheal tube will need to be advanced beyond the injury, then the tear repaired surgically.

Lung Transplantation

Induction

Lung transplants are scheduled with little notice by nature. Therefore, patients are rarely appropriately nil *per os* (NPO). Preoxygenation is critical in patients about to undergo lung transplantation. Supplemental oxygen should be administered via face masks to denitrogenize the lungs prior to creating apnea. If the patient requires supplemental oxygen at baseline, a longer preoxygenation time should be prepared for [20].

If the patient has significant hemodynamic risk factors, such as pulmonary hypertension or heart failure, consider awake fiberoptic intubation [21].

Cardiopulmonary collapse can occur during the transition from negative pressure to positive pressure ventilation. It is important to have inotropes and vasopressors immediately available to augment vascular tone and cardiac function [21].

Intraoperative Management

Traditionally, CPB has been used as the mechanical support method of choice for lung transplantation. However, venoarterial ECMO (VA-ECMO) is often used as an alternative. The downside to CPB is the increased blood–air interface of the venous reservoir, which requires a much higher dose of anticoagulation than ECMO. ECMO has less systemic inflammation, and therefore less coagulopathy and bleeding than CPB [20].

Indications for Mediastinoscopy

The most challenging aspect of patient care is the potential presence of an anterior mediastinal mass and the possibility of catastrophic airway obstruction or cardiovascular collapse after induction of general anesthesia. Mediastinoscopy can open a window to observe the subdivisions of the mediastinum. Typically, this procedure is used to biopsy mediastinal lymph nodes, and the most common indication is bronchogenic carcinoma; other indications for mediastinoscopy include lymphadenopathy associated with lymphoma and sarcoidosis, and a biopsy of the tissue for diagnosis.

While relative contraindications include previous mediastinoscopy and radiation, this is due to risk of adhesion and increased bleeding. Mortality has been reported as <0.1%, and morbidity includes bleeding, pneumothorax, vocal cord paralysis, esophageal perforation, pleural perforation, and tracheal laceration. Specific indications for potential mediastinoscopy and/or surgical interventions for pleural disease are described in Table 16.9.

Postoperative Analgesia

Most thoracic surgery programs adopt multimodal analgesia (MMA) due to postoperative analgesia being critical to a successful thoracic procedure, especially when an enhanced recovery protocol is implemented. MMA involves using IV analgesics such as nonsteroidal antiinflammatory drugs, acetaminophen, opioids, and other pharmaceuticals, as well as thoracic neuraxial approaches, such as thoracic epidural analgesia, intercostal blocks, and truncal blocks.

Table 16.9 Surgical considerations for specific pleural diseases

Pleural effusion [22]		*Interventions*
Excessive collection of fluid in the pleural space (transudative versus exudative)	Classified as either a transudate or an exudate, based on Light's criteria:	Thoracentesis:

Pleural effusion [22]

Excessive collection of fluid in the pleural space (transudative versus exudative)

- Fluid accumulates in the pleural space → external mass effect limits lung expansion → leads to ineffective ventilation, increased work of breathing, atelectasis, and hypoxemic shunting

Classified as either a transudate or an exudate, based on Light's criteria:

- *Transudative* – either net increase in hydrostatic pressure OR decrease in oncotic pressure across intact capillary beds (e.g., CHF or liver cirrhosis)
- *Exudative* – either decreased lymphatic drainage OR increased capillary permeability that results in fluid leakage into pleural space (e.g., pneumonia, malignant pleural disease, PE)
- Most common malignant etiologies: lung cancer (37.5%) > breast cancer (16.8%) > lymphoma (11.5%) > genitourinary (9.4%)

Interventions

Thoracentesis:

- Generally safe but can lead to some degree of pneumothorax in up to 39% of cases
- Other complications: hemothorax, solid organ puncture, ineffective aspiration of fluid → minimize with US guidance

Large-volume drainage can alleviate symptoms and/or assess reexpandability if pleurodesis is being considered:

- If lung is reexpandable: insertion of an indwelling → pleural drainage catheter and/or pleurodesis (induced adherence of visceral and parietal pleura through scarification) is recommended
- If lung is not reexpandable (occurs in 30% of cases) → placement of an indwelling catheter alone is preferred over attempting pleurodesis

For patients dealing with chronic malignant pleural effusion either refractory to pleurodesis or with lung entrapment:

- Pleurperitoneal shunting (palliative) → minimizes fluid accumulation in the thorax as one-way valves permit drainage into peritoneal cavity → *important risk of procedure is possibility of malignant cells seeding into the abdomen*

Chylothorax [23]

Intrathoracic leakage of chyle

Causes

- Congenital, neoplastic, or traumatic processes (video-assisted thoracoscopic lung resections, esophageal surgery)

Classifications

- Low volume (<500 mL over 24 hours)
- High volume (>1000 mL over 24 hours) → increased risk of malnutrition, immunosuppression, infection, and respiratory disorders
- Left untreated → 30% risk of mortality [25]

Interventions

- Dietary fat restriction → if high volume still elevated after 5–7 days, surgical management is indicated
- Surgical options: pleurodesis, thoracic duct ligation, and noninvasive intravascular thoracic duct embolization

Empyema [24]

Exudative collection of purulent fluid that results from infection within the pleural space

- Three stages of development
- Earlier stages (I and II) → similar rate of mortality whether managed with or without surgery, but surgery associated with shorter hospital stays

Nonsurgical interventions

- Success of nonsurgical management has been attributed to administration of fibrinolytic agents into the thoracostomy drainage tube

Table 16.9 (cont.)

Surgical interventions

- Thoracoscopic delocculation and decortication may be performed
- Depending on the stage of development, entrapped lung segments may also require resection
- If there are larger lung segments that are not reexpandable, the pleural space may be obliterated by insertion of muscle flaps or silicone implants, so as to obliterate voided pleural space
- Patients with comorbid conditions that compromise their survivability after one of these interventions → establishing a temporary open-window thoracotomy can be attempted to enable drainage of infected material

---

Hemothorax [25]

Blood accumulated in pleural space

Causes

- Blunt or penetrating chest trauma, surgery, coagulopathy, vascular disease, or vascular-invasive or angio-proliferative, neoplastic processes or from a variety of other less common etiologies

Initial management

- Placement of a thoracostomy drain

Factors that suggest further surgical intervention

- Initial release of 1500 mL or more of bloody fluid
- Sustained release of 200 mL for >4 hours
- Unstable hemodynamics that are refractory to nonsurgical treatment

Pneumothorax [26]

Gas entering the pleural space

Mechanisms

- Spontaneous pneumothorax, in both the presence or absence of underlying lung pathology, traumatic chest wall injury, and iatrogenic procedural complication

Conditions resulting from chest wall defects may require specific early intervention to close the defect; however, in general, whether or not to primarily manage medically or place a thoracostomy drain tube is based on:

- The presence of concurrent lung disease
- Pleural-to-chest wall distance >2 cm on coronary chest radiograph
- Degree of respiratory insufficiency

- For prolonged pleural leaks that do not abate within 3–5 days → surgical intervention is warranted
- For patients unwilling or unable to undergo surgery → nonoperative chemical pleurodesis injection into the thoracostomy drain may be attempted
- Surgical options include → pleurodesis and resection of associated diseased lung segments

Table 16.9 (cont.)

		Treatment
Malignant mesothelioma [27] Highly aggressive cancer that involves mesothelial tissues, including the pleura	• Highly invasive locally and produces malignant pleural effusion	• Usually involves chemotherapy, along with radiation therapy • Surgical debridement is often performed for palliation • Surgical options: talc pleurodesis, pleurectomy with or without decortication, and extrapleural pneumonectomy • Infiltrative spread of the cancer renders any surgical option technically challenging and high risk
Bronchopleural or alveolopleural fistulae [28] • Bronchopleural fistulae – communications between either a mainstem or a lobar bronchus, or a segmental bronchus, and the pleural space • Alveolopleural fistulae – connect the pleural space to the airway that is distal to the segmental bronchus	• Bronchopleural fistulae occur in as many as 4–5% of patients after pneumonectomy and are associated with an increased risk of mortality • Alveolopleural fistulae are more likely to occur across staple line defects after performing pulmonary wedge resections	• Management of airway fistulae is based on the severity of the leak and the likelihood of recovery with nonsurgical care • Severity of air leak can be graded into four classes → ranging from air leak only with forced expiration to continuous air leak • Prolonged air leak (>5 days) are more central sources of leak and more likely to require surgical correction • In general: bronchopleural fistulae – often require surgical intervention; alveolopleural fistulae – more amenable to spontaneous recovery

CHF, congestive heart failure; PE, pulmonary embolism; US, ultrasound.

References

1. Salati M, Brunelli A. Risk stratification in lung resection. *Curr Surg Rep*. 2016;4(11):37.

2. Mehrotra M, Jain A. Single lung ventilation. In: *StatPearls*. Treasure Island, FL: StatPearls Publishing; 2021. Available from: www.ncbi.nlm.nih.gov/books/NBK538314/.

3. Blank RS, Colquhoun DA, Durieux ME, *et al*. Management of one-lung ventilation: impact of tidal volume on complications after thoracic surgery. *Anesthesiology*. 2016;124(6):1286–95.

4. Colquhoun DA, Naik BI, Durieux ME, *et al*. Management of one lung ventilation– variation and trends in clinical practice: a report from the Multicenter Perioperative Outcomes Group (MPOG). *Anesth Analg*. 2018;126(2):495–502.

5. Karzai W, Schwarzkopf K. Hypoxemia during one-lung ventilation: prediction, prevention, and treatment. *Anesthesiology*. 2009;110(6):1402–11.

6. Inoue S, Nishimine N, Kitaguchi K, Furuya H, Taniguchi S. Double lumen tube location predicts tube malposition and hypoxaemia during one lung ventilation. *Br J Anaesth*. 2004;92(2):195–201.

7. Kaye AD, Urman RD, eds. *Thoracic Anesthesia Procedures*. New York, NY: Oxford University Press; 2021.

8. Licker M, Triponez F, Ellenberger C, Karenovics W. Fluid therapy in thoracic surgery: a zero-balance target is always best! *Turk J Anaesthesiol Reanim*. 2016;44 (5):227–9.

9. Feng S, Yang S, Xiao W, Wang X, Yang K, Wang T. Effects of perioperative goal-directed fluid therapy combined with the application of alpha-1 adrenergic agonists on postoperative outcomes: a systematic review and meta-analysis. *BMC Anesthesiol*. 2018;18(113). Available from: www.ncbi.nlm.nih.gov/pmc/articles/PMC6098606/.

10. American Society of Anesthesiologists. Standards for basic anesthetic monitoring. 2020. Available from: www.asahq.org/standards-and-guidelines/standards-for-basic-anesthetic-monitoring.

11. Tacconi F, Pompeo E. Non-intubated video-assisted thoracic surgery: where does evidence stand? *J Thorac Dis*. 2016;8(Suppl 4):S364–75.

12. Kiss G, Castillo M. Nonintubated anesthesia in thoracic surgery: general issues. *Ann Transl Med*. 2015;3(8):110.

13. Blank RS, de Souza DG. Anesthetic management of patients with an anterior mediastinal mass: continuing professional development. *Can J Anaesth*. 2011;58 (9):853–9, 860–7.

14. Stricker PA, Gurnaney HG, Litman RS. Anesthetic management of children with an anterior mediastinal mass. *J Clin Anesth*. 2010;22(3):159–63.

15. Bergman NA. Reduction in resting end-expiratory position of the respiratory system with induction of anesthesia and neuromuscular paralysis. *Anesthesiology.* 1982;57(1):14–17.

16. Narang S, Harte BH, Body SC. Anesthesia for patients with a mediastinal mass. *Anesthesiol Clin North Am.* 2001;19(3):559–79.

17. Hackett S, Jones R, Kapila R. Anaesthesia for pneumonectomy. *BJA Educ.* 2019;19 (9):297–304.

18. Slinger P. Update on anesthetic management for pneumonectomy. *Curr Opin Anaesthesiol.* 2009;22(1):31–7.

19. Durkin C, Schisler T, Lohser J. Current trends in anesthesia for esophagectomy. *Curr Opin Anaesthesiol.* 2017;30(1):30–5.

20. Javidfar J, Brodie D, Iribarne A, *et al.* Extracorporeal membrane oxygenation as a bridge to lung transplantation and recovery. *J Thorac Cardiovasc Surg.* 2012;144 (3):716–21.

21. Ius F, Kuehn C, Tudorache I, *et al.* Lung transplantation on cardiopulmonary support: venoarterial extracorporeal membrane oxygenation outperformed cardiopulmonary bypass. *J Thorac Cardiovasc Surg.* 2012;144(6):1510–16.

22. Feller-Kopman DJ, Reddy CB, DeCamp MM, *et al.* Management of malignant pleural effusions: an official ATS/STS/STR clinical practice guideline. *Am J Respir Crit Care Med.* 2018;198(7):839–49.

23. Morabito J, Bell MT, Montenij LJ, *et al.* Perioperative considerations for chylothorax. *J Cardiothorac Vasc Anesth.* 2017;31(6):2277–81.

24. Redden MD, Chin TY, van Driel ML. Surgical versus non-surgical management for pleural empyema. *Cochrane Database Syst Rev.* 2017;3:CD010651.

25. Broderick SR. Hemothorax: etiology, diagnosis, and management. *Thorac Surg Clin.* 2013;23(1):89–96, vi–vii.

26. He J, Liu J, Zhu C, *et al.* Expert consensus on spontaneous ventilation video-assisted thoracoscopic surgery in primary spontaneous pneumothorax (Guangzhou). *Ann Transl Med.* 2019;7(20):518.

27. Woolhouse I, Maskell NA, Introducing the new BTS guideline: the investigation and management of pleural malignant mesothelioma. *Thorax.* 2018;73:210–12.

28. Poulin V, Vaillancourt R, Somma J, Gagné N, Bussières JS. High frequency ventilation combined with spontaneous breathing during bronchopleural fistula repair: a case report. *Can J Anaesth.* 2009;56(1):52–6.

Chapter 17

Neuroanesthesia

Lakshmi N. Kurnutala and Vishal Yajnik

Introduction

Anesthesia for neurosurgical procedures is challenging. Understanding of neuroanatomy, physiology, and pharmacology gives anesthesiologists the opportunity to optimize patient care. Tailoring anesthesia, including medications, monitoring techniques, and physiologic manipulation, relates closely to the patient's pathology and surgical procedure. Maintaining cerebral perfusion pressure (CPP), controlling the intracranial pressure (ICP), and preventing the progression of neurologic insults are an integral part of perioperative neuroanesthesia care.

Neuroanatomy and Physiology

The central nervous system (CNS) comprises the brain and spinal cord. The brain, which includes the cerebral cortex (composed of the gray and white matter), brainstem (midbrain, pons, and medulla), and cerebellum, is covered by protective layers of the meninges (pia, arachnoid, and dura mater). The cerebral cortex is divided into frontal, parietal, temporal, and occipital lobes. While the cortex is responsible for processing information and thinking, the brainstem is responsible for vital functions of the body, including respiratory and hemodynamic control. The cerebrospinal fluid (CSF) in the subarachnoid (SA) space surrounds the brain and spinal cord, providing nutrition, waste management, and protection. It is produced by the choroid plexus in the lateral ventricles and absorbed by the arachnoid villi in cerebral venous sinuses. The CSF flows from the lateral ventricles to the third ventricle through the interventricular foramen (foramen of Monro), and then enters the fourth ventricle via the cerebral aqueduct. From the fourth ventricle, it reaches the SA space (foramina of Luschka and Magendie) to surround the brain and spinal cord.

The Monro–Kellie hypothesis states that the sum of the intracranial volumes (CSF, blood, and brain) and ICP are in equilibrium. An increase in one volume should cause a decrease in the other, with significant implications in the management of cerebral blood flow (CBF) and ICP (see Figure 17.1). The ICP is determined by several intracranial elements,

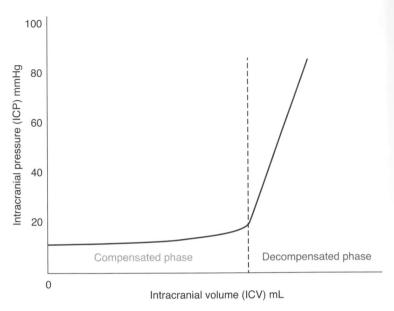

Figure 17.1 Intracranial pressure–volume curve. During a compensated phase, an increase in intracranial volume is compensated for, with minimal or no change in the ICP. Once it reaches the elbow of the ICP curve, this physiologic compensation is exhausted and a minimal increase in volume causes a significant and sharp rise in ICP.

including the CBF and CSF, and other intracranial contents, including space-occupying lesions and cerebral edema. The ICP can be increased by factors such as increase in intrathoracic pressure or intraabdominal pressure, pain, and shivering. It is often measured with an external ventricular drainage (EVD) catheter through a ventriculostomy or through an intraparenchymal catheter. Maintenance of a stable ICP is important, and while not routinely measured intraoperatively, it can often be gauged by neurosurgeons while operating. The anesthesiologist's goal is to provide a "relaxed" brain, without sudden increases in intracranial pressure that can compromise operating conditions as well as the CPP. Maintenance of an adequate CPP is a critical and primary anesthetic goal, and it is defined as the mean arterial pressure (MAP) minus the ICP (or central venous pressure (CVP), whichever is higher). Through autoregulation, maintained by MAP, end-tidal carbon dioxide ($ETCO_2$), and PaO_2, the CBF is maintained relatively constant over a CPP of 50–150 mmHg (see Figure 17.2).

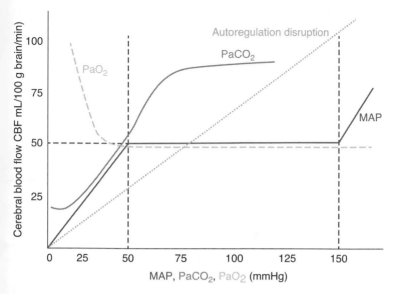

Figure 17.2 Cerebral autoregulation. The CBF is maintained constant with the MAP (50–150 mmHg). An increase in $PaCO_2$ causes a marked increase in CBF (10 mmHg increase in CO_2 = 10 mL CBF increase/100 mg brain). The PaO_2 has minimal effect on the CBF (<50 mmHg PaO_2, higher CBF).

Monitoring – ASA Monitors, Neuromonitoring (EEG, ECoG, EMG, SSEP, MEP, BERA, VEP)

Monitoring of patients undergoing neurosurgical procedures depends on the complexity of the patient's condition, surgical procedure, duration, blood loss, and intraoperative events. Standard American Society of Anesthesiologists (ASA) monitors, including ECG, SpO_2, $ETCO_2$, blood pressure, and temperature, are monitored for all neurosurgical procedures. Neuromuscular blockade is monitored closely and invasive arterial pressure (IAP) monitoring also facilitates frequent blood gas analysis. A CVP catheter is placed for fluid therapy and aspiration of air if a venous air embolus (VAE) arises, and for administration of vasopressors or other necessary medications. A urinary catheter is vital in guiding fluid management in many neurosurgical procedures, especially in patients receiving osmotic diuretics.

The anesthetic management of patients undergoing intraoperative neuromonitoring (IONM) requires close collaboration with neurosurgeons, neurophysiologists, and neurologists. Neuromonitoring assesses the functional integrity of structures (brain, brainstem, spinal cord, cranial nerves, and peripheral nerves) through the localization of anatomical structures, and reduces postoperative deficits. IONM is based on gauging spontaneous electrical activity through electromyography (EMG), EEG (electroencephalography), EcoG (electrocorticography), and evoked responses, through the stimulation of neural pathways. Evoked potentials (EPs) are divided into sensory (somatosensory evoked potentials (SSEPs), brainstem evoked response audiometry (BERA) or auditory evoked potentials (AEPs), visual evoked potentials (VEPs)) and motor (MEPs), based on stimulation and the recording site. The decision regarding the optimal type of IONM is based on the type of surgery and neural structures involved. Intraoperative EEG monitoring is primarily used for seizure surgery, whereas ECoG involves mapping the functional cortex, useful in cerebrovascular and CNS tumor surgery. Intraoperatively, anesthesiologists need to consider both physiologic and pharmacologic factors that affect IONM. Such physiologic factors include hypoxia, hypotension, hypothermia, and carbon dioxide (CO_2) levels. Pharmacologically, inhalational agents tend to affect EPs more than intravenous agents do. The most sensitive EPs to inhalational anesthetics are visual, whereas those the least affected are auditory (VEP > MEP > SSEP > AEP). Based on baseline IONM, inhalational agent use is typically limited (<0.3–0.5 minimum alveolar concentration (MAC)) and total intravenous anesthesia (TIVA) is commonly used during anesthetic management. Any changes in intraoperative monitoring (amplitude, latency, frequency, morphology, and threshold) should prompt evaluation as to whether the changes are localized or global, as well as prompt amelioration of insults to prevent postoperative neurological deficits.

Effects of Anesthetic Agents on Neurophysiology

The anesthesiologist plays a major role in maintaining optimal neurophysiology and facilitating optimal operating conditions, with a smooth anesthetic emergence that allows for a timely neurological examination postoperatively. In general, intravenous anesthetic agents decrease CBF and cerebral metabolic rate of oxygen ($CMRO_2$) in relative parallel, whereas the inhaled gases decrease $CMRO_2$, with a relative increase in CBF, with some nuances and exceptions discussed below.

Inhalational Agents

Inhalational anesthetics have the potential to increase ICP and reduce $CMRO_2$, with the exception of nitrous oxide (N_2O). The effect of inhalational anesthetics on CBF is a balance between a reduction in CBF caused by $CMRO_2$ suppression and increased CBF secondary to direct cerebral vasodilation.

N_2O is shown to increase CBF and ICP, with a variable effect on $CMRO_2$. Furthermore, it can enlarge potential air space, and for this reason, N_2O is suboptimal for use in patients with the potential for intracranial or intravascular air. Sevoflurane tends to produce less vasodilation than isoflurane or desflurane, and preserves $PaCO_2$ reactivity the best. Its purported neuroprotective effect is similar to that seen with isoflurane. Moreover, its lower solubility in blood makes it a desirable choice for more rapid emergence from anesthesia. Desflurane is comparable to the aforementioned halogenated compounds in its potential neuroprotection, and while its low solubility in blood favors more rapid emergence from anesthesia, it tends to produce elevation in ICP, especially in patients with supratentorial lesions.

Intravenous Anesthetic Agents

Most of these medications will decrease both CBF and $CMRO_2$, and thus provide a favorable profile for ICP control and optimal neurosurgical conditions. Barbiturates offer neuroprotection, but ensuring stable hemodynamics can prove challenging, as can facilitation of an early postoperative neurological examination, given their slow metabolism and tissue accumulation. As such, propofol emerged with a better profile, dose-dependent 50–60% reduction in CBF, and a shorter context-sensitive half-life, as compared with barbiturates. Currently, propofol is a preferred choice in balanced neurosurgical anesthesia and it preserves CO_2 reactivity. Etomidate produces minimal cardiac side effects, with a parallel decrease of approximately 30–50% in CBF and $CMRO_2$, while largely preserving CO_2 vascular reactivity. Etomidate use is limited by the potential adverse effects of adrenocortical suppression and seizure activity in neurologically compromised patients. Ketamine increases CBF and ICP, and thus vigilance with CO_2 control is important as this can mitigate such issues to some extent. It has not traditionally been a first choice for anesthetic induction or maintenance for patients with reduced intracranial compliance, but has found a role for such patients who also have hemodynamic instability. Benzodiazepines, specifically midazolam, have a relatively similar effect to propofol on CBF and $CMRO_2$, and provide relative hemodynamic neutrality. Judicious use is recommended, as reversal with flumazenil in delayed emergence can risk the induction of seizures, increasing CBF and $CMRO_2$. As such, benzodiazepines do not typically form a core element of maintenance neuroanesthesia. Dexmedetomidine in animal models reduced global and regional CBF without a significant concomitant reduction in $CMRO_2$, raising concerns for reduced brain tissue oxygenation, but these results have not been clinically reproduced. Moreover, perioperative dexmedetomidine use has been shown to reduce intraoperative opioid consumption and reduces the odds of postoperative delirium in neurosurgical patients, so careful use of the medication may prove beneficial.

Opioids

The effects of opioids on CBF, $CMRO_2$, and ICP are variable, often dependent on other medications and elements. Fentanyl is one of the most commonly used perioperative opioids and, along with sufentanil, largely produces neutral effects on neurophysiology. It is important to consider the dosing of these medications, given their potentially prolonged effects resulting in delayed anesthetic emergence. Postoperative nausea, vomiting, and hypercarbia from respiratory depression can thus lead to increased ICP. Remifentanil is a commonly used synthetic opioid in neuroanesthesia, with a rapid-onset and -offset mechanism, particularly conducive as the analgesic component for TIVA. While its μ-receptor agonism can elicit nausea and vomiting, like other opioids, its ultrashort duration of action makes it a good choice for rapid emergence. Special attention should be paid to prevent postoperative hyperalgesia.

Neuromuscular Blockers

Succinylcholine, useful in the management of rapid sequence induction and difficult airway, is often avoided as a neuromuscular blocking agent (NMBA) in neurologically injured patients, given its tendency to increase ICP transiently through fasciculations. This can be attenuated through pretreatment with a nondepolarizing agent and careful control of $PaCO_2$ by ventilation. Nondepolarizing NMBAs (e.g., rocuronium, vecuronium) are the typical choice in neuroanesthetic care, with minimal effect on CBF, $CMRO_2$, and ICP. Rocuronium enjoyed widespread use, given its rapid onset of action and reversibility with sugammadex. Adequate depth of muscle relaxation during surgery is typically monitored with a train-of-four twitch monitor.

Anesthetic Management of Acute Brain Trauma

The focus in caring for an acute head trauma patient should be on protecting airway, breathing, and circulation. Traumatic brain injury is managed nonoperatively, but certain conditions warrant neurosurgical intervention. Craniotomy for evacuation of large or rapidly expanding subdural, epidural, and intraparenchymal hematomas, as well as decompressive craniotomy for refractory cerebral edema, is often performed early in the course of the acute brain trauma patient. Anesthesia care is centered on continuing the initial resuscitation and minimizing secondary brain injury, which can manifest as ischemia, hemorrhage, cerebral edema, or herniation, and is a process which begins within minutes after the initial trauma, continuing to evolve over subsequent hours and days. Systemically, it is vital to avoid hypoxemia, hypotension, fever, and derangements in $PaCO_2$ and glucose control.

For airway management, it is important to recognize that intubation for patients with a neurologic inability (Glasgow coma scale (GCS) score ≤8) to protect their airway and optimize oxygenation and ventilation is a critical first step. As the cervical spine may be unstable, it is important to maintain in-line stabilization while performing airway intubation and exercising caution to minimize manipulation of the head and neck.

Maintaining adequate CPP should be a key objective in neuroanesthesia for the head trauma patient. CPP is usually maintained between 50 and 70 mmHg prior to dural opening, and derangements, such as coughing, that can raise ICP should be avoided. A reduced CPP can result in cerebral ischemia in early critical periods and result in long-term deleterious consequences.

Anesthesia is maintained using predominantly intravenous anesthetic agents that can reduce $CMRO_2$ to maintain CPP. Benzodiazepines, opioids, and minimal use of low-dose (<0.5–1.0 MAC) inhalational anesthetics are used to supplement the anesthetic. Avoidance of hypotension is achieved, in part, through maintaining euvolemia, with special attention paid to the patient's concomitant injuries. Appropriate and balanced transfusion is used to ensure adequate perfusion and cardiac output, and thus oxygen delivery to all tissues, helping to preserve any remaining cerebral autoregulation. Hypothermia, acidosis, and coagulopathy are to be avoided, as they can exacerbate bleeding, delay recovery, and extend the time spent in the operating room, shown to be detrimental in trauma patients. Furthermore, the anesthesiologist should ensure that iatrogenic injury is minimized and all IV lines and tubes, including chest tubes, are functioning appropriately.

Postanesthetic care involves safe transport of the patient to the neurocritical care unit, usually intubated and mechanically ventilated. Maintenance of sedation and analgesia to avoid pain, coughing, and significant ventilator dyssynchrony is important to reduce derangements in neurophysiology. With prudent care, the anesthesiologist can maintain the continuum of neurocritical care and optimize the opportunity for a good patient outcome.

Anesthetic Management for Intracranial Mass Surgery

Anesthesia for intracranial mass surgery should focus on facilitating good operating conditions by maximizing brain elastance, while preserving neurophysiology and being prepared to address intraoperative crises unique to these procedures.

A new, fast-growing supratentorial mass can profoundly raise ICP and alter the brain's compensatory mechanisms, threatening herniation as the most dire consequence (see Figure 17.1). The edema surrounding the mass can contribute to this, often mitigated by the perioperative use of steroid therapy. Moreover, a mass can potentially be epileptogenic, and it is vital for the anesthesiologist to be prepared with antiepileptic medications, in discussion with the neurosurgical team.

Good preoperative preparation and adequate IV access are important. If the intracranial mass is especially vascular or compresses the venous sinuses, a CVP catheter, vasoactive agents, and transfusion products should be considered. A smooth induction and intubation are important to avoid significant fluctuations in blood pressure that can affect cerebral autoregulation. Ventilation allows for control of $PaCO_2$, which largely dictates cerebral arteriolar dilation and constriction. An arterial line is a useful tool in facilitating these goals, especially if arterial blood gases are frequently monitored. Maintenance of general anesthesia is best approached primarily with IV medications, such as propofol and opioid infusions, commonly forming the core of balanced neuroanesthesia.

The administration of osmotic agents, such as mannitol ($0.25–1$ g kg^{-1}) or hypertonic saline (variable dosing; goal serum osmolality should be maintained at <320 mOsm kg^{-1}), is often recommended prior to dural opening, to facilitate brain elastance. Adequate neuromuscular blockade is important to reduce the incidence of ventilator dyssynchrony or coughing, which can increase the ICP and reduce brain elastance intraoperatively. Intraoperative ICP can be managed with adequate anesthesia and analgesia, and with controlled CSF drainage if an EVD or lumbar drain is present. Venous drainage from the brain is facilitated with a slight head-up position, while ensuring that intrathoracic and intraabdominal pressures are minimized to aid in ICP management. Lastly, hyperventilation, thereby reducing $PaCO_2$, can be used to reduce the ICP, but this comes at the cost of reducing cerebral perfusion through cerebral arteriolar vasoconstriction; thus, it is reserved for when other means of ICP reduction have been exhausted.

Anesthetic Management of Vascular Malformations (Aneurysms, Arteriovenous Malformations): Interventional Neurosurgical Procedures

Most intracranial aneurysms occur in the anterior circulation (90%) of the brain, with a yearly incidence of 1 in 10,000 persons and half of these patients bearing a history of an associated congenital etiology or a connective tissue disorder. Other common risk factors include hypertension and smoking, and the diagnosis of an aneurysm is based on history, physical examination, and imaging (CT scan). In the case of ruptured aneurysms resulting in subarachnoid hemorrhage (SAH), rerupture is at its highest risk in the first 24–48 hours following the initial rupture, with the risk of cerebral vasospasm peaking at 4–14 days after the initial rupture.

Endovascular or surgical management can be performed emergently to control bleeding from a ruptured aneurysm or as elective surgery to prevent rupture. During the preoperative assessment, it is important to consider coexisting disease and congenital malformations. Anesthetic management should focus on providing optimal surgical conditions, hemodynamics, and maintenance or reduction of the ICP to minimize transmural pressure across the aneurysm, and thus the risk of rupture. Standard ASA monitors, a urinary catheter, large-bore IV access, and an arterial line for close hemodynamic monitoring are all important considerations. Most intracranial aneurysms are managed with an endovascular approach, facilitating concurrent imaging and neurosurgical management. Some of these procedures are performed under general anesthesia but are increasingly managed with local anesthesia and sedation. Endovascular procedures are often performed with several team members and bear radiation risk, so good communication between the anesthesiologist and the intervention team is vital. Intraoperative EEG monitoring is often used during aneurysm surgery to identify ischemia. Communication of neuromonitoring findings can help in titration of anesthesia and hemodynamics, for which rapid-onset, short-acting, and infusion-titratable calcium channel blockers, such as nicardipine or clevidipine, are preferred. Smooth, timely emergence from anesthesia is important to facilitate early postoperative neurological assessment.

Arteriovenous malformations (AVMs) are congenital abnormalities with abnormal connections between veins and arteries, which can result in rupture and intraparenchymal hemorrhage or SAH. They are seen in nearly all age groups, mainly in patients aged 10–30 years. Common presentation includes headache and seizures, with cerebral angiography serving as the gold standard for diagnosis. Management can involve a combination of endovascular embolization, stereotactic radiosurgery, or surgical resection, and anesthetic management of these patients is similar to that discussed for aneurysm surgery.

Anesthetic Management of Carotid Endarterectomy (Regional versus General Anesthesia)

Patients presenting for carotid endarterectomy (CEA) are often elderly, with associated coronary artery disease (CAD) and/or peripheral arterial disease (PVD). Carotid artery stenosis (CAS) is a common cause of transient ischemic attack (TIA) or acute ischemic stroke. These conditions are usually treated with endovascular intervention, such as balloon angioplasty or carotid stent placement or, alternatively, open intervention and CEA. During CEA, the carotid artery is cross-clamped, and thus brain ischemia is an intraoperative concern. To this end, regional anesthesia is often considered, allowing for a more accurate intraoperative neurological examination as a standard for neuromonitoring. Multiple studies have shown no difference in outcomes between general and regional anesthesia for CEA. Regional anesthesia (superficial cervical plexus block or deep cervical plexus block, or both) reduces intraoperative blood loss and postoperative pulmonary complications, but does not prevent embolic events during surgery. Standard ASA monitors and IAP monitoring are recommended. Maintenance of CPP and normocapnia is important during surgery to reduce the risk of cerebral ischemia. If CEA is performed under general anesthesia, neuromonitoring with EEG can signal reduction in cerebral perfusion and potentially a need for temporary carotid shunt placement. Cerebral oximetry (near-infrared spectroscopy (NIRS)), jugular venous oxygen saturation, and stump pressure are useful for intraoperative neuromonitoring. Postoperatively, these patients are observed in intensive care or high-dependency units for neurological assessment (stroke, cranial nerve palsies, hyperperfusion syndrome), cardiovascular abnormalities (hypertension, myocardial infarction, arrhythmias), postoperative bleeding, and airway compression secondary to hematoma.

Anesthetic Management of Sitting Position Neurosurgical Procedures

The sitting position provides excellent surgical conditions for posterior fossa (tumors, AVMs, aneurysms, subtemporal approach for intracranial fossa) and posterior cervical spine surgery (see Table 17.1). Nevertheless, it can present significant challenges for anesthesiologists related to positioning, pressure injuries, and VAE. Most neurosurgeons avoid the sitting position due to the significantly higher risk of VAE, and instead perform these surgeries either in the prone or lateral position. Preoperative preparation may involve transesophageal echocardiography (TEE) or transthoracic echocardiography, to help evaluate for an intracardiac shunt, and thus the risk of a paradoxical air embolism. A discussion involving the patient, neurosurgeon, and anesthesiologist regarding the risks, benefits, and alternatives can improve the outcome (see Tables 17.2 and 17.3).

Table 17.1 Contraindications for sitting position neurosurgery

Contraindications
• *Absolute*: ventriculoatrial shunt, intracardiac shunt with right heart pressure higher than left heart pressure
• *Relative*: extremes of age group, uncontrolled hypertension, severe chronic obstructive pulmonary disease, intracardiac shunt with left heart pressure higher than right heart pressure

Table 17.2 Advantages and disadvantages of sitting position

Advantages	Disadvantages
• Improved surgical exposure • Better anatomical orientation, with less manipulation of the brainstem and cranial nerves • Improved venous drainage • Superior hemostasis • Gravitational drainage of CSF, with reduction in ICP • Better access to patient's face, airway, and chest • Improved respiratory dynamics (caudal movement of diaphragm)	• Systemic hypotension (vasodilation, reduced venous return) • Peripheral nerve damage (related to positioning) • Macroglossia • Subdural hematoma • Cranial nerve damage, quadriplegia • Tension pneumocephalus • Venous air embolism (pulmonary, paradoxical systemic air embolism)

CSF, cerebrospinal fluid; ICP, intracranial pressure.

Table 17.3 Monitoring and management during sitting position neurosurgery

Monitoring	Management of complications
• Standard ASA monitors • Invasive arterial pressure • Multiorifice CVP catheter • Urinary catheter • Pericardial Doppler • TEE (optional) • Transcranial Doppler (optional) • PCWP (optional)	• Pressure point padding and proper positioning of extremities to prevent nerve injury • Optimal fluid load, vasopressors to maintain CPP • VAE – if any suspected VAE, notify the surgeon immediately, flood the surgical field with saline, bone wax over bony edges, hemostasis of open vessels, 100% oxygen, administration of intravenous fluids and vasopressors to maintain blood pressure, jugular venous compression, lower the head and turn the patient to the left if possible, aspiration of air through CVP catheter. Be ready to position the patient supine for CPR in case of cardiac arrest

CVP, central venous pressure; TEE, transesophageal echocardiography; PCWP, pulmonary capillary wedge pressure; CPP, cerebral perfusion pressure; VAE, venous air embolism; CPR, cardiopulmonary resuscitation.

Anesthesia for Awake Craniotomy

Awake craniotomies can be used very efficiently for epilepsy, brain tumor, and AVMs, and in surgeries where lesions are close to eloquent areas (speech, motor, and visual centers) of the brain. It facilitates intraoperative neurological assessment, providing an opportunity for maximal tumor resection and preservation of the functional area of the brain. Patient considerations for success in this approach include minimal comorbidities, especially those relating to airway obstruction or significant cardiac disease. Intraoperative monitoring includes standard ASA monitors, IAP monitoring, and a urinary catheter, as well as neuromonitoring (EEG, ECoG, SSEP, and MEP). An asleep–awake–asleep (AAA) method or monitored anesthesia care with bilateral scalp block are preferred techniques, and sedation is usually managed with propofol or dexmedetomidine, with remifentanil. Proper positioning to reduce pressure injuries while maintaining access to the patient is critical, and the anesthesiologist should prepare for complications, including nausea, vomiting, seizures, airway compromise, and VAE. Deep brain stimulation (DBS) surgery is done for movement disorders, often with a combination of sitting craniotomy and awake craniotomy positioning, and the anesthesiologist should pay special attention to the patient's preoperative Parkinson's disease medications, while carefully minimizing intraoperative involuntary movements.

Anesthetic Management of Spinal Cord Trauma

The spinal cord is a continuation of the brainstem, which begins at the foramen magnum of the skull and ends as the conus medullaris in adults at L2 vertebral level. Below this level, lumbar and sacral nerve roots form the cauda equina. The anterior two-thirds of the spinal cord (motor function) is supplied by one anterior spinal artery, and the posterior third (sensory) is supplied by two posterior spinal arteries. Autoregulation of the spinal cord is maintained at a MAP of 50–150 mmHg, with the curve shifting to the right in chronic hypertensive patients. $PaCO_2$ and PaO_2 affect autoregulation of the spinal cord, similar to that seen in the brain. Perioperative care of patients with acute spine injury should focus on airway maintenance and oxygenation, stabilizing the spine, reducing spinal cord edema, and maintaining spinal cord perfusion, thereby helping to improve postoperative functional outcome (see Tables 17.4 and 17.5). Patients with acute spine trauma may present with significant associated problems, including head injury, traumatic brain injury, facial injuries, and thoracic, abdominal, and vascular injuries. A quick systemic assessment, as well as good communication with the trauma team and neurosurgeon, improves perioperative morbidity and mortality. If the patient has a cervical spine injury, with a cervical collar or halo traction, it is imperative to carefully plan for a difficult airway intubation and surgeon availability for potential emergency tracheostomy.

Table 17.4 Anesthetic considerations in acute spinal cord injury

If patient in respiratory distress	If respiration adequate
• Secure the airway with manual in-line stabilization of the neck • Full stomach precautions • Video laryngoscopy versus fiberoptic • May need a surgical airway if the above fails • Radiological assessment of the spine • Maintain hemodynamic stability (heart rate, blood pressure) • Temperature control (prevents hypothermia)	• Radiological assessment of the spine (X-ray, CT, MRI) • Continuous monitoring of vitals and neurological assessment (consciousness, motor, sensory, and cranial nerves) • Temperature control (prevents hypothermia)

Table 17.5 Anesthetic considerations in chronic spinal cord injury

System– issues	Management
• CVS – hypovolemia, hypotension • Autonomic dysreflexia (if spinal cord injury at T6 and above) • Respiratory – depending on the level of spinal cord injury, involvement of the phrenic nerve (C3–C5 nerve roots), aspiration risk, and pneumonia • Neurological – chronic pain • Muscular – weakness, pressure sores, increased extrajunctional receptors • Gastrointestinal – gastroparesis • Vascular system – DVT	• Optimal fluid management, control of vitals • Intraoperatively – inform the surgeon, stop the stimulus, check the depth of anesthesia, increase FiO_2, short-acting antihypertensive • Prolonged intubation and ventilation • Multimodal analgesia • Management of pressure points, change of patient positioning; avoid succinylcholine to prevent hyperkalemia • More susceptible to aspiration • Pressure stockings, DVT prophylaxis

DVT, deep vein thrombosis.

Anesthetic Management of Spine Surgery

Anesthetic management of spine surgery can involve both elective and emergency situations. Emergency spine surgery is performed in patients with trauma of the vertebral column (discussed above) or spinal cord compression by tumor, hematoma, disc, bone, or abscess. Elective surgery for degenerative spine disease and tumors is performed in the supine, prone, lateral, and sitting positions. Standard ASA monitors are often sufficient for minor spine surgery, but for major, multilevel spine surgery with the potential for significant bleeding or even spinal cord injury, more considerations are warranted. In these cases, an arterial line for close hemodynamic monitoring, a urinary catheter and a CVP catheter to monitor and maintain euvolemia, and preparation for transfusion are important considerations. Careful positioning of these patients depending on the type of surgery, with attention to the alignment of the cervical spine, pressure points, face, eyes (high risk of postoperative visual loss if malpositioned), abdomen, and extremities, are critical. IONM is commonly performed for spine surgery to assess baseline function and detect/prevent intraoperative spinal cord injury. Anesthetic management (TIVA versus balanced anesthesia using inhalational anesthetics) is tailored to provide optimal conditions for IONM and to facilitate early neurological assessment following extubation.

Further Reading

Gritti P, Akeju O, Lorini FL, Lanterna LA, Brembilla C, Bilotta FA. Narrative review of adherence to subarachnoid hemorrhage guidelines. *J Neurosurg Anesthesiol*. 2018;30 (3):203–16.

Gupta A, Gelb A, Duane D, Adapa R, eds. *Gupta and Gelb's Essentials of Neuroanesthesia and Neurointensive Care*, 2nd ed. Cambridge: Cambridge University Press; 2018.

Kurnutala LN, Soghomonyan S, Bergese SD. Perioperative acute hypertension-role of clevidipine butyrate. *Front Pharmacol*. 2014;5:197.

Kurnutala LN, *et al*. Semisitting position and venous air embolism in neurosurgical patients with patent foramen ovale: a systematic analysis. *Int J Anesth Res*. 2016;4 (8):305–12.

Pasternak JJ. Neuroanesthesiology update. *J Neurosurg Anesthesiol*. 2020;32(2):97–119.

Soghomonyan S, *et al*. Neurophysiological monitoring during surgery on the central nervous system: the role of evoked responses. *Int J Anesth Res*. 2015;3(6):119–29.

Zuleta-Alarcon A, Castellon-Larios K, Moran KR, Soghomonyan S, Kurnutala LN, Bergese SD. Anesthesia-related perioperative seizures: pathophysiology, predisposing factors and practical recommendations. *Austin J Anesth Analg*. 2014;2(4):9.

Chapter

18

Renal Anesthesiology in Clinical Practice

Pankaj Thakur, Harish Bangalore Siddaiah,
Vijay Kata, Shilpadevi S. Patil, Naina Singh,
and Alan David Kaye

Basic Renal Physiology

Kidneys are paired organs, the primary function of which is to excrete metabolic byproducts involving physiologic processes of filtration, reabsorption, secretion, and excretion. The nephron forms the basic functional unit of kidneys and is primarily involved in urine production, excretion of metabolic waste, maintaining serum osmolality, and acid–base homeostasis. All these physiologic processes involve neurohormonal mechanisms and transporters.

The nephron has its origin in the cortex at the glomeruli and ends at the papilla by joining the collecting ducts. The glomeruli of the nephron contain afferent and efferent capillary tufts where the ultrafiltrate flows into the proximal convoluted tubule (PCT), all of which lie in the cortex. The loop of Henle (LOH), distal convoluted tubule (DCT), and collecting duct lie in the medulla. Nephrons are anatomically classified into cortical and juxtamedullary nephrons. Juxtamedullary nephrons extend into the medulla and play an indispensable role in urine concentration [1]. Approximately 99% of the filtrate is reabsorbed as it moves down the nephron tubules.

Juxtaglomerular Complex

The juxtaglomerular complex is a small structure within each nephron involved in the regulation of the nephron, and has three different cell types:

1. Macula densa: specialized cells of the DCT that regulate the juxtaglomerular apparatus (JGA) via paracrine regulation of sodium and chloride sensing
2. Juxtaglomerular cells: innervated by sympathetic nerves and secrete renin, based on afferent arteriolar pressure and chloride concentration
3. Extraglomerular mesangial cells: contractile cells that help regulate vascular tone.

Renal Blood Supply

The kidneys represent only 0.5% of body weight but receive approximately 20–25% of cardiac output via the renal arteries. The renal arteries arise from

287

the aorta, dividing into segmental, interlobar, and arcuate arteries. These further give rise to afferent arterioles, forming a network or glomerulus, and then evolve into efferent arterioles. Efferent arterioles form the vasa recta and eventually drain into the renal veins via peritubular capillaries.

Renal Blood Flow

Renal blood flow is measured by use of para-aminohippuric acid.

$$\text{Renal blood flow} = \text{renal plasma flow}/(1 - \text{hematocrit})$$

Renal blood flow is 600 mL min^{-1}, and renal plasma flow is 1200 mL min^{-1}.

Regulation of Renal Blood Flow

Although renal blood flow is determined by arteriovenous pressure difference, it is renal autoregulation that ensures sustainable blood flow with blood pressure fluctuation, involving myogenic and neurohumoral mechanisms [1]. Autoregulation of renal blood flow normally occurs at mean arterial blood pressures of 80–180 mmHg, via afferent arteriolar tone and myogenic autoregulation.

1. *Renin–angiotensin–aldosterone system (RAAS) axis*: This is a neurohormonal feedback system that regulates blood pressure and maintains body fluid balance by regulating renal blood flow, which involves renin, angiotensin II, and aldosterone. Any cause leading to renal hypoperfusion is detected by the afferent arteriole, hyponatremia is detected by the macula densa, or increased renal beta-1 receptor sympathetic activation; leads to renin secretion by the juxtaglomerular cell. Renin then converts angiotensinogen produced by the liver to angiotensin I, which is then converted to angiotensin II in the lungs via angiotensin-converting enzyme. Angiotensin II acts as potent vasoconstrictor and maintains the glomerular filtration rate (GFR) via efferent arteriole vasoconstriction, and stimulates thirst by secretion of antidiuretic hormone (ADH) from the posterior pituitary. Angiotensin II also induces aldosterone secretion from the adrenals, which increases sodium and water reabsorption. This aids in restoring blood volume and blood pressure, and stimulates secretion of hydrogen ions and potassium to maintain a homeostatic milieu.

2. *Tubuloglomerular feedback*: This feedback system communicates between the tubules and the glomeruli, and maintains the GFR over a wide range of fluctuating blood pressures. The macula densa in the JGA responds to sodium concentration in the DCT as an indicator of the GFR. Sodium chloride is sensed by apical Na–K–2Cl cotransporters. Sodium chloride concentration in the tubular fluid leads to increased or decreased GFR via reflex changes in afferent arteriolar vascular tone. Hypotonic urine leads to vasodilation of the afferent arteriole, leading to increased GFR.

Hypertonic urine leads to vasoconstriction of the afferent arteriole, leading to decreased GFR.

a. Factors increasing tubuloglomerular feedback: adenosine, thromboxane, aldosterone, angiotensin II, and prostaglandins.

b. Factors decreasing tubuloglomerular feedback: atrial natriuretic peptide, cyclic adenosine monophosphate, nitric oxide, and prostacyclin.

Autonomic Autoregulation

Sympathetic innervation to the kidneys is through the celiac and renal plexuses, which carry T4–L1 outflow. Sympathetics innervate the JGA via beta-1 and renal vessels via alpha-1 receptors. Norepinephrine binds to alpha-1 receptors, leading to vasoconstriction of arterioles and decreased blood flow. Dopamine binds to D1 receptors and causes arteriolar vasodilation, which increases blood flow.

Hormonal Regulation via Natriuretic Peptides

1. Atrial natriuretic peptide (ANP): secreted in response to overextension of the atrium secondary to volume overload.

2. Brain natriuretic peptide (BNP): secreted in response to overextension of the ventricles secondary to volume overload.

Increased volume overload leads to increased sodium and water excretion. These peptides also increase the GFR via dilation of afferent arterioles and inhibit adrenocorticotrophic hormone (ACTH), renin, and aldosterone secretion.

Glomerular Filtration Rate and Creatinine Clearance

Glomerular filtration is the process by which the kidney filters blood primarily based on the hydrostatic and osmotic pressure difference. The GFR is used as a surrogate marker of kidney function and for staging of chronic kidney disease (CKD). Normal GFR varies according to body habitus, sex, and age – males: 120 mL/(min 1.73 m^2). A GFR of < 60 mL min^{-1} denotes the stage when CKD complications start to arise. Creatinine clearance is the rate of clearance of creatinine by the kidneys and is used clinically to estimate the GFR.

Creatinine Clearance (Urine Creatinine × Urine Flow Rate/Serum Creatinine)

Ultrafiltration is a vital step in urine formation in the glomeruli of the nephron at a glomerular filtration rate (GFR) of 125 mL min^{-1}. The basement membrane lies between the glomerulus and Bowman's capsule and acts as the only barrier within

Table 18.1 Reabsorbed substances and transporters

Reabsorbed substance	Segment	Transporters
Water	• Proximal convoluted tubule • Thin descending loop of Henle • Collecting duct	• Osmotic gradient • Aquaporins
Sodium	• Proximal convoluted tubule • Thick ascending loop of Henle • Distal convoluted tubule • Collecting duct	• Na^+/K^+ ATPase • Na^+/glucose symporter • $Na^+/K^+/2Cl^-$ • Na^+/Cl^- cotransporter
Chloride	• Proximal convoluted tubule • Thick ascending loop of Henle • Distal convoluted tubule • Collecting duct	• $Na^+/K^+/2Cl^-$ • Na^+/Cl^- cotransporter
Calcium	• Proximal convoluted tubule • Loop of Henle • Collecting duct	• Na^+/Ca^{2+} antiporter • Ca^{2+} ATPase
Bicarbonate	• Proximal convoluted tubule • Collecting duct	• Na^+ symporter
Phosphate	• Proximal convoluted tubule	• Na^+/PO4 cotransporter
Glucose	• Proximal convoluted tubule	• GLUT transporter • Na^+/glucose transporter

the nephron. This ultrafiltration leads to high filtration pressure called the hydrostatic pressure (see Table 18.1). The glomcruli selectively filter the substrate, despite greater permeability compared to the regular capillaries [1]. It is impermeable to larger-sized plasma proteins but effectively filters dissolved substances [1]. Water, electrolytes, and glucose are reabsorbed, along with amino acids. The nephron tubules accompany peritubular capillaries that allow movement of various solutes from the tubules to peritubular capillaries [1]. Transport of these solutes occurs via active transport that requires energy consumption, as in the case of sodium reabsorption (see Table 18.1). If active transport is coupled with another substrate, for example, sodium and glucose,

Table 18.2 Secreted substances and transporters

Secreted substance	Segment	Transporters
Potassium	• Distal convoluted tubule • Collecting ducts	• Na⁺/K⁺ ATPase • Na⁺/K⁺/2Cl⁻ cotransporter • H⁺/K⁺ antiporter
Hydrogen ions	• Thick ascending loop of Henle • Collecting ducts	• Na⁺/H⁺ antiporter • H⁺ ATPase
Urea	• Loop of Henle	• Urea transporters

then it is termed cotransport. When positive ions are actively transported, negative ions follow to maintain electrical neutrality, such as chloride and urea (see Table 18.2) [1]. Passive mechanism moves solutes across their gradients.

Anesthesia for Kidney Transplant

With advances in immunosuppression and use of immunoglobulins since the 1960s, use of allografts has had more successful outcomes with living donor grafts than with cadaver donors. End-stage renal disease (ESRD) (with the most common etiologies being diabetes mellitus, hypertension, and glomerular diseases) affects multisystem physiology, and its effects on the cardiovascular system account for approximately 50% mortality. Thorough knowledge of changes in multisystem physiology is important [2]. A comprehensive preoperative examination, laboratory tests, human leukocyte antigen (HLA) typing and crossmatching, hemodialysis within 24 hours, volume status, and evaluation of cardiac function are of prime importance. Intraoperatively, standard American Society of Anesthesiologists (ASA) monitors, with invasive blood pressure and central venous pressure (CVP) monitoring, are routinely utilized. Intraoperative arteriovenous fistula monitoring is done every 15 minutes. Propofol is utilized as a standard induction agent and cisatracurium is a mainstay muscle relaxant. Succinylcholine should be used for rapid sequence induction only if a patient has a recent normal potassium level. Fentanyl is the main opioid utilized, whereas morphine, hydromorphone, and meperidine are avoided due to accumulation of secondary metabolites. Desflurane, isoflurane, and total intravenous anesthesia (TIVA) are commonly utilized; however, sevoflurane is also commonly utilized, even though there is a theoretical risk of compound A resulting in renal injury in a dose-dependent manner, as shown in animal models [3]. Potassium-containing fluids are generally avoided. Postoperatively, patients can be extubated and rarely require critical care unit monitoring unless indicated [2]. Numerous drugs have been utilized for immunosuppression to revert graft rejection, namely cyclosporin, sirolimus, interleukin 2, daclizumab, and azathioprine. Induction (first phase) of immunosuppressants is started a week before transplant, and maintenance (second phase) is utilized to prevent graft rejection for 3–6 months. Long-term immunosuppression (third phase) is utilized lifelong. A commonly used regimen includes tacrolimus as the prime drug for maintenance and mycophenolate for adjunctive oral maintenance. Methylprednisolone is used as an adjunct to the induction regimen. Thymoglobulin is used both for induction and for acute rejection, and basiliximab is utilized in the immediate period following transplantation [2].

Regional Anesthesiology for End-Stage Renal Disease and Chronic Kidney Disease

Given hematologic abnormalities in ESRD, including abnormal coagulation profile, dysfunctional platelets, heparin use, electrolyte abnormalities, and acid–base abnormalities, regional anesthesia for transplant is commonly utilized [2]. A combined spinal epidural technique can provide supplemental analgesia, but most facilities have utilized general anesthesia for predictable anesthetic depth during renal transplant [2]. There is also a potential for local anesthetic toxicity, especially in plexus volume blocks where larger doses of local anesthetic are utilized. No difference has been found in patients with ESRD and normal individuals with regard to optimally placed nerve block duration and quality. Brachial plexus blocks are commonly utilized for arteriovenous fistula surgery. At the authors' institution, a combination of 15 mL of 0.5% ropivacaine and 15 mL of 1.5% mepivacaine is commonly utilized for preoperative supraclavicular block in arteriovenous fistula surgery. If the block is patchy or incomplete, general anesthesia is reverted to with use of endotracheal tube placement or TIVA, with similar goals and concerns for general anesthesia in renal transplant patients.

Perioperative Management in Clinical Renal Conditions

End-Stage Renal Disease

High morbidity and mortality rates constantly plague ESRD patients, decreasing successful health or surgical outcomes. In comparison to those with normal-functioning kidneys, ESRD patients who undergo dialysis have longer mechanical ventilation times, longer intensive care unit (ICU) stays, and increased stays at the hospital [4]. Before taking the patient to surgery, dialysis should be performed typically on the previous day and blood work should corroborate (if possible) hemodynamic stability. Hyperkalemia, volume overload, and glycemic control should be monitored prior to surgery, and clinicians should take note of changes in laboratory values [4]. ESRD patients have decreased renal filtration and excretion of metabolites, so pharmacokinetics and pharmacodynamics should be monitored by the anesthesiologist perioperatively [5]. Perioperative management of ESRD patients under general anesthesia should also take into account disease pathophysiology, involving cardiovascular dysfunction, fluid levels, electrolyte imbalances, anemia, and other complications [6]. The anesthetic technique that is implemented depends on the functional status of the patient, coagulation changes, surgical necessity, and the preferences of the multidisciplinary team [5]. Postoperative problems increase with age, signaling that the condition deteriorates due to the patient's physical status and overall health. Restarting dialysis postoperatively and administering medications, such as heparin for blood clotting, help to restore normal functions and reduce the risk of bleeding, pain, or other complications [5].

Nephrectomy

Depending on the progression of the disease, the physician may opt to perform a partial or radical nephrectomy. A preoperative evaluation of current medical conditions, such as cardiovascular, pulmonary, or cerebrovascular disease, is necessary for standard treatment [7]. Estimating kidney function before and after partial/total nephrectomy remains vital towards patient outcomes. Preoperative considerations involve examining anticoagulation medications, blood type, kidney damage/localization, method of attack, and other pertinent factors [8]. Intraoperative outcomes aim to provide a minimally invasive technique that utilizes accurate regional/general anesthesia dosages. Throughout the surgery, perioperative management helps to reduce the rates of pressure sores, nerve damage, venous congestion, and blood loss [7]. Patients may require mechanical ventilation postoperatively and need to be watched for any further complication, but the use of a laparoscopic nephrectomy procedure leads to shorter hospital stays, reduced painful episodes, and rapid convalescence [7].

Bladder

The primary care physician, nephrologist, surgeon, urologist, and anesthesiologist determine the patient's physical state and prognosis regarding bladder dysfunction within ESRD [9]. Urinary tract infections (UTIs) are common in ESRD patients, leading to more pain and progressive weakening of the bladder [10]. Bladder complications can inflame the tissue and provide a range of abnormalities, such as distension of, or defects in, the bladder wall [10]. Renal protection and other intraoperative techniques maintain the body's physiologic parameters and avoid nephrotoxicity through natural and pharmacologic protection [9]. The anesthesiologist and surgical staff should monitor the rates of hemorrhaging, infection from bacteremia, and any urinary/bladder abnormalities that arise [10]. Postoperative care entails analyzing a variety of factors, such as blood volume and electrolyte levels. A multidisciplinary team continues to observe the patient's postoperative bladder function for the duration of the hospital stay.

Prostate/Transurethral Resection of the Prostate

Men with ESRD who possess an enlarged prostate may require a transurethral resection of the prostate (TURP) to relieve ongoing pressure towards the urethra and bladder. Preoperative measures that track the patient's age, comorbidities, prostate volume, urea and creatinine levels, electrolyte concentrations, and abdominal/genital pain provide a better picture of renal function [11]. TURP operates in a narrow surgical field and utilizes an irrigating fluid that modifies intravascular volume and osmolality [7]. The anesthesiologist observes the patient's intraoperative reactions to either a general or a spinal anesthetic. During the surgical procedure, the surgeon must not perforate the prostatic capsule and should maintain high alertness for different symptoms, such as dyspnea, arrhythmia, hypotension, and seizures, even though the patient is sedated [7]. Common postoperative complications to track during the TURP procedure include bleeding, completeness of the resection, transurethral resection (TUR) syndrome, sexual dysfunction, and stress urinary incontinence [12]. Postoperative care should entail routine monitoring until the patient becomes suitable for discharge.

Nephrolithiasis

Medical research has illustrated that kidney stones can increase the risk of ESRD and contribute to poorer health outcomes. Recurrent stone formation often exacerbates kidney damage, so preoperative measures should monitor patients' age, gender, diet, fluid intake, medications, and family history [13]. General anesthesia for nephrolithotomy has its advantages in securing the airway while prone and decreasing pleural injury through tidal volume manipulation [7]. General anesthesia in nephrolithotomy requires prone placement and can damage the ears, eyes, and nose [7]. Spinal anesthesia, on the other hand, reduces recovery time and does not affect the ears, eyes, and nose [7].

Renal Effects of Anesthetic Drugs

The principal route of elimination for anesthetic drugs after undergoing biotransformation is via renal excretion. Failure to excrete anesthetic drugs in a timely fashion can result in prolonged duration of action, systemic alterations in hemodynamic factors, and potentiation or attenuation of co-administered agents (see Table 18.3).

Table 18.3 Renal effects of anesthetic agents

Anesthetic agent	Effect in compromised renal function
Induction agents	
Propofol	Elimination of inactive metabolites independent of renal function
Etomidate	Decreased protein binding due to hypoalbuminemia, prolonged pharmacodynamic effect
Ketamine	Elimination of active metabolites dependent on renal function, prolonged pharmacodynamic effect
Dexmedetomidine	Decreased protein binding due to hypoalbuminemia, prolonged pharmacodynamic effect
Opioids	
Fentanyl, alfentanil, sufentanil	Elimination of inactive metabolites unaltered with impaired renal function
Remifentanil	Elimination of inactive metabolites unaltered with impaired renal function
Morphine, codeine, hydrocodone	Elimination of active metabolites dependent on renal function, prolonged pharmacodynamic effect
Meperidine	Elimination of active metabolites dependent on renal function, prolonged pharmacodynamic effect, lower seizure threshold
Volatile anesthetics	
Methoxyflurane	Renal metabolism yields fluoride ions, nephrotoxic
Sevoflurane	Elimination independent of renal function, unaltered pharmacokinetics and pharmacodynamic effect
Isoflurane	Elimination independent of renal function, unaltered pharmacokinetics and pharmacodynamic effect
Desflurane	Elimination independent of renal function, unaltered pharmacokinetics and pharmacodynamic effect
Adjuvants	
Benzodiazepines: diazepam, midazolam	Elimination of active metabolites dependent on renal function, prolonged pharmacodynamic effect

Table 18.3 (cont.)

Anesthetic agent	Effect in compromised renal function
	Muscle relaxants
Succinylcholine	Risk of inducing hyperkalemia due to prolonged elimination
Atracurium, cisatracurium	Elimination independent of renal function
Rocuronium, vecuronium	Elimination partially dependent on renal function, prolonged pharmacodynamic effect
Pancuronium	Elimination primarily dependent on renal function, prolonged pharmacodynamic effect
	Reversal drugs
Neostigmine	Elimination dependent on renal function, prolonged elimination half-life
Sugammadex	Elimination dependent on renal function, prolonged elimination of drug complexes

Induction Drugs

Propofol

Propofol predominantly undergoes hepatic glucuronidation and metabolism via cytochrome P450 isoforms, followed by renal clearance of inactive metabolites within 5 days. The pharmacokinetics of propofol are unaffected by impaired renal function; thus, propofol does not accumulate in patients with CKD. Hemodynamics of renal blood flow is maintained with propofol infusion; however, patients with diminished renal perfusion secondary to decreased cardiac output are at increased risk of renal injury during the perioperative period, as propofol causes a dose-dependent decrease in cardiac output [14].

Etomidate

Etomidate is primarily protein-bound and metabolized via hepatic and plasma ester hydrolysis, followed by renal excretion of inactive metabolites. In patients with decreased renal function with concurrent hypoproteinemia, etomidate can exhibit a prolonged pharmacodynamic effect [15].

Dexmedetomidine

Dexmedetomidine is predominantly protein-bound, and patients who have renal disease with concomitant hypoalbuminemia can experience prolonged sedation as more free drug is available to cross the blood–brain barrier [16].

Ketamine

Ketamine is metabolized via hepatic cytochrome P450 isoforms to its active metabolite norketamine, which undergoes further metabolism, followed by renal excretion. Renal elimination accounts for the excretion of 2% of unchanged ketamine, 2% of norketamine, and the rest as secondary metabolites. Excretion of norketamine can be delayed in renal disease; however, it is less potent than ketamine and dose adjustments are not needed in patients with renal failure [17–19].

Benzodiazepines

Benzodiazepines are protein-bound, have a large volume of distribution due to their lipophilicity, and undergo hepatic metabolism, followed by renal elimination of pharmacologically active metabolites. Delayed renal elimination can subsequently prolong sedation due to active metabolites, notably with midazolam and diazepam [20].

Opioids

Fentanyl, Alfentanil, and Sufentanil

Fentanyl, alfentanil, and sufentanil undergo hepatic metabolism, followed by renal excretion of inactive metabolites. Excretion of inactive metabolites is unaltered in patients with renal failure [21, 22].

Remifentanil

Remifentanil is metabolized via blood esterases, followed by renal excretion of inactive metabolites. The production and excretion of their inactive metabolites are unaltered in renal disease and thus, remifentanil can be used in patients with renal failure [21, 22].

Morphine, Codeine, and Hydrocodone

Pharmacologically active metabolites of morphine, codeine, and hydrocodone accumulate in patients with renal disease, cause prolonged respiratory depression, and are therefore not advisable [21, 22].

Meperidine

Meperidine metabolism produces normeperidine, an active metabolite that lowers the seizure threshold. To mitigate the accumulation of active metabolites, decreasing the dose frequency or avoiding its use in patients with renal compromise are effective [21, 22].

Volatile Anesthetics

Metabolism of methoxyflurane occurs in the liver and kidneys. Production of fluoride metabolites during renal metabolism causes nephrotoxicity, as they damage the proximal tubule; therefore, its use is avoided in renal failure and this drug has not been utilized in the past few decades because of its high metabolism [23, 24].

Sevoflurane, isoflurane, desflurane, and nitric oxide undergo minimal biotransformation and are not dependent on renal excretion; thus, they are preferred for use in patients with renal impairment [23, 24].

Neuromuscular Blocking Agents

Succinylcholine

Succinylcholine induces hyperkalemia with repeated doses, as there is increased depolarization of acetylcholine receptors. In patients with existing renal failure who are normokalemic preoperatively, a single dose of succinyl-choline for rapid sequence intubation can be used safely, with close monitoring of potassium levels and hemodynamic parameters [22].

Atracurium and Cisatracurium

Atracurium and cisatracurium are the preferred nondepolarizing neuromus-cular blocking agents in patients with renal failure, as they are metabolized via plasma esterases and Hofmann degradation, and do not yield active metabo-lites. Also, their elimination is independent of renal function [22].

Rocuronium and Vecuronium

In addition to biliary excretion, elimination of rocuronium and vecuronium is dependent on renal function, and increased doses can accumulate in patients with renal failure. Renal failure patients undergoing maintenance with these agents for more lengthy procedures require close monitoring [22].

Pancuronium

Pancuronium use is avoided in patients with renal disease, as it relies primarily on renal function to eliminate its active metabolite [22].

Reversal Medications

Neostigmine

Neostigmine is predominantly dependent on renal function for elimination; therefore, renal failure patients can experience prolonged half-life.

Decreased clearance of neostigmine does not directly affect the rate of reversal of neuromuscular blockade, and dose adjustment is not needed [25–27].

Sugammadex

Upon encapsulating neuromuscular blocking agents, sugammadex relies on renal function to rapidly eliminate the drug complexes. Patients with renal failure experience delayed elimination, as the drug complexes accumulate [25, 28]. At present, sugammadex can been used for patients with significant renal disease; however, there are no clinical studies in patients with renal failure.

References

1. Preuss HG. Basics of renal anatomy and physiology. *Clin Lab Med*. 1993;13 (1):1–11.

2. Baxi V, Jain A, Dasgupta D. Anaesthesia for renal transplantation: an update. *Indian J Anaesth*. 2009;53(2):139–47.

3. Mittel AM, Wagener G. Anesthesia for kidney and pancreas transplantation. *Anesthesiol Clin*. 2017;35(3):439–52.

4. Akdemir AO, Oztekin CV, Doluoglu OG, *et al*. The effects of transurethral resection of the prostate on morbidity and mortality in patients with nondialysis-requiring renal insufficiency. *Ther Adv Urol*. 2012;4(2):51–6.

5. Carlo JO, Phisitkul P, Phisitkul K, Reddy S, Amendola A. Perioperative implications of end-stage renal disease in orthopaedic surgery. *J Am Acad Orthop Surg*. 2015;23 (2):107–18.

6. Dhondup T, Kittanamongkolchai W, Vaughan LE, *et al*. Risk of ESRD and mortality in kidney and bladder stone formers. *Am J Kidney Dis*.2018;72(6):790–7.

7. Domi R, Huti G, Sula H, *et al*. From pre-existing renal failure to perioperative renal protection: the anesthesiologist's dilemmas. *Anesthesiol Pain Med*. 2016;6 (3):e32386.

8. Kanda H, Hirasaki Y, Iida T, *et al*. Perioperative management of patients with end-stage renal disease. *J Cardiothorac Vasc Anesth*. 2017;31(6):2251–67.

9. Kefer JC, Desai MM, Fergany A, Novick AC, Gill IS. Outcomes of partial nephrectomy in patients on chronic oral anticoagulant therapy. *J Urol*. 2008;180 (6):2370–4.

10. Koo C, Ryu J. Anesthetic considerations for urologic surgeries. *Korean J Anesthesiol*. 2020;73(2):92–102.

11. Nasr R, Chilimuri S. Preoperative evaluation in patients with end-stage renal disease and chronic kidney disease. *Health Serv Insights*. 2017;10:117863291771302.

12. Olanipekun T, Effoe V, Turner J, Flood M. Bladder necrosis and perforation in end-stage renal disease and recurrent urinary tract infection: a rare medical emergency. *Int J Crit Illn Inj Sci.* 2019;9(2):101–4.

13. Teo JS, Lee YM, Ho HS. An update on transurethral surgery for benign prostatic obstruction. *Asian J Urol.* 2017;4(3):195–8.

14. Sahinovic MM, Struys MMRF, Absalom AR. Clinical pharmacokinetics and pharmacodynamics of propofol. *Clin Pharmacokinet.* 2018;57(12):1539–58.

15. Erdoes G, Basciani RM, Eberle B. Etomidate – a review of robust evidence for its use in various clinical scenarios. *Acta Anaesthesiol Scand.* 2014;58(4):380–9.

16. Zhong W, Zhang Y, Zhang MZ, *et al.* Pharmacokinetics of dexmedetomidine administered to patients with end-stage renal failure and secondary hyperparathyroidism undergoing general anaesthesia. *J Clin Pharm Ther.* 2018;43 (3):414–21.

17. Aroni F, Iacovidou N, Dontas I, Pourzitaki C, Xanthos T. Pharmacological aspects and potential new clinical applications of ketamine: reevaluation of an old drug. *J Clin Pharmacol.* 2009;49(8):957–64.

18. Mion G, Villevieille T. Ketamine pharmacology: an update (pharmacodynamics and molecular aspects, recent findings). *CNS Neurosci Ther.* 2013;19 (6):370–80.

19. Zanos P, Moaddel R, Morris PJ, *et al.* Ketamine and ketamine metabolite pharmacology: insights into therapeutic mechanisms. *Pharmacol Rev.* 2018;70 (3):621–60

20. Cornett EM, Novitch MB, Brunk AJ, *et al.* New benzodiazepines for sedation. *Best Pract Res Clin Anaesthesiol.* 2018;32(2):149–64.

21. King S, Forbes K. A systematic review of the use of opioid medication for those with moderate to severe cancer pain and renal impairment: a European Palliative Care Research Collaborative opioid guidelines project. *Palliat Med.* 2011;25 (5):525–52.

22. Alizadeh R, Fard ZA. Renal effects of general anesthesia from old to recent studies. *J Cell Physiol.* 2019;234(10):16944–52.

23. Ong Sio LC, Dela Cruz RG, Bautista A. Sevoflurane and renal function: a meta-analysis of randomized trials. *Med Gas Res.* 2017;7(3):186–93.

24. Dayan AD. Analgesic use of inhaled methoxyflurane. *Hum Exp Toxicol.* 2016;35 (1):91–100.

25. Isik Y, Palabiyik O, Cegin BM, Goktas U, Kati I. Effects of sugammadex and neostigmine on renal biomarkers. *Med Sci Monit.* 2016;22:803–9.

26. Luo J, Chen S, Min S, Peng L. Reevaluation and update on efficacy and safety of neostigmine for reversal of neuromuscular blockade. *Ther Clin Risk Manag.* 2018;14:2397–406.

27. Craig RG, Hunter JM. Neuromuscular blocking drugs and their antagonists in patients with organ disease. *Anaesthesia*. 2009;64(Suppl. 1):55–65.

28. Staals LM, Snoeck MMJ, Driessen JJ, *et al.* Reduced clearance of rocuronium and sugammadex in patients with severe to end-stage renal failure: a pharmacokinetic study. *Br J Anaesth*. 2010;104(1):31–9.

Chapter 19

Anesthesia for General Surgical Procedures

Julie A. Gayle and Alan David Kaye

Introduction

General surgical procedures encompass a multitude of surgical types. For the purposes of this chapter, the focus will be on anesthetic considerations for different types of esophageal, abdominal, intestinal, and peritoneal surgery, as well as colorectal surgery. In addition, common surgical techniques used for general surgical procedures to include in open, endoscopic, laparoscopic, and robotic surgery will be discussed.

Laparoscopic General Surgery

Many general surgical procedures lend themselves to a laparoscopic approach and resultant benefits, including smaller incisions, less postoperative pain, shorter recovery times, and reduced postoperative stress response. Typical laparoscopic surgical procedures include cholecystectomy, appendectomy, inguinal hernia repair, esophageal fundoplication, bowel resection, and splenectomy. Laparoscopic-assisted colorectal surgery requires an additional small incision to exteriorize the intestine and access the mesentery to create an anastomosis. General endotracheal anesthesia is utilized for most laparoscopic surgeries and is required for laparoscopic surgeries in the Trendelenburg position to achieve adequate ventilatory control. Use of intraperitoneal carbon dioxide provides insufflation for the surgeon to visualize and to perform surgical maneuvers without the need for extensive incision and exposure. Insufflation of carbon dioxide into the peritoneal cavity, or pneumoperitoneum, results in an increase in intraabdominal pressure and absorption of carbon dioxide. Pneumoperitoneum, coupled with extremes of patient positioning to facilitate surgical exposure, results in predictable cardiovascular and pulmonary physiologic changes (see Table 19.1).

Preoperative preparation for laparoscopic general surgical procedures is similar to that for anesthesia for open general surgical procedures. Focus should be placed on evaluation and optimization of medical conditions that will affect the response to the physiologic changes that occur with the laparoscopic technique and the surgery itself. Induction of general endotracheal

Table 19.1 Physiologic changes in pneumoperitoneum

	CNS	CV	Respiratory	GI	Endocrine	Renal	Other
Increase	ICP CBF IOP	SVR MVO_2 MAP	V/Q mismatch Peek airway pressure Airway resistance, PVR	IAP	Circulating catecholamines, activation of RAS	RVR	Edema – face and airway, VAE, gastric regurgitation, brachial plexus injury, ETT dislodgement
Decrease		HR (vagal stimulation)	Airway compliance FRC			GFR UOP	

ICP, intracranial pressure; CBF, cerebral blood flow; IOP, intraocular pressure; SVR, systemic vascular resistance; MVO_2, myocardial oxygen consumption; MAP, mean arterial pressure; V/Q, ventilation/perfusion; PVR, pulmonary vascular resistance; IAP, intraabdominal pressure; RAS, renin–angiotensin system; RVR, renal vascular resistance; VAE, venous air embolism; ETT, endotracheal tube; HR, heart rate; FRC, functional residual capacity; GFR, glomerular filtration rate; UOP, urine output.

anesthesia is achieved with typical induction drugs, as dictated by patient comorbidities, aspiration risk, and airway examination.

Maintenance of general endotracheal anesthesia involves inhalational agents, intravenous agents, or a combination of the two. Standard American Society of Anesthesiologists monitoring applies and invasive monitoring may be indicated, depending upon patient condition, duration of surgery, and expected blood loss. Ensuring adequate intravenous access prior to positioning is necessary if the arms are inaccessible during surgery. The extent of muscle relaxation with neuromuscular blockade depends on the clinical situation and surgical needs. Controlled ventilation is modified to maintain oxygenation (saturation >90%) and normocarbia (end-tidal carbon dioxide 40 mmHg) during insufflation. Intraoperative ventilatory strategies to protect the lungs include tidal volumes of 6–8 mL kg^{-1} of ideal body weight and 5–10 cmH$_2$O of positive end-expiratory pressure. Depending on positioning and the degree of insufflation, allowing mild hypercarbia may be necessary to avoid barotrauma. Hypercarbia that does not correct with hyperventilation should prompt suspicion of subcutaneous emphysema (see Table 19.2).

Techniques to improve oxygenation during insufflation include increasing the fraction of inspired oxygen, performing recruitment maneuvers, and increasing positive end-expiratory pressure. Refractory hypoxemia and/or high peak airway pressures in patients in the Trendelenburg position often respond to decreasing the Trendelenburg position or slightly reducing the insufflation pressure.

Laparoscopic surgery typically causes less postoperative pain than open surgical procedures. Use of multimodal analgesia works well for postoperative pain control and minimizes systemic opioid needs. Typical combinations include acetaminophen and nonsteroidal antiinflammatory drugs, in addition

Table 19.2 Risk factors and treatment options for subcutaneous emphysema caused by CO$_2$ insufflation during laparoscopy

Risk factors	Treatment[a]
Age >65 years	Visualization by laryngoscopy to assess edema prior to emergence and extubation
Use of six or more surgical ports	Extubation over a tube exchanger
Surgical time >200 minutes	Delayed extubation, head-up position for several hours to allow reabsorption of CO$_2$
Nissen fundoplication surgery	

[a] When external swelling is severe and persists after deflation of the abdomen.

to infiltration of local anesthetic at the incision sites by the surgeon prior to emergence. Transversus abdominis plane (TAP) block may be useful in laparoscopic procedures with longer incisions.

Given the high incidence of postoperative nausea and vomiting (PONV) in patients undergoing laparoscopy, antiemetics play an important role in PONV prophylaxis. All patients benefit from intravenous dexamethasone 4–8 mg after induction, and ondansetron administration prior to emergence. For patients with multiple risk factors for PONV, a preoperative scopolamine patch is recommended. Total intravenous anesthesia with propofol is a good option for patients at high risk of PONV who are undergoing laparoscopic surgery.

Laparoscopic surgery may be converted to laparotomy for a variety of reasons. Inability to define the anatomy, presence of dense adhesions, disease acuity, and other surgical conditions may result in conversion to open to complete surgery in a timely and effective manner. In these cases, postoperative pain management includes multimodal analgesia, regional block, neuraxial analgesia, and supplemental intravenous opioids.

Robotic General Surgery

Robotic-assisted surgery has become commonplace in many hospitals. Both robotic and laparoscopic surgery are considered minimally invasive; however, robotic-assisted surgery offers specific advantages over laparoscopic surgery. Robotic systems give surgeons greater control and vision during surgery. Robotic-assisted surgery allows the surgeon to sit at a console equipped with two master controllers that maneuver four robotic arms. The console displays a high-definition, three-dimensional image that allows precise, computer-controlled movements. Robotic arms have the highest level of dexterity, rotating 360 degrees, with flexibility beyond that of the human hand. Robotic-controlled instruments can access areas of the body previously inaccessible. Like with laparoscopic surgery, potential patient benefits of minimally invasive robotic surgery include shorter hospital stay, significantly less postoperative pain, quicker recovery and return to normal activities, smaller incisions, fewer complications, and less risk of infection.

Robotic-assisted surgery is used in a wide range of specialties, including gynecology, urology, gastrointestinal, colorectal, endocrine, cardiac, and thoracic surgeries. Preoperative evaluation and optimization considerations are similar to those used in preparing the patient for laparoscopic surgery. Focus is on medical conditions that affect response to the physiologic impact of robotic-assisted surgery, including extremes of positioning (i.e., steep Trendelenburg, reverse Trendelenburg, and lateral decubitus). General endotracheal anesthesia is necessary for optimal surgical conditions. Patient comorbidities, aspiration risk, and airway examination determine the choice of induction technique.

Maintenance of anesthesia includes a balance of inhaled agents, intravenous agents, or both, along with continuous muscle relaxation to provide safe surgical conditions. In addition to standard monitoring, the need for invasive lines and invasive monitoring depends upon patient condition, duration of surgery, and expected blood loss. Patient positioning and padding require close attention. Patient extremities and shoulders, eyes, and face are of particular concern due to robotic arm movement. Once the robot is docked, there is limited access to the patient. Therefore, proper positioning of the patient and provider access to intravenous lines and monitors must be secured prior to robot docking.

Physiologic changes related to extremes of positioning in robotic-assisted surgery are similar to those in laparoscopic-assisted surgery and often result in exaggerations of common physiologic changes. The addition of carbon dioxide pneumoperitoneum can amplify these changes even more. Techniques to maintain oxygenation and ventilation during robotic-assisted surgery include those used for laparoscopic-assisted surgery.

Postoperative pain management following robotic-assisted surgery includes use of multimodal analgesia to minimize systemic opioid needs. Just like with laparoscopic-assisted surgery, useful medication combinations include acetaminophen and nonsteroidal antiinflammatory drugs, in addition to infiltration of local anesthetic at the incision sites by the surgeon. Regional anesthesia techniques, such as TAP or erector spinae blocks, are options for longer abdominal incisions.

Prevention of PONV with prophylactic agents is important. Risk factors for PONV include female sex, history of motion sickness and/or PONV, nonsmoker, volatile anesthetic use, and need for postoperative opioids. A preoperative scopolamine patch, intravenous dexamethasone 4–8 mg after induction of general endotracheal anesthesia, and ondansetron administration prior to emergence are routinely used for PONV prevention. Total intravenous anesthesia with propofol should be considered for patients who are at high risk of PONV.

Esophageal Surgery

Most esophageal surgery requires general endotracheal anesthesia. Neuraxial or regional nerve block may be performed to supplement surgical anesthesia, as well as to provide postoperative analgesia. Common esophageal surgeries include esophagectomy, esophagostomy, and esophagogastric fundoplasty. Patients presenting for esophageal surgery are frequently elderly and have comorbidities associated with a history of tobacco and alcohol use, including cardiac and pulmonary disease.

Patients requiring esophageal surgery (i.e., patients with esophageal mass or stricture) are often at risk of pulmonary aspiration during induction and intubation; therefore, appropriate antacid medications and rapid sequence intubation should be employed as indicated. In patients with potential difficult intubation, awake intubation and/or video laryngoscopy are recommended to secure the airway. Esophageal surgery utilizing a thoracic approach or a combined thoracic–abdominal approach requires a double-lumen tube and the ability to provide one-lung ventilation during surgery. For surgical procedures such as transhiatal esophagectomy, a single-lumen tube is adequate. Typically, a nasogastric tube is placed to maintain gastric decompression.

The intraoperative anesthetic technique for esophageal surgery, such as esophagectomy, is general endotracheal anesthesia, which may be used in combination with continuous neuraxial analgesia (thoracic epidural analgesia) or other regional anesthetic techniques. Maintenance of anesthesia involves inhalational agents, intravenous agents, or a combination of these. Invasive monitoring, including an arterial catheter for continuous blood pressure readings, is useful to monitor frequent hemodynamic fluctuations, guide fluid administration, and patient response to treatments. While insertion of a central venous catheter may be warranted, large-bore intravenous catheters are important for fluid resuscitation. Goals of fluid management are to maintain normovolemia, oxygen, and blood flow to tissues while avoiding excessive fluid administration. Urine output measurements via a Foley catheter assist with fluid management. Depending upon cardiopulmonary status and the extent of the surgical procedure, the patient may be extubated when criteria for level of consciousness, oxygenation, ventilation, and muscle strength are met.

Postoperative pain management for esophageal surgery performed by the open thoracotomy or laparotomy approach includes neuraxial analgesia such as thoracic epidural analgesia or regional nerve block (i.e., paravertebral and erector spinae blocks) (see Table 19.3).

Table 19.3 Postoperative neuraxial and regional nerve blocks for pain control in esophageal surgery

Open thoracotomy/ upper abdominal laparotomy	Thoracoscopic approach	Laparoscopic approach
Thoracic epidural	Erector spinae block	Thoracic or lumbar epidural
Paravertebral nerve block	Intercostal nerve block	Paravertebral nerve block
Intercostal nerve block	Serratus anterior nerve block	Transversus abdominis plane block
Transversus abdominis plane block	Erector spinae nerve block	Erector spinae nerve block

Neuraxial analgesia provides superior pain control to systemic opioids, decreases supplemental opioid requirements, and reduces intravenous opioid-associated complications. Patients undergoing laparoscopic esophageal surgery usually experience less postoperative pain than those requiring thoracotomy and/or laparotomy. TAP block, local infiltration, and nonopioid analgesics with supplemental intravenous opioids provide adequate analgesia following laparoscopic esophageal surgery in most patients. PONV prophylactic agents should be administered as risk factors dictate.

Stomach Surgery

Common general surgical procedures involving the stomach include gastric resection and repair of gastric or duodenal perforation. Total or partial gastrectomy for gastric cancer includes resection of gastric tumor, the omentum, lymph nodes, and affected adjacent organs. Restoration of intestinal continuity follows gastric resection by joining a Roux limb of the jejunum to the distal esophagus in the case of total gastrectomy or gastrojejunostomy (Billroth II) for partial gastrectomy. Patients presenting with gastric or duodenal perforation require emergency surgery due to peritonitis. A midline open approach or a laparoscopic approach may be used to apply an omental patch, known as a Graham's patch.

Preoperative evaluation and optimization are necessary for patients undergoing gastric resection. Gastric carcinoma and gastrointestinal stromal tumors are associated with comorbidities seen in patients with a history of tobacco and alcohol use and related disease processes. Emergency surgery for patients presenting with perforation or gastrointestinal bleeding requires rapid preoperative assessment and treatment for hemodynamic instability with fluid resuscitation and possibly blood products. Patients in need of gastric resection or perforation repair should be considered at risk of aspiration, and treated with appropriate prophylaxis medications and rapid sequence intubation.

Intraoperative management of patients undergoing gastric resection and perforation repair requires general endotracheal anesthesia. For planned gastric resection, general anesthesia may be combined intraoperatively with neuraxial analgesia, which may also be used to provide postoperative analgesia. Maintenance of anesthesia involves inhalational agents, intravenous agents, or both, in conjunction with neuraxial anesthesia if epidural placement is not contraindicated. Standard monitoring is appropriate. The decision to use invasive monitoring (arterial catheter, central venous catheter) is based on patient status, presence of, or anticipated, hemodynamic instability, and expected blood loss. Large third space losses are common; therefore, adequate intravenous access is important. A nasogastric or orogastric tube allows for gastric decompression. At the conclusion of surgery, the decision to extubate prior to leaving the operating room requires evaluation of the patient's cardiopulmonary status, as well as the magnitude of the surgical procedure. If deemed appropriate, the patient may be extubated once criteria are met.

Postoperative pain management for gastric surgery includes neuraxial analgesia, such as thoracic or lumbar epidural analgesia, or regional block (i.e., TAP and erector spinae blocks). Supplemental systemic opioids may be necessary, in which case patient-controlled analgesia is frequently prescribed in the immediate postoperative period. PONV prophylaxis should be considered and administered as appropriate and in accordance with risk factor stratification.

Intestinal and Peritoneal Surgery

Common surgical procedures of the intestine include small bowel resection, ileostomy pouch, intraabdominal and retroperitoneal tumor excision, and subphrenic abscess drainage. Peritoneal surgery includes surgeries such as exploratory and staging laparotomy, as well as inguinal, femoral, and incisional hernia repair, and repair of abdominal dehiscence. For intestinal and peritoneal surgery, for example laparotomy, general endotracheal anesthesia is typically required. Uncomplicated hernia repair may be done safely under general, regional, or local anesthesia, with intravenous sedation as needed.

Preoperative preparation for patients undergoing planned intestinal and peritoneal surgery should include evaluation and optimization of underlying medical conditions. In cases of abdominal and/or intestinal pathology, obstruction, or strangulation, aspiration risk is high. Preoperative aspiration prophylaxis should be administered, and rapid sequence intubation should be considered to secure the airway if general endotracheal anesthesia is the anesthetic approach indicated.

Maintenance with balanced anesthesia of inhaled agents, intravenous agents, or both is appropriate for intestinal surgery. Local anesthetic, with or without opioids, via an epidural may be used in combination with general anesthesia for intestinal surgery, to supplement analgesia and optimize surgical conditions. Orogastric or nasogastric tube insertion facilitates gastric decompression. Standard monitoring is applicable and invasive monitoring may be indicated, depending on patient condition, length of surgery, and anticipated blood loss. Adequate intravenous access is necessary, as large fluid shifts should be expected. Continuous muscle relaxation contributes to ideal surgical conditions.

The intraoperative anesthetic technique for peritoneal surgery varies, based on patient condition and the surgical procedure. For patients undergoing hernia repair (inguinal, femoral, incisional) without incarceration, strangulation, or obstruction, anesthetic options include general anesthesia (endotracheal tube, laryngeal mask airway), neuraxial anesthesia (spinal, epidural), and regional nerve block (peripheral nerve block, local infiltration). The choice of anesthesia depends on the surgical approach, size and type of hernia, and preferences of the surgeon and patient. Standard monitoring is typically adequate, as is peripheral intravenous access.

Postoperative pain management for intestinal and peritoneal surgery varies. Surgeries such as open small bowel resection and exploratory laparotomy have more extensive pain control requirements. Epidural analgesia provides pain control for intestinal and peritoneal surgery requiring large abdominal incisions. Regional nerve block (i.e., TAP and erector spinae blocks) is also a good option for postoperative pain management. If supplemental systemic opioids are necessary, patient-controlled analgesia is frequently used in the immediate postoperative period. The need for postoperative pain control in peritoneal surgery, such as uncomplicated hernia repair, is usually satisfied with oral pain medications, with or without regional nerve block. PONV prophylaxis should be administered according to the number of risk factors present.

Colorectal Surgery

Colorectal procedures are performed using open, laparoscopic, or laparoscopic-assisted techniques. Enhanced recovery after colorectal surgery involves use of evidence-based protocols to standardize medical care and improve outcomes and cost savings. Clinically, Enhanced Recovery After Surgery (ERAS) protocols strive to maintain normal physiologic function, augment the recovery process, and reduce postoperative complications. Colorectal conditions requiring colectomy are commonly treated surgically using ERAS protocols and laparoscopic techniques (see Table 19.4).

Patients with cancer and inflammatory bowel disease may present for large bowel procedures such as total and partial colectomy, colostomy, stoma closure, and peristomal hernia repair. General endotracheal anesthesia, with or without epidural placement, is required for colon resection. Many of these procedures are performed with a hand-assisted laparoscopic approach. Anesthetic techniques for rectal surgery, such as repair of rectal prolapse and anal fistula, hemorrhoidectomy, and anal sphincteroplasty for fecal incontinence, include general anesthesia (endotracheal tube or laryngeal mask airway), spinal anesthesia, and intravenous sedation with local infiltration.

Patients undergoing colorectal surgery benefit from preoperative evaluation and optimization. Patients with colorectal conditions may present with poor oral intake, vomiting, and diarrhea, resulting in hypovolemia and electrolyte abnormalities that should be addressed prior to planned surgery. In addition, previous steroid use should be treated accordingly with supplementation (i.e., stress dose) on the day of surgery. For patients at risk of aspiration, preoperative prophylaxis and rapid sequence intubation are indicated.

Intraoperative balanced anesthesia of inhaled agents and/or intravenous agents is used for large bowel surgery. For open procedures, general

Table 19.4 Common elements of ERAS protocols

Preoperative	Intraoperative	Postoperative
Preadmission evaluation and education	Use of laparoscopic surgical techniques	Multimodal analgesia, minimizing opioid use
Early discharge planning	Active warming	Glucose control
Avoid prolonged fasting; clear liquids allowed until 2 hours prior to anesthesia (clear carbo-hydrate drink encouraged)	Opioid-sparing techniques; rapid awakening anesthetic	Avoid excessive postoperative fluid administration
Avoid bowel prep	Avoid nasogastric tubes and drains	Early ambulation
Prewarming	Goal-directed perioperative fluid management	Early oral nutrition
Venous thromboembolism prophylaxis	Nausea and pain management	Early catheter removal
Avoid long-acting sedative medications		Prevention of postoperative ileus
Antibiotic prophylaxis within 60 minutes of incision		Defined discharge criteria

endotracheal anesthesia, combined with thoracic epidural local anesthesia, provides adequate surgical anesthesia and options for postoperative analgesia with neuraxial opioids. For laparoscopic large bowel surgery, general endotracheal anesthesia is also required; however, surgical exposure and postoperative pain needs do not typically require supplementation with neuraxial analgesia. Standard monitoring is required. Patient condition, length of surgery, and anticipated blood loss dictate the need for invasive monitoring. Third space losses may be significant; therefore, adequate intravenous access is necessary and allows for a route to restoring and maintaining euvolemia. Lung-protective ventilation with tidal volumes of 6–8 mL kg^{-1} and positive end-expiratory pressure of 5 cmH$_2$O (10 cmH$_2$O during laparoscopy) provide optimal, nonharmful conditions for oxygenation and ventilation.

Intraoperative anesthetic techniques for patients undergoing anorectal surgery depend upon patient condition and the surgical procedure and positioning needs. Patients are often placed in the prone jackknife, lithotomy, or lateral decubitus position. While general anesthesia (endotracheal tube, laryngeal mask airway), neuraxial anesthesia (spinal), or intravenous sedation with local infiltration are all options, securing the airway with an endotracheal tube may be advantageous for patients in the prone position. Peripheral intravenous access and standard monitors are usually all that is necessary for patients having anorectal surgery.

Postoperative pain management for intestinal and peritoneal surgery varies. Surgeries such as open small bowel resection and exploratory laparotomy have more extensive postoperative pain control requirements. Epidural analgesia provides pain control for intestinal and peritoneal surgery requiring large abdominal incisions. Regional nerve block (i.e., TAP and erector spinae blocks) is also an option for postoperative pain management. If supplemental systemic opioids are necessary, patient-controlled analgesia is frequently used in the immediate postoperative period. Oral pain medications, with or without regional nerve block, usually provide adequate postoperative pain control following peritoneal surgery, such as uncomplicated hernia repair. PONV prophylaxis should be administered according to the number of risk factors present.

Postoperative pain management for large bowel surgery depends upon the surgical approach. For patients undergoing open colon surgery, pain management options include epidural analgesia or regional block (i.e., TAP and erector spinae blocks). Patient-controlled analgesia is frequently used in the immediate postoperative period, as needed. Postoperative pain management for laparoscopic large bowel surgery is customized to patient needs and clinical conditions. ERAS protocols aim to prevent and relieve pain, nausea, and vomiting. ERAS protocols utilize multimodal analgesia, including preoperative preemptive analgesia (i.e., ultrasound-guided nerve blocks, gabapentinoid agents, acetaminophen, and cyclooxygenase 2 inhibitors), intraoperative analgesia (i.e., ketamine, dexmedetomidine, acetaminophen, etc.), and postoperative nonopioid analgesia (i.e., nonsteroidals, gabapentinoid agents, etc.). Oral multimodal analgesia usually fulfills postoperative pain control needs for anorectal surgery, such as hemorrhoidectomy, repair of rectal prolapse and anal fistula, and anal sphincteroplasty. A concerted effort to avoid PONV should be made by assessing for patient risk factors and administering PONV prophylaxis accordingly. In summary, a solid understanding of surgical procedures and utilization of preparation and anesthetic management strategies throughout the perioperative process are key components in delivering excellent acute pain management.

Further Reading

Andersen LPH, Hansen EG, Gögenur I, Rosenberg J. Optimized anesthesia and analgesic regimen for robotic colorectal surgery. *J Anesth Clin Res*. 2014;5:2.

Assad OM, El Sayed AA, Khalil MA. Comparison of volume-controlled ventilation and pressure-controlled ventilation volume guaranteed during laparoscopic surgery in Trendelenburg position. *J Clin Anesth*. 2016;34:55–61.

Baldini G, Fawcett WJ. Anesthesia for colorectal surgery. *Anesthesiol Clin*. 2015;33 (1):93–123.

Brandão JC, Lessa MA, Motta-Ribeiro G, *et al*. Global and regional respiratory mechanics during robotic-assisted laparoscopic surgery: a randomized study. *Anesth Analg*. 2019;129(6):1564–73.

Carney A, Dickinson M. Anesthesia for esophagectomy. *Anesthesiol Clin*. 2015;33 (1):143–63.

Lee JR. Anesthetic considerations for robotic surgery. *Korean J Anesthesiol*. 2014;66 (1):3–11.

Peden C, Scott MJ. Anesthesia for emergency abdominal surgery. *Anesthesiol Clin*. 2015;33(1):209–21.

Russo A, Di Stasio E, Scagliusi A, *et al*. Positive end-expiratory pressure during laparoscopy: cardiac and respiratory effects. *J Clin Anesth*. 2013;25(4):314–20.

Végh T. Anesthesia for esophageal surgery. In: M Granell Gil, M Şentürk, eds. *Anesthesia in Thoracic Surgery: Changes of Paradigms*. Cham: Springer; 2020. DOI: 10.1007/978-3-030-28528-9_22.

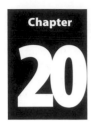

Chapter 20

Anesthesia for Endocrine Diseases

Alex D. Pham, James L. Dillon, Gregory M. Tortorich, Stuart H. Brown, Gopal Kodumudi, Oren Cohen, Joshua J. Hurley, Brittni M. Lanoux, Elyse M. Cornett, and Alan David Kaye

Introduction

Although anesthesiology and endocrinology are two distinct branches of medicine, some recent breakthrough treatments have brought together both medical specialties, particularly those concerned with surgical sciences and critical care. Related to the use of various traditional surgical techniques, the lack of newer and safer drugs, the lack of monitoring tools, and the scarcity of critical care services in the past, managing patients with various endocrine disorders has always been perceived as being more difficult by practicing anesthesiologists.

Patients with diverse endocrinopathies provide anesthesiologists with a variety of challenges during the perioperative phase. As such, a multidisciplinary strategy involving endocrinologists, anesthesiologists, intensivists, and surgeons is required today for a better perioperative patient outcome. The effect of endocrine abnormalities on perioperative outcome cannot be overstated, no matter how modest. Thus, it is critical to have a thorough understanding of the many anesthetic and nonanesthetic medicines that influence neurotransmitter and hormone production, to minimize perioperative morbidity and death. Among the primary endocrinologic illnesses, those affecting the thyroid, parathyroid, pancreatic, adrenal, and pituitary glands have a considerable impact on surgical results and anesthetic methods.

Hypothalamus/Posterior Pituitary

To understand these diseases, we must first remind ourselves of the role of antidiuretic hormone (ADH). ADH is produced in the hypothalamus and stored in the posterior pituitary where it is released in response to high plasma osmolality. Plasma osmolality is sensed in the hypothalamus by osmoreceptors. Once ADH is released, it has its primary effect in the distal convoluted tubule and collecting duct of the kidney by regulating the release of aquaporin channels, which allow the movement of water across cell membranes [1].

Syndrome of Inappropriate Diuretic Hormone

SIADH occurs when the posterior pituitary continues to release ADH despite normal or low plasma osmolality. This high circulating level of ADH results in the production of concentrated urine due to water retention. Although ADH does cause water retention, SIADH results in a euvolemic, hyponatremic state. As the levels of ADH increase, the concentration of urine also increases. This results in high urine osmolality and high urine sodium concentration. Due to high water retention, patients will have decreasing sodium concentration, which is the ultimate cause of the symptoms seen with this disease. Early signs of SIADH are nonspecific such as fatigue, muscle weakness, nausea, confusion, and headaches. As sodium imbalance worsens, patients can experience life-threatening seizures and cerebral edema. SIADH has a large host of etiologies, including, but not limited to, central nervous system (CNS) disturbances, malignancy, pulmonary disease, drug toxicity, and surgery. To properly treat SIADH in the long term, healthcare workers must first localize the source of the syndrome and correct it. However, in the acute setting, first-line management is fluid restriction (<800 mL per day), unless the patient has subarachnoid hemorrhage as this can cause cerebral vasospasm. Intravenous (IV) hypertonic saline and salt tablets (salt tablets are known to cause nausea) can be used in severe cases of hyponatremia. Care must be taken not to correct faster than 8 mEq L^{-1} in a 24-hour period, as this can result in osmotic demyelination, a potentially lethal complication. A loop diuretic can be used in cases where urine osmolality is over twice the plasma osmolality. Vasopressin receptor antagonists, such as tolvaptan, are less commonly used due to their costs and side effect profile (e.g., hepatotoxicity and excessive thirst) [2].

Cerebral Salt Wasting

Cerebral salt wasting (CSW) is a somewhat controversial distinction from SIADH in which severe CNS injuries result in inability of the body to retain salt, leading to a hypovolemic, hyponatremic state. One possible mechanism is loss of sympathetic regulation, and therefore decreased release of aldosterone and renin. Another source is decreased B-type natriuretic peptide (BNP), which impairs sodium reabsorption in the renal tubules. The resulting sodium loss will lead to increased ADH circulation, increased urinary sodium concentration, increased urine osmolality, and decreased plasma sodium concentration. Signs and symptoms of CSW include hypotension, decreased skin turgor, elevated hematocrit, and eventually more life-threatening outcomes such as seizures and cerebral edema. The difficulty in distinguishing SIADH from CSW lies in the difficulty in truly measuring body volume. CSW would theoretically respond to isotonic saline by releasing more dilute urine; however, this is generally not recommended, as patients can have concurrent

SIADH, which will cause worsening of hyponatremia and possible fatal outcomes. As CSW is associated with CNS injuries, the first-line therapy is usually hypertonic saline until a safe plasma sodium concentration is reached [3].

Diabetes Insipidus

Two forms of diabetes insipidus (DI) exist: central and nephrogenic. Central DI occurs when the body is unable to produce ADH, resulting in polyuria, polydipsia, and nocturia. Nephrogenic DI occurs when the kidney fails to respond to ADH, with similarly resulting symptoms. The key difference is that central DI will have low ADH levels, whereas nephrogenic DI will have high ADH levels. You can tell the difference clinically using a water deprivation test. Urine osmolality will increase in response to an ADH analog in central DI. The mainstay of treatment in central DI is desmopressin. In nephrogenic DI, the mainstay of treatment is hydrochlorothiazide (HCTZ). In both forms of DI, it is important for the patient to remain hydrated at all times and not ignore their thirst mechanism [4].

Thyroid: Pathophysiology, Differential Diagnosis, Treatment, and Perioperative Management

Hypothyroidism

Etiology

- Primary – $\uparrow$ thyroid-stimulating hormone (TSH) and $\downarrow$ free thyroxine (T_4); >90% of hypothyroidism cases: Hashimoto thyroiditis (+ antithyroid peroxidase (TPO), antithyroglobulin (Tg)), iatrogenic (thyroidectomy, radioactive iodine, amiodarone, lithium), iodine deficiency.
- Secondary ($\downarrow$ free T_4 and $\uparrow$, $\downarrow$, or normal TSH): central, due to hypothalamic or pituitary failure.
- Subclinical hypothyroidism.

Clinical Manifestations

See references [5] and [6].

- *Early*: fatigue, weakness, depression, weight gain, headache, myalgia, arthralgia, cold intolerance, dry skin, coarse and brittle hair, brittle nails, delayed deep tendon reflexes, carpal tunnel syndrome, constipation, menorrhagia, hyperlipidemia, diastolic hypertension.
- *Late*: slow speech, hoarseness, periorbital puffiness, myxedema (nonpitting edema), bradycardia, atherosclerosis, pleural, pericardial and peritoneal effusions.

- *Myxedema crisis and coma*: profound hypothyroidism, with high mortality rate (50–75%), even with treatment. Often precipitated by trauma, infection, illness, or narcotics. Hallmark – hypothermia and change of mental status (confusion, lethargy, obtundation, psychotic features, and coma). Hypotension, hypoventilation, hyponatremia, and hypoglycemia frequently present.

Management

See reference [7].

- Levothyroxine 1.5–1.7 µg kg^{-1} per day → titrate until euthyroid, rechecking TSH every 5–6 weeks.
- Decreased starting dose 0.3–0.5 µg kg^{-1} per day if elderly or risk of ischemic heart disease.
- Increased dose if poor gastrointestinal (GI) absorption (celiac, inflammatory bowel disease), pregnancy, drugs (proton pump inhibitor (PPI), iron, calcium, colestyramine, phenytoin, phenobarbital).
- *Myxedema coma*: load with 5–8 µg kg^{-1} T$_4$ intravenously (IV), then 50–100 µg IV once daily. May give 5–10 µg T$_3$ IV every 8 hours if unstable with bradycardia and/or hypothermia (peripheral conversion T$_4$ → T$_3$ impaired). Must give empiric glucocorticoid replacement (e.g., IV hydrocortisone 100 mg every 8 hours). Correction takes time – supportive care to maintain blood pressure and respiration, electrolytes and glucose correction, and passive rewarming.

Myxedema Coma and Glucocorticoid Replacement

See reference [7].

- Primary hypothyroidism (most cases of myxedema coma): associated with primary autoimmune-mediated adrenal insufficiency.
- Central hypothyroidism associated with hypopituitarism, secondary adrenal insufficiency, and impaired pituitary adrenocorticotrophic hormone (ACTH) response to stress.

Anesthetic Considerations in Hypothyroidism
Preoperative

- Confirm euthyroid status in patients with known hypothyroidism.
- Thyroid replacement therapy should be continued in the perioperative period.
- Subclinical and mild disease: not at increased risk of complications.

- Moderate to severe disease: consider delaying elective surgery. If emergent, consider pretreatment with IV thyroxine ± T_3 and corticosteroids.
- Airway evaluation: enlarged tongue, mucinous edema of the pharynx and larynx (myxedema).

Intraoperative

- ↑ sensitivity and exaggerated response to anesthetics, sedatives, and opioids. Consider etomidate and ketamine for induction.
- ↓ myocardial function → ↑ risk of hemodynamic instability or myocardial ischemia.
- ↓ response to α- and β-adrenergic agents → larger doses of vasopressors may be needed.
- Hypoventilation (↓ respiratory drive and ↓ respiratory muscle strength).
- ↓ Red blood cell (RBC) mass and anemia.
- Hypothermia (↓ metabolic rate, ↓ Na^+/K^+ ATPase pumps).
- Myxedema coma (see above).

Postoperative

- ↑ risk of delayed emergence and prolonged ventilatory support (hypothermia, slow drug metabolism, and respiratory depression).
- Consider hypothyroidism in respiratory failure with difficulty to wean off ventilator → weaning aided by treatment.
- ↓ Gut motility can lead to constipation and ileus.

Pathophysiology
Cardiovascular

See references [8] and [9].

- ↓ Myocardial function (↓ cardiac output, ↑ systemic vascular resistance, ↓ or normal systolic blood pressure, ↑ diastolic blood pressure, ↓ contractility, ↓ heart rate) → ↑ risk of hemodynamic instability or myocardial ischemia.
- Diminished response to α- and β-adrenergic agents → larger doses of vasopressors needed.
- Can induce or worsen arrhythmias.
- Pericardial effusion.

Respiratory

See references [10] and [11].

- ↓ Hypoxic respiratory drive and ↓ hypercapnic respiratory drive (severe diagnosis), and ↓ respiratory muscle strength → alveolar hypoventilation.
- ↑ Obstructive sleep apnea (OSA) (2/2 to ↓ respiratory drive or airway narrowing due to enlarged tongue and mucinous edema of the pharynx and larynx).
- Exudative pleural effusions.
- Minimum alveolar concentration (MAC) not affected by hypothyroidism.
- ↑ risk of delayed emergence and prolonged ventilatory support.
- Consider hypothyroidism in respiratory failure with difficulty to wean off ventilator → weaning aided by treatment.

Metabolic

- ↓ Renal and hepatic clearance of medications (antiepileptics, anticoagulants, opioids, and hypnotics).
- Hypothermia: ↓ metabolism and thermogenesis; associated with mortality.
- Hyponatremia: ↓ free water clearance (excess ADH, renal impairment, adrenal insufficiency).
- Hypoglycemia: ↓ gluconeogenesis and glycogenolysis; adrenal insufficiency can contribute.
- ↓ RBC mass → normochromic, normocytic anemia.
- ↓ clearance of vitamin K-dependent factors – coumadin dose adjustment.

Hyperthyroidism

Etiology

See reference [12].

- Primary (↓ TSH, ↑ free T_4 and T_3): Graves' disease (60–80% of cases), thyroiditis, and toxic adenomas.
- TSH-secreting tumors and pituitary resistance: very rare (↑ TSH, ↑ free T_4).
- Human chorionic gonadotrophin (hCG)-secreting tumor, metastatic follicular thyroid cancer.
- Subclinical hyperthyroidism.

Clinical Manifestations

See reference [13].

- Restlessness, sweating, tremor, hyperreflexia, most warm skin, heat intolerance, fine hair, tachycardia, palpitations, atrial fibrillation, weight loss, ↑ bowel movement frequency, menstrual irregularities, osteoporosis, stare, and lid lag. Graves' disease-specific: ophthalmopathy and infiltrative dermopathy (myxedema). Elderly patients can present with lethargy only.

- Thyroid storm (20–30% mortality): massive release of T_4. Presents with fever, delirium, tachycardia, systolic hypertension with wide pulse pressure and $\downarrow$ mean arterial pressure (MAP), and GI symptoms. Unlike malignant hyperthermia, there is no increase in CO_2 that is unresponsive to increased minute ventilation, no $\uparrow$ in creatine kinase (CK), and no muscle rigidity or acidosis.

Management of Thyroid Storm

See reference [14].

- Beta-blocker ($\downarrow$ adrenergic tone) – propranolol 60–80 mg every 4–6 hours; adjust for heart rate and blood pressure control.
- Propylthiouracil (PTU) 200 mg every 4 hours or methimazole 20 mg every 4–6 hours (to block new hormone synthesis). PTU > methimazole due to its inhibition of peripheral $T_4 \rightarrow T_3$ conversion.
  o Propranolol, PTU, and methimazole can be given through a nasogastric tube.
- Iopanoic acid or iodine >1 hour after PTU (Wolff–Chaikoff effect).
- Iodinated radiocontrast (inhibits peripheral $T_4 \rightarrow T_3$ conversion).
- Glucocorticoid ($\downarrow$ peripheral $T_4 \rightarrow T_3$ conversion, $\uparrow$ vasomotor stability, $\downarrow$ autoimmune process in Graves' disease or treatment-associated adrenal insufficiency) – IV hydrocortisone 100 mg every 8 hours.
- Bile acid sequestrants (severe cases; $\downarrow$ enterohepatic recycling of thyroid hormones – cholestyramine 4 g orally four times daily).
- Aggressive management of hyperpyrexia with cooling blankets and acetaminophen.

Anesthetic Considerations in Hyperthyroidism
Preoperative

- Confirm euthyroid status – risk of thyroid storm.
- Continue antithyroid medications and beta-blockers to the day of surgery.
- Airway evaluation: check for compression and tracheal deviation.
- Benzodiazepines for preoperative sedation.

Intraoperative

- $\uparrow$ Sensitivity to catecholamines $\rightarrow$ consider direct-acting vasoconstrictors (phenylephrine).
- $\uparrow$ Risk of hemodynamic instability and myocardial ischemia.

- Slower induction and ↑ concentrations of inhaled anesthetics may be needed due to ↑ cardiac output (effects on uptake and redistribution) and rate of drug metabolism.
- No change in MAC requirement.
- Thyroid storm: intraoperatively or in first 18 hours postsurgery. Watch for hyperthermia, tachycardia, and changes in blood pressure (see above for more details).
- Normochromic, normocytic anemia (↑ in plasma volume > ↑ in RBC mass).

Postoperative

- Thyroid storm: intraoperatively or in first 18 hours postsurgery. Watch for hyperthermia, tachycardia, and changes in blood pressure (see above for more details).
- May need postoperative mechanical ventilation support after general anesthesia.

Pathophysiology
Cardiovascular
See reference [15].

- ↑ Cardiac output, ↑ contractility, ↑ peripheral oxygen consumption, ↑ heart rate, ↑ pulse pressure, ↓ systemic vascular resistance, ↑ systolic blood pressure → ↑ risk of hemodynamic instability or myocardial ischemia.
- Prone to sinus tachycardia and atrial fibrillation, coronary spasms, and development of cardiomyopathy.

Respiratory
See reference [16].

- ↑ Ventilation due to ↑ oxygen consumption and carbon dioxide production (hypoxemia and hypercapnia).
- ↓ Respiratory muscle strength.
- Tracheal obstruction due to goiter.
- ↑ Pulmonary artery systolic pressure.

Metabolic

- Hyperglycemia (impaired glucose tolerance).

Complications of Thyroid Surgery

- *Hypocalcemia* (most common complication): 24–72 hours postoperatively. Symptoms range from mild (paresthesia) to moderate (muscle twitching and cramping) and severe (trismus or tetany). Management: calcium carbonate

1250–2500 mg daily in 2–4 doses. If on PPI, give calcium citrate. If persistent hypocalcemia and symptoms despite oral calcium, consider IV calcium and magnesium. Calcitriol if very low parathyroid hormone (PTH) [17].

- *Hypoparathyroidism*: parathyroid gland damage or accidental removal. Can be transient (days, weeks, or months) or permanent.
- *Hoarseness* (common): transient (24–48 hours) due to vocal cord edema caused by endotracheal tube; resolves spontaneously. Persistent or severe hoarseness is rare and can be due to arytenoid dislocation or nerve injury causing cord dysfunction → laryngoscopy and neurolaryngeal evaluation [18].
- *Nerve injury and vocal cord paresis or paralysis*: nerves affected include superior laryngeal (voice changes), recurrent laryngeal (difficulty swallowing and ↑ risk of aspiration) and vagus (sensory and motor deficits of larynx; ↑↑ risk of aspiration) [19].
- *Dysphagia*: uncertain etiology; may be related to postoperative adhesions, decreased laryngeal elevation, cricothyroid trauma/inflammation, or nerve damage [20].
- *Horner syndrome*: associated with lateral neck dissection, ischemic nerve damage, or stretching of cervical sympathetic chain.
- *Cervical hematoma*: immediate or delayed (days). Cessation of anticoagulation prior to surgery can prevent hematoma formation. If it occurs, manage with evacuation in the operating room. Hematoma must be evacuated prior to intubation, as the mass can compress the larynx, complicating intubation.
- *Seroma*: resolves without intervention.
- *Chyle leak or fistula*: injury to the thoracic duct most common during lateral node dissection. It can lead to severe fluid loss and electrolyte imbalance → <500 mL per day; manage with fasting, and high-output leaks require surgical repair.
- *Tracheal injury*: necrosis due to cautery damage to small branches of the inferior thyroid artery. Can result in air leak or subcutaneous emphysema. Requires surgical repair or tracheostomy.

Parathyroid: Hyperparathyroidism versus Hypoparathyroidism – Pathophysiology, Signs and Symptoms, Differential Diagnosis, and Management

Hyperparathyroidism

The parathyroid gland is essential in maintaining proper calcium homeostasis. It secretes PTH, which acts on receptors in osteoclast cells in bone to increase bone resorption and subsequently calcium and PTH levels. Calcium-sensing receptors in the parathyroid gland regulate the amount of PTH secretion in response to calcium levels [21].

Ninety years ago, primary hyperparathyroidism (PHPT) was first discovered simultaneously in the United States and Europe. Since that time, the medical understanding of this disease process has drastically changed – initially, it was seen as being only characterized by severe symptoms of "bones, stones, groans" (e.g., osteoporosis, osteitis fibrosa cystica, nephrolithiasis, abdominal pain, and other GI symptoms); PHPT is now understood to encompass also characteristic biochemical changes of hypercalcemia and increased or inappropriately normal PTH levels, even when patients are asymptomatic [21]. Subclinical skeletal disease and osteoporosis have been observed through dual-energy X-ray absorptiometry (DEXA).

PHPT results from increased PTH secretion by abnormal parathyroid glands. The causes and respective incidences of PHPT are as follows: parathyroid adenoma (approximately 80%); parathyroid hyperplasia (10–15%); multiple adenomas (5%); and parathyroid carcinoma (<1%) [21]. It can also be seen in familial syndromes such as multiple endocrine neoplasia type 1 (MEN 1) and 2a (MEN 2a). PHPT is more commonly seen in postmenopausal women (nearly half of all patients) and African Americans.

Secondary hyperparathyroidism (SHPT) is associated with hypocalcemia and elevated PTH. Common etiologies include vitamin D deficiency, chronic kidney disease (CKD), and malabsorption. Parathyroid hyperplasia occurs in response to the hypocalcemic stimulus [22]. In CKD, the kidneys cannot convert vitamin D to its active form and thus have reduced absorption of calcium from the GI tract; increased phosphate levels are due to inadequate excretion by the kidneys.

Tertiary hyperparathyroidism (THPT) occurs as a sequela of protracted, severe SHPT; the parathyroid gland becomes autonomous and secrete excessively high levels of PTH, resulting in hypercalcemia and hypophosphatemia. THPT is often seen in renal transplant patients with SHPT after they continue to have high PTH levels.

Management and Treatment

Parathyroidectomy is the only definitive therapy for PHPT. It is pursued in symptomatic cases (including those with cognitive or psychiatric symptoms) and in asymptomatic cases where subclinical end-organ renal or skeletal effects have been confirmed. Medical management includes HCTZ (decreased urinary calcium excretion), estrogen replacement therapy, bisphosphonates, and cinacalcet.

Management of SHPT is typically medical and involves maintenance of normal serum calcium levels, normal phosphate levels, and control of PTH and vitamin D levels. Phosphate binders (aluminum hydroxide, sevalamer, lanthanum carbonate) and dietary restriction of phosphate-rich foods (meat, cheese, certain beverages) are used to maintain normophosphatemia. Calcimimetics such as cinacalcet or etelcalcetide improve the sensitivity of calcium-sensing receptors in the parathyroid gland and decrease PTH production. Cinacalcet is frequently used in dialysis patients [23]. Vitamin D analogs are used to decrease PTH levels and have multiple benefits in CKD patients, including improved mortality, reduced hospitalizations, and reduced inflammation [24]. Surgical treatment with subtotal or total parathyroidectomy is used in cases where medical therapy has been unsuccessful or in those with severe features such as severe hypercalcemia (>10.2 mg dL^{-1}), calciphylaxis, osteoporosis, fractures, or recalcitrant pruritus [25]. Subtotal parathyroidectomy has been associated with less postoperative hypocalcemia. Parathyroidectomy is also the cornerstone of treatment for THPT.

Anesthetic Considerations for Hyperparathyroidism

The anesthetic provider should consider a potentially difficult airway due to mass effect from the goiter or osteopenic bone that could result in fractures of the mandible and vertebral bodies. Physiologic changes due to hypercalcemia include confusion, psychiatric changes, hypertension, hypovolemia, conduction blockade, potential respiratory muscle weakness, renal failure, and nephrolithiasis. From a GI standpoint, nausea, vomiting, pancreatitis, and increased aspiration can occur. Although hypercalcemia can result in weakness, hypercalcemia may also antagonize neuromuscular blockers, so they should be carefully titrated to effect. Careful positioning is necessary to prevent any pathologic fractures.

Calcium levels and ECG should be monitored perioperatively The ECG may show a shortened PR or QT interval. Calcium levels can be reduced by increasing the intravascular fluid volume and administering furosemide [26]. Hemodialysis should be utilized in the case of life-threatening hypercalcemia or acute renal failure.

Postoperative airway obstruction can occur after parathyroidectomy due to recurrent laryngeal nerve injury, hematoma, hypocalcemia, tracheomalacia, or mandibular fracture [26].

Hypoparathyroidism

Hypoparathyroidism is an endocrine disease with defective PTH secretion. Primary causes are genetic, rare, and numerous; some causes include familial idiopathic syndromes, X-linked agenesis of the parathyroid gland, Sanjad–Sakati syndrome, and hypoparathyroidism–retardation–dysmorphism syndrome. Hypoparathyroidism causes hypocalcemia related to decreased bone resorption and decreased calcium absorption from the GI tract [27]. Diagnosis is made with the biochemical findings of hypocalcemia, hyperphosphatemia, and low PTH levels. Secondary causes include ablation of the parathyroid gland during surgery, metal overload (iron, copper, or aluminum), and transient and neonatal hypoparathyroidism.

Anesthetic Considerations for Hypoparathyroidism

Preoperative evaluation must include full history and exploration of the associated syndrome, especially in rare primary causes. The anesthesia provider should evaluate for Chvostek and Trousseau signs, both of which indicate neuromuscular irritability from chronic hypocalcemia. In the acute setting, calcium levels should be repleted with calcium chloride or calcium gluconate. Calcium carbonate and vitamin D should have been given to correct the chronic form.

Hypocalcemia can result in arrhythmias, so the ECG should be monitored in the preoperative, perioperative, and postoperative periods. The genetic causes of primary hypothyroidism can have facial abnormalities, so the provider should be aware of possible difficult intubation [28]. QT-prolonging agents should be avoided. Neuromuscular blockers have increased efficacy in hypocalcemic patients.

Endocrine Pancreas: Diabetes – Pathophysiology, Signs and Symptoms, Differential Diagnosis, Treatment, and Management Perioperatively

Endocrine Pancreas

Pathophysiology

- In a normal adult pancreas, approximately 50 units of insulin are secreted each day from the pancreas, specifically the beta cells located in the islets of Langerhans. The rate of secretion is largely determined by plasma glucose concentration. Insulin promotes glycogenesis, protein synthesis, glucose transport, triglyceride storage, and fatty acid absorption into fat cells.

- Type 1: autoimmune destruction of beta cells, which leads to insulin deficiency; development occurs in genetically susceptible individuals following one or more environmental factors, and develops over several months or years.

- Type 2: development involves a multitude of factors, including genetic, metabolic, and environmental. In brief, there is malfunctioning of feedback loops between insulin and insulin secretion, which results in high blood glucose levels. Beta cells are dysfunctional and insulin secretion is reduced, thus limiting the body's capacity to maintain physiologic glucose levels. Insulin resistance is also a contributing factor, leading to increased glucose production in the liver and decreased uptake by muscle, the liver, and adipose tissue [29].

Signs and Symptoms

- Type 1: polydipsia, polyuria, enuresis in children with no such prior history, polyphagia, nausea, vomiting, unintended weight loss, irritability and other mood changes, fatigue and weakness, blurred vision.
- Type 2: polyuria, polydipsia, polyphagia, fatigue, blurred vision, increased time of wound healing, frequent infections, numbness or tingling in the hands or feet.

Differential Diagnosis

- Metabolic syndrome, hyperthyroidism, Cushing's syndrome, glucagonoma, iatrogenic (glucocorticoids, thiazides, phenytoin), alcohol use disorder, cirrhosis, hemochromatosis.

Treatment

- Type 1: basal–bolus regimens are recommended for most patients; basal insulins include glargine, detemir, and isophane insulin (NPH); bolus insulins include regular, lispro, glulisine, and aspart. Basal insulins are given once daily, and bolus doses are given with meals, as carbohydrate intake, or for hyperglycemia correction.
- Type 2: medications include glucagon-like peptide 1 (GLP-1) receptor agonists (dulaglutide, exenatide), biguanides (metformin), sodium–glucose cotransporter 2 (SGLT-2) inhibitors (canagliflozin, dapagliflozin), dipeptidyl peptidase 4 (DPP-4) inhibitors (sitagliptin, saxagliptin), thiazolidinediones (rosiglitazone, pioglitazone), sulfonylureas (glyburide, glipizide, glimepiride), and insulin. The choice of medication is based upon the extent of disease, comorbidities, current medication regimen, and response to previous medications.

Diabetic Autonomic Dysfunction

- Gastric motility/emptying: gastric emptying is abnormally slow in up to 50% of diabetic patients, causing nausea and vomiting and affecting postprandial glucose control. Emptying is slower during hyperglycemia, when compared to euglycemia. Regarding anesthetic management, patients with gastroparesis may have unanticipated full stomach, which could lead to reflux or aspiration, so premedication with an antacid and metoclopramide is suggested.

- Neuropathy: diabetic patients are predisposed to neuropathy, meaning they may be unaware of prior myocardial ischemia or infarction, so preoperative ECG is indicated to rule out abnormalities. These patients are also prone to reflex dysautonomia, limiting their ability to compensate for intravascular volume changes with tachycardia and increased peripheral resistance, predisposing to cardiovascular instability [30].

Perioperative Management

- The goal of glucose management is to avoid hypoglycemia while keeping glucose below 180 mg dL^{-1}, as either extreme may worsen postoperative outcomes. The most common method of perioperative insulin management is continuous infusion of regular insulin, which leads to more precise control of insulin delivery than can be achieved with subcutaneous administration. Infusion rate can be adjusted in accordance with blood glucose levels. Supplemental dextrose can be given if the patient becomes hypoglycemic.

- If a patient is taking an oral hypoglycemic agent, it can be continued until the day of surgery. Due to longer half-life of metformin and sulfonylurea, they should be discontinued 24–48 hours preoperatively.

- Insulin requirements intraoperatively for noninsulin-dependent type 2 diabetics vary, depending on the length of surgery; however, given their insulin resistance, they may respond differently and require hourly glucose monitoring.

- Type 1 diabetics on insulin pumps can continue their basal setting if undergoing a short procedure; however, if the procedure is extensive, IV insulin should be used, and the pump suspended [29].

Diabetic Crises

- Diabetic ketoacidosis (DKA): decreased insulin activity, along with a precipitating factor (most common causes – infection, infarction, insulin noncompliance, and impregnation), leads to catabolism of free fatty acids into ketone bodies (acetoacetate and beta-hydroxybutyrate). Accumulation of ketone bodies results in an anion gap metabolic acidosis known as DKA. The goal for decreasing blood glucose concentration should be 10% per hour. Therapy begins with IV insulin at 0.1 units/(kg hr). Potassium should be monitored due to intracellular shift, so potassium should be repleted as necessary. Lactated Ringer's solution should also be initiated at a rate of approximately 250 mL hr^{-1}, as patients are usually dehydrated. Once plasma glucose concentration reaches <250 mg dL^{-1}, 5% dextrose in water (D5W) infusion should be started to avoid hypoglycemia. Once the anion gap is closed and bicarbonate concentration is >18, long-acting insulin should be started and the infusion should be discontinued 4 hours later.

- Hyperosmolar nonketotic coma: this is hyperglycemia-induced diuresis, leading to dehydration and hyperosmolality. This hyperosmolality induces dehydration of neurons, causing altered mental status and seizures. Ketoacidosis does not occur, likely because there is enough insulin to prevent ketone body formation. Extreme hyperglycemia leads to factitious hyponatremia (each 100 mg dL^{-1} increase in plasma glucose concentration lowers plasma sodium concentration by 1.6 mEq L^{-1}). Treatment involves fluid resuscitation with lactated Ringer's solution, small doses of insulin, and potassium repletion [31].

Glucagonoma

- Glucagonoma is a tumor of pancreatic alpha cells which results in over-production of the hormone glucagon. Glucagon acts on the liver to increase amino acid oxidation and gluconeogenesis. Signs and symptoms include the same as those of diabetes mellitus, along with weight loss, normochromic anemia, hypolipidemia, and necrolytic migratory erythema.
- Surgical resection is the gold standard for localized disease, and chemotherapy for metastatic disease. Octreotide injections partially suppress glucagon; however, it also leads to glucose intolerance due to decreased insulin secretion. Theoretically, problems with glucose homeostasis and myocardial function could be anticipated following resection, so management should be prepared accordingly with beta-blockade and dextrose [32].

Adrenal Glands: Role, Addison's/Hypocortisolism – Pathophysiology, Primary versus Secondary, Signs and Symptoms, Differential Diagnosis, and Management

Adrenal Glands

The adrenal gland is divided into the cortex and medulla. The cells of the medulla produce epinephrine and norepinephrine, whereas the cells of the cortex secrete steroid hormones, including mineralocorticoids, glucocorticoids, and androgens [33].

The release of epinephrine and norepinephrine is regulated by the sympathetic nervous system, which can be activated by various stimuli (e.g., hypotension, hypothermia, hypoglycemia, hypoxia, pain). These catecholamines then act on various receptors to exert physiologic effects such as vasoconstriction (α1 receptors), bronchodilation (β2 receptors), and increased heart inotropy and chronotropy (β1 receptors).

The mineralocorticoid aldosterone stimulates sodium reabsorption from the distal convoluted tubule of the kidneys, in exchange for potassium and hydrogen ions, which are excreted in the urine. Reabsorption of sodium results in water retention and expansion of the extracellular fluid. Cortisol is a glucocorticoid that promotes gluconeogenesis to ensure appropriate fasting blood glucose levels, and it is also necessary for normal cardiovascular response to catecholamines during physiologic stress [34]. Aldosterone release is regulated by the renin–angiotensin–aldosterone system, whereas cortisol release is controlled by the hypothalamic–pituitary–adrenal (HPA) axis [34].

Adrenal Insufficiency

Primary adrenal insufficiency occurs as a result of adrenal gland dysfunction and results in decreased cortisol and aldosterone production. The most common form of primary adrenal insufficiency is Addison's disease, an autoimmune disease in which autoantibodies against the 21-hydroxylase enzyme destroy adrenal cortical cells. Primary adrenal insufficiency can also be caused by adrenal hemorrhage, cancer, infection (e.g., HIV, tuberculosis), and certain drugs such as etomidate, which inhibits 11-beta hydroxylase, an enzyme responsible for cortisol production [35]. Nonspecific symptoms of primary adrenal insufficiency include fatigue, nausea, vomiting, abdominal pain, weight loss, and myalgias. More specific signs and symptoms include skin hyperpigmentation (from overproduction of melanocyte-stimulating hormone), hypoglycemia (glucocorticoid deficiency), and dehydration, hypotension, and salt craving from mineralocorticoid deficiency [35].

Secondary and tertiary adrenal insufficiency is due to pathology (tumors, Sheehan syndrome, prior surgery, or radiation) of the anterior pituitary and hypothalamus, respectively, or due to HPA axis suppression from prolonged glucocorticoid use. These patients will have similar symptoms to those with primary adrenal insufficiency, but an important distinction is that they typically maintain mineralocorticoid function, as mineralocorticoid levels are maintained by the renin–angiotensin–aldosterone system. Thus, these patients will not have dehydration, hypotension, or salt craving. Hyperpigmentation also will be absent in these patients. Patients with pituitary or hypothalamic tumors may additionally have symptoms of mass effect such as headache or visual field deficits [36].

Anesthetic Management

Anesthetic management of patients with known adrenal insufficiency starts with preoperative measurement of glucose and electrolyte concentrations, with correction of volume deficits, hypoglycemia, and electrolyte disturbances (hyponatremia, hyperkalemia, acidosis). Etomidate should be avoided for induction in these patients, given its ability to cause transient adrenal insufficiency [37]. Stress of surgery in these patients can trigger acute adrenal insufficiency (Addisonian crisis) where a lack of circulating glucocorticoids and/or mineralocorticoids results in shock, hypoglycemia, electrolyte disturbances (hyponatremia, hyperkalemia, acidosis), convulsions, and arrhythmias. Perioperative steroid dosing is controversial, given currently limited evidence, but patients with known adrenal insufficiency or those with a potentially suppressed HPA axis (on doses equivalent to 20 mg prednisone daily for >2 weeks within the past year) can be given perioperative steroids following a variable dosing strategy:

- Minor procedures (e.g., hernia repair): patients receive a one-time dose of 25 mg hydrocortisone IV preoperatively.
- Moderate surgical stress (total knee arthroplasty, revascularization procedures): patients receive a total of 50–75 mg hydrocortisone daily for 1–2 days.
- Major surgery (open heart surgery, colectomy): patients receive 100–150 mg hydrocortisone daily for 2–3 days, followed by steroid tapering back down to their maintenance steroid dose [38].

Ovaries and Testes

Polycystic Ovarian Syndrome

This is a syndrome characterized by hyperandrogenism and an irregular menstrual cycle in women. While the pathophysiology is still being discovered to this day, it is believed to evolve from both genetic and environmental features. We know that most cases are caused by excess androgen production by the ovaries. This results in many of the clinical features associated with this syndrome, including acne, hirsutism, and male pattern balding. Abnormal follicular maturation occurs due to dysregulation of the hypothalamic hormonal feedback response system. This causes an imbalance in the luteinizing hormone (LH):follicle-stimulating hormone (FSH) ratio, leading to anovulation, another key clinical finding in polycystic ovary syndrome (PCOS). Finally, transvaginal ultrasound can reveal characteristic-appearing cysts. If clinicians note two of these three findings, this means that the Rotterdam criteria have been met. A key feature in many patients with PCOS is insulin resistance/hyperinsulinemia. This results in many of the metabolic symptoms, such as weight gain and cardiovascular disease, and causes ovarian theca cells to produce more androgen, propagating hyperandrogenism [39].

The mainstay of treatment in PCOS is weight loss. Even modest weight loss has been proven to decrease the risk of adverse metabolic side effects and even help promote regular menstrual cycles. In women who do not seek pregnancy, oral contraceptive pills are a very common treatment strategy, as they help suppress the hyperandrogenism effects and regulate menstrual cycles. If the patient does seek pregnancy, letrozole (an aromatase inhibitor) or clomiphene citrate are recommended to help induce ovulation.

Anesthesia practitioners must consider complications that can arise from insulin resistance in PCOS. Diabetes is a common complication in PCOS. Diabetes can lead to many complications for anesthetic providers, including silent myocardial ischemia, poor intrinsic compensation, reduced joint mobility, infection, poor wound healing, and increased mortality. A reasonable goal for intraoperative blood glucose level is 85–180 mg dL^{-1}. Providers should certainly avoid hypoglycaemia, as this can have deadly outcomes [40].

Functional Neuroendocrine Pathophysiology – Pheochromocytoma/Paragangliomas

Background

Pheochromocytomas and paragangliomas (PPGL) are rare catecholamine-secreting neuroendocrine tumors. When they occur in adrenal glands, they are referred to as pheochromocytomas. Extra-adrenal tumors are called paragangliomas. However, they are histologically identical [41]. PPGL may occur spontaneously or in association with hereditary disorders such as von Hippel–Lindau disease or multiple endocrine neoplasia type 2 (MEN 2).

Signs, Symptoms, and Diagnosis

Patients often present with nonspecific symptoms such as headache, diaphoresis, tachycardia, and chronic or paroxysmal hypertension. These vague symptoms often result in delayed diagnosis. Occasionally, the presentation can be quite dramatic, with the initial presentation being myocardial infarction, stroke, or other manifestations of a hypertensive emergency [42]. Of particular concern to the anesthesiologist is catecholamine-induced cardiomyopathy. Approximately 10–13% of patients will have cardiac involvement. Diagnosis of PPGL is made with urinary and plasma fractionated catecholamines and metanephrines, with subsequent radiologic evaluation once biochemical confirmation is made.

Preoperative Management

Preoperative management includes evaluation, medical management, and a high-salt diet to restore catecholamine-induced volume depletion. An ECG and transthoracic echocardiography will help identify signs of ischemia and/or cardiomyopathy, so that appropriate medical optimization can be initiated.

Medical management typically involves 2–3 weeks of α-adrenergic blockade to minimize the risk of hypertensive crises in the operating room. Phenoxybenzamine or doxazosin are typically used and are equally as efficacious. Their use has been called into question, however, as several studies have failed to show efficacy of preoperative blockade versus no blockade. Calcium channel blockers are commonly used as adjuncts if additional blood pressure control is necessary. β-adrenergic blockade may be necessary but should only be initiated after α-adrenergic blockade.

Intraoperative Management

An arterial line is necessary for continuous monitoring of blood pressure. A central line is recommended. Surgical resection is divided into two phases. Phase 1 begins at induction and ends after clamping of the adrenal veins. This period is defined by periods of hemodynamic lability and hypertensive episodes. Quick-acting, short-duration vasodilators should be used such as sodium nitroprusside, phentolamine, nicardipine, or clevidipine.

Phase 2 is characterized by prolonged hypotension. Management includes volume administration and vasoactive medications such as phenylephrine and norepinephrine.

Postoperative Management

Often the patient can be extubated and taken to the postanesthesia care unit (PACU) prior to going to a medical floor. However, admission to the intensive care unit (ICU) may be warranted if ongoing pressor support is necessary.

Gastrointestinal: Carcinoid Syndrome/Carcinoid Tumors – Pathophysiology, Signs and Symptoms, Differential Diagnosis, and Management

Carcinoid Tumors

Careful consideration should be made in the intraoperative management of a patient with known carcinoid tumor. Most commonly originating in the GI tract or bronchial tree, the tumors are prone to metastases that can secrete bioactive substances or hormones, causing deleterious reactions to a patient's hemodynamic stability in the intraoperative setting. These tumors are known to secrete vasoactive substances such as serotonin, histamine, prostaglandins, bradykinins, ACTH, etc. The term "carcinoid syndrome" has been coined to describe symptoms caused by these substances. Given the broad range of hormones that may be secreted, symptoms vary from hypertension or hypotension to diarrhea, flushing, bronchoconstriction, wheezing, and more. The syndrome occurs when the tumor resides in a location where its secreted mediators bypass the portal system, and thus enter the circulation prior to metabolization by the liver [43].

Carcinoid crisis refers to a life-threatening exaggeration of the symptoms described in carcinoid syndrome. This usually occurs during surgical manipulation of the tumor, in tumor necrosis (such as from chemotherapy), or during induction of anesthesia. Typical reactions include dramatic changes in blood pressure (both hypotension and hypertension), cardiac arrhythmias, and mental status changes [44].

Preoperative Management

Extensive preoperative consideration should be made, including a thorough history and physical examination to determine the patient's severity of symptoms, ECG, and echocardiography [43]. Serotonin release can lead to tricuspid stenosis and right heart failure.

History should include an investigation of the patient's exacerbations and triggers. The clinician should also enquire about history of asthma, wheezing, flushing, diarrhea, and palpitations. Physical examination should include an extensive cardiac examination to evaluate for symptoms of heart failure or murmurs that may indicate valvular abnormalities. Chronic diarrhea may present with vitamin and electrolyte abnormalities and, commonly, symptoms of pellagra. Pellagra is a niacin deficiency that typically presents with symptoms, including angular stomatitis, scaly skin, oral lesions, glossitis, and encephalopathy [45].

Labs should include liver function and 24-hour urinary 5-hydroxyindoleacetic acid (5-HIAA). The goal of preoperative evaluation is to determine the patient's symptoms and triggers, and to optimize the patient using a combination of drugs that block the various hormones released. Octreotide has become the mainstay treatment for endocrine tumors. This somatostatin analog has been found to reduce flushing and diarrhea symptoms in >70% of patients.

Use of octreotide in the management of carcinoid tumors is effective in reducing symptoms. However, a standardized regimen has not been agreed upon yet and management varies across facilities [44]. Suggestions include 100 μg octreotide subcutaneously three times daily for 2 weeks prior to surgery, followed by 100 μg prior to induction of anesthesia [44]. Many facilities will start octreotide 24–48 hours prior to surgery, and begin an infusion prior to induction that is weaned off over a period of 3 days to a week [44].

Intraoperative Considerations

At a minimum, intraoperative monitoring should include standard American Society of Anesthesiologists (ASA) monitors such as noninvasive blood pressure (NIBP), pulse oximetry, and ECG. The patient should also have an arterial line prior to induction for timely blood pressure monitoring. Central venous pressure (CVP) monitoring may also assist in assessing fluid balance and management in the setting of hypotension [44].

Release of vasoactive substances by the tumor are exacerbated by sympathetic stimulation, extreme fluctuations in blood pressure, and surgical manipulation. Thus, anxiolytics should be given prior to surgery. Premedication with benzodiazepines and antihistamines is useful for reducing the perioperative stress response [44]. It is important to avoid any histamine-releasing medications. Propofol is an adequate induction agent to blunt the sympathetic response and minimize the release of hormones. Succinylcholine used to be thought of as an exacerbator of symptoms due to transient increase of intraabdominal pressure, but researchers have not found any evidence supporting this. It is important to avoid opioids associated with histamine release. Similarly, some nondepolarizing muscular blocking agents have been shown to release histamine. Thus, vecuronium and rocuronium are good choices for maintenance of blockade [44].

Treatment of vasoactive symptoms in the operating room can commonly be rectified with use of IV octreotide boluses, sometimes at 1 mg doses. Hydrocortisone may also be used to blunt these responses. Vasopressors, such as phenylephrine, may be used. However, any vasopressors with β-adrenergic stimulation can cause release of vasoactive substances from the tumor. Because of this, epinephrine should be avoided in these patients. The mainstay of blood pressure management should include IV fluids, octreotide, and phenylephrine [44].

Conclusion

Endocrinopathies can lead to adverse perioperative events. It is paramount that clinicians have a comprehensive understanding of endocrine diseases, as this may lead to a reduction in morbidity and mortality. Understanding the relationship between the disciplines of anesthesiology and endocrinology is tantamount. In summary, we have attempted to provide an in-depth understanding of the signs, symptoms, diagnoses, and perioperative treatment of endocrinopathies encountered in anesthesiology. Continued learning about these complex and interesting diseases is warranted to ensure the best possible outcome for your patients, especially given continued advances in management and treatment.

References

1. Palmer BF. Hyponatremia in patients with central nervous system disease: SIADH versus CSW. *Trends Endocrinol Metab*. 2003;14(4):182–7.

2. Verbalis JG, Greenberg A, Burst V, *et al.* Diagnosing and treating the syndrome of inappropriate antidiuretic hormone secretion. *Am J Med*. 2016;129(5):537.e9–23.

3. Sterns RH, Silver SM. Cerebral salt wasting versus SIADH: what difference? *J Am Soc Nephrol*. 2008;19(2):194–6.

4. Gubbi S, Hannah-Shmouni F, Koch CA, Verbalis JG. Diagnostic testing for diabetes insipidus. In: KR Feingold, B Anawalt, A Boyce, *et al.*, eds. *Endotext*. South Dartmouth, MA: MDText.com, Inc.; 2019. Available from: www.ncbi.nlm.nih.gov /books/NBK537591/.

5. McDermott MT. In the clinic: hypothyroidism. *Ann Intern Med*. 2009;151(11): ITC61.

6. Ono Y, Ono S, Yasunaga H, Matsui H, Fushimi K, Tanaka Y. Clinical characteristics and outcomes of myxedema coma: analysis of a national inpatient database in Japan. *J Epidemiol*. 2017;27(3):117–22.

7. Bigos ST, Ridgway EC, Kourides IA, Maloof F. Spectrum of pituitary alterations with mild and severe thyroid impairment. *J Clin Endocrinol Metab*. 1978;46 (2):317–25.

8. Klein I, Danzi S. Thyroid disease and the heart. *Circulation*. 2007;116(15):1725–35.

9. Sachdev Y, Hall R. Effusions into body cavities in hypothyroidism. *Lancet*. 1975;305 (7906):564–6.

10. Wilson WR, Bedell GN. The pulmonary abnormalities in myxedema. *J Clin Invest*. 1960;39(1):42–55.

11. Sadek SH, Khalifa WA, Azoz AM. Pulmonary consequences of hypothyroidism. *Ann Thorac Med*. 2017;12(3):204.

12. De Leo S, Lee SY, Braverman LE. Hyperthyroidism. *Lancet*. 2016;388 (10047):906–18.

13. Angell TE, Lechner MG, Nguyen CT, Salvato VL, Nicoloff JT, LoPresti JS. Clinical features and hospital outcomes in thyroid storm: a retrospective cohort study. *J Clin Endocrinol Metab*. 2015;100(2):451–9.

14. Akamizu T, Satoh T, Isozaki O, *et al.* Diagnostic criteria, clinical features, and incidence of thyroid storm based on nationwide surveys. *Thyroid*. 2012;22 (7):661–79.

15. Osuna PM, Udovcic M, Sharma MD. Hyperthyroidism and the heart. *Methodist DeBakey Cardiovasc J*. 2017;13(2):60–3.

16. McElvaney GN, Wilcox PG, Fairbarn MS, *et al.* Respiratory muscle weakness and dyspnea in thyrotoxic patients. *Am Rev Respir Dis*. 1990;141(5 Pt 1):1221–7.

17. Lopes MP, Kliemann BS, Bini IB, *et al.* Hypoparathyroidism and pseudohypoparathyroidism: etiology, laboratory features and complications. *Arch Endocrinol Metab*. 2016;60(6):532–6.

18. Cooper MS, Gittoes NJL. Diagnosis and management of hypocalcaemia. *BMJ*. 2008;336(7656):1298–302.

19. Dralle H, Sekulla C, Lorenz K, Brauckhoff M, Machens A; German IONM Study Group. Intraoperative monitoring of the recurrent laryngeal nerve in thyroid surgery. *World J Surg.* 2008;32(7):1358–66.

20. Lombardi CP, Raffaelli M, De Crea C, *et al.* Long-term outcome of functional post-thyroidectomy voice and swallowing symptoms. *Surgery.* 2009;146 (6):1174–81.

21. Walker MD, Silverberg SJ. Primary hyperparathyroidism. *Nat Rev Endocrinol.* 2018;14(2):115–25.

22. Muppidi V, Meegada SR, Rehman A. Secondary hyperparathyroidism. In: *StatPearls.* Treasure Island, FL: StatPearls Publishing; 2022. Available from: www .ncbi.nlm.nih.gov/books/NBK557822/.

23. Cozzolino M, Galassi A, Conte F, Mangano M, Di Lullo L, Bellasi A. Treatment of secondary hyperparathyroidism: the clinical utility of etelcalcetide. *Ther Clin Risk Manag.* 2017 1(13):679–89.

24. Gravellone L, Rizzo MA, Martina V, Mezzina N, Regalia A, Gallieni M. Vitamin D receptor activators and clinical outcomes in chronic kidney disease. *Int J Nephrol.* 2011;2011:419524.

25. Pitt SC, Sippel RS, Chen H. Secondary and tertiary hyperparathyroidism, state of the art surgical management. *Surg Clin North Am.* 2009;89(5):1227–39.

26. Bajwa SJS, Sehgal V. Anesthetic management of primary hyperparathyroidism: a role rarely noticed and appreciated so far. *Indian J Endocrinol Metab.* 2013;17 (2):235–9.

27. Hans SK, Levine SN. Hypoparathyroidism. In: *StatPearls.* Treasure Island, FL: StatPearls Publishing; 2022. Available from: www.ncbi.nlm.nih.gov/books/NB K441899/.

28. Bissonnette B, Luginbuehl I, Marciniak B, Dalens BJ. Hypoparathyroidism. In: B Bissonnette, I Luginbuehl, B Marciniak, BJ Dalens, eds. *Syndromes: Rapid Recognition and Perioperative Implications.* New York, NY: McGraw-Hill; 2006. Available from: https://accessanesthesiology.mhmedical.com/content.aspx? aid=58080446.

29. Maker AV, Sheikh R, Bhagia V; Diabetes Control and Complications Trial (DCCT) Research Group. Perioperative management of endocrine insufficiency after total pancreatectomy for neoplasia. *Langenbecks Arch Surg.* 2017;402 (6):873–83.

30. Vinik AI, Maser RE, Mitchell BD, Freeman R. Diabetic autonomic neuropathy. *Diabetes Care.* 2003;26(5):1553–79.

31. Dogra P, Jialal I. Diabetic perioperative management. In: *StatPearls.* Treasure Island, FL: StatPearls Publishing; 2022. Available from: www.ncbi.nlm.nih.gov/bo oks/NBK540965/.

32. Cao X, Wang X, Lu Y, *et al.* Spleen-preserving distal pancreatectomy and lymphadenectomy for glucagonoma syndrome. *Medicine (Baltimore).* 2019;98 (38):e17037.

33. Willenberg HS, Bornstein SR. Adrenal cortex; development, anatomy, physiology. In: KR Feingold, B Anawalt, A Boyce, *et al.*, eds. *Endotext.* South Dartmouth, MA: MDText.com, Inc.; 2017. Available from: www.ncbi.nlm.nih.gov/books/NB K278945/.

34. Burford NG, Webster NA, Cruz-Topete D. Hypothalamic–pituitary–adrenal axis modulation of glucocorticoids in the cardiovascular system. *Int J Mol Sci.* 2017;18 (10):2150.

35. Neary N, Nieman L. Adrenal insufficiency: etiology, diagnosis and treatment. *Curr Opin Endocrinol Diabetes Obes.* 2010;17(3):217–23.

36. Hahner S, Ross RJ, Arlt W, *et al.* Adrenal insufficiency. *Nat Rev Dis Primer.* 2021;7 (1):1–24.

37. Thompson Bastin ML, Baker SN, Weant KA. Effects of etomidate on adrenal suppression: a review of intubated septic patients. *Hosp Pharm.* 2014;49 (2):177–83.

38. Salem M, Tainsh RE, Bromberg J, Loriaux DL, Chernow B. Perioperative glucocorticoid coverage. A reassessment 42 years after emergence of a problem. *Ann Surg.* 1994;219(4):416–25.

39. Witchel SF, Oberfield SE, Peña AS. Polycystic ovary syndrome: pathophysiology, presentation, and treatment with emphasis on adolescent girls. *J Endocr Soc.* 2019;3 (8):1545–73.

40. Williams T, Mortada R, Porter S. Diagnosis and treatment of polycystic ovary syndrome. *Am Fam Physician.* 2016;94(2):106–13.

41. Fishbein L. Pheochromocytoma and paraganglioma: genetics, diagnosis, and treatment. *Hematol Oncol Clin North Am.* 2016;30(1):135–50.

42. Vindenes T, Crump N, Casenas R, Wood K. Pheochromocytoma causing cardiomyopathy, ischemic stroke and acute arterial thrombosis: a case report and review of the literature. *Conn Med.* 2013;77(2):95–8.

43. Melnyk DL. Update on carcinoid syndrome. *AANA J.* 1997;65(3):265–70.

44. Mancuso K, Kaye AD, Boudreaux JP, *et al.* Carcinoid syndrome and perioperative anesthetic considerations. *J Clin Anesth.* 2011;23(4):329–41.

45. Castiello RJ, Lynch PJ. Pellagra and the carcinoid syndrome. *Arch Dermatol.* 1972;105(4):574–7.

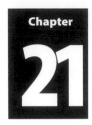

Anesthesia for Neuromuscular and Collagen Vascular Diseases

Erin Yen and Timothy Martin

Introduction

Neuromuscular and collagen vascular diseases comprise a wide array of disorders that bear a broad range of implications for anesthetic management throughout the perioperative period. Thorough preanesthetic evaluation is essential, with focus on the airway, pulmonary, and cardiovascular systems paramount, in addition to close attention to anticipated special positioning needs intraoperatively. Specific anesthetic medications may be contraindicated in some conditions, and a number of these patients may require perioperative glucocorticoid supplementation due to chronic steroid use. Some patients are susceptible to postoperative cardiopulmonary compromise and may require increased or extended postoperative monitoring.

Tables 21.1 and 21.2 summarize the principal perioperative anesthetic considerations of neuromuscular and collagen vascular diseases.

Neuromuscular Diseases

Myasthenia Gravis

Myasthenia gravis (MG) is an autoimmune disorder that results from antibody formation against either acetylcholine receptors (75% of cases) or related macromolecules known as muscle-specific kinase or lipoprotein receptor-related protein (remaining cases). The antibodies result in complement-mediated degradation of the target receptors or proteins, leading to impaired neuromuscular transmission in striated muscle [1]. Women are more often affected in young adulthood, whereas men are more likely affected in later decades. Patients with MG may have generalized or localized weakness that typically improves with rest, and in >50% of patients, there are ocular or other bulbar findings such as diplopia and ptosis [2]. Although several classification schemes have been devised over the years, currently, the model of the Myasthenia Gravis Foundation of America that recognizes five groups according to the severity of symptoms is widely employed [1].

Table 21.1 Neuromuscular diseases of importance to anesthesia providers, with principal features and considerations

Disease	Physical and diagnostic findings	Preoperative considerations	Intraoperative/anesthetic considerations	Postoperative considerations
Myasthenia gravis (MG)	• Generalized or localized weakness; improves with rest • Assess for bulbar findings and respiratory compromise	• Assess medical management, including pyridostigmine dose quantification, steroids, and immunosuppressants • Assess for thymoma or "mediastinal mass"	• Provide perioperative glucocorticoid coverage if patient on steroids • Regional anesthetic techniques optimal • Avoid succinylcholine due to possible resistance and prolongation of effect by pyridostigmine • Reduce dose or avoid nondepolarizing muscle relaxants; monitor depth of blockade closely	• Monitor closely for ventilatory insufficiency if extubated • May require postoperative mechanical ventilation • Monitor for myasthenic and cholinergic crises
Lambert–Eaton myasthenic syndrome (LEMS)	• Autoantibodies against presynaptic calcium channels • Muscle weakness that improves with repeated use • Paraneoplastic syndrome; most often associated with small	• Autonomic dysfunction can occur • Consider PFTs • Review any available chest imaging, particularly CXR	• Sensitive to depolarizing and nondepolarizing neuromuscular blockade (decreased dose requirement) • Closely monitor neuromuscular function • Consider regional anesthesia technique if applicable	• May require postoperative mechanical ventilation

Table 21.1 (cont.)

Disease	Physical and diagnostic findings	Preoperative considerations	Intraoperative/anesthetic considerations	Postoperative considerations
	cell lung cancer or other malignancy • Clinical diagnosis; confirmed by electrophysiologic testing and the presence of antibody • Treatment: 3,4-diaminopyridine, treatment of underlying neoplasm			
Guillain–Barré syndrome (GBS)	• Autoimmune demyelinating ascending peripheral neuropathy • Usually associated with GI or respiratory infection/illness prior to symptoms • Treatment: plasmapheresis, IVIG, supportive	• Consider PFTs	• Avoid succinylcholine; can cause life-threatening hyperkalemia • Autonomic dysfunction may occur with drastic changes in BP and HR	• May require post-operative mechanical ventilation
Muscular dystrophies and congenital myopathies; Duchenne and Becker muscular dystrophies	• X-linked lack of dystrophin gene (Duchenne) or reduction in functional dystrophin (Becker)	• Cardiac workup (echocardiography, MRI) for underlying cardiomyopathy • PFTs	• Sensitive to nondepolarizing neuromuscular blockade • Closely monitor neuromuscular function	• May require post-operative mechanical ventilation

	• Muscle weakness, CHF, and scoliosis are commonly seen • Average lifespan is 30 years (Duchenne) • Treatment: corticosteroids, supportive	• Avoid succinylcholine and halogenated agents, which may induce "AIR" (anesthesia-induced rhabdomyolysis) • Consider regional anesthesia technique if applicable	
Mitochondrial myopathy	• Hypotonia, developmental delay, possible seizures • Cardiac and endocrine dysfunction; consider preoperative ECG and echocardiography	• Limit preoperative fasting; consider placing peripheral IV catheter and beginning glucose-containing IV fluids when NPO • Limit stress and hypothermia	• Nearly all anesthetics have inhibitory effects on the respiratory chain • Low-dose inhalational anesthetics, ketamine, and short-acting opioids are ideal • Avoid propofol, or use in single dose for short period • Carefully monitor any neuromuscular blockade, or avoid use if possible • Monitor intraoperative glucose • Maintain normovolemia	• Possible delayed emergence • Maintain hydration and avoid hypoglycemia • May require postoperative ventilation

PFT, pulmonary function test; GI, gastrointestinal; IVIG, intravenous immunoglobulin; BP, blood pressure; HR, heart rate; CHF, congestive heart failure; NPO, nil per os.

Table 21.2 Collagen vascular diseases of importance to anesthesia providers, with principal features and considerations

Disease	Physical and diagnostic findings	Preoperative considerations	Intraoperative/anesthetic considerations	Postoperative considerations
• Rheumatoid arthritis (RA) and juvenile idiopathic arthritis (JIA)	• Chronic autoimmune inflammatory symmetric polyarthritis • Highly variant systemic effects	• Elucidate cervical spine involvement; review imaging • Cardiac and pulmonary workup: echocardiography, PFTs • Patients receiving corticosteroids may need supplementation in perioperative period	• Possible difficult tracheal intubation • Extra caution when positioning • Consider advanced monitoring (e.g., arterial line) with cardiopulmonary involvement • Antiinflammatory drugs may impact clotting • Biologic agents can increase risk of infection • Regional techniques may be more technically difficult	• May require postoperative mechanical ventilation with severe pulmonary involvement
Systemic lupus erythematosus (SLE)	• Autoimmune multisystem disease with variable symptoms	• CXR, PFTs, and echocardiography if cardiopulmonary involvement	• Laryngeal involvement can make tracheal intubation difficult	• Postextubation stridor may occur; IV steroids often effective

	and organ involvement • Can be induced by certain drugs • Most commonly seen in women of childbearing age	• Labs to assess renal function • Careful medication reconciliation (interactions with many anesthetic drugs) • Patients receiving corticosteroids may need supplementation in perioperative period	• Careful use of depolarizing and nondepolarizing neuromuscular blockade (possible drug interactions)	• Monitor for respiratory compromise
Systemic sclerosis (SSc)	• Multisystemic changes in microvasculature causing fibrosis and inflammation • Widely variant clinical presentation	• Most commonly affects pulmonary system: PFTs, echocardiography to evaluate right heart function and pulmonary hypertension • CXR	• Taut skin can lead to reduced mouth opening; can complicate airway management • Consider advanced cardiovascular monitoring • Increased sensitivity to muscle relaxants (decrease dose) • Consider regional anesthesia; may have prolonged response to local anesthetics	• May require postoperative mechanical ventilation • Consider ICU postoperatively if use of advanced monitoring required

Table 21.2 (cont.)

Disease	Physical and diagnostic findings	Preoperative considerations	Intraoperative/anesthetic considerations	Postoperative considerations
Dermatomyositis (DM) and polymyositis (PM)	• Noninfectious muscle inflammation and weakness • Most commonly affects proximal musculature (DM)	• ECG, echocardiography, CXR, and PFTs to evaluate cardiopulmonary function • Careful medication reconciliation (interactions with many anesthetic drugs) • Patients receiving corticosteroids may need supplementation in perioperative period	• Esophageal dysmotility increases the risk of aspiration pneumonia and pneumonitis • Variable response to neuromuscular blockade; closely monitor neuromuscular function if paralysis required • Consider regional anesthesia	

PFTs, pulmonary function tests; IV, intravenous; ICU, intensive care unit.

Physostigmine, a cholinesterase inhibitor in the same drug class as neostigmine, is the primary medical treatment as it acts to increase the concentration of acetylcholine at the neuromuscular junction (NMJ). Due to their effects in attenuating the immune response, corticosteroids may also be employed. Immunosuppressants (e.g., azathioprine, methotrexate, etanercept) are required in some patients, and in the setting of acute disease, patients may require intravenous (IV) immunoglobulins or plasma exchange. Thymectomy, either thoracoscopic or via median sternotomy, is often provided [2].

Anesthetic Considerations

Preoperative evaluation should focus on the extent of muscle weakness, particularly involving the bulbar and respiratory muscles, and optimization of medical therapy. The presence of thymoma or thymic hyperplasia and resultant tracheal compression ("mediastinal mass") should be assessed with CT or MRI. Patients may have cardiac conduction disturbances and signs of autonomic instability, including blood pressure lability and gastroparesis. Patients should be assessed for evidence of other autoimmune and endocrine disorders, including thyroid dysfunction, rheumatoid arthritis (RA), and systemic lupus erythematosus (SLE) [1]. Pyridostigmine should be continued in the perioperative period, including intravenous (IV) administration intraoperatively. Due to high first-pass extraction of orally administered pyridostigmine, a conversion ratio of IV to oral doses of 1:30 is recommended [2]. Patients who have been receiving chronic glucocorticoid therapy should receive "stress dose" steroid coverage perioperatively.

Anesthetic management considerations include use of regional anesthetic techniques whenever the nature of the surgical procedure allows, and for general anesthesia, avoidance of neuromuscular blocking agents when practical. Succinylcholine is generally avoided as patients with MG are thought to be relatively resistant to its effects and pyridostigmine would be expected to prolong its duration of action. When nondepolarizing muscle relaxants are required, conventional practice is to employ reduced doses and either no or lengthened redosing intervals. Sugammadex has generally proven successful in reversing nondepolarizing relaxant (rocuronium and vecuronium only) effects in patients with MG, although one case report demonstrated perceived failure of sugammadex to antagonize rocuronium blockade [3, 4]. Other medications, such as potent inhalation anesthetics and various antimicrobials, that are known to interfere with neuromuscular function (e.g., ciprofloxacin, erythromycin, aminoglycosides) should be avoided when possible. Total intravenous anesthetic techniques that employ continuous infusions of propofol and short-acting opioids, such as remifentanil, may be ideal [5].

Postoperatively, patients may require mechanical ventilation and, if extubated, should be monitored for respiratory insufficiency for an extended period. Both myasthenic and cholinergic crises may be encountered postoperatively.

Lambert–Eaton (Myasthenic) Syndrome

Lambert–Eaton syndrome is a rare immune-mediated disease associated with antibodies against the presynaptic calcium channel at the NMJ. It is associated with malignancy in many cases [2]. Patients often complain of weakness, which can be mistaken for MG. Of note, patients with Lambert–Eaton syndrome do not respond to anticholinesterases or steroids but do improve with repeated activity [6]. The pathophysiology of Lambert–Eaton syndrome involves a presynaptic defect that interferes with the release of acetylcholine. Patients are particularly sensitive to all neuromuscular blocking agents, and these should be avoided if possible [7, 8].

Anesthetic Considerations

Patients with Lambert–Eaton syndrome are sensitive to the effects of both depolarizing and nondepolarizing neuromuscular blockers (NDNMBs). Recovery of neuromuscular function should be closely monitored. The most common and serious perioperative complications are respiratory in nature and some patients might require postoperative mechanical ventilation.

Guillain–Barré Syndrome

Guillain–Barré syndrome (GBS) is an autoimmune disease that is thought to be triggered by viral or bacterial infection [9]. The infectious agent produces a substance that resembles a host neural component and causes the formation of autoantibodies that attack the host peripheral nervous system. Patients with GBS have antibodies against gangliosides in the peripheral nerves. Most patients with GBS have a history of respiratory or gastrointestinal illness or infection within 4 weeks of the appearance of neurological symptoms [9, 10]. GBS is characterized by weakness that occurs in an ascending pattern, beginning in the lower extremities and progressing more cephalad. Paresthesias may precede skeletal muscle weakness in some patients.

Anesthetic Considerations

Autonomic nervous system dysfunction may occur with GBS, and stimulation (e.g., direct laryngoscopy, positioning, tracheal intubation, etc.) may lead to drastic and wide changes in heart rate and blood pressure [11]. Succinylcholine should be avoided in patients with GBS due to the risk of hyperkalemia. Intermediate-acting NDNMBs, such as rocuronium, have been used safely in patients with GBS. The most serious threat to GBS patients is respiratory insufficiency and the need for mechanical ventilation postoperatively.

Muscular Dystrophies and Congenital Myopathies

Muscular dystrophies and congenital myopathies are a group of genetic muscle disorders characterized by skeletal muscle weakness, although cardiac and smooth muscle can also be affected. This broad group of disorders differs in the specific muscle groups affected, age of onset, and severity of symptoms.

Duchenne muscular dystrophy (DMD) is the most common childhood muscular dystrophy and is caused by the complete absence of dystrophin [12]. Dystrophin is a large protein found on skeletal muscle membranes and is responsible for regulating the integrity of the sarcolemma on striated muscle [13]. DMD is a progressive neuromuscular disease, with degeneration of skeletal, cardiac, and smooth muscle beginning at 3–5 years of age [12]. Rapid progression of muscle weakness leads to failure to walk by adolescence and eventual death from respiratory failure. Becker muscular dystrophy (BMD) is caused by a reduction in functional dystrophin and these patients have a similar, but milder, course of disease than those with DMD [14].

Anesthetic Considerations

Perioperative evaluation and management of patients with muscular dystrophies depend on the particular disease and speed of its progression. The most pressing complications in these patients are cardiac involvement and respiratory muscle function. Surveillance with echocardiography and cardiac MRI is recommended by most for evaluation of left ventricular function and arrhythmia [12–14]. Preoperative review of these studies will assist in anesthetic planning. Patients with severely diminished left ventricular function may require invasive hemodynamic monitoring in the perioperative period. DMD patients are especially sensitive to succinylcholine, as well as to halogenated inhaled agents. Their use can lead to rhabdomyolysis and severe hyperkalemia, and thus should be avoided. It was previously thought patients with muscular dystrophies were at increased risk of malignant hyperthermia (MH). However, there is no evidence the risk is greater than in the general population [12–13]. Patients with muscular dystrophies are sensitive to NDNMBs and neuromuscular function should be closely monitored. Patients may also require postoperative mechanical ventilation due to respiratory muscle weakness.

Mitochondrial Myopathies

The "mitochondrial myopathies" (MM) are a relatively recently recognized group of congenital disorders of energy metabolism in the mitochondria that primarily affect tissues with high energy requirements, including muscle – hence the term "mitochondrial myopathies." However, these inborn errors of metabolism typically involve also other organs and tissues with increased energy requirements, including the nervous, cardiovascular, and endocrine systems [15]. Defects in any of the five enzyme/protein complexes (I–V) that make up the "respiratory chain" may result in a mitochondrial energy production disorder, including myopathy. The estimated prevalence of these disorders is 1 in 5000 live births [16].

Presentation in childhood tends to portend more severe disease, and may include encephalopathy with developmental delay and skeletal muscle weakness with hypotonia. Diagnosis is confirmed by various histologic and electron microscopic studies of biopsied muscle tissue. Plasma creatine kinase concentrations are typically normal, although lactic acid may be elevated. Although the genetic transmission patterns are complex and there is often an overlap of symptoms and signs of MM, members of this group of disorders are referred to as Leigh syndrome, Kearns–Sayre syndrome, and MELAS (mitochondrial encephalopathy, lactic acidosis, and stroke-like episodes) syndrome.

Anesthesia for patients with MM is challenging for several reasons, including often varied and contrary responses of different patients to the same anesthetic agents and the reality that many anesthetic medications inhibit or interfere with one or more enzyme functions of the respiratory chain [16]. Due to baseline lactic acidosis or a propensity to develop lactic acidosis, avoidance of prolonged fasting, dehydration, and hypothermia, as well as early supplementation with IV glucose (energy substrate), is often recommended to minimize perioperative flares of MM symptoms and complications, while also avoiding IV solutions containing lactate. Inhalational anesthetics and propofol inhibit complexes I and II of the respiratory chain, and propofol has also several other suppressive effects on the mitochondria. With prolonged or repeated propofol exposure, some MM patients develop a clinical picture resembling propofol infusion syndrome (PRIS) [17]. While some anesthesiologists avoid administration of propofol altogether in patients with known or suspected MM, others indicate that the use of propofol for brief procedures is reasonable, particularly if the patient has had previous good experience with this medication [16]. Review of past anesthetic records and patient outcomes, and listening closely to the input and experiences described by parents of pediatric MM patients are invaluable. Because both sensitivity and resistance to nondepolarizing neuromuscular blocking agents have been reported, it is essential that neuromuscular transmission be objectively monitored during muscle relaxant use and reversal. Any association between MM and MH has generally been dismissed [18].

Collagen Vascular Diseases

Rheumatoid Arthritis and Juvenile Idiopathic Arthritis

RA is a chronic autoimmune inflammatory condition, without clear etiology and with diverse clinical manifestations. Juvenile idiopathic arthritis

(JIA) is a diagnosis of exclusion, with all other causes of arthritis being excluded in a patient with symptoms that started before the age of 16 years [19]. RA can be characterized by synovial cellular hyperplasia leading to the destruction of cartilage and articular surfaces of any joint [20]. The most commonly affected joints are the metacarpophalangeal and interphalangeal joints of the hands, with the knee being the most commonly affected joint in the lower extremity [21–22]. The extra-articular symptoms of RA are broad and can affect the cardiovascular, pulmonary, nervous, and hematological systems.

Anesthetic Considerations

The clinical manifestations of RA are diverse and must be elucidated for each patient on an individual basis. The presence and severity of systemic dysfunction must be identified prior to anesthetic and surgical planning. Arthritis involving the cervical spine and cricoarytenoid joints may complicate direct laryngoscopy and tracheal intubation. Video laryngo-scopy and flexible fiberoptic bronchoscopes should be available for use, if necessary. Systemic arthritic changes may complicate positioning. Extremities must be positioned with caution to minimize the risk of neu-rovascular injury and prevent further damage to the joint. The extent of cardiopulmonary involvement may necessitate advanced cardiovascular monitoring, as well as postoperative mechanical ventilation [23]. Patients may be taking chronic corticosteroid therapy and require supplementation in the perioperative period. Regional anesthesia should be considered in patients with RA. However, regional techniques may be more technically difficult, secondary to altered anatomy from joint damage, potential platelet dysfunction, and the ability for the patient to lay still in one position for prolonged periods.

Systemic Lupus Erythematosus

SLE is a chronic autoimmune connective tissue disorder with a heterogenous presentation affecting multiple organ systems. The exact pathogenesis of SLE is unclear, but the various clinical manifestations are influenced by the many genes that affect the immune system [24]. SLE can affect almost any organ system in the body but most commonly affects the joints and the integumen-tary, renal, cardiovascular, central nervous, and hematologic systems (see Table 21.2). SLE is most common in women of childbearing age, and antiDNA, antiphospholipid, and anticardiolipin antibodies, as well as lupus anticoagulant, may be detected in many patients with SLE [25–27]. Although SLE is most commonly an autoimmune disorder, causation has also been associated with specific drugs (hydralazine, isoniazid, procainamide, methyl-dopa, enalapril, and captopril) [24].

Anesthetic Considerations

Preoperative assessment of a patient with SLE depends on the clinical history and symptoms of each individual patient. Choice of the anesthetic technique should consider pharmacologic interactions with anesthetic drugs, immunosuppression of patients, increased thrombotic risk, and unexpected difficult airway with laryngeal edema, among other patient factors. Patients on corticosteroids should receive a perioperative dose of corticosteroids. Drugs for treatment of SLE can influence the choice of anesthetic drugs. Azathioprine can increase the dose requirement for NDNMBs, and cyclophosphamide may prolong the duration of action of succinylcholine by inhibiting cholinesterase [24–25].

Systemic Sclerosis (Scleroderma)

Systemic sclerosis (SSc) is a progressive systemic disease characterized by changes in the microvasculature that cause fibrosis and inflammation of the skin, blood vessels, cardiovascular and pulmonary systems, kidneys, and gastrointestinal tract [24, 28–31]. Most commonly, SSc affects the pulmonary system, with >80% of patients developing interstitial lung disease, eventually leading to pulmonary hypertension and right-sided heart failure [24]. The patient's skin becomes thickened and eventually fibrotic and taut, leading to reduced joint mobility, as well as limited mouth opening if the face is involved. Treatment is aimed at immunosuppression with agents such as cyclophosphamide, mycophenolate, and methotrexate.

Anesthetic Considerations

SSc has diverse clinical manifestations, and preoperative assessment should be tailored to the individual patient's symptoms and disease course. Thorough cardiopulmonary physical examination, as well as pulmonary function testing, preoperative CXR, and echocardiography, may be considered to determine the severity of organ dysfunction. Tracheal intubation can often be difficult due to reduced motion of the temporomandibular joint, requiring an awake fiberoptic technique. Esophageal dysmotility can increase the risk of aspiration and pulmonary pneumonitis during general anesthesia [28, 29]. Involvement of the cardiovascular system (e.g., coronary arteriosclerosis, depressed myocardial function) may necessitate advanced hemodynamic monitoring during surgery, including arterial catheterization and central venous cannulation. Placement of these lines may be difficult with deposition of fibrotic material within blood vessels. Regional anesthesia may be an appropriate alternative to general anesthesia, although individual patient factors must be considered. Patients with SSc have shown prolonged response to local anesthetics [32].

Dermatomyositis and Polymyositis

Dermatomyositis (DM) and polymyositis (PM) are idiopathic inflammatory myopathies characterized by severe muscle weakness and noninfectious muscle inflammation [24, 33]. Presenting features of DM include proximal muscle (shoulder and pelvic girdle) weakness and a distinct skin rash. The skin rash is described as periorbital edema, heliotrope rash (purple discoloration of the eyelids), and Gottron papules (scaly lesions on the knuckles) [24]. DM may be associated with malignancies, whereas PM is often associated with other connective tissue diseases [33]. Treatment for both diseases includes corticosteroids followed by immunosuppressants (azathioprine, methotrexate, cyclosporine, mycophenolate, etc.).

Anesthetic Considerations

There is considerable overlap between the inflammatory myopathies. However, the most important clinical consideration in this patient population is the potential involvement of the cardiac and pulmonary systems. DM and PM patients have esophageal dysmotility and are at higher risk of aspiration pneumonitis. They can also have cardiac conduction abnormalities and cardiomyopathies. Response to muscle relaxants may be variable in this patient population, and neuromuscular function should be monitored closely if neuromuscular blockers are used.

References

1. JP Cata, JD Lasala, W Williams, *et al.* Myasthenia gravis and thymoma surgery: a clinical update for the cardiothoracic anesthesiologist. *J Cardiothorac Vasc Anesth.* 2019;33:2537–45.

2. P Turakhia, B Barrick, J Berman. Patients with neuromuscular disorder. *Med Clin N Am.* 2013;97:1015–32.

3. HD deBoer, MO Shields, LHDJ Booij. Reversal of neuromuscular blockade with sugammadex in patients with myasthenia gravis – a case series of 21 patients and review of the literature. *Eur J Anaesthesiol.* 2014;31:708–21.

4. H Dos Santos Fernandes, JL Saraiva Ximenes, D Ibanhes Nunes, *et al.* Failure of reversion of neuromuscular block with sugammadex in patient with myasthenia gravis: case report and brief review of literature. *BMC Anesthesiol.* 2019;19:160–3.

5. L Blichfeldt-Lauridsen, BD Hansen. Anesthesia and myasthenia gravis. *Acta Anaesthesiol Scand.* 2012;56:17–22.

6. TN Weingarten, CN Araka, ME Mogenson, *et al.* Lambert–Eaton myasthenic syndrome during anesthesia: a report of 37 patients. *J Clin Anesth.* 2014;26(8):648–53.

7. JA Katz, GS Murphy. Anesthetic consideration for neuromuscular diseases. *Curr Opin Anaesthesiol.* 2017;30(3):435–40.

8. B Schoser, B Eymard, J Datt, *et al.* Lambert–Eaton myasthenic syndrome (LEMS): a rare autoimmune disorder often associated with cancer. *J Neurol.* 2017;264:1854–63.

9. RAC Hughes, DR Cornblath. Guillain–Barré syndrome. *Lancet.* 2005;366 (9497):1653–66.

10. S Hocker, E Nagarajan, M Rubin, *et al.* Clinical factors associated with Guillain–Barré syndrome following surgery. *Neurol Clin Pract.* 2018;8(3):201–6.

11. GD Jones, JM Wilmshurst, K Sykes, *et al.* Guillain–Barré syndrome: delayed diagnosis following anaesthesia. *Pediatr Anesth.* 1999;9:539–42.

12. J Hayes, F Veyckemans, B Bissonnette. Duchenne muscular dystrophy: an old anesthesia problem revisited. *Pediatr Anesth.* 2008;18:100–6.

13. LG Segura, JD Lorenz, TN Weingarten, *et al.* Anesthesia and Duchenne or Becker muscular dystrophy: review of 117 anesthetic exposures. *Pediatr Anesth.* 2013;23:855–64.

14. LH Cripe, JD Tobias. Cardiac considerations in the operative management of the patient with Duchenne or Becker muscular dystrophy. *Pediatr Anesth.* 2013;23:777–84.

15. J Niezgoda, PG Morgan. Anaesthetic considerations in patients with mitochondrial defects. *Pediatr Anesth.* 2013;23(9):785–93.

16. J Lerman. Perioperative management of the paediatric patient with coexisting neuromuscular disease. *Br J Anaesth.* 2011;107(S1):i79–89.

17. JJ Driessen. Neuromuscular and mitochondrial disorders: what is relevant to the anaesthesiologist? *Curr Opin Anaesthesiol.* 2008;21:350–5.

18. AK Ross. Muscular dystrophy versus mitochondrial myopathy: the dilemma of the undiagnosed hypotonic child (editorial). *Pediatr Anesth.* 2007;17:1–6.

19. N Fanaras, NS Parry, NS Matthews. Multidisciplinary approach in the management of absolute trismus with bilateral temporomandibular joint replacements for a patient with juvenile idiopathic arthritis. *J Oral Maxillofac Surg.* 2014;72(11):2262–72.

20. EM Vieira, S Goodman, PP Tanaka. Anesthesia and rheumatoid arthritis. *Braz J Anesthesiol.* 2011;61(3):367–75.

21. D Tokunaga, H Hase, Y Mikami, *et al.* Atlantoaxial subluxation in different intraoperative head positions in patients with rheumatoid arthritis. *Anesthesiology.* 2006;104(4):675–9.

22. KJ Lyssy, A Escalante. Perioperative management of rheumatoid arthritis. Areas of concern for primary care physicians. *Postgrad Med.* 1996;99(2):191–206.

23. EM Galvin, D O'Donnell, IE Leonard. Rheumatoid arthritis: a significant but often underestimated risk factor for perioperative cardiac morbidity. *Anesthesiology.* 2005;103(4):910–11.

24. SF Dierdorf, JS Walton, AF Stasic, *et al.* Rare coexisting diseases. In: PG Barash, BF Cullen, RK Stoelting, eds. *Clinical Anesthesia.* Philadelphia, PA: Wolters Kluwer; 2017, pp. 612–44.

25. E Ben-Menachem. Systemic lupus erythematosus. *Anesth Analg.* 2010;111 (3):665–76.

26. JS Paranjpe, RJ Thote. Perioperative considerations of systemic lupus erythematosus and antiphospholipid syndrome. *Med J DY Patil Univ.* 2016;9:91–4.

27. S Rajagopalan. Systemic lupus erythematosus. In: S Mankowitz, ed. *Consults in Obstetric Anesthesiology.* New York, NY: Springer International; 2018, pp. 575–8.

28. F Ye, G Kong, J Huang. Anesthetic management of a patient with localized scleroderma. *SpringerPlus.* 2016;5:1507.

29. C D'Eramo, P Zuccoli, M Monica, *et al.* [Anesthesiologic management in scleroderma patients. Presentation of a clinical case]. *Acta Biomedica de L'ateneo Parmense.* 1986;57(1–2):33–7.

30. T Bansal, S Hooda. Emergency surgery in a patient with scleroderma – anaesthetic challenges: a case report. *Indian Anaesthetists' Forum.* 2013;14(7):1–4.

31. Y Shionoya, H Kamiga, G Tsujimoto, *et al.* Anesthetic management of a patient with systemic sclerosis and microstomia. *Anesth Prog.* 2020;67(1):28–34.

32. GB Lewis. Prolonged regional analgesia in scleroderma. *Can Anaesth Soc J.* 1974;21 (5):495–7.

33. DC Adams, EJ Heyer. Problems of anesthesia in patients with neuromuscular disease. *Anesthesiol Clin North Am.* 1997;15(3):673–89.

Anesthesia for Ocular, Ear, and Throat Diseases

Sheriza L. Hussain and Graham T. Lubinsky

Ocular

Factors that Influence Intraocular Pressure

Normal intraocular pressure (IOP) ranges between 10 and 22 mmHg. This pressure represents a balance between aqueous humor production and drainage [1]. An increase in IOP is harmful because it can decrease blood supply to the optic nerve [2]. Special care must be taken if the globe is open during surgery, as increased IOP in a patient with an open globe can lead to expulsion of ocular contents and permanent damage or blindness [2]. Surgeries in which there is an open globe include cataract extraction, corneal laceration repair, corneal transplant, trabeculectomy, vitrectomy, and ruptured globe repair. Other complications of increased IOP include acute glaucoma and retinal hemorrhage [1].

Most anesthetic drugs, including nondepolarizing neuromuscular blocking drugs (NMBDs), lead to decreased IOP. Exceptions include succinylcholine and ketamine [1].

During induction, increased IOP can be caused by straining, coughing, mask ventilation, laryngoscopy, and intubation, whereas it is less likely with laryngeal mask airway (LMA) placement. This response can be attenuated by administering lidocaine (1.5 mg kg^{-1}), a beta-blocker, or an opioid prior to laryngoscopy. Intubation should not occur under light anesthesia or inadequate muscle relaxation. The Trendelenburg position can increase IOP by preventing drainage of aqueous humor. Hypoxemia, hypercarbia/hypoventilation, and systemic hypertension can also increase IOP [1].

Choosing Pharmacologic Agents

Succinylcholine transiently increases IOP by 5–10 mmHg for <10 minutes, due to prolonged contracture of the extraocular muscles (EOMs) [2]. While this effect is transient, care must be taken in patients with pathology leading to an elevated preinduction IOP.

The effect of ketamine on IOP is controversial. While the classic teaching is that ketamine should be avoided in ocular cases due to a theoretical increase in IOP, studies have shown that this effect is not clinically significant unless doses of >4 mg kg^{-1} are used [3].

The ophthalmologist may inject a gas bubble, such as sulfur hexafluoride (SF6) or perfluoropropane (C3F8), into the posterior chamber during vitreo-retinal surgery. Nitrous oxide (N$_2$O) is 35 times more soluble in blood than in nitrogen. Thus, it can expand this bubble, leading to increased IOP. If used during vitreoretinal surgery, it should be turned off 15 minutes before injection of the gas bubble, and should not be used for at least 7–10 days after SF6 or 1 month after C3F8 injection [4]. The safest practice is to provide patients with a wristband stating this restriction.

Ophthalmologic Drugs

Topical eye drops have some degree of systemic absorption. Epinephrine eye drops can cause hypertension, tachycardia, and arrhythmias, whereas timolol eye drops can cause bradycardia. Atropine eye drops may cause central anti-cholinergic syndrome, especially in the elderly.

Topical echothiophate, which is used for glaucoma, is an irreversible acetylcholinesterase inhibitor. Systemic absorption reduces plasma cholines-terase activity, leading to prolonged duration of action of succinylcholine. This effect can last up to 3–7 weeks [1].

Regional Anesthesia

Benefits/Drawbacks

Benefits of regional anesthesia include akinesia (immobility) and analgesia of the eye, suppression of the oculocardiac reflex, lower incidence of postopera-tive nausea and vomiting (PONV), significant postoperative analgesia, and faster recovery leading to shorter stay in the postoperative care unit (PACU). Regional anesthesia may not be a good choice for patients who are very anxious and unable to lie still for the nerve block and/or surgery. Additionally, the oculocardiac reflex can be elicited during placement of regional nerve blocks [2].

Types of Blocks

Retrobulbar and peribulbar blocks (see Table 22.1) are the most common regional blocks used for eye surgery. In a retrobulbar block, local anesthetic is injected into the orbital cone formed by the EOMs, whereas in a peribulbar block, it is injected outside the muscle cone. Since retrobulbar blocks involve direct injection into the muscle cone, they are associated with a more rapid onset and more complete akinesia and anesthesia, requiring a smaller volume of local anesthetic, but are also associated with a higher risk of complications [1].

Table 22.1 Bulbar anesthesia

	Retrobulbar block	Peribulbar block
Location of injection	*Inside* orbital cone (aka INTRAconal block)	*Outside* orbital cone (aka EXTRAconal block)
Onset and density	Faster onset and denser block	Slower onset and less dense block
Local anesthetic volume	Small volume	Large volume
Advantages	Faster onset and denser block	• Lower risk of penetration of globe or optic nerve • Lower risk of hemorrhage • Less pain on injection • Less technical difficulty
Complications	• Retrobulbar hemorrhage → proptosis + CRAO • Globe perforation • Seizures • Respiratory arrest due to brainstem anesthesia • Elicitation of oculocardiac reflex	• Periorbital ecchymosis • Transient blindness (complications listed under "Retrobulbar block" can also be seen with peribulbar block, but are much less likely)
Contraindications	Extreme myopia (elongated globe increases the risk of globe perforation)	

| Contraindications to EITHER | • Uncontrolled cough or tremors
• Excess anxiety
• Altered mental status
• Bleeding disorders (risk of retrobulbar hemorrhage)
• Open eye injury (risk of extrusion of intraocular contents) |

See reference [1].

Oculocardiac Reflex

The oculocardiac reflex manifests as sudden bradycardia, in response to traction on the EOMs or pressure on the globe. The afferent limb is the ophthalmic division (V1) of the trigeminal nerve (CN5). The efferent limb is the vagus nerve (CN10). Eliciting the oculocardiac reflex can lead to bradycardia, atrioventricular (AV) block, ventricular ectopy, ventricular fibrillation, and asystole. It is more likely to occur in children, particularly during strabismus surgery.

If this reflex occurs, the first step in management is to alert the surgeon, so that they can temporarily stop causing traction on the eye muscles or pressure on the eye. Typically, this will resolve the bradycardia. If bradycardia persists, then after assessing for other causes of bradycardia, including inadequate ventilation and oxygenation, intravenous (IV) atropine (10 μg kg^{-1}) can be given. Local anesthetic infiltration of the EOMs, via a retrobulbar block, also prevents this reflex. However, the reflex can also be elicited during placement of a retrobulbar block [5].

Postoperative Eye Injuries

Painful

Corneal abrasion is the most common cause of postoperative eye pain. Other symptoms include foreign body sensation and tearing. It is caused by direct trauma from objects touching the cornea, such as surgical drapes or the anesthetic mask. It can be prevented by taping the eyelids carefully, using an ocular lubricant, and preventing patients from rubbing their eyes as they emerge from anesthesia. Although bothersome, corneal abrasions usually heal spontaneously within 24–72 hours. Antibiotic ointment may be given to prevent infection [1].

Acute glaucoma presents with painful vision loss, which may be associated with the appearance of halos around lights, headache, nausea, and vomiting. This is an ophthalmic emergency, requiring time-sensitive evaluation by an ophthalmologist to prevent blindness [1].

Painless

Postoperative vision loss (POVL) is usually painless. It is predominantly caused by ischemic optic neuropathy (ION), but can be caused also by central retinal artery occlusion (CRAO) [2]. It is more likely to occur during spine surgery in the prone position, as well as in cardiac surgery. Risk factors include hypotension, significant blood loss, administration of large volumes of crystalloid, and anemia. Patient risk factors include smoking, diabetes, and obesity [4].

Ophthalmology consultation should be obtained as soon as possible [1].

Surgeries

Strabismus Surgery

Strabismus surgery is the most common eye procedure in children. Strabismus is a condition in which there is eye misalignment. It often occurs in healthy children, but there is a higher incidence in Down syndrome and cerebral palsy. It can also be associated with other myopathies, which increases the risk of malignant hyperthermia. Strabismus surgery is associated with severe PONV and frequent triggering of the oculocardiac reflex [2].

Cataract Extraction

Cataract surgery is one of the most common surgical procedures. Cataracts are lens opacifications, which may cause blurred vision or even blindness. Surgery involves removal of the patient's lens, with subsequent insertion of an intra-ocular lens (IOL) implant. Removal of the lens may include phacoemulsification, in which ultrasound energy is used to break the lens into fragments to allow easier removal. This procedure is most commonly performed using only topical local anesthetics, without sedation [4].

Trabeculectomy

Glaucoma is prolonged elevation in IOP leading to hypoperfusion of the optic nerve, which can lead to blindness. Trabeculectomy allows drainage of aqueous humor, which relieves IOP. Topical anesthesia or a subtenon block may be used [4].

Retina Surgery

Retinal detachment may be caused by diabetes, retinopathy of prematurity, and trauma, including open globe injury. It often requires urgent surgery. If associated with an open globe injury, care must be taken to avoid increases in IOP. As discussed in "Choosing Pharmacologic Agents," N_2O should be avoided during and after vitreoretinal surgery. Most retinal procedures can be done under MAC with a regional block [4].

Ear, Nose, and Throat

Choosing Pharmacologic Agents

Muscle relaxation is often necessary to prevent coughing and bucking, which may lead to postoperative bleeding, and to immobilize the vocal cords during laryngeal surgery. On the other hand, avoidance of muscle relaxation may be needed if intraoperative nerve monitoring is used by the surgical team, such as during facial nerve dissection or thyroidectomy [4].

Airway surgery often includes periods of intense sympathetic stimulation due to use of the suspension laryngoscope, which is particularly worrisome in patients with cardiovascular disease [2]. Short-acting medications, such as esmolol and remifentanil, can be used to help prevent hemodynamic instability. Total intravenous anesthesia (TIVA) is a popular technique for endoscopic surgery. It has the benefits of improving recovery time and hemodynamic stability, and decreasing PONV. Postoperative airway edema can be prevented with high doses of dexamethasone. Ear, nose, and throat (ENT) surgeries have a high incidence of PONV, and antiemetics, such as ondansetron, dexamethasone, and propofol, may be beneficial [4].

Difficult Airway

ENT patients often have a compromised airway. A thorough preoperative airway examination should be conducted, and factors for difficult mask ventilation and difficult intubation should be identified. If there is a known difficult airway, awake intubation with fiberoptic bronchoscopy should be considered. If an asleep intubation is planned, a difficult airway cart, as well as alternate methods of intubation, such as video laryngoscopy, should be readily available. Transnasal humidified rapid insufflation ventilatory exchange (THRIVE) should be considered during intubation to help achieve apneic oxygenation and ventilation [4]. Communication with the surgical team is necessary in order to form a joint plan in case loss of an airway occurs, which may include tracheostomy by the surgical team.

Shared Airway

Airway surgery presents a unique circumstance in which the airway must be shared with the ENT team. Several strategies exist for ventilation, which will depend on the surgical procedure, airway anatomy, oxygen reserve of the patient, and access to specialized endotracheal tubes (ETTs) (see Table 22.2). A popular technique used when visualization or access of the surgical field requires the patient not to be intubated is to combine TIVA with jet ventilation. If intubation is warranted, an intermittent apnea technique with a small ETT (5.0 mm internal diameter (ID) or smaller) is often utilized. This technique involves frequent removal and replacement of the ETT throughout the surgery. Although volatile agents are used in this scenario, an adjunct infusion is often added to ensure adequate depth of anesthesia when the ETT is removed. Remifentanil is an especially good choice as an adjunct infusion because it can prevent tachycardia and hypertension from sympathetic stimulation caused by the suspension laryngoscope, as well as blunt tracheal reflexes [4].

Table 22.2 Specialized endotracheal tubes

	Standard ETT	Microlaryngoscopy tube (MLT)	Ring–Adair–Elwyn (RAE)	Armored (reinforced)	Parker Flex-Tip
Features	Single-lumen ETT made of PVC with left-facing bevel and Murphy eye	Small-diameter ETT (4–6 mm ID) with length suitable for adults	Preformed ETT with acute bend	Reinforced with metal coils	Flexible, curved, tapered tip with two Murphy eyes
Advantages		• Small diameter improves surgical visualization/access • Longer tube allows adequate depth	Directs ETT away from surgical field	• Minimizes kinking, even if severely angled • Less likely to be compressed by metal tools (e.g., rigid bronchoscope)	Lower risk of trauma during intubation – flexes and slides gently past protruding structures (e.g., arytenoids, nasal turbinates)
Useful for		Vocal cord surgery	Oral RAE: • T&A • Facial surgery Nasal RAE: • Oral and maxillofacial surgery	• Tracheostomy • Facial surgery • Rigid bronchoscopy • T&A	Fiberoptic intubation

ETT, endotracheal tube; PVC, polyvinyl chloride; ID, internal diameter; T&A, tonsillectomy and adenoidectomy. See reference [6].

Laser Surgery

Laser surgery allows precision, while minimizing postoperative edema and pain. Carbon dioxide (CO_2) lasers are the most commonly used. As the laser wavelength increases, tissue penetration decreases. For example, a CO_2 laser has a longer wavelength (10,600 nm), so it is better for superficial structures versus a Nd:YAG laser, which has a short wavelength (1064 nm) [2]. Precautions need to be taken during laser airway surgery. These include, but are not limited to: FiO_2 below 30%; avoidance of N_2O; utilization of specialized ETTs (see Table 22.3); preparing a backup ETT; having saline and wet towels on hand in case of fire; allowing adequate time for alcohol-based prep to dry; and protective equipment focusing on the safety of those in the room and those passing by in the hall [1].

Complications

Airway Fire

For an airway fire to occur, there must be a triad of:

1. Fuel (e.g., ETT, drapes, alcohol skin preps)
2. Oxidizer (oxygen, N_2O)
3. Ignition source (e.g., laser, cautery).

In the event of an airway fire:

1. Turn off all anesthetic gases, including oxygen, and detach the ETT from the anesthesia circuit.

Table 22.3 Laser-resistant endotracheal tubes

	Mallinckrodt Laser-Flex	Xomed Laser-Shield II	Sheridan Laser-Trach	Laser tubes
Features	Stainless steel corrugated spiral ETT with double cuff	Silicone rubber ETT wrapped in aluminum foil and Teflon	Red rubber ETT wrapped in copper foil, covered by absorbent fabric	Soft white rubber ETT wrapped in copper foil and absorbent sponge with double cuff designed as a cuff within a cuff
Compatible with	CO_2 or KTP lasers	CO_2 or KTP lasers	CO_2 or KTP lasers	All types of lasers (CO_2, Nd:YAG, argon, etc.)

2. Remove the ETT and pour saline into the airway to extinguish the fire.
3. Proceed with bag–mask ventilation with 100% oxygen.
4. Airway examination via rigid or fiberoptic bronchoscopy – examine the extent of the burns and look for foreign bodies, such as ETT fragments and other debris.
   a. Extensive burns may require reintubation and admission to the intensive care unit (ICU). Treatment with steroids and antibiotics should be considered.

Note: In patients with a known difficult airway, the risk of removing the ETT during the fire must be weighed against the risk of losing the airway. One method that can be used in this scenario is to use an airway exchange catheter to replace the ETT. In the event of a failed reintubation in this case, the exchange catheter would still allow ventilation, giving the anesthesiologist time to coordinate further methods of reintubation, such as fiberoptic bronchoscopy or a surgical airway [2].

Laryngospasm

Laryngospasm refers to forceful spasm of the laryngeal muscles due to stimulation of the superior laryngeal nerve (SLN). This can lead to complete occlusion of the vocal cords. This reflex can be triggered by secretions, blood, intubation, and extubation. It usually occurs if a patient is extubated during stage 2 of anesthesia, which is a transitional excitement phase that may include disconjugate gaze, breath-holding, or coughing. Infants and children are at increased risk, especially if there was a recent viral upper respiratory infection or second-hand smoke exposure. Desflurane use increases the risk of laryngospasm due to its pungency. IV or topical lidocaine can help prevent laryngospasm. It can present with high-pitched inspiratory stridor but may be silent if there is complete vocal cord occlusion. Initial treatment consists of bilateral jaw thrust (Larson's maneuver) with continuous positive airway pressure (CPAP) and 100% oxygen. If this is unsuccessful at breaking the laryngospasm, the patient should be deepened with anesthetics, such as with small doses of propofol. Succinylcholine (0.1–1 mg kg^{-1} IV or 4 mg kg^{-1} intramuscular) is a last resort [1].

Negative Pressure Pulmonary Edema

Negative pressure pulmonary edema (NPPE) is a rare consequence of upper airway obstruction, which typically occurs after extubation. It is a transudative edema caused by exaggerated negative inspiratory pressure against an obstructed airway. This exaggerated negative pressure leads to increased pulmonary venous pressure, which causes fluid to transudate into the lung. Muscular healthy patients are more susceptible because of their ability to generate a large negative inspiratory pressure. The most common cause of

NPPE is laryngospasm. It presents with hypoxemia, tachypnea, tachycardia, and respiratory distress, which usually occurs approximately 90 minutes after the airway obstruction is relieved. Bilateral pulmonary edema may be seen on CXR. Supportive treatment includes supplemental oxygen and diuretics. If hypoxemia and respiratory distress are severe, positive pressure ventilation may also be necessary [1].

Surgeries

Tonsillectomy and Adenoidectomy

Tonsillectomy and adenoidectomy is a common procedure in children. Indications include chronic infection, obstructive sleep apnea (OSA), cancer, and peritonsillar abscess. This procedure requires intubation. The surgeon will place a metal mouth gag during the case. Use of an armored ETT, which has reinforced metal coils that make it less likely to be obstructed by the mouth gag, should be considered. Patients may have an increased risk of a difficult airway due to enlarged tonsils or redundant pharyngeal tissue. Increased bleeding risk may occur due to hypertrophied adenotonsillar tissue; thus, extra care should be taken during laryngoscopy. Standard IV induction with propofol and fentanyl and maintenance with volatile anesthetic are usually done. If the patient has OSA, less narcotics may be used due to increased sensitivity [4].

Bronchoscopy

Bronchoscopy involves using a camera to examine the trachea and bronchi. Rigid bronchoscopy has the advantage of allowing forceps to be used to obtain biopsies or to remove a foreign body. Flexible bronchoscopy with a fiberoptic bronchoscope is more commonly used; it allows suction and irrigation. Muscle relaxation is important because it prevents bucking or straining while the bronchoscope is in the trachea or bronchi. Topical lidocaine can help blunt hemodynamic responses to airway stimulation by the bronchoscope. Glycopyrrolate may be considered to help reduce secretions that may obstruct the provider's view.

For rigid bronchoscopy, patients can be intubated, although this is commonly done with jet ventilation. If planning on intubation, an armored ETT should be considered because it can help prevent compression of the ETT by the rigid bronchoscope. For flexible bronchoscopy, a large ETT (7.5–8 mm ID) is needed to allow space for the bronchoscope to fit into the ETT. Alternatively, an endoscopy mask, such as the Patil–Syracuse mask, may be used to avoid intubation. This mask has a special port that allows a fiberoptic bronchoscope to be inserted while bag–mask ventilation occurs [4].

Direct Laryngoscopy

Laryngoscopy involves using a camera to examine the pharynx, hypopharynx, and larynx. Microlaryngoscopy is used to remove lesions such as papillomas, polyps, and tumors. General anesthesia with intubation and muscle relaxation is usually required due to the high degree of stimulation caused by the suspension laryngoscope, and also to prevent movement of the vocal cords. Propofol is a good induction agent. Fentanyl is not necessary since there is minimal postoperative pain. A microlaryngeal tube (MLT), which has a small diameter (4–6 mm ID), but of adult length, may be helpful in improving surgical visualization and access. Jet ventilation can be used to avoid intubation, which is especially helpful for posterior vocal cord lesions. Jet ventilation may be less favorable for laser resection of papillomas due to the risk of viral spread to personnel of the operating room (OR). An intermittent apnea technique, in which the ETT is removed and replaced several times during the surgery, can also be used but can be distracting and time-consuming.

Microlaryngoscopy for procedures such as papilloma removal may also include laser therapy. As discussed above, precautions for laser surgery and prevention of airway fires should be maintained.

TIVA with propofol (± remifentanil) is often utilized, although volatile agents can also be used. Sympathetic stimulation from the laryngoscope can be blunted with remifentanil and esmolol. Full muscle relaxation is usually required to prevent vocal cord movement. Towards the end of the surgery, this can be accomplished by deepening the anesthesia, rather than giving additional neuromuscular blockers. Laryngoscopy increases the risk of postoperative airway edema, which can be prevented with high doses of dexamethasone (4–8 mg) [4].

Ear Surgery

Common ear surgeries include myringotomy, tympanomastoidectomy, and cochlear implantation.

Myringotomy is a procedure in which an incision is made through the tympanic membrane to help control recurrent ear infections. Ear tubes are usually placed at the same time to allow drainage of the middle ear. This is a very short procedure, which is usually done under general anesthesia with mask ventilation. In children, it may more often be accompanied with tonsillectomy or adenotonsillectomy, in which intubation is usually required.

Tympanomastoidectomy is a combination procedure that includes mastoidectomy and tympanoplasty. The mastoid bone is located behind the ear. Removal of the mastoid bone is indicated for mastoiditis, as well as for cholesteatoma, which is a keratinized epithelial cyst. Tympanoplasty is done to fix structural changes that were caused by chronic infection or cholesteatoma. This surgery is usually performed under general endotracheal anesthesia.

Cochlear implantation is indicated for severe sensorineural hearing loss. The procedure includes a mastoidectomy, which is used as an access point to the inner ear.

Most ear surgeries require the surgeon to use a microscope; thus, the OR table is usually turned 180°. With the exception of myringotomy, muscle relaxation is very important to prevent trauma to the ear. N_2O should be avoided because it can increase middle ear pressure. PONV is common with ear surgery, and should be preempted with dexamethasone and ondansetron [4].

Laryngectomy/Neck Dissection

Laryngeal squamous cell carcinoma can be treated via radiation, chemoradiation, or partial/total laryngectomy. Along with removal of laryngeal tissue, a tracheostomy is also performed. Neck dissection may be included if there are cervical metastases. Free flap placement may also be done. Partial laryngectomy patients will require a temporary tracheostomy with a cuffed tracheostomy tube. Total laryngectomy patients usually do not require a tracheostomy tube or an ETT.

Laryngeal tumors and former radiation therapy may distort the airway. Cervical metastases and radiation fibrosis can also limit head and neck mobility. A difficult airway should be anticipated and discussed with the surgical team. Preoperative endoscopic airway examination findings should be reviewed. Awake fiberoptic intubation may be a good option, although standard induction is possible if airway compromise is minimal. THRIVE should be considered during intubation. If there is severe stridor and a high likelihood of failed intubation, an awake tracheostomy can be performed at the beginning of the procedure.

If a neck dissection is included, muscle relaxation should be held until nerves are identified, to facilitate intraoperative nerve monitoring. Moderate hypotension is favorable during the procedure to prevent bleeding. Dissection near the carotid sinus may cause bradycardia and hypotension, which should resolve with cessation of stimulation. Atropine or lidocaine infiltration by the surgeon can be given if this effect is sustained [4].

Obstructive Sleep Apnea Surgery

The purpose of OSA surgery is to relieve upper airway obstruction during sleep. Examples of OSA surgery include uvulopalatopharyngoplasty (UPPP), laser midline glossectomy (LMG), and maxillomandibular osteotomy (MMO).

In UPPP, the tonsils and part of the soft palate are removed, including the uvula. Asleep intubation can be done, but patients with OSA are at increased risk of desaturation. Adequate preoxygenation in a semi-upright position with CPAP helps prolong apnea time. TIVA with propofol and remifentanil is beneficial in preventing hemodynamic instability during stimulating parts of the procedure. Opioids and benzodiazepines should be minimized due to increased sensitivity, and multimodal analgesia with nonnarcotic pain medications and local anesthesia should be employed. To prevent desaturation on extubation, full reversal of neuromuscular blockade should be demonstrated and the patient should be extubated in a semi-upright position. Patients who use CPAP at home should be extubated to CPAP [4].

Surgical Airways – Cricothyrotomy and Tracheostomy

Cricothyrotomy

Cricothyrotomy is usually performed in emergency situations in which intubation is difficult or impossible. An incision is made in the cricothyroid membrane, in which a small ETT or tracheostomy tube can be inserted. This is usually done as a temporizing measure, until a tracheostomy can be performed.

Tracheostomy

Indications for tracheostomy include upper airway obstruction, major head and neck surgery, and the need for prolonged mechanical ventilation. An incision is made in the trachea, with the formation of a tracheal flap inferior to this point.

The induction plan for tracheostomy depends on its indication. ICU patients on prolonged mechanical ventilation will simply need to be switched from IV to inhalational agents and connected to the anesthesia machine. If the patient is not intubated, a plan should be in place in anticipation of a difficult airway. Full muscle relaxation is required during the procedure. 100% FiO_2 should be given until the tracheostomy tube is inserted. ICU patients may also require a higher level of positive end-expiratory pressure [4].

References

1. Pardo MC, Miller RD. *Basics of Anesthesia*, 7th ed. Philadelphia, PA: Saunders/Elsevier; 2017.

2. Miller RD. *Miller's Anesthesia*, 8th ed. Philadelphia, PA: Elsevier/Saunders; 2015.

3. Drayna PC, Estrada C, Wang W, *et al*. Ketamine sedation is not associated with clinically meaningful elevation of intraocular pressure. *Am J Emerg Med*. 2012;30:1215–18.

4. Jaffe RA. *Anesthesiologist's Manual of Surgical Procedures*, 6th ed. Philadelphia, PA: Lippincott Williams & Wilkins; 2019.

5. Butterworth IV JF, Mackey DC, Wasnick. JD. *Morgan & Mikhail's Clinical Anesthesiology*, 6th ed. New York, NY: McGraw-Hill; 2018.

6. Hagber CA, Artime CA, Aziz MF. *Benumof and Hagberg's Airway Management*. Philadelphia, PA: Elsevier; 2018.

Chapter 23

Orthopedic Anesthesia

Adrienne Mejia, Paul C. DeMarco,
Erik Helander, and Jinlei Li

Upper Extremity

Shoulder and Proximal Upper Extremity Procedures

Shoulder surgery can be accomplished arthroscopically or open, and is usually performed in either a lateral decubitus (LDP) or beach-chair (BCP) position. The LDP involves placing the patient on their side on a padded table on top of a bean bag to support the pelvis and lower torso. For the BCP, the patient is placed on a table with a headrest and the bed is positioned in Trendelenburg, with the feet elevated to 15 degrees and the knees flexed to 30 degrees. Some potential advantages of the BCP over the LDP include shorter surgical times, less difficult conversion to an open procedure, and a lower incidence of neuropathies. The BCP can present a unique challenge for the anesthesia provider in accessing the airway and has been associated with rare, but catastrophic, neurologic complications, including transient visual loss, spinal cord ischemia, and strokes. These complications have been suggested to be from the gravitational effects of the sitting position and the blunting of cerebral autoregulation under general anesthesia (GA). There is some evidence that patients in the BCP have diminished cerebral autoregulation and lower regional cerebral oxygenation when compared to the LDP. This, however, does not relate to cognitive outcomes. It is still considered prudent to take into consideration the difference in where the blood pressure is measured (brachial or popliteal artery) in relation to the external auditory meatus. If not, significant cerebral hypotension may occur. From where the blood pressure is measured, there is a decrease of 0.77 mmHg in arterial blood pressure for every 1-cm elevation [1].

Traditionally, most shoulder surgeries are performed under GA, but can be performed using regional anesthesia as the primary anesthetic. Pain, especially dynamic pain, can be a significant factor after shoulder surgery impeding discharge and recovery, and is often managed using multimodal analgesia, including nerve blocks. Enhanced Recovery After Surgery (ERAS) protocols are becoming commonplace for total shoulder arthroplasties. Regional anesthesia utilized for shoulder surgeries includes cervical paravertebral, interscalene, supraclavicular, infraclavicular, superficial cervical plexus, suprascapular, axillary, and potentially erector spinae plane blocks. Interscalene blocks (ISBs) are the most effective and widely used, and are currently the gold standard. ISBs have 100% involvement of the ipsilateral phrenic nerve, so they may not be suitable for patients with underlying respiratory disease. The type and combination of regional anesthesia used for shoulder surgery should be based upon the type of surgery and patient comorbidities.

Interscalene brachial plexus block as a single-injection or continuous block is frequently used for perioperative analgesia in a variety of procedures, such as arthroplasty, Latarjet, proximal humerus osteosynthesis, acromioclavicular resection, shoulder luxation, clavicle osteosynthesis, rotator cuff repair, arthrolysis, acromioplasty, and Bankart's repair, as well as various arthroscopic shoulder procedures. When combined with cervical plexus block, the ISB can be used to provide complete surgical anesthesia for the shoulder/proximal humerus and clavicle. Furthermore, to provide surgical analgesia for the entire shoulder for certain procedures with significant axilla involvement such as biceps tenodesis, the intercostobrachial nerve can be separately targeted, as discussed in "Distal Upper Extremity Procedures" (see Table 23.1). The phrenic nerve is almost always blocked during the ISB. The ISB is associated with hemidiaphragmatic paralysis (HDP). Alternative diaphragm-sparing nerve blocks include the suprascapular nerve block (SSB) and axillary nerve block [2].

Distal Upper Extremity Procedures

Minor soft tissue operations of the hand, such as carpal tunnel release, can be done with local infiltration or intravenous (IV) regional anesthesia (or Bier block). However, for operations lasting >1hour, such as invasive procedures involving bones or joints, the brachial plexus block is the preferred regional anesthesia technique. The supraclavicular approach to the brachial plexus block (SCB) is commonly used for arm surgery at, or distal to, the elbow, including forearm and hand surgery. The SCB provides blockade to the musculocutaneous, radial, ulnar, and median nerves but fails to block the medial aspect of the upper arm supplied by the intercostobrachial nerve, which should be blocked separately. Special consideration also needs to be taken for the risk of phrenic nerve palsy, Horner syndrome, and recurrent laryngeal nerve palsy with the SCB. The infraclavicular and axillary approaches to the brachial plexus block share similar indications to the SCB, and target the cord and terminal peripheral nerves of the brachial plexus, respectively. The musculocutaneous nerve is often missed during the axillary block, as the nerve branches off the plexus prior to branching of the radial, ulnar, and median nerves. Under ultrasound guidance, the musculocutaneous

Table 23.1 Brachial plexus blocks for the upper extremity

Type	Major indications	Alternative indications	Anatomy and sonoanatomy	Choice of ultrasound transducer	Considerations
Interscalene brachial plexus block	Upper arm surgeries: shoulder, proximal humerus, lateral two-thirds of the clavicle	Has been used in surgery of the arm or forearm; may have ulnar nerve-sparing effects	Around the superior and middle trunks of the brachial plexus. Roots C5–7 are most densely blocked	Linear probe positioned transverse on the neck, 3–4 cm superior to the clavicle, over the external jugular vein	Phrenic nerve blockade, respiratory function compromise in patients with pulmonary pathologies
Supraclavicular brachial plexus block	Arm surgical sites, including elbow, forearm, wrist, and hand	Can be used in combination with other blocks for shoulder surgery when ISB is contraindicated	Injection of local anesthetic surrounding the divisions of the brachial plexus within the brachial plexus sheath, lateral and posterior to the subclavian artery	Linear probe transverse on the neck, superior to the clavicle, over the midpoint of the supraclavicular fossa	Risk of subclavian artery puncture and pneumothorax, especially in the absence of direct visualization via ultrasound. Risk of phrenic nerve palsy is lower than with ISB

Table 23.1 (cont.)

Type	Major indications	Alternative indications	Anatomy and sonoanatomy	Choice of ultrasound transducer	Considerations
Infraclavicular brachial plexus block	Surgical procedures at, or distal to, the elbow	Upper extremity surgery for patients who cannot tolerate impaired respiratory function	Local anesthetic spread around the axillary artery in a U-shaped pattern, cephalad, caudal, and posterior blocks all three cords	Curvilinear probe or high-frequency linear probe placed in parasagittal plane over the point 2 cm medial, and 2 cm caudal, to the coracoid process inferior to the clavicle. The medial, lateral, and posterior cords will appear as hyperechoic bundles caudal, cephalad, and posterior to the axillary artery, respectively	Pneumothorax is rare with infraclavicular block. The deepest location of all brachial plexus block approaches; in the event of bleeding, it cannot be easily stopped by pressure
		Useful alternative approach for patients with an indwelling catheter in the subclavian region or with a transcutaneous pacemaker			

| Axillary brachial plexus block | Upper extremity procedures at, or distal to, the elbow | Can be used in conjunction with SSB for shoulder surgery | The axillary nerve traversing quadrangular space with the posterior circumflex artery and vein | Linear probe positioned posteriorly on the arm in a sagittal plane to the humeral head. The axillary artery and vein are visualized in cross-section | The musculocutaneous nerve needs to be blocked separately
Higher risk of local anesthetic systemic toxicity than with other approaches of brachial plexus block |

ISB, interscalene block; SCB, supraclavicular brachial plexus block; SS3, suprascapular nerve block.

nerve can be visualized laterally between the fascial planes of the biceps brachii and the coracobrachialis muscle, and can be traced distally with the probe turned longitudinally along the coracobrachialis muscle (see Table 23.1). Distal upper extremity surgeries can be performed under brachial plexus block with sedation as needed, or under GA with or without brachial plexus block.

Lower Extremity

Lower extremity surgeries can be performed under GA [3] with or without peripheral nerve blocks, or under neuraxial anesthesia, including spinal anesthesia for procedures of relatively short duration of a couple of hours, and epidural anesthesia or combined spinal and epidural anesthesia for procedures of relatively longer duration. Neuraxial anesthesia, when compared with general anesthesia, has been shown to be associated with less blood loss and transfusion requirement, decreased infection risk [3], less risk of deep vein thrombosis (DVT) and pulmonary embolism (PE), and decreased length of stay and postoperative cognitive decline. The lower extremity is innervated by the lumbar and sacral plexuses. The lumbar plexus is formed by the ventral rami of L1–4, with variable contribution from T12. Three major nerves that arise from the lumbar plexus are the femoral (L2–4), lateral femoral cutaneous (L1–3), and obturator (L2–4) nerves. The femoral nerve provides sensory innervation to the anterior thigh, and motor innervation to the flexor muscles of the hip and thigh. The adductor canal block is primarily a sensory nerve block involving the nerve to the vastus medialis, the saphenous nerve (the terminal sensory branch of the femoral nerve), and the articular branches of the obturator nerve; it has increasingly replaced the femoral nerve block for quadriceps-sparing effects. The sacral plexus arises from L4–5 and S1–4 (see Table 23.2). The sciatic nerve is a major nerve originating from the lumbosacral trunk and innervates the skin of the foot, as well as most of the lower leg (except for its medial side). Small branches of the sciatic nerve can be blocked in a motor-sparing block utilizing infiltration between the popliteal artery and the capsule of the knee. Infiltration Between Popliteal Artery and Capsule of Knee (iPACK), which has proven to be an effective analgesic in knee surgeries without adverse effects, such as lower extremity weakness or foot drop [4]. Perioperative pain control protocols for knee procedures typically include the adductor canal block and iPACK; protocols for foot and ankle procedures commonly include the popliteal sciatic nerve block and adductor canal block, and protocols for hip procedures can include the traditional femoral, infrainguinal fascia iliaca, lateral femoral cutaneous, obturator nerve, and emerging fascia plane blocks, such as suprainguinal fascia iliaca block, quadratus lumborum block, and erector spinae plane block, which are promising but need further study for definitive efficacy and safety [4].

Table 23.2 Peripheral nerve blocks for the lower extremity

Type	Major indications	Alternative indications	Anatomy and sonoanatomy	Choice of ultrasound transducer	Considerations
Femoral nerve block	Procedures involving the anterior aspect of the lower extremity, such as hip procedures including hip fracture		Lateral to the femoral artery, below the fascia lata and fascia iliaca	Located superficially around the inguinal grease; linear transducer	Profound quadriceps muscle weakness, need falls precaution
Adductor canal block	Lower leg surgeries, total procedures at or below the knee, such as knee arthroplasty, ACL repair, meniscal reconstruction, ankle and foot procedures	Alternative to femoral nerve block, can be combined with sciatic nerve block for complete analgesia below the knee for ankle surgery	Lateral aspect of the superficial femoral artery, into the plane to fill the adductor canal, anesthetizing the saphenous nerve and the nerve to the vastus medialis	Linear probe Midpoint of the patella and inguinal crease, on the medial aspect of the thigh over the sartorius muscle Alternatively, place the probe at the inguinal crease, scanning caudally until visualizing the	Produces comparable analgesia to femoral nerve block in lower extremity procedures at or below the knee, sparing most of the motor fibers to the quadriceps muscle

Table 23.2 (cont.)

Type	Major indications	Alternative indications	Anatomy and sonoanatomy	Choice of ultrasound transducer	Considerations
				femoral artery becomes the superficial femoral artery and the sartorius muscle is in the view	
Saphenous nerve block	Analgesia for knee surgery and used in conjunction with sciatic nerve block for complete coverage below the knee	Supplemental block to sciatic block for medial foot and ankle surgeries Supplemental block in multimodal approach to analgesia in total knee arthroplasty	Local anesthetic spread lateral to the femoral artery and deep to the sartorius muscle for the proximal approach, or more distal below the knee adjacent to the saphenous vein	Linear probe transverse on the anteromedial thigh, at the junction between the middle and distal third of the thigh, identify the junction between the sartorius, vastus medialis, and adductor muscles in cross-section just distal to the adductor canal	Lower falls risk in ambulation than with femoral nerve block; nonetheless, this can result in partial modal block of the vastus medialis due to block of the femoral nerve branch to the vastus medialis muscle

Sciatic nerve block	Hip, thigh, knee, lower leg, and foot surgeries	Analgesia for knee surgery involving the posterior compartment Popliteal approach provides coverage for foot, ankle, and Achilles tendon surgeries	Local anesthetic spread within the sciatic epineural sheath	Transducer positioning in: • Anterior approach – transverse on the proximal medial thigh • Transgluteal approach – transverse on the posterior buttock, between the ischial tuberosity and the greater trochanter • Subgluteal approach – transverse on the gluteal crease	The distal approach can be done below the level of the knee at the level of the tibial tuberosity	Anterior approach useful for patients who cannot be positioned in the lateral position due to pain, trauma, and the presence of external fixation hardware impacting positioning Sparing of the hamstring muscle enables lifting of the foot with knee flexion, facilitating earlier ambulation

Table 23.2 (cont.)

Type	Major indications	Alternative indications	Anatomy and sonoanatomy	Choice of ultrasound transducer	Considerations
				• Popliteal approach – transverse over the popliteal fossa	
Infiltration between the popliteal artery and the capsule of the knee (iPACK)	Analgesic coverage of the posterior aspect of the knee for knee surgeries, namely total knee arthroplasty, ACL repair, and knee arthroscopy	Often used in conjunction with anterior knee block such as femoral nerve block or adductor canal block, and neuraxial anesthesia (spinal/epidural)	Interspace between the popliteal artery and the femur towards the joint capsule	In the popliteal fossa, visualize the femoral condyle and popliteal artery; moving 1 cm cephalad, the space between the femur and the popliteal artery can be seen The popliteal artery should be kept in view for the entirety of the block	Spares significant sciatic motor block Targets terminal branches of the sciatic nerve only; aim is to reduce the risk of foot drop

Obturator nerve block	Knee surgery, ACL repair with gracilis tendon harvest for reconstruction, prevention of tourniquet pain in lower leg surgery, hip surgery	Often combined with femoral, lateral femoral cutaneous, and sciatic blocks	The anterior branch of the obturator nerve in the fascial plane between the adductor longus and brevis / Fascial plane between the adductor brevis and magnus for the posterior branch of the obturator nerve	Curved or linear probe, depending on the patient's body habitus / Transverse orientation on the inguinal crease over the femoral artery. After identifying the femoral artery, scan medially to visualize the adductor muscles: adductor brevis, longus, and magnus	Reduced risk of lower extremity weakness/falls risk
Lateral femoral cutaneous nerve block	Hip surgery, regional blocking for skin grafts/muscle biopsy of the proximal lateral thigh, supplemental block for ACL repair, tourniquet pain control	Commonly used as a component of multimodal regional block group. Provides improved analgesia when	Needle placement lateral to the medial trajectory through the subcutaneous tissue in plane: passing through the tensor fascia lata and sartorius	Place the probe inferior to the ASIS, parallel to the inguinal ligament. Identify the tensor fascia lata and sartorius muscle; in between these, the nerve will	Can be used as a diagnostic tool to differentiate between spinal radiculopathy and local lateral femoral cutaneous nerve entrapment

Table 23.2 (cont.)

Type	Major indications	Alternative indications	Anatomy and sonoanatomy	Choice of ultrasound transducer	Considerations
	when used in combination with femoral, sciatic, and obturator nerve blocks	incision is over the lateral thigh	muscle, spreading local anesthetic through the fascial plane	appear as a hyperechoic structure	

ACL, anterior cruciate ligament: ASIS, anterior superior iliac spine.

Chest

There are not many orthopedic surgeries involving the ribs, chest, or chest wall, but one of the most significant is repair of pectus excavatum or pectus carinatum. The same principles from this surgery can be carried over to other surgeries. Pectus excavatum and carinatum are repaired electively to improve body image and contour. There are some controversial data that point towards improvement in cardiopulmonary function after the repair and specifically no significant change in resting pulmonary function, but a larger change in maximal exercise tolerance. Pectus excavatum repair involves removal of 4–6 pairs of costal cartilage, depending on the age of the patient and severity of the defect, with possible sternal fixation. Pectus carinatum is a similar repair, but the approach and exact technique are more varied due to the rotational defect that accompanies the anterior–posterior displacement [5]. Newer minimally invasive techniques involve smaller incisions and little resection, but significant manipulation of the sternum and surrounding cartilage [5]. These surgeries last about 2–3 hours; patients are supine, and expected estimated blood loss is 100–150 mL. Patients usually head to the intensive care unit (ICU) postoperatively.

Typically, this surgery is performed in patients aged 5–10 years; occasionally, this is performed in teenage years, and very rarely for adult patients. In terms of preoperative evaluation, very little is needed for patients with mild deformities. However, patients with severe pectus can have restrictive lung disease and thus CXRs and pulmonary function tests (PFTs) are warranted. Similarly, severe pectus can displace the heart and compress it, leading to arrhythmias and right ventricular outflow tract obstruction. ECG and echocardiography are often necessary in this case. Routine laboratory tests are mainly needed based on the patient's other history. Young patients often benefit from premedication with short-acting benzodiazepines prior to surgery. For anesthesia, general endotracheal anesthesia (GETA) is indicated, along with standard IV or inhaled induction. However, it is necessary to avoid myocardial depressants and tachycardia if the patient has underlying cardiac issues. Standard inhaled anesthetic maintenance is used, along with emergence and extubation typically occurring in the operating room (OR). Blood loss is usually not very high during these cases, but at least one large-bore IV access should be maintained throughout the case. As with induction, standard monitors are used and an arterial line may be used if the patient has the above-listed cardiac issues. Pain management for these patients is best accomplished with an epidural catheter delivering epidural opioids with or without local anesthetics [4]. A similar plan can be used for other semi-related surgeries, such as rib fracture stabilization, flail chest stabilization, and chest wall resection (for tumor or infection). One-sided surgeries/injuries or minimally invasive pectus repair may be amenable to other pain management techniques, such as single-shot epidurals, paravertebral blocks/catheters, and rib blocks [5].

Pelvis

Orthopedic surgeries involving the pelvis can be roughly broken down into three categories: traumatic injuries, tumors/cancers, and congenital/ acquired instability. Pelvic fractures are commonly associated with major trauma, motor vehicle/motorcycle accidents, falls, and crush injuries. Patients who suffer these often require open reduction internal fixation (ORIF) of the pelvis or acetabulum. Given the amount of force required to cause these injuries, keep in mind that these patients often have multiple other injuries [6]. Repair of these injuries can take a while (1–6 hours) and involves large-volume blood loss of ≥1000 mL. During these operations, the patient may be in various positions – supine, lateral, or prone – and may need to be repositioned multiple times during surgery. Given these requirements, these patients will need to be intubated and paralyzed during the case. A related surgery is closed reduction and external fixation of the pelvis. Since the principle is to stabilize an unstable fracture so that the patient's other injuries can be addressed without worsening their condition, this surgery is much shorter than ORIF (1–1.5 hours). There is generally little blood loss from this surgery, but likely the patient has already suffered massive blood loss. Lastly, fractures of the acetabulum are similar to pelvic fractures because the acetabulum is part of the pelvis bony structure. However, ORIF of the acetabulum is unique because of the requirement of preserving hip function. From an anesthetic standpoint, the requirements are similar due to a similar variety of surgical approaches, similar surgical duration (2–5 hours), and similar range of estimated blood loss of 100–2000 mL.

Instability of the pelvis can be due to trauma but can also be caused by congenital or acquired mechanisms. Acetabular insufficiency or dysplasia is a cause of pelvic/hip instability and dysfunction. It results from trauma to the growth plate, neuromuscular disorders, or congenital hip dysplasia. This issue is generally addressed with osteotomy and bone graft augmentation of the pelvis. These patients are often kept supine during surgery but still require GETA and paralysis during the case. Surgical procedures such as these last about 3 hours and patients lose, on average, 500 mL of blood. Sacroiliac (SI) joint pathology is another cause of pelvic pain or instability. SI joint dysfunction is often preceded by trauma, but also may be due to septic arthritis of the SI joint. Surgical fixation of the SI joint is accomplished through anterior or posterior exposure of the joint, excision of the cartilage, and grafting/packing of cancellous bone (from the iliac crest) into the space that is created. The joint is then fixed with screws and possibly plates. This can be a shorter pelvis surgery, requiring about 2–3 hours, and these patients will sustain about 200–500 mL of blood loss.

Severe trauma, malignant tumors, and aggressive uncontrollable infections could necessitate one of two thankfully rare, but often lifesaving, operations: disarticulation of the hip or hindquarter amputation. Hip disarticulation is accomplished via amputation through the hip joint, detachment of all muscle groups crossing the hip, and isolation and ligation of multiple nerves and vessels (femoral nerve/artery/vein, obturator vessels, sciatic nerve, and other deep vessels). Hindquarter amputations are more proximal, involving excision of a portion of the pelvis and often ligation of either the common or external iliac vessels. In the end, a gluteal flap is brought forward to cover the defect and these surgeries usually require about 3–5 hours. Like many of the other pelvic surgeries, estimated blood loss ranges from 1000 to 3000 mL.

Pelvic surgeries can be either very large and highly involved cases in incredibly unstable patients or quite straightforward elective surgeries. Because of the range of cases and patients, there is a large range of anesthetic considerations. During preoperative evaluation, CXRs and other studies, if available, must be reviewed to look for respiratory or cardiac injuries and compromise. ECG and labs, such as cardiac enzymes, can evaluate for cardiac trauma that should be taken into consideration. X-rays and CT of the head, neck, and spine are important if trauma to these areas is known or suspected. Renal injury is common when there has been pelvic trauma; thus, urine analysis is important, along with blood urea nitrogen and creatinine levels. Other important labs include complete blood count and electrolyte panels. As always, good physical examination and history are important prior to any anesthesia. Premedication can be helpful, especially anxiolysis with midazolam for healthy/stable patients having elective or semi-urgent surgery. Other patients may require IV opioids, such as hydromorphone, if their pain is severe prior to surgery. Unstable patients, especially those with cardiovascular or respiratory compromise, should be carefully evaluated before being given opioids.

As mentioned earlier, patients undergoing a variety of pelvic surgeries will require GETA. Patients undergoing elective surgery may undergo standard IV or inhaled induction, but often trauma patients require a rapid sequence induction. Maintenance of anesthesia is often best accomplished with inhaled anesthetics and lung-protective ventilation. The vast majority of elective cases will be extubated at the end of the case awake, with their protective airway reflexes intact. Trauma and cancer cases may be treated in the same way; however, worsening of the patient's respiratory status or pulmonary conditions, such as aspiration, PE, fat embolism, or pulmonary contusions, may necessitate transporting these patients to the ICU, intubated and sedated for further monitoring. Due to the likelihood of significant blood loss during many of these cases, be prepared to deal with this by having large-bore peripheral IV access (14 or 16 G IVs, rapid infusion catheters). Use fluid warmers to infuse crystalloids and blood products as needed, including having 2–4 units of packed red blood cells available at the beginning of the case. Standard American Society of Anesthesiologists (ASA) monitors are always necessary, and to this should be added an arterial line, the ability to measure urine output, and possibly intraoperative echocardiography. Pain management can be accomplished with use of a multimodal approach, including acetaminophen, ketamine, and hydromorphone or other IV opioids. Epidural analgesia is another useful technique that can be added to the management of these patients. Epidurals can be placed in the mid-lumbar region, similar to labor epidurals, given the similar range of spinal nerve roots that need to be covered. The epidural infusion is often somewhat based on institutional norms and comfort. In general, a standard epidural infusion includes bupivacaine 0.0625–0.125%, with hydromorphone 6–10 μg mL^{-1} or fentanyl 2 μg mL^{-1} at a rate of 4–8 mL hr^{-1} [6, 7].

References

1. Johnson S, Rishi R, Andone A, *et al*. Determinants and functional significance of renal parenchymal volume in adults. *Clin J Am Soc Nephrol*. 2011;6(1):70–6.

2. Neuts A, Stessel B, Wouters PF, *et al*. Selective suprascapular and axillary nerve block versus interscalene plexus block for pain control after arthroscopic shoulder surgery: a noninferiority randomized parallel-controlled clinical trial. *Reg Anesth Pain Med*. 2018;43(7):738–44.

3. Zorrilla-Vaca A, Grant MC, Mathur V, Li J, Wu CL. The impact of neuraxial versus general anesthesia on the incidence of postoperative surgical site infections following knee or hip arthroplasty: a meta-analysis. *Reg Anesth Pain Med*. 2016;41(5):555–63.

4. Li J, Lam D, King H, Credaroli E, Harmon E, Vadivelu N. Novel regional anesthesia for outpatient surgery. *Curr Pain Headache Rep*. 2019;23(10):69.

5. Aydin G, Sahin AT, Gencay I, *et al*. Which is more effective for minimally invasive pectus repair: epidural or paravertebral block? *J Laparoendosc Adv Surg Tech A*. 2020;30(1):81–6.

6. van den Berg JC. Imaging and endovascular management of traumatic pelvic fractures with vascular injuries. *Vasa*. 2019;48(1):47–55.

7. Molnar R, Emery G, Choong PF. Anaesthesia for hemipelvectomy – a series of 49 cases. *Anaesth Intensive Care*. 2007;35(4):536–43.

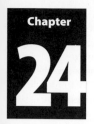

Obstetric and Gynecologic Anesthesia

Ankit Bhatia and Reine Zbeidy

Physiologic Changes of Pregnancy

The pregnant patient undergoes various physiologic changes which allow them to adapt to the stress of pregnancy, labor, and delivery. The physiologic changes of pregnancy are summarized in Table 24.1.

Neurologic System

Elevated progesterone levels in pregnancy cause a decrease in minimum alveolar concentration (MAC) by up to 40%. Pregnant patients are also more sensitive to neuraxial local anesthetics and require a lower dose compared to nonpregnant patients.

Cardiovascular System

Cardiac output increases in pregnancy secondary to an increase in stroke volume and heart rate. Cardiac output is highest immediately after delivery of the fetus due to autotransfusion of uteroplacental blood as the evacuated uterus contracts. A mild decrease in blood pressure typically accompanies pregnancy due to a decrease in systemic vascular resistance related to the vasodilatory effects of progesterone. Central venous pressure (CVP) and capillary wedge pressure do not change during pregnancy. After about 20 weeks of gestation, the parturient may also experience supine hypotension syndrome when lying flat due to the gravid uterus compressing the inferior vena cava (IVC) and decreasing venous return. Management involves placing the patient in left uterine displacement, which displaces the uterus off the IVC and increases venous return.

Airway and Respiratory System

Pregnancy is associated with an increased incidence of difficult airway and mask ventilation, compared to the general population. As pregnancy progresses, there is an increase in airway edema and capillary engorgement, leading to higher Mallampati scores. Increased friability of the oral mucosa

Table 24.1 Summary of physiologic changes of pregnancy

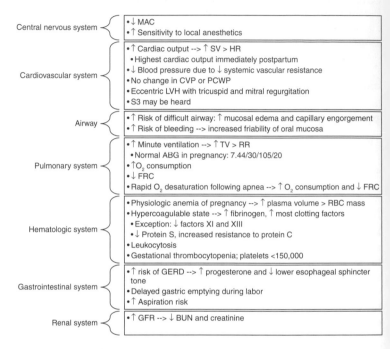

Central nervous system	• ↓ MAC • ↑ Sensitivity to local anesthetics
Cardiovascular system	• ↑ Cardiac output --> ↑ SV > HR • Highest cardiac output immediately postpartum • ↓ Blood pressure due to ↓ systemic vascular resistance • No change in CVP or PCWP • Eccentric LVH with tricuspid and mitral regurgitation • S3 may be heard
Airway	• ↑ Risk of difficult airway: ↑ mucosal edema and capillary engorgement • ↑ Risk of bleeding --> increased friability of oral mucosa
Pulmonary system	• ↑ Minute ventilation --> ↑ TV > RR • Normal ABG in pregnancy: 7.44/30/105/20 • ↑O_2 consumption • ↓ FRC • Rapid O_2 desaturation following apnea --> ↑ O_2 consumption and ↓ FRC
Hematologic system	• Physiologic anemia of pregnancy --> ↑ plasma volume > RBC mass • Hypercoagulable state --> ↑ fibrinogen, ↑ most clotting factors • Exception: ↓ factors XI and XIII • ↓ Protein S, increased resistance to protein C • Leukocytosis • Gestational thrombocytopenia; platelets <150,000
Gastrointestinal system	• ↑ risk of GERD --> ↑ progesterone and ↓ lower esophageal sphincter tone • Delayed gastric emptying during labor • ↑ Aspiration risk
Renal system	• ↑ GFR --> ↓ BUN and creatinine

MAC, minimum alveolar concentration; SV, stroke volume; HR, heart rate; CVP, central venous pressure; PCWP, pulmonary capillary wedge pressure; LVH, left ventricular hypertrophy; TV, tidal volume; RR, respiratory rate; ABG, arterial blood gas; FRC, functional residual capacity; RBC, red blood cell; GERD, gastroesophageal reflux disease; GFR, glomerular filtration rate; BUN, blood urea nitrogen.

predisposes these patients to an increased risk of bleeding from airway manipulation. Pregnant patients also have decreased functional residual capacity and increased oxygen consumption, making them more prone to rapid desaturation after preoxygenation. Minute ventilation is increased primarily due to an increase in tidal volume.

Hematologic System

In pregnancy, plasma volume increases disproportionately compared to red blood cell mass, resulting in physiologic anemia of pregnancy. Normal hemoglobin values during pregnancy are between 10.5 and 12 g dL^{-1}. Pregnancy is a hypercoagulable state, with increased production of all clotting factors, except factors XI and XIII. The anticoagulant factor protein S is decreased, and increased resistance to protein C develops. A significant increase in fibrinogen is also seen, with normal values in pregnancy of >400 g dL^{-1}. Thrombocytopenia also develops due to dilution, as well as increased consumption.

Gastrointestinal System

Increased progesterone during pregnancy reduces lower esophageal sphincter tone and slows gastric emptying and gastrointestinal (GI) motility, predisposing pregnant patients to increased reflux symptoms and higher aspiration risk. Pregnant patients also have an increase in gastric volume and acidity, with a volume of >25 mL and pH <2.5, respectively. All pregnant patients beyond the first trimester are considered to have a full stomach and be at increased risk of regurgitation and aspiration; thus, they should all receive a nonparticulate antacid to reduce the risk of pneumonitis, should aspiration occur.

Stages of Labor and Anatomy of Labor Pain

Labor is divided into three stages:

The first stage of labor commences with maternal perception of regular uterine contractions and ends with complete cervical dilation of approximately 10 cm, through which the fetus can be expelled. Pain during this stage is primarily visceral and is transmitted via afferent C fibers accompanying sympathetic nerve fibers to enter the spinal cord at T10–L1 spinal segments. Pain during this stage is caused by uterine contractions, accompanied by dilation of the cervix and stretching of the lower uterine segment.

The second stage of labor commences with complete cervical dilation and ends with delivery of the fetus. Pain during this stage is primarily somatic, caused by distension of the vaginal vault and perineum, and is transmitted via the pudendal nerve to the S2–S4 spinal segments.

The third stage of labor involves delivery of the placenta. Pain during this stage is also transmitted via sacral somatic fibers via the pudendal nerve (S2–S4).

Methods of Labor Analgesia

Pharmacologic

Systemic opioids can be used for labor analgesia. However, the risk of maternal sedation, respiratory depression, and loss of protective airway reflexes, and the proximity to the time of delivery warrant their judicious use. Maternal side effects of opioids include nausea/vomiting, pruritus, and decreased gastric motility. All opioids readily cross the placenta and can have effects on the neonate, including decreased fetal heart rate variability and dose-related neonatal respiratory depression after birth.

Fentanyl is a highly lipid-soluble synthetic opioid, commonly used for labor analgesia due to its short half-life and no active metabolites. Doses of 50–100 μg hr^{-1} can be used with no significant effect on neonatal Apgar scores and respiratory effort compared to mothers not receiving fentanyl.

Morphine is seldomly used for labor analgesia due to significant maternal sedation and accumulation of its active metabolite (morphine-6-glucuronide). Maternal side effects include histamine release causing pruritus and rash, and an increased risk of respiratory depression.

Remifentanil patient-controlled analgesia (PCA), although less efficacious than epidural analgesia, offers superior pain relief, with a decreased risk of neonatal side effects compared to other intravenous opioid analgesics. Metabolism depends on plasma and tissue esterases, and it is rapidly metabolized in both mother and fetus. The primary risk associated with use of remifentanil is respiratory depression, and thus careful oxygenation and ventilation monitoring are required throughout treatment.

Nitrous oxide can be used for labor analgesia and is typically administered via self-inhalation just before and during contractions in a 50:50 blended mixture with oxygen. Although inferior to epidural analgesia, it is a safe and effective method to provide labor analgesia without resultant hypoxia, unconsciousness, or loss of protective airway reflexes in the parturient who desires a less invasive approach or has contraindications to neuraxial techniques. Its use requires appropriate scavenging equipment in labor and delivery rooms to prevent occupational exposure.

Regional Techniques

Regional techniques provide excellent analgesia, with minimal depressant effects on the mother and fetus. Commonly employed regional techniques in obstetric anesthesia include central neuraxial blocks – spinal, epidural, combined spinal/epidural (CSE). Paracervical, pudendal, and lumbar sympathetic blocks are less commonly employed due to unfamiliarity with the technique and an increased risk of both maternal and fetal side effects. During the first stage of labor, visceral pain impulses from T10 to L1 must be blocked. In the second stage of labor, analgesia must be extended to also include somatic pain impulses from S2 to S4.

Neuraxial analgesia is the most reliable and effective method for reducing pain during labor, and is the only form of analgesia that provides complete analgesia for both stages of labor. Contraindications to neuraxial block include patient refusal or inability to cooperate, increased intracranial pressure secondary to mass lesion, uncorrected maternal hypovolemia or shock, infection at the site of needle insertion, and coagulopathy.

Lumbar Epidural Analgesia

Lumbar epidural analgesia is a safe, effective, and versatile technique that can be used to provide pain relief during labor and vaginal delivery, while also allowing flexibility to make the block denser, prolong its duration, and convert to epidural anesthesia if operative delivery is required. Epidural analgesia is typically initiated after an epidural catheter is inserted into the epidural space between the L2 and L5 intervertebral space. Analgesia is typically maintained with a continuous infusion of local anesthetic and opioid through the catheter. Addition of opioids, such as fentanyl or sufentanil, to the local anesthetic solution allows the administration of a more dilute local anesthetic to minimize side effects and complications from each drug. Long-acting amide local anesthetics, such as bupivacaine 0.25% or ropivacaine 0.1%, are typically administered as they provide excellent sensory analgesia while also minimizing motor blockade.

Spinal Analgesia

In spinal analgesia, a single injection in the subarachnoid or intrathecal space for labor analgesia is quick to perform and offers the advantage of a fast and reliable onset of neural blockade. However, because of its limited duration of action and unpredictable duration of labor, this technique may not be useful for most laboring women. A single-shot spinal injection is typically utilized for labor analgesia in a parturient who is unable to hold still, to facilitate placement of an epidural, and is usually reserved for when the duration of labor can be reasonably estimated, such as in multiparous women with advanced dilation or in the second stage of labor.

Continuous Spinal Analgesia

Continuous spinal analgesia with a spinal catheter can be utilized in the case of accidental dural puncture. However, the high incidence of postdural puncture headache (PDPH) precludes the elective placement of spinal catheters through epidural needles in most patients. When utilized, continuous spinal analgesia provides excellent analgesia and the ability to convert to surgical anesthesia in the event cesarean delivery is required.

Combined Spinal/Epidural

CSE has become an increasingly popular technique in obstetric anesthesia for labor analgesia. It combines the rapid, reliable onset of profound labor analgesia with minimal motor blockade from the spinal injection, with the flexibility and duration associated with a continuous epidural technique. The needle-through-needle technique is most commonly utilized, which involves identification of the epidural space, followed by insertion of a 25–27 G spinal needle into the intrathecal space. Upon confirmation of free-flowing cerebrospinal fluid (CSF), an opioid or a local anesthetic, or a combination of both, is administered. The spinal needle is removed, and a catheter is threaded into the epidural space for continuous analgesia.

Other Regional Techniques
Paracervical, Lumbar Sympathetic, and Pudendal Nerve Blocks

Lumbar sympathetic, paracervical, and pudendal nerve blocks can be used to block specific nerve plexuses for pain relief during labor. Unfavorable risk–benefit profiles of these blocks have limited their use when other options are available for labor analgesia.

Paracervical Block

Paracervical block can be used to provide analgesia for the first stage of labor. Bilateral paracervical blocks interrupt transmission of pain impulses from the uterus and cervix. Although effective for pain relief during the first stage of labor, its use has fallen out of favor due to its association with fetal bradycardia and maternal local anesthetic toxicity.

Lumbar Sympathetic Block

Lumbar sympathetic block can also be used to provide analgesia during the first stage of labor, as it interrupts painful transmission of cervical and uterine impulses. Its use has fallen out of favor due to difficulty in the block technique and the risk of intravascular injection.

Pudendal Block

The pudendal nerves are derived from the S2–S4 sacral nerve roots and supply the vaginal vault, perineum, rectum, and parts of the bladder. Pudendal nerves can be blocked using a transvaginal or transperitoneal approach to treat pain during the second stage of labor. High rates of block failure, local anesthetic toxicity, and ischiorectal or vaginal hematoma have caused this technique to fall out of favor.

Anesthesia for Cesarean Delivery

Cesarean delivery is the most common surgical procedure performed. Indications for cesarean delivery include nonreassuring fetal status, arrest of labor, malpresentation, cephalopelvic disproportion, prior cesarean delivery, and prior uterine surgery involving the corpus. The decision to use general anesthesia or neuraxial anesthesia for cesarean delivery is determined by various factors, including the condition of the mother and fetus, the urgency of delivery, maternal comorbidities, the presence of a previously placed epidural for labor analgesia, surgical considerations, and maternal preferences.

Neuraxial anesthetic techniques (spinal, epidural, CSE) are generally preferred in patients undergoing cesarean delivery, as they offer several advantages over general anesthesia, including: avoidance of airway manipulation; decreased risk of gastric aspiration; reduced neonatal exposure to maternal anesthetics; the mother allowed to remain awake during delivery; less operative blood loss; and improved postoperative pain.

Neuraxial Anesthesia

To perform cesarean delivery, blockade to the T4 dermatome level is required.

Spinal Anesthesia

Spinal anesthesia is the most common neuraxial technique used for cesarean delivery due to its simplicity, speed of onset, and reliability. Hyperbaric bupivacaine (10–15 mg) is most commonly used. Adding fentanyl 10–25 µg, or sufentanil 5–10 µg, to the intrathecal local anesthetic solution enhances the intensity of the spinal block and prolongs its duration without adversely affecting neonatal outcome. Addition of preservative-free morphine 0.1–0.3 mg can prolong postoperative analgesia to up to 24 hours but requires monitoring for delayed respiratory depression. Hypotension commonly accompanies initiation of spinal anesthesia and can be prevented or reduced by placing the patient in left uterine displacement, and giving intravenous (IV) fluid administration, IV boluses of ephedrine (5–10 mg) and/or phenylephrine (40 120 µg), and a phenylephrine infusion. Nausea and vomiting may also accompany initiation of spinal anesthesia and may be related to hypotension or increased vagal tone from the sympathectomy. Drawbacks to spinal anesthesia include limited duration of anesthesia and inability to titrate the extent of sensory blockade.

Epidural Anesthesia

Epidural anesthesia is associated with a slower onset of action and a larger drug requirement to achieve an adequate sensory block compared to spinal anesthesia. Lidocaine 2% (typically with 1:200,000 epinephrine) or chloroprocaine 3% are most commonly used. The addition of fentanyl 50–100 µg, or sufentanil 10–20 µg, greatly enhances analgesic intensity and prolongs its duration without adversely affecting neonatal outcome. Sodium bicarbonate (7.5% or 8.4% solution) can be added to the local anesthetic solution (1 mEq sodium bicarbonate/10 mL of lidocaine) to increase the concentration of the nonionized free base and produce faster onset and more rapid spread of epidural anesthesia. Advantage of epidural anesthesia over single-shot spinal anesthesia is the ability to titrate the level, density, and duration of anesthesia.

The degree of hypotension is also attenuated, compared to spinal anesthesia, due to a slower onset of sympathetic blockade, which may be beneficial to patients in whom hypotension is poorly tolerated.

Combined Spinal/Epidural

CSE combines the rapid, intense, and reliable block of spinal anesthesia with the flexibility of an epidural catheter, to allow supplementation of anesthesia and provide postoperative analgesia.

General Anesthesia for Cesarean Delivery

General anesthesia is typically indicated for emergency cases or when contraindications to neuraxial techniques exist. Indications for emergency cesarean section include massive bleeding, umbilical cord prolapse, and severe fetal distress. Advantages of general anesthesia include very rapid and reliable onset, controlled airway and ventilation, and potentially more hemodynamic control compared to neuraxial anesthesia. Its principal disadvantages are the risk of pulmonary aspiration, the potential for failed endotracheal intubation, and drug-induced fetal depression.

Pregnant patients are considered to have a full stomach and are at increased risk of aspiration of gastric contents. All parturients presenting for cesarean delivery should receive aspiration prophylaxis with a nonparticulate antacid 30–45 minutes prior to induction. Patients with additional risk factors for aspiration, such as obesity, history of gastroesophageal reflux disease, anticipated difficult airway, and emergent surgical delivery without an elective fasting period, should receive additional pharmacotherapy with ranitidine and/or metoclopramide to prevent aspiration pneumonitis. A rapid sequence induction and intubation with cricoid pressure are also standard due to increased risk of aspiration.

Patients presenting for cesarean delivery should be placed in the supine position with left uterine displacement. Pregnant patients are prone to rapid desaturation due to their decreased functional residual capacity, and should be adequately preoxygenated with 100% oxygen for 3–5 minutes. A rapid sequence induction and intubation with cricoid pressure is performed, with use of propofol 2 mg kg^{-1} and succinylcholine 1.5 mg kg^{-1}. Alternatively, ketamine 1–2 mg kg^{-1} can be used for induction in volume-depleted patients. Anesthesia is typically maintained with 1 MAC of volatile agent until the infant is delivered. Upon delivery, volatile concentration is reduced to 0.5% MAC and anesthesia is supplemented with up to 70% nitrous oxide and IV opioid to help ensure amnesia and prevent uterine relaxation. A benzodiazepine may also be administered to prevent recall and awareness. Prior to emergence, an oral gastric tube should be placed, and gastric contents aspirated to decrease the risk of pulmonary aspiration. Upon completion of surgery, complete reversal of neuromuscular blockade, with the patient fully awake and following commands, prior to extubation is required to reduce the risk of aspiration.

Complications of Neuraxial Anesthesia

Pruritus

Pruritus is the most common side effect of neuraxial opioid administration. Intrathecal opioid administration is associated with a higher incidence of pruritus, compared to epidural opioid administration. Pruritus is mediated through central μ-opioid receptors and is unrelated to histamine release. Pruritus is typically self-limiting and usually resolves within an hour following neuraxial opioid administration. For continued pruritus, preferred management consists of nalbuphine (partial agonist–antagonist), as it is less likely to reverse the analgesia produced by intrathecal or epidural opioids compared to the centrally acting μ-opioid antagonists naloxone and naltrexone.

Nausea and Vomiting

Nausea and vomiting are common during labor and delivery, and may be related to epidural and intrathecal opioid administration or neuraxial-induced hypotension.

Hypotension

Neuraxial-induced hypotension primarily occurs secondary to sympathetic blockade, leading to decreased peripheral vascular resistance and increased venous capacitance. The incidence of neuraxial-induced hypotension can be decreased by preventing aortocaval compression when in the supine position, administering 1V crystalloid solutions at the time of block placement, and vasopressor use with either phenylephrine or ephedrine.

Postdural Puncture Headache

PDPH develops after unintentional or intentional dural puncture, with resultant loss of CSF. PDPH is primarily located in the frontal or occipital region and is orthostatic in nature, with increase in severity in the sitting position and relief in the supine position. Associated symptoms may include neck pain/stiffness, cranial nerve palsies, tinnitus, and nausea/vomiting. The risk of developing PDPH is higher in patients who are young and thin, in those with a history of headaches, and when large-gauge cutting needles are used. The majority of cases of PDPH resolve spontaneously within 1 week but may persist longer. Management is typically conservative with hydration, analgesics, and oral caffeine. An epidural blood patch is curative and typically performed when conservative management fails, and involves autologous administration of blood into the epidural space to "patch" the dural hole with clot and prevent further CSF leakage. Typically, 15–20 mL of blood is given; however, the development of back or neck pain with injection may limit the volume of blood administered. Further workup is indicated when PDPH fails to respond to epidural blood patch or is associated with fever or other neurologic abnormalities.

Neuraxial Hematoma

Neuraxial hematoma is a rare event that can lead to compression of the spinal cord or cauda equina. Risk factors include traumatic or difficult epidural placement, coagulopathy, and anticoagulant use. It typically presents with motor weakness, with or without back pain, that persists or worsens despite discontinuation of local anesthesia. Imaging should be obtained upon suspicion and the neurosurgical team should be consulted for immediate decompression.

Neuraxial Infection

Neuraxial infection is a rare occurrence that may manifest as meningitis or abscess. Sterile preparation, draping, and use of a surgical mask during neuraxial block placement help prevent iatrogenic infection.

Total Spinal Anesthesia

A high or total spinal blockade may occur in several circumstances, such as unintentional and/or unrecognized intrathecal injection of local anesthetic, migration of an epidural catheter into the subarachnoid space, or an overdose of local anesthetic in the epidural space. Catheter aspiration and administration of an appropriate local anesthetic test dose with careful assessment of the patient's response may help attenuate the risk of unintentional subarachnoid injection. High or total spinal blockade presents with agitation, hypotension, bradycardia, dyspnea, loss of phonation, and loss of consciousness. Unconsciousness is due to brain and brainstem hypoperfusion. If total spinal blockade occurs, oxygenation, ventilation, and circulation must be supported. Immediate management consists of avoidance of aortocaval compression, administration of 100% oxygen, tracheal intubation, fluid resuscitation, and use of vasopressors to maintain blood pressure as needed.

Intravascular Injection of Local Anesthetic

The risk of systemic local anesthetic toxicity during epidural analgesia and anesthesia is minimized by performing intermittent aspiration for blood, slowly administering dilute solutions for labor pain and by fractionating the total dose administered for cesarean section into 5-mL increments.

Management of High-Risk Parturients

Hypertensive Disorders in Pregnancy

Hypertensive disorders in pregnancy are a common cause of maternal and neonatal morbidity and mortality worldwide. Hypertension during pregnancy can be classified into four categories:

- Chronic hypertension: preexisting hypertension or hypertension that develops prior to 20 weeks of gestation.
- Gestational hypertension: systolic blood pressure >140 mmHg and/or diastolic blood pressure >90 mmHg that develops after 20 weeks of gestation in the absence of significant proteinuria or severe features of preeclampsia.
- Preeclampsia: systolic blood pressure >140 mmHg and/or diastolic blood pressure >90 mmHg that develops after 20 weeks of gestation, accompanied by significant proteinuria (>300 mg day^{-1}) or evidence of organ dysfunction, which may include thrombocytopenia, impaired liver function, new-onset renal insufficiency (creatinine >1.1 mg dL^{-1}), pulmonary edema, and new-onset visual or cerebral disturbances. Its pathophysiology involves endothelial dysfunction leading to an increase in production of the vasoconstrictor thromboxane A2 and a decrease in production of the vasodilator prostaglandin I2 (prostacyclin), resulting in a primarily vasoconstricted state. Preeclampsia is associated with an increased risk of cerebral hemorrhage. Current guidelines recommend initiating treatment when systolic blood pressure is >160 mmHg to prevent intracerebral hemorrhage, while also minimizing fetal risk of decreased uteroplacental perfusion. Recommended antihypertensives include IV labetalol, hydralazine, and oral nifedipine.
- Preeclampsia with severe features: systolic blood pressure >160 mmHg or diastolic blood pressure >100 mmHg, with evidence of end-organ dysfunction, which may include proteinuria, renal dysfunction, pulmonary edema, new-onset visual or cerebral disturbance, thrombocytopenia, subcostal pain, liver dysfunction, and development of HELLP syndrome.

HELLP syndrome is preeclampsia associated with hemolysis, elevated liver enzymes, and low platelet count.

Eclampsia is preeclampsia complicated by seizures.

Anesthetic Management of the Preeclamptic Patient

In the absence of coagulopathy or HELLP syndrome, neuraxial techniques are preferred for labor analgesia and operative anesthesia, as they avoid the risk of pulmonary aspiration, difficult airway management, and increased bleeding associated with airway manipulation during general anesthesia. Benefits of neuraxial techniques include decreased release of catecholamines with improved blood pressure control and resultant improvement in uteroplacental perfusion as long as hypotension is avoided. Thrombocytopenia and/or coagulopathy must be ruled out, and hypovolemia corrected prior to performing any neuraxial procedure in a preeclamptic patient.

General anesthesia may be warranted when contraindications to neuraxial techniques exist. A rapid sequence induction and intubation with cricoid pressure are typically employed with use of propofol and succinylcholine.

Laryngoscopy and tracheal intubation in preeclamptic patients may lead to acute elevations in blood pressure that significantly increase the risk of cerebral hemorrhage and pulmonary edema. This risk may be attenuated with use of short-acting agents, such as esmolol, fentanyl, lidocaine, or nitroglycerin, to reduce the hypertensive response to laryngoscopy. Anesthesia is typically maintained with a combination of volatile agent, nitrous oxide, and neuromuscular blockade, as needed. Magnesium sulfate potentiates neuromuscular blockade, and lower doses of nondepolarizing agents may be required. In the event of uterine atony and postpartum hemorrhage, it is recommended to avoid ergot alkaloids, such as methylergonovine/methergine, as they may worsen hypertension.

Obstetric Hemorrhage

Obstetric hemorrhage is the leading cause of maternal mortality worldwide. Causes of obstetric hemorrhage can be placed into four categories: abnormal tone, abnormal placentation, abnormal coagulation, and trauma.

Antepartum Hemorrhage

Common causes of antepartum hemorrhage include placenta previa and abruptio placentae.

Placenta Previa

Placenta previa occurs when the placenta implants within the lower uterine segment, resulting in partial to complete occlusion of the cervical os. It typically presents as painless, bright red vaginal bleeding, and diagnosis is confirmed by ultrasound. Risk factors include previous cesarean delivery, prior uterine surgery or pregnancy termination, multiple gestation, advanced maternal age, and smoking. Expectant management occurs if the fetus is immature and maternal and fetal status is stable with minimal bleeding. Immediate cesarean delivery is indicated if the fetus is mature at onset of symptoms, hemorrhage is severe, or the fetal status is nonreassuring, regardless of gestational age. Adequate IV access and cross-matched blood should always be available due to potentially massive blood loss. If the mother is hemodynamically stable, neuraxial anesthesia may be performed for delivery.

Abruptio Placentae

Abruptio placentae is premature separation from the uterine wall after 20 weeks of gestation and before delivery. It typically presents as uterine tenderness and painful vaginal bleeding. Risk factors include smoking, cocaine abuse, trauma, preeclampsia, and advanced maternal age. Bleeding may be concealed or apparent, and range in severity from mild to severe. Emergent cesarean section is indicated for maternal or fetal distress. Anesthetic management involves ensuring adequate venous access and availability of blood product. General anesthesia is typically performed due to hypovolemia, risk of coagulopathy, and surgical urgency.

Postpartum Hemorrhage

Postpartum hemorrhage is defined as blood loss of >500 mL after vaginal delivery and of >1000 mL after cesarean delivery. Uterine atony is the most common cause of postpartum hemorrhage. Management of uterine atony involves bimanual uterine massage, use of uterotonic agents, discontinuation of drugs that impair uterine contraction, such as volatile anesthetics, and hysterectomy when atony is unresponsive to therapy.

Obesity

Obesity in pregnancy is associated with an increased risk of poor obstetric and neonatal outcomes. The risk of developing hypertensive disorders, diabetes, fetal macrosomia, shoulder dystocia, dysfunctional labor, and intrauterine fetal demise, as well as cesarean delivery, is increased in the obese patient population. The obese parturient also presents various challenges to the anesthesia provider. Decreased lung volumes, increased work of breathing and oxygen consumption, and redundant tissues make them prone to complications during induction and airway management. These patients have a high risk of difficult mask ventilation, endotracheal intubation, and aspiration of gastric contents. Neuraxial analgesia is generally preferred to decrease the risk of general anesthesia. However, neuraxial techniques can be challenging and may require the use of ultrasound to facilitate proper block placement.

Review Questions

1. Which of the following statement(s) is/are true about changes to the hematological system during pregnancy?

   (a) The increase in clotting activity is highest during the second trimester
   (b) All coagulation factors increase during pregnancy
   (c) Platelet count is often <150 × 10^9 L^{-1}
   (d) Fibrinolysis is reduced
   (e) Neuraxial hematomas are common in obstetric anesthesia

2. Which of the following statement(s) is/are true about pregnancy?

   (a) Gastrointestinal motility and stomach acidity are unchanged during labor
   (b) Resuscitation of pregnant patients should follow appropriate guidelines, which include left lateral tilt to avoid supine hypotension

(c) Pregnancy-induced changes in lung volumes cause desaturation to occur more rapidly than in nonpregnant patients during induction of general anesthesia

(d) The stomach is pushed up against the left hemidiaphragm by the gravid uterus in late pregnancy, which contributes to a risk of aspiration during induction of general anesthesia

(e) There is a reduced risk of difficult airway in pregnant patients who undergo general anesthesia for emergency surgery

Answers

1 (d) Plasminogen and antiplasmin concentrations rise during pregnancy but systemic fibrinolytic activity, is markedly depressed during pregnancy; the reduced fibrinolytic activity returns to non-pregnant values very soon after delivery. The loss of fibrinolytic activity is presumed to be due to the loss of the plasminogen activator.

2 (b) The enlarging uterus can produce increased afterload through compression of the aorta and decreased cardiac return through compression of the inferior vena cava, starting at ≈12 to 14 weeks of gestational age. As a result, the supine position, which is most favorable for resuscitation, can lead to hypotension.

2 (c) Functional residual capacity decreases by 10% to 25% during pregnancy as the uterus enlarges and elevates the diaphragm. Oxygen consumption increases because of the demands of the fetus and maternal metabolic processes, reaching a level 20% to 33% above baseline by the third trimester. The reduced functional residual capacity reservoir and increased consumption of oxygen are responsible for the rapid development of hypoxemia in response to hypoventilation or apnea in the pregnant woman.

Further Reading

Arent KW. The 2015 Gerard W. Ostheimer lecture: what's new in labor analgesia and cesarean delivery. *Anesth Analg.* 2016;122:1524.

Blumenfeld YJ, Reynolds-May MF, Altman RB, *et al.* Maternal–fetal and neonatal pharmacogenomics: a review of current literature. *J Perinatol.* 2010;30:571–9.

Shnol H, Paul N, Belfer I. Labor pain mechanisms. *Int Anesthesiol Clin* 2014; 52:1–17.

Wong CA, Scavone BM, Peaceman AM, *et al.* The risk of cesarean delivery with neuraxial analgesia given early versus late in labor. *N Engl J Med.* 2005;352:655.

Chapter 25

Pediatric Anesthesia

Elyse M. Cornett, Alan David Kaye, and Sonja A. Gennuso

Introduction

Pediatric anesthesiology is a distinct subspecialty of anesthesia. It focuses on the perioperative care of preterm and term neonates, infants, children, and teenagers. The pediatric population is vastly different from adults, as the clinician must recognize variations in anatomy, physiology, pharmacodynamics, and pharmacokinetics. For example, infants and children under 3 years old have a greater rate of morbidity and mortality associated with anesthesia than adults [1, 2]. The American Society of Anesthesiologists Closed Claims Project reports almost half of malpractice litigation involving pediatric injuries have been related to adverse respiratory events associated with improper oxygenation and/or ventilation. It is important for anesthesiologists caring for children to have a detailed knowledge of the distinctions between pediatric and adult patients. This chapter will discuss anatomic, physiologic, and pharmacologic distinctions, as well as infection prevention and anesthetic considerations, in the pediatric population.

Anatomy

Head and Neck

When compared to adults, neonates and infants have a comparatively big head and tongue, but a relatively small body, necessitating a particular neutral shoulder roll for anesthesia induction [3, 4]. The "sniffing position" is less advantageous for bag–mask ventilation or glottic visualization because of an infant's relatively large head. Neonates have a more cephalad and anterior larynx, situated at the C3–4 vertebrae, rather than at the C6 vertebral level in adults [2, 3]. The epiglottis is narrow, omega-shaped, and angled away from the axis of the trachea, thus obscuring the vocal cords [2]. Whereas an adult's larynx is cylindrical in nature, a child's larynx is funnel-shaped [5]. Additionally, the cricoid cartilage is the narrowest portion of the airway in children aged 5 years or younger; the glottis is the narrowest section of the airway in older children and adults [5]. The cricoid cartilage reaches adult proportions at the age of 10–12 years. Neonates are obligate nasal breathers until the age of 3–5 months. Prior to this age, the delicate nasal passages can be obstructed or compromised by secretions, nasal congestion, stenosis, canal atresia, endotracheal tubing, or even the tongue [6].

Physiology

Respiratory

Oxygen consumption in a full-term neonate is twice that of an adult. In preterm neonates, oxygen consumption is three times an adult's oxygen consumption. In comparison to adult patients, infants have the most resistance to airflow in small airways and the bronchi. The relatively smaller diameter of the neonatal airway and greater compliance of the trachea, bronchi, and chest wall provide less support to maintain negative intrathoracic pressure. Combined with low lung compliance (stiff lungs), increased chest wall compliance results in diminished functional residual capacity (FRC). Neonates and infants are more susceptible to hypoxia and respiratory failure because of a lower proportion of type 1 muscle fibers in the diaphragm and other respiratory muscles [2, 5]. Type 1 fibers allow prolonged, repetitive movement and the percentage of these muscle fibers increases with age. Therefore, preterm neonates have significantly fewer type 1 fibers, compared to even a 2-year-old child.

Loss of tone in pharyngeal and laryngeal structures is responsible for airway obstruction during sedation and anesthesia. This occurs in a dose-dependent fashion. The greater the depth of sedation, the greater the loss of airway muscle tone. Continuous positive airway pressure (CPAP), chin lift, and jaw thrust, as well as lateral positioning, improve airway patency and ventilation.

Cardiovascular

Newborns have a different cardiovascular physiology than older children and adults. Throughout growth, the cardiovascular system undergoes constant shifts in preload, afterload, contractility, loading, and flow patterns [7]. There are characteristic differences in cytoarchitecture, metabolism, and function between the immature neonatal myocardium and the adult myocardium. For example, the neonatal myocardium has poorly formed T tubules and fewer mitochondria and sarcoplasmic reticulum, and depends on extracellular calcium for contractility. Carbohydrates and lactate serve as its primary energy source. However, the neonatal myocardium is parasympathetic-dominant, and has limited cardiac output increase with increased preload, as well as decreased compliance. Therefore, contractility cannot be enhanced to improve stroke volume with increased fluid volume. As a result, blood pressure is increased by increasing the heart rate [8]. Anesthetic overdose can quickly result in bradycardia, which decreases cardiac activity. The neonatal heart is more vulnerable to unpredictable anesthetics and narcotics than the adult heart [2]; however, the neonatal myocardium can tolerate ischemia much better than the adult myocardium. Of note, cardiovascular events, such as bradycardia and asystole, frequently occur following inadequate oxygenation and ventilation. Thus, the origin of cardiovascular events seems to be secondary to respiratory complications.

Renal

Renal function is immature at birth and approaches adult values by the age of 2 years [9, 10]. At birth, the newborn is in a condition of hypofiltration, with 20% of an adult's glomerular filtration rate [11, 12]. Renal blood flow doubles in the first 2 weeks after birth and will reach adult values by the age of 2 years. As a result, the glomerular filtration rate parallels renal blood flow, and also doubles in the first 2 weeks following birth and increases until it reaches adult values, occurring at the age of between 1 and 2 years [2, 12].

Fluid and volume management is an important task by the anesthesiologist because the neonatal kidney cannot conserve or excrete water in the same manner compared to older children and adults. Neonates are less efficient at excreting potassium and tend to have a higher normal serum value of potassium than adults. Neonates are also limited in their ability to respond to an acid load and tend to maintain a slightly acidic pH (7.37) and decreased plasma bicarbonate concentration, compared to older children and adults.

Kidney function impairment throughout adolescence has an impact on opioid clearance, intake, delivery, and metabolism [10].

Hepatic

A major function of the liver is to transform lipid-soluble drugs into water-soluble metabolites that are excreted by the kidney. At birth, the liver is structurally and physiologically immature. Hepatic blood supply is decreased in neonates and gradually improves as heart activity increases [10]. Drug-metabolizing enzymes, delivery mechanisms, and protein-binding systems are also impaired [2, 10]. At birth, cytochrome P450 enzyme levels are 30% of adult levels [13]. Cytochrome P450 enzymes are responsible for drug biotransformation. In neonates, phase I behavior is decreased but eventually increases to adult levels by late puberty [14]. Due to physiologic immaturity of neonatal hepatic metabolism, medications administered to neonates remain metabolically active for extended amounts of time, raising their susceptibility to general anesthetics, barbiturates, and opioids [2]. Furthermore, impaired liver function raises the likelihood of hypoglycemia, hyperbilirubinemia, and coagulopathy [13].

Hematologic

Fetal hemoglobin (HbF) accounts for 70–90% of hemoglobin molecules in new-borns, but is replaced by adult hemoglobin (HbA) at the age of 3 months [13]. Thus, physiologic anemia is observed in preterm infants at 3–6 postnatal weeks and in term infants aged 8–12 weeks. HbF has a greater affinity for oxygen, which shifts the oxygen–hemoglobin dissociation curve to the left, thus shielding red blood cells from sickling [13]. Due to an inactive liver during the first few months of development, there is a deficiency of vitamin K-dependent clotting factors II, VII, IX, and X. As a result, preterm and term neonates have prolonged pro-thrombin time (PT) and activated partial thromboplastin time (aPTT).

Central Nervous System

Children are more vulnerable to head and spinal trauma than adults due to poor neck muscles and ligaments and a comparatively big head in comparison to body height [15]. Additionally, the neonate's spinal cord and dural sac stretch to the L3 and S4 vertebral levels, respectively. Since weak blood vessels and an abnormal cerebral autoregulation system predispose neonates born before 32 weeks' gestation to intraventricular hemorrhage, up to 20% of children born before 32 weeks' gestation suffer from interventricular hemor-rhage [16]. Neonatal blood–brain barriers are immature, which increases resistance to lipid-soluble medications, and immature myelination reduces the influence of local anesthetics on the central nervous system [13].

Glucose Regulation

The perinatal period is marked by improvements in endocrine activity, glu-cose homeostasis, and gluconeogenic enzyme levels [17]. Hypoglycemia is a serious, but common, complication in neonatal growth [18, 19]. Preterm infants have depleted liver glycogen reserves, premature gluconeogenic enzymes, and immature hormonal responses [19]. Children who are preterm and/or small-for-gestational age are more likely to experience hypoglycemia when fasting. This is particularly true for children under the age of 3 [18, 19]. Prolonged hypoglycemia has been linked to long-lasting neurologic complica-tions [17–20]. However, glucose supplementation is not likely for healthy infants undergoing surgical procedures. This is likely due to hormonal stress decreasing glucose uptake and anesthetic agents decreasing metabolic demands. Children who are critically ill do require blood glucose monitoring and possibly intraoperative glucose supplementation.

Thermoregulation

Increased heat flow in preterm and term infants and its surroundings is facili-tated by a large surface area-to-body volume ratio, narrow-diameter and pro-minent curvatures of body parts, low subcutaneous fat, and a thin and easily permeable epidermis [21, 22]. Related to their underdeveloped shivering processes, these patients depend heavily on nonshivering thermogenesis, a phase in which brown adipose tissue found in the spine, scapulae, kidneys, and adrenal glands is metabolically active [2, 22, 23]. It is important to maintain normal body temperature in children undergoing anesthetic agents. Lack of shivering in infants leads to their inability to recognize hypothermia [23]. Covering the child's head can significantly reduce temperature loss. Forced air warming units have been shown to help maintain normothermia. Other measures, such as warming the operating room and adding humidity to the ventilator circuit, assist in maintaining normal physiologic temperatures in neonates and children.

Pharmacokinetics

Absorption

Volatile anesthetics enter the body by inhalation through lung alveoli where they enter the capillary beds. Owing to their increased alveolar airflow and comparatively poor functional residual potential, neonates and young children absorb volatile anesthetics more rapidly [24, 25]. Drugs administered enterally in pediatric patients are usually absorbed more slowly than drugs administered in adults. This is because of narrower gastrointestinal tract, sluggish gastric emptying, immature secretion, and fewer protein transporters in children, as well as higher gastric pH in early childhood [26, 27].

Distribution

Factors affecting drug distribution include rate of blood flow, molecular size and solubility of the medication, and drug binding to plasma proteins and tissues. Pediatric patients usually have lower levels of plasma protein, lower body fat level, and a higher body water content, all of which affect the intensity of opioid delivery [27]. Reduced plasma protein levels result in an increase of free opioid molecules, while reduced body fat content results in an increase in drug level in the bloodstream due to lower volume for drug delivery [28]. On the other hand, higher amounts of overall body water increase the amount of drug delivery. The immature neonatal blood–brain barrier often affects opioid distribution, leading to heightened susceptibility to anesthetic agents in neonates [29].

Metabolism

While the liver is the primary site of anesthetic agent metabolism, other sites of drug metabolism include the kidney, bowel, lung, and skin [27]. The cytochrome P450 pathway is largely responsible for completing drug metabolism in the liver. These enzymes are found at the cellular level within the endoplasmic reticulum and mitochondrial membranes. Drugs may remain in their prodrug form, from which the biologically active form is synthesized, but most drugs are inactivated during metabolism. Neonates have slightly lower hepatic enzyme levels and blood supply, which results in medications being metabolically active over a more prolonged period than in adult patients.

Excretion

Drug metabolites are excreted from the body via water, saliva, or exhaled breath. The liver excretes metabolites into bile, which then travels through the gastrointestinal tract to the intestines before excretion in the feces. Certain metabolites are reabsorbed from the gastrointestinal tract and eventually excreted in the urine via the kidneys. Children's slower gastrointestinal activity lengthens the time required for metabolites to be reabsorbed from the intestines. The kidneys are not fully functioning before the 20th week of life, with decreased glomerular filtration rates, thus resulting in metabolites being excreted more slowly [29].

Infection Prevention

Hospital-acquired infections are a significant source of morbidity and mortality in the healthcare setting. Infections cost billions of dollars per year and lead to extended hospital stays and higher mortality [30–32]. Infection prevention and transmission should be a major goal in the organizational mission. Safety programs for both patients and healthcare workers should be implemented, with specifically designed accident prevention policies and procedures. Anesthesiologists are critical to the prevention of perioperative infections. Handwashing and decontamination are well-known means of infection prevention. Prophylactic antibiotics administered on time and temperature regulation in the operating room also decrease infection rates and are within the anesthesiologist's control [33–35].

Implementing best-practice bundles in pediatric intensive care units can decrease catheter-associated bloodstream infection rates, with maintenance bundles playing a critical role in infection reduction [36]. These bundles provide measures to maintain the highest possible seal, sterile and clean dressings, and skincare before catheter insertion. Central line insertion bundles are considered standard of care.

Another consideration for anesthesiologists is the risk of contamination of peripherally inserted central lines after airway modulation. The oral cavity contains over 500 bacteria species, including *Staphylococcus* and *Streptococcus* strains [37]. The anesthesiologist's mask breathing, oral airway positioning, and endotracheal tube placement all provide the potential for bacterial infection and dissemination to other locations; these are also more likely to occur concurrently with, or before obtaining, vascular access in pediatric anesthesia, in contrast to adult anesthesia where vascular access is usually obtained before induction with anesthetic agents [38].

Perioperative Anesthesia

Preoperative

Preoperative assessment is a mostly outpatient examination performed either by a nurse over the phone or through an online survey. However, the anesthesiologist anesthetizing the child should perform the preoperative assessment. Complete medical, surgical, and family history should be reviewed. Prior medical records and laboratory and imaging studies should also be reviewed in depth. Preoperative evaluation aims to obtain diagnostic evidence that might signal the need for further preoperative testing before the surgical day, build rapport between patient and physician, outline the anesthetic complications, and review the detailed anesthesia schedule, including any postoperative analgesia [39]. Proper preoperative treatment can improve patient outcomes and minimize morbidity and mortality. The anesthesiologist should assess prescriptions, allergies, and prior medical background. Prescriptions should also be checked and updated as required.

Medical history evaluation should include cardiopulmonary review, genetic abnormalities, obstructive sleep apnea syndrome, bronchopulmonary dysplasia, complicated airway, upper respiratory tract inflammation, asthma, epilepsy disorders, and sickle cell disease [40]. Additionally, particular care must be extended to children who have a history of psychological or behavioral disorders such as autism or depression [41]. Child life specialists are very helpful in preparing the child and family for anesthesia and surgery. Booklets, videotapes, and hospital tours can be used to assist in the preparation of the child and families.

It is also important to consider patients who have ongoing medical care. Chronic pain patients are typically advised to continue their analgesic regimens with nonsteroidal antiinflammatory drugs (NSAIDs) perioperatively to improve postoperative pain management [30, 42]. Withholding any psychiatric medication must be decided on an individual basis (cost–benefit analysis). Food allergies should also be addressed appropriately since they often correlate with anesthetic agent reactions (e.g., peanut allergies and propofol, seafood allergies and contrast dyes, vaccination allergies and topical thrombotic agents) [42].

Finally, perioperative settings may be frightening for children and their families, and this is particularly true for pediatric patients on the autism spectrum. As a result, anesthesiologists must invest time in developing a close rapport with patients and providers by establishing reasonable goals and adhering to perioperative timelines [40]. Physical examination should include the cardiovascular, respiratory, and neurologic systems. Any missing teeth or congenital defects should be noted [32]. Finally, the patient should be assessed for anxiety and preoperative medication, such as midazolam or dexmedetomidine, may be employed to ease the transition of the child away from familiar caregivers to the foreign operating room.

Intraoperative

Preparation for induction requires preparation of warming devices and any emergency medications (e.g., succinylcholine, atropine, albuterol, epinephrine). After emphasizing to the parent that this time may cause discomfort, they may be permitted to be present during induction. There are several pharmacologic agents eligible for pediatric sedation/anesthesia, which can be narrowly classified as inhaled anesthetics, intravenous anesthetics, antidepressants, and neuromuscular blocking agents. Inhalation mask induction is the standard of care in pediatric communities since needles and injections can traumatize children and have a detrimental effect on postoperative pain treatment [42]. Sevoflurane, isoflurane, desflurane, and halothane are all inhaled anesthetics that are often supplemented with 70% nitrous oxide, leading to a faster rate of induction [43]. In practice, sevoflurane is the preferred inhalational agent for pediatric anesthesia. It is the least pungent of all agents and facilitates quick induction of anesthesia. Intravenous induction is an alternative to inhalational induction. Patients who are at risk of cardiovascular dysfunction, already have an intravenous access, or have contraindications to inhaled anesthetics can be induced with intravenous agents. Ketamine, etomidate, and propofol are examples of intravenous agents. Case studies indicate that ketofol (a mixture of propofol and ketamine) has improved favorability for brief and unpleasant pediatric procedures [44, 45]. Notably, recent publications have shown an increased protection profile when sedation plans are limited to single-agent pharmacy, rather than using multidrug regimens. Anesthesia maintenance is typically accomplished with inhaled anesthetics but may also be accomplished with intravenous substances, such as propofol. Other requirements for pediatric maintenance include neuromuscular blocking agents, where necessary, opioids, and antiemetics [2].

Postoperative

The final stages in pediatric anesthesia include emergence and extubation, with proper postoperative care unit treatment/recovery. The aim of this time period is to ensure regulated and smooth emergence from anesthesia without oxygen desaturation, coughing, vomiting, laryngospasm, or bronchospasm.

Before extubating, it is typical to ensure spontaneous and regular breathing, with conjugate eye/pain grimacing to oropharyngeal suctioning [46]. Emergence delirium, a cluster of visual hallucinations and psychomotor agitation, is of particular concern in the immediate postoperative phase. Pediatric emergence delirium is estimated to occur in 10–80% of cases [47]. Recent clinical studies have validated a single dose of dexmedetomidine (1–2 μg kg^{-1}) as a highly successful means for reducing delirium emergence [48, 49].

Conclusion

Pediatric anesthesia is significantly different from adult anesthesia. These pertinent distinctions in anatomy, physiology, and pharmacology are important for anesthesiologists to consider. Additionally, anesthesia is a traumatic process for pediatric patients and their parents, and distress associated with anesthesia can raise stress hormone levels and impair postoperative wound healing. Medication complications are a significant problem when administering anesthesia to pediatric patients. As a result, it is important for anesthesiologists to follow evidence-based protocols to minimize errors. These procedures involve carefully reading legibly labeled syringes before administration, organizing drawers and workspaces in a systematic manner, doing two-person tests before administration of medications, and carefully measuring the patient's weight.

References

1. Tay CLM, Tan GM, Ng SBA. Critical incidents in pediatric anaesthesia: an audit of 10 000 anaesthetics in Singapore. *Pediatr Anesth.* 2001;11(6):711–18.

2. Kaye AD, Fox CJ, Padnos IW, *et al.* Pharmacologic considerations of anesthetic agents in pediatric patients: a comprehensive review. *Anesthesiol Clin.* 2017;35(2): e73–94.

3. Höhne C, Haack M, Machotta A, Kaisers U. [Atemwegsmanagement in der kinderanästhesie]. *Anaesthesist.* 2006;55:809–19.

4. Dalal PG, Murray D, Messner AH, Feng A, McAllister J, Molter D. Pediatric laryngeal dimensions: an age-based analysis. *Anesth Analg.* 2009;108(5):1475–9.

5. Butterworth JF, Mackey DC, Wasnick JD, eds. *Morgan & Mikhail's Clinical Anesthesiology*, 5th ed. New York, NY: McGraw Hill; 2013.

6. Trabalon M, Schaal B. It takes a mouth to eat and a nose to breathe: abnormal oral respiration affects neonates' oral competence and systemic adaptation. *Int J Pediatr.* 2012;2012:1–10.

7. Vrancken SL, van Heijst AF, de Boode WP. Neonatal hemodynamics: from developmental physiology to comprehensive monitoring. *Front Pediatr.* 2018;6:87.

8. Miller RD, Pardo MC, Jr, eds. *Basics of Anesthesia*, 6th ed. Philadelphia, PA: Elsevier; 2011.

9. Bueva A, Guignard J-P. Renal function in preterm neonates. *Pediatr Res.* 1994;36:572–7.

10. Rodieux F, Wilbaux M, van den Anker JN, Pfister M. Effect of kidney function on drug kinetics and dosing in neonates, infants, and children. *Clin Pharmacokinet.* 2015;54:1183–204.

11. Musso CG, Ghezzi L, Ferraris J. Renal physiology in newborns and old people: similar characteristics but different mechanisms. *Int Urol Nephrol.* 2004;36(2):273–5.

12. Sulemanji M, Vakili K. Neonatal renal physiology. *Semin Pediatr Surg.* 2013;22 (4):195–8.

13. Doherty TM, Salik I. Physiology, neonatal. In: *StatPearls.* Treasure Island, FL: StatPearls Publishing; 2022. Available from: www.ncbi.nlm.nih.gov/books/NB K539840/.

14. Hines RN. Developmental expression of drug metabolizing enzymes: impact on disposition in neonates and young children. *Int J Pharm.* 2013;452:3–7.

15. Figaji AA. Anatomical and physiological differences between children and adults relevant to traumatic brain injury and the implications for clinical assessment and care. *Front Neurol.* 2017;8:685.

16. Szpecht D, Szymankiewicz M, Nowak I, Gadzinowski J. Intraventricular hemorrhage in neonates born before 32 weeks of gestation – retrospective analysis of risk factors. *Childs Nerv Syst.* 2016;32(8):1399–404.

17. Beardsall K, Dunger D. The physiology and clinical management of glucose metabolism in the newborn. *Endocrine Rev.* 2007;12:124–37.

18. Zijlmans WCWR, van Kempen AAMW, Serlie MJ, Sauerwein HP. Glucose metabolism in children: influence of age, fasting, and infectious diseases. *Metabolism.* 2009;58:1356–65.

19. Bester K, Pretorius T. Intraoperative glucose management in children < 1 year or < 10 kg: an observational study. *South Afr J Anaesth Analg.* 2017;23(5):119–22.

20. Cowett RM, Loughead JL. Neonatal glucose metabolism: differential diagnoses, evaluation, and treatment of hypoglycemia. *Neonatal Netw.* 2002;21:9–19.

21. Tourneux P, Libert JP, Ghyselen L, *et al.* [Échanges thermiques et thermorégulation chez le nouveau-né]. *Arch Pediatr.* 2009;16:1057–62.

22. Soll RF. Heat loss prevention in neonates. *J Perinatol.* 2008;28:S57–9.

23. Kumar V, Shearer JC, Kumar A, Darmstadt GL. Neonatal hypothermia in low resource settings: a review. *J Perinatol.* 2009;29:401–12.

24. Stoelting RK, Hines RL, Marschall KE. *Stoelting's Anesthesia and Co-existing Disease.* Philadelphia, PA: Saunders/Elsevier; 2012.

25. Olsson GL. Inhalational anaesthesia at the extremes of age: paediatric anaesthesia. *Anaesthesia*. 1995;50(s10):34–6.

26. Edginton AM, Fotaki N. Oral drug absorption in pediatric populations. In: JB Dressman, C Reppas, eds. *Oral Drug Absorption: Prediction and Assessment*, 2nd ed. (Vol. 193) (Drugs and the Pharmaceutical Sciences). Informa Healthcare; 2010, pp. 108–26.

27. Lu H, Rosenbaum S. Developmental pharmacokinetics in pediatric populations. *J Pediatr Pharmacol Ther*. 2014;19:262–76.

28. Kaye AD, Fox CJ, Padnos IW, *et al.* Pharmacologic considerations of anesthetic agents in pediatric patients: a comprehensive review. *Anesthesiol Clin*. 2017;35(2):e73–94.

29. Pardo MC, Jr, Miller RD, eds. *Basics of Anesthesia*, 7th ed. Philadelphia, PA: Elsevier; 2018.

30. Brooks MR, Golianu B. Perioperative management in children with chronic pain. *Pediatr Anesth*. 2016;26(8):794–806.

31. Coté CJ, Lerman J, Anderson BJ. The practice of pediatric anesthesia. In: CJ Coté, J Lerman, BJ Anderson, eds. *A Practice of Anesthesia for Infants and Children*, 6th ed. Philadelphia, PA: Elsevier; 2019, pp. 1–7.

32. Macfarlane F. Paediatric anatomy and physiology and the basics of paediatric anaesthesia. 2005. Available from: https://resources.wfsahq.org/atotw/paediatric-anatomy-and-physiology-and-the-basics-of-paediatric-anaesthesia/.

33. Bratzler DW, Dellinger EP, Olsen KM, *et al.* Clinical practice guidelines for anti-microbial prophylaxis in surgery. *Am J Health Syst Pharm*. 2013;70(3):195–283.

34. Sessler DI. Perioperative thermoregulation and heat balance. *Lancet*. 2016;387:2655–64.

35. Morse J, Blackburn L, Hannam JA, Voss L, Anderson BJ. Compliance with perio-perative prophylaxis guidelines and the use of novel outcome measures. *Pediatr Anesth*. 2018;28(8):686–93.

36. Miller MR, Griswold M, Harris JM, *et al.* Decreasing PICU catheter-associated bloodstream infections: NACHRI's quality transformation efforts. *Pediatrics*. 2010;125:206–13.

37. Samaranayake L, Matsubara VH. Normal oral flora and the oral ecosystem. *Dent Clin North Am*. 2017;61(2):199–215.

38. Martin LD, Kallile M, Kanmanthreddy S, Zerr DM. Infection prevention in pedi-atric anesthesia practice. *Paediatr Anaesth*. 2017;27:1077–83.

39. Tobias JD. Preoperative anesthesia evaluation. *Semin Pediatr Surg*. 2018;27 (2):67–74.

40. Ghazal EA, Vadi MG, Mason LJ, Coté CJ. Preoperative evaluation, premedication, and induction of anesthesia. In: CJ Coté, J Lerman, BJ Anderson, eds. *A Practice of*

Anesthesia for Infants and Children, 6th ed. Philadelphia, PA: Elsevier; 2019, pp. 35–68.

41. Swartz JS, Amos KE, Brindas M, Girling LG, Ruth Graham M. Benefits of an individualized perioperative plan for children with autism spectrum disorder. *Pediatr Anesth*. 2017;27(8):856–62.

42. Lerman J, Becke K. Perioperative considerations for airway management and drug dosing in obese children. *Curr Opin Anaesthesiol*. 2018;31(3):320–6.

43. Khurmi N, Patel P, Kraus M, Trentman T. Pharmacologic considerations for pediatric sedation and anesthesia outside the operating room: a review for anesthesia and non-anesthesia providers. *Paediatr Drugs*. 2017;19:435–46.

44. Jalili M, Bahreini M, Doosti-Irani A, Masoomi R, Arbab M, Mirfazaelian H. Ketamine-propofol combination (ketofol) vs propofol for procedural sedation and analgesia: systematic review and meta-analysis. *Am J Emerg Med*. 2016;34 (3):558–69.

45. Roback MG, Carlson DW, Babl FE, Kennedy RM. Update on pharmacological management of procedural sedation for children. *Curr Opin Anaesthesiol*. 2016;29: S21–35.

46. Lien C, Koff H, Malhotra V, Gadalla F. Emergence and extubation: a systematic approach. *Anesth Analg*. 1997;85(5):1177.

47. Moore AD, Anghelescu DL. Emergence delirium in pediatric anesthesia. *Paediatr Drugs*. 2017;19(1):11–20.

48. Whitman TM. Emergence delirium in children. *J Pediatr Surg Nurs*. 2018;7(2):41–6.

49. Di M, Han Y, Yang Z, *et al*. Tracheal extubation in deeply anesthetized pediatric patients after tonsillectomy: a comparison of high-concentration sevoflurane alone and low-concentration sevoflurane in combination with dexmedetomidine pre-medication. *BMC Anesthesiol*. 2017;17(1):28.

50. Cravero JP, Agarwal R, Berde C, *et al*. The Society for Pediatric Anesthesia recommendations for the use of opioids in children during the perioperative period. *Paediatr Anaesth*. 2019;29(6):547–71.

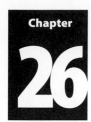

Chapter

26

Geriatric Anesthesia

Zhuo Sun and Anterpreet Dua

Introduction

The World Health Organization predicts that the number of people aged 60 years and over will grow to an estimated 1.2 billion by 2025 and to 2 billion by 2050. In parallel, the number of both elective and emergent surgeries on elderly people also will increase. It is of key importance that anesthesiologists understand the fundamental characteristics of physiology, anatomy, and pharmacology associated with aging, as well as have the ability to optimize care to improve outcomes in this population.

Age-Related Physiological Changes

Aging is associated with a decline in all organ functions, with an associated reduction in reserve capacity. This overall functional reduction puts the geriatric population at increased risk during anesthesia and surgery.

Nervous System

Normal aging is accompanied by decreased brain mass, reduced neuronal density, decreased cerebral blood flow proportional to neuronal loss, increased ventricular volume, and widening of sulci in the central nervous system. In the peripheral nervous system, there is a reduction in myelinated fibers, with potential alterations in pain perception. In addition, there is a decrease in the number of neuroreceptors and a reduction in neurotransmitter synthesis. The glial cells increase in number to compensate for the loss in neuronal mass. These functional changes correlate with an increased incidence of postoperative delirium and cognitive dysfunction and longer recovery from general anesthesia, as well as increased sensitivity to inhaled anesthetic agents and centrally acting anticholinergic drugs (see Table 26.1).

Cardiovascular System

Significant structural changes in the cardiovascular system among aging adults include left ventricular hypertrophy with decreased wall compliance, increased vascular rigidity, decreased compliance of vessels from gradual loss

Table 26.1 Physiologic changes in the nervous system and anesthetic implications

System	Structural changes	Functional changes	Anesthetic implications
Nervous	↓ Brain mass ↓ Neuronal density ↑ Ventricular volume ↓ Myelinated fibers	↓ Cerebral blood flow ↓ Cerebral metabolic rate ↓ Neuroreceptors ↓ Neurotransmitter synthesis ↑ BBB permeability	↑ Postoperative delirium ↑ POCD ↓ MAC (↓ 6% per decade) ↑ Sensitivity to anesthetic agents ↑ Recovery time from GA

BBB, blood brain barrier; POCD, postoperative cognitive dysfunction; MAC, minimum alveolar concentration; GA, general anesthesia.

of elastin, deposition of collagen, and calcification of valves and vasculature. Consequences of these changes include increased systolic pressure, increased mean arterial pressure, and decreased diastolic function.

Fatty infiltration of pacemaker cells, decreased conduction fiber density, and sinoatrial node cell number may increase the susceptibility to arrhythmias, such as sick sinus syndrome, atrial fibrillation, premature atrial contractions, and exaggerated bradycardia, after opioid administration in the elderly population.

Autonomic changes include increased sympathetic activity and decreased parasympathetic tone. Combined with increased vascular stiffness, this leads to greater lability in blood pressure. Decreased sensitivity of beta receptors results in limited ability to increase the heart rate pharmacologically, leading to dependence on preload and vascular tone. Decreased cardiac reserve may manifest as exaggerated hypotension upon induction of general anesthesia (see Table 26.2).

Pulmonary System

Overall, pulmonary reserve decreases with aging. Increased chest wall stiffness, decreased elasticity of the lung parenchyma, flattening of the diaphragm, and reduction of respiratory muscle strength are predictable changes during aging which may lead to diaphragmatic fatigue, a predisposition to respiratory failure during the postoperative period, and difficulty in weaning from mechanical ventilation.

Alveolar gas exchange is negatively impacted by decreased functional alveolar surface area, decreased diffusing capacity of carbon monoxide, ventilation–perfusion mismatch, and an increase in dead space. The elderly population has decreased expiratory reserve volume, vital capacity, functional vital

Table 26.2 Physiologic changes in the cardiovascular system and anesthetic implications

System	Structural changes	Functional changes	Anesthetic implications
Cardiovascular	↑ LV hypertrophy ↑ Vascular rigidity ↓ SA node cell number ↓ Conduction fiber density	↑ MAP ↑ LV filling pressure ↓ Contractility ↑ Diastolic dysfunction ↓ Vascular compliance ↓ Beta-adrenergic receptor response	↓ SV and CO ↑ SVR and SBP ↑ Labile BP ↑ Risk of arrhythmias ↑ CHF ↑ Autonomic dysfunction

LV, left ventriclular; SA, sinoatrial; MAP, mean arterial pressure; SV, stroke volume; CO, cardiac output; SVR, systemic vascular resistance; SBP, systolic blood pressure; BP, blood pressure; CHF, congestive heart failure.

Table 26.3 Physiologic changes in the pulmonary system and anesthetic implications

System	Structural changes	Functional changes	Anesthetic implications
Pulmonary	↑ Chest wall stiffness ↓ Elastic tissue ↑ Flattened diaphragm ↓ Small airway diameter ↑ Central airway size	↓ VC, FVC, FEV$_1$, ERV ↑ RV, CC ↓ DLCO ↓ Central response to hypoxia ↑ PAP ↑ V/Q mismatch	↑ Risk of hypoxia and hypercarbia ↑ Risk of desaturation ↑ Atelectasis ↑ Postoperative pulmonary complication ↑ Difficulty in weaning from ventilator

VC, vital capacity; FVC, forced vital capacity; FEV$_1$, forced expiratory volume in 1 second; ERV, expiratory reserve volume; RV, residual volume; CC, closing capacity; DLCO, diffusing capacity of carbon monoxide; PAP, pulmonary arterial pressure; V/Q, ventilation–perfusion.

capacity, and arterial oxygen tension, as well as increased residual volume (RV), RV/TLC (total lung capacity) ratio, closing volume, and closing capacity (CC). By the age of 65 years, CC exceeds functional residual capacity, which, in turn, leads to closure of small airways, thus resulting in hypoxemia and an increased incidence of respiratory adverse events (see Table 26.3).

Renal System

Aging causes a variable decline in renal blood flow, glomerular filtration rate (GFR), creatinine clearance, renal mass, tubular function, concentrating ability, and diluting capacity. Other changes include impaired fluid handling, decreased drug excretion, decreased responsiveness of the renin–angiotensin–aldosterone system, and impaired potassium excretion. Plasma concentrations of renally excreted drugs may be elevated and/or prolonged (see Table 26.4).

Gastrointestinal and Hepatic System

Esophageal motility decreases and gastric emptying time becomes prolonged, putting older adults at increased risk of perioperative aspiration.

Aging causes a decline in liver mass and hepatic blood flow, hence diminishing hepatic function, resulting in slower metabolism of medications. There is decreased protein synthesis, resulting in increased free drug fractions of highly protein-bound drugs, including benzodiazepines and propofol. Impaired hepatic function influences the synthesis of coagulation factors, thus putting older patients at increased risk of perioperative bleeding (see Table 26.5).

Age-Related Pharmacological Changes

Geriatric patients are more sensitive to anesthetic agents than younger patients, a fact attributed to declining organ function, reserve, and metabolic processes.

In the gastrointestinal (GI) tract, transmucosal absorption of medications is usually preserved. Absorption in the GI tract can be altered by changes in

Table 26.4 Physiologic changes in the renal system and anesthetic implications

System	Structural changes	Functional changes	Anesthetic implications
Renal	↓ Renal mass ↓ Renal blood flow	↓ GFR ↓ Tubular function ↓ Concentrating ability ↓ Diluting capacity ↓ Response to RAAS ↓ Ability of fluid handling ↓ Potassium excretion	↑ Fluid overload ↑ Dehydration ↑ Perioperative acute renal failure ↑ Potassium derangements ↑ Nephrotoxicity with contrast and NSAIDs

GFR, glomerular filtration rate; RAAS, renin–angiotensin–aldosterone system; NSAID, nonsteroidal antiinflammatory drug.

Table 26.5 Physiologic changes in the gastrointestinal and hepatic system and anesthetic implications

System	Structural changes	Functional changes	Anesthetic implications
Gastrointestinal and hepatic	↓ Liver mass ↓ Intestine surface	↓ Hepatic metabolism ↓ Coagulation factors ↑ Free drug fractions ↓ Gastric acid secretion ↓ Gastrointestinal motility	↑ Risk of drug toxicity ↑ Risk of bleeding ↑ Risk of aspiration ↑ Risk of constipation

gastric motility, decreased peristalsis, and increased gastric emptying time. Additionally, decreased gastric blood flow and acid secretion may play a role in preventing effective drug ionization and uptake. Drug absorption through other routes can also be impacted. For example, reduced gas exchange across the alveolar membrane in the aging respiratory system alters the translocation of inhaled anesthetics, impacting both induction and emergence, which is presented as decreased minimum alveolar concentration.

Total body water decreases by 10–15% in the elderly, as compared to their younger counterparts, which can lead to an increase in initial plasma concentration following intravenous administration of drugs. Therefore, a decreased parenteral loading dose of 10–20% is recommended in older adults. Body fat increases up to 20–40% with aging, so the loading dose of lipid soluble drugs (most anesthetic drugs) may be increased by 10–20%.

In elderly adults, plasma albumin levels decrease by up to 20%, whereas the level of α1-acid glycoprotein increases. These changes predominantly affect highly protein-bound acidic drugs, resulting in increased circulating free drug concentrations.

Decreased hepatic blood flow affects the hepatic metabolism of drugs. The age-related reduction in liver mass decreases the amount of hepatic microsomal enzymes and prolongs the half-life of drugs, including anesthetics.

The GFR decreases by approximately $1 \text{ mL/min}/1.73 \text{ m}^2$ per year after the age of 40 years, prolonging the plasma half-life and increasing the steady-state concentration of renally excreted drugs. Additionally, renal blood flow decreases by 10% with each decade of life, warranting dose reduction in the elderly.

Pharmacodynamic factors play a major role in opioid dosing, as pharmacokinetics are not significantly affected by age. An increase in sensitivity warrants a 50% decrease in the dosage requirement of fentanyl, alfentanil, and sufentanil in the geriatric population. Theoretically, remifentanil is ideal for this age group, as it has a very short half-life and is independent of liver and renal function for clearance. Because of increased responsiveness, a remifentanil bolus dose should be decreased by 50% and the infusion rate should be about one-third that for younger patients.

Increased brain sensitivity and decreased clearance of opioids can put older patients at higher risk of severe hypoventilation and apnea. Increased sensitivity in the elderly and synergism between opioids and benzodiazepines, even in low doses, can result in adverse respiratory events. Etomidate, dexmedetomidine, and ketamine are better choices in the setting of aged adults, with a reduced incidence of respiratory depression as compared to propofol or benzodiazepines.

The pharmacodynamics of neuromuscular blocking drugs are unchanged with age; however, the pharmacokinetics of these drugs are significantly altered. Nondepolarizers, such as vecuronium and rocuronium, may have a prolonged duration of action. The recovery indices (time from 75% to 25% block) are increased by as much as 200% for these drugs. Cisatracurium is a muscle relaxant of choice in the elderly, as its metabolism is not dependent on renal or hepatic function. Here is a summary of medication-related anesthetic implications in the geriatric population (see Table 26.6).

Table 26.6 Medication-related anesthetic implications in the geriatric population

Medication	Anesthetic implications
ACEI	Hypotension
Scopolamine	Delirium, confusion
Midazolam	Ataxia, sedation, and cognitive impairment (↓ dose by 50–75%)
Benadryl	Delirium
Ketorolac	Renal injury
Opioids	Respiratory depression (↓ dose by up to 50%)
Inhalation agents	Decreased MAC
Induction agents	Increased sensitivity
NMBs	Prolonged duration of action
Cholinesterase inhibitor	Prolonged succinylcholine effects

ACEI, angiotensin-converting enzyme inhibitor; MAC, minimum alveolar concentration; NMB, neuromuscular blocker.

Preoperative Assessment

Preoperative evaluation could be challenging for the elderly because of diminished physiologic function and comorbidities. Investigative and laboratory tests should be based on patients' medical history and the type of surgery, rather than as a function of age. Routine chest radiography and ECG are not indicated preoperatively in the absence of suggestive symptoms. Instead, evaluation of elderly patients should include age-related geriatric syndromes.

Cognitive Function Evaluation

Preexisting cognitive impairment is one important predictor of postoperative delirium and possibly postoperative cognitive dysfunction (POCD). The American Society of Anesthesiologists Brain Health Initiative guidelines recommend evaluating baseline cognition in patients older than 65 years. There are no universally accepted cognitive screening tools; however, the Animal Fluency Test, Montreal Cognitive Assessment, and Mini-Cog are options.

Definitive strategies can be used to mitigate the risk of postoperative psychological complications in cognitively impaired adults. Dementia patients are sensitive to the adverse effects of anticholinergic medications, which should be avoided. Antipsychotic medications should be used with extreme caution preoperatively in patients who have dementia with Lewy bodies, to avoid untoward reactions such as neuroleptic malignant syndrome, irreversible Parkinsonism, and impaired consciousness.

Medication Evaluation

Multimorbidity and accompanying polypharmacy are common in the geriatric population, increasing the risk of adverse drug-related events. Accurate medication history taking is vital preoperatively. The duration of succinylcholine may be prolonged with reduced plasma cholinesterase levels in Alzheimer's disease and dementia patients who are being treated concomitantly with cholinesterase inhibitors. Cholinesterase inhibitors may also interfere with anticholinesterase agents, resulting in unpredictable responses. Monoamine oxidase inhibitors can cause a potentially fatal cholinergic interaction with meperidine. It is recommended that angiotensin-converting enzyme inhibitors be held prior to surgery to avoid significant hypotension during induction of anesthesia. Anticoagulants should be reviewed preoperatively to ensure adherence to guidelines before regional procedures, so that surgery can be performed more safely.

Institutionalized Patient Evaluation

Preoperative evaluation of an institutionalized patient is particularly challenging due to extensive comorbidities. Dementia is estimated to be present in 40–60% of nursing home residents. Malnutrition varies between 14% and 50%

among patients in nursing homes, hospitals, and rehabilitation facilities. Frailty rates range from 23% to 69% in institutionalized patients in developed countries. Coexisting conditions increase the risk of postoperative morbidity, and even mortality, thus requiring additional attention. The Comprehensive Geriatric Assessment is the cornerstone of geriatric evaluation and is recommended during the preoperative assessment to achieve a strategic plan of evaluation for older patients.

Intraoperative Management

Anesthetic Mode

There is no single best anesthetic mode for elderly patients. There is no difference in postoperative morbidity, mortality, and rates of rehospitalization/hospitalization costs in geriatric patients who undergo general versus regional anesthesia for noncardiac surgery. Neuraxial or regional anesthesia may reduce the risk of pulmonary complications. Monitored anesthesia care, combined with regional techniques, is becoming increasingly popular in older patients. Age-adjusted doses for sedation should be carefully titrated, while instituting vigilant monitoring. Anesthesiologists should choose an anesthetic mode based on patients' preferences, comorbidities, and potential perioperative complications.

Fluid Management

The objective of intraoperative fluid management in elderly patients is to maintain an effective circulating volume and prevent inadequate tissue perfusion. There is currently insufficient evidence to recommend a best practice in fluid management. In general, restrictive or goal-directed strategies are preferred over fixed-volume strategies. Goal-directed management using fluids or vasoactive medication may significantly improve global blood flow but may not be effective in decreasing mortality rates. The multifactorial effects of aging, comorbidities, anesthetic agents, volume status, and tissue perfusion need to be considered during decision-making and should be individualized.

Temperature Management

Hypothermia is more pronounced in older adults due to a compromised thermoregulatory ability because of decreased muscle mass, metabolic rate, and vascular reactivity, thus increasing the risk of wound infection, impaired coagulation function, reduced medication metabolism, cardiac ischemia, arrhythmias, and morbid cardiac events. Therefore, it is recommended that temperature monitoring should be done and forced air warmers and/or warmed intravenous fluids should be utilized in older patients undergoing procedures lasting for >30 minutes.

Positioning

Older patients are more susceptible to intraoperative nerve and pressure point injury due to poor circulation, skin atrophy, and decreased skin integrity. Therefore, it is imperative to ensure proper positioning and padding of bony prominences.

Postoperative Management

Postoperative Delirium

Delirium is among the most significant age-related postoperative complications, as it is associated with higher mortality, longer intensive care unit (ICU) and hospital lengths of stay, and worse outcomes for the patient in general. Early postoperative delirium screening of high-risk patients with validated screening instruments could trigger early optimal delirium treatment. Possible precipitating causes of delirium include uncontrolled pain, hypoxia, pneumonia, infection, electrolyte abnormalities, hypoglycemia, urinary retention, fecal impaction, and polypharmacy. After addressing the underlying causes, multicomponent nonpharmacologic intervention is preferred and pharmacologic treatment is reserved only for patients who might harm themselves or others with agitated, hyperactive delirium behaviors.

Pulmonary Complications

The most common pulmonary complications are atelectasis, pneumonia, respiratory failure, and exacerbation of underlying chronic lung disease. In addition to optimizing the pulmonary status during the preoperative and intraoperative windows, postoperative strategies are also important to prevent pulmonary complications. These include aspiration precautions, incentive spirometry, chest physical therapy, deep breathing exercises, and use of regional anesthesia.

Postoperative Nausea and Vomiting

Though advanced age is not a risk factor per se, prophylactic intervention should be applied to elderly adults at moderate or high risk of postoperative nausea and vomiting. Appropriate risk stratification is important in the geriatric population to avoid medications, such as scopolamine, that may precipitate confusion and postoperative delirium.

Urinary Tract Infection

Older adults are at particular risk of urinary tract infection. Urinary catheterization should not be used as a substitute for incontinent geriatric patients. Thoracic epidural anesthesia and analgesia are not an indication to place a urinary catheter. If an older patient has a catheter placed, daily assessment and early removal are warranted.

Postoperative Pain Management

Postoperative pain management in older adults can be challenging. While they may have decreased pain perception, elderly patients are nevertheless often undertreated for pain. Inadequate pain relief is also associated with severe adverse effects. An appropriate analgesic plan, multimodal in nature, should always be developed before surgery for older adults.

For mild pain, acetaminophen may be given via the intravenous, oral, or rectal route. Other nonopioid alternatives include nonsteroidal antiinflammatory drugs (NSAIDs), acupuncture, music therapy, and massage therapy. Regional techniques and neuraxial or peripheral nerve blocks can be utilized in the perioperative period to reduce the need for systemic opioids. When indicated, a reduced dose of opioids should be considered, with appropriate monitoring in the postanesthetic care unit (PACU). Patient-controlled analgesia (PCA) should be considered if additional intravenous analgesia is needed to improve pain score and better patient satisfaction.

Future Direction of Geriatric Anesthesia

The field of medicine is becoming more personalized and care is currently being reframed as patient-centered care. Physicians are expected to provide care to improve the patient's quality of life. Keeping the patient's realistic expectation in view, a comprehensive interdisciplinary and multidisciplinary team approach is important during the perioperative period. Informed consent should be tailored for each patient. In addition to discussions on the benefits versus risks from surgeries, the burden of treatment, and risks of postoperative cognitive and functional impairment, consideration should also be given to postoperative support, rehabilitation, home care, and family support. Hence, the shared decision-making model, allowing both the clinician and the patient to have input and meaningful discussion in the perioperative setting, could be more appropriate.

At the environmental level, innovations in engineering and technology may reshape the perioperative care for aging patients. Age- and/or dementia-friendly initiatives and the Hospital Elder Life Program have been developed to encourage early mobilization, prevent constipation, and ensure the use of hearing and visual aids for earlier recovery. Also, virtual medical units could be used in the perioperative setting by anesthesiologists to monitor and manage discharged patients in the community by using a mobile multidisciplinary system to reduce postoperative complications in aging patients.

The goal of anesthetic care will focus more on quality-of-life outcomes for elderly patients. High-quality studies are needed to provide evidence-based care in the geriatric population and move in the direction of precision medicine.

Acknowledgments

We would like to thank Nadine Odo and Ashraar Dua for their contribution in editing this book chapter.

Review Questions

1. Which of the following parameters can be increased by aging?

    (a) Coagulation factors
    (b) Vital capacity
    (c) Forced expiratory volume in 1 second (FEV_1)
    (d) Closing capacity

2. Mr. XX is an 82-year-old man who is taking memantine for Alzheimer's disease. He has arrived to the operating room for a total hip replacement. Which of the following medications is the first choice as a muscle relaxant?

    (a) Succinylcholine
    (b) Pancuronium
    (c) Cisatracurium
    (d) Rocuronium

Answers

1 (d) Closing capacity is increased in elderly adults. By the age of 65 years, closing capacity exceeds functional residual capacity, which will lead to closure of small airways, causing hypoxemia. Obesity and pregnancy usually do not change closing capacity.

2 (c) Cisatracurium is a muscle relaxant of choice in the elderly, as its metabolism is not dependent on renal or hepatic function. The recovery index (time from 75% to 25% block) is increased by as much as 200% for neuromuscular blocking drugs. The recovery index for vecuronium is 15 minutes in younger patients, as compared to nearly 50 minutes in elderly patients; the recovery index for rocuronium varies from 13 to 22 minutes, whereas that of pancuronium increases from approximately 40 to 60 minutes. Patients with Alzheimer's

disease or dementia are commonly treated with cholinesterase inhibitors. The reduced plasma cholinesterase level may prolong the duration of succinylcholine.

Further Reading

Andres TM, McGrane T, McEvoy MD, Allen BFS. Geriatric pharmacology: an update. *Anesthesiol Clin.* 2019;37(3):475–92.

Barnett SR. Preoperative assessment of older adults. *Anesthesiol Clin.* 2019;37 (3):423–36.

Butterworth JF, Mackey DC, Wasnick JD. Geriatric anesthesia. In: JF Butterworth, DC Mackey, JD Wasnick, eds. *Morgan & Mikhail's Clinical Anesthesiology*, 5th ed. New York, NY: McGraw Hill; 2013, pp. 907–17.

Khan KT, Hemati K, Donovan AL. Geriatric physiology and the frailty syndrome. *Anesthesiol Clin.* 2019;37(3):453–74.

Lim BG, Lee IO. Anesthetic management of geriatric patients. *Korean J Anesthesiol.* 2020;73(1):8–29.

Mohanty S, Rosenthal RA, Russell MM, Neuman MD, Ko CY, Esnaola NF. Optimal perioperative management of the geriatric patient: a best practices guideline from the American College of Surgeons NSQIP and the American Geriatrics Society. *J Am Coll Surg.* 2016;222(5):930–47.

Ryan-Barnett S. Elderly patients. In: RD Miller, MC Pardo, Jr, eds. *Basics of Anesthesia*, 6th ed. Philadelphia, PA: Elsevier; 2011, pp. 568–79.

Chapter

Anesthesia for Ambulatory Surgical Procedures

Sandra N. Gonzalez, Olga C. Nin, and Sonia D. Mehta

Anesthesia for Ambulatory Surgery

Ambulatory surgery centers (ASCs) have become the place of choice for an increasing number of diagnostic and surgical procedures. Improvements in anesthesia and pain control, minimally invasive surgical techniques, patient expectations, and economic factors have driven this increase in number and complexity of procedures performed at ASCs. Patients with significant comorbidities are also making up an increasing proportion of the population undergoing ambulatory procedures. There are multiple advantages with performing same-day surgical procedures in this setting – the cost of care is lower in comparison with same-day procedures performed in hospital; waiting times and ease of access are also more convenient for patients and caretakers; and physicians can maximize the use of their operating room time by having efficient scheduling practices. At the same time, and in order to maintain the viability of ASCs, it is fundamental to understand the factors that make for a successful ambulatory surgical practice, such as optimal patient and procedure selection, preoperative preparation, anesthesia management and pain control strategies, management of postanesthesia care unit (PACU) complications, appropriate staffing and management of human resources, and contingency plans in the event of changes in patient condition that require hospital admission for further diagnosis or treatment. Multiple factors must be considered to make the decision of carrying out a procedure at an ASC: patient factors such as age and comorbidities; social factors, as the patient will recover at home and will need someone to assist during the postoperative period; type of surgical procedure and expectation that postoperative pain can be treated with oral analgesics or a peripheral nerve block (PNB); and factors related to the ASC in terms of equipment, staff, and ability to transfer the patient to a higher level of care, should that be necessary.

Preoperative Care

Patient Selection

Appropriately choosing patients who are undergoing surgeries at ASCs is the first step in increasing the likelihood of successful perioperative outcomes. Morbidity and mortality for ambulatory surgeries are very low (<0.1%), confirming the safety of same-day surgeries. While many times the decision to perform ambulatory surgery in a patient with significant comorbidities is made empirically by anesthesiologists and surgeons, there is some evidence that specific conditions may influence perioperative outcomes and are increasingly common in patients presenting to ASCs:

- Age – while perioperative mortality increases with age, particularly for major surgery and emergency procedures, the risk of death is low for elderly patients in the outpatient setting, with a 7-day mortality rate of 25 per 100,000 procedures at ASCs, compared to 50 per 100,000 procedures at outpatient hospitals, in patients older than 65 years. Elderly patients have a higher incidence of intraoperative cardiovascular events, but not of postoperative events. Patients aged 85 years and older have a higher rate of readmission after ambulatory surgery. Transurethral resection of bladder tumor (TURBT), commonly performed in older adults, is associated with high admission rates.

- Hypertension (HTN) – commonly present in the elderly and independently associated with an increased rate of intraoperative cardiovascular events. Blood pressure (BP) values measured in clinic should be 160/100 mmHg or below, and appropriate control and treatment of HTN are recommended. For patients noncompliant with therapy or with unknown baseline BP measurements, or who remain hypertensive despite maximum therapy, a measurement of 180/110 mmHg and below is acceptable, understanding that the period to achieve cardiovascular risk reduction is longer than what is needed for HTN control. If surgery is delayed for HTN control, it is advisable to do it in conjunction with the primary care physician and to allow a period of 6–8 weeks for regression of vascular changes.

- Obesity – patients with obesity frequently present with coexisting comorbidities, including HTN, congestive heart failure (CHF), and obstructive sleep apnea (OSA). The prevalence of cardiovascular disease increases as the body mass index (BMI) increases. Obese patients have an increased rate of perioperative respiratory events, although high BMI per se does not increase the risk of difficult intubation. Despite this increase in respiratory events, the rate of unanticipated admission is not higher in obese patients. Performing PNBs is also not free of problems, as block failure rate is higher when obesity is present.

- Smoking – associated with an increased risk of postoperative respiratory complications and also with impaired wound healing. Cessation of smoking 4 weeks prior to surgery has been shown to improve outcomes.

- Asthma – intraoperative events, such as bronchospasm, occur in approximately 2% of asthma patients. For patients who present with symptoms of asthma, the increase in postoperative respiratory complications is almost fivefold; therefore, it is prudent to ensure that asthmatic patients are medically optimized, and with minimal to no respiratory symptoms before undergoing elective procedures.

- Chronic obstructive pulmonary disease (COPD) – patients with COPD have an increased risk of perioperative lower airway events. Patients who have COPD and are asymptomatic do not have longer PACU length of stay, suggesting that respiratory events might be minor. Patients experiencing symptoms are the ones at highest risk of pulmonary complications and should be optimized prior to elective surgery.

- Obstructive sleep apnea (OSA) – patients with OSA are more likely to be difficult to intubate and have a higher rate of PACU complications such as HTN, arrhythmias, desaturation, airway obstruction, and need for reintubation. The use of opiates may play a role in the incidence of complications; therefore, judicious use of these agents is advised. If the patient receives treatment with continuous positive airway pressure (CPAP), they need to be proficient in their use. Patients identified at risk of OSA during preoperative assessment should be referred for further assessment with polysomnography.

- Coronary artery disease (CAD) – the incidence of perioperative myocardial infarction (MI) in the ambulatory setting is low. Patients with intermediate clinical predictors, including mild ischemic heart disease, acute coronary event over 1 month old, compensated CHF, diabetes mellitus, and renal insufficiency, can undergo low-risk surgical procedures without further testing. Intermediate-risk surgery can proceed without further testing in patients who have functional capacity >4 METS.

- Transient ischemic attack (TIA)/cerebrovascular accident (CVA) – the risk of adverse outcomes and postoperative morbidity and mortality is higher in patients with a history of stroke. This risk does not return to baseline but stabilizes 9 months after the event.

Preoperative Assessment

With the increasing number of comorbidities with which patients present when scheduled for ambulatory procedures, an effective way to avoid cancellations on the day of surgery, and to identify patients who need optimization, is to perform a preoperative in-person or over-the-phone consultation, if possible. In terms of preoperative testing, routine tests are not recommended and the approach to perioperative testing should rather focus on what tests are needed to assess specific aspects of the patient's condition (e.g., HbA1c for diabetic patients) plus reviewing of testing that the patient has undergone as part of follow-up of baseline comorbidities (e.g., ECG for patients with a history of CAD). Additional testing may be requested if the results will change anesthetic management or if testing is needed to make decisions about postponing surgery to optimize baseline conditions. Table 27.1 summarizes the most important questions to ask during preoperative phone assessment.

Table 27.1 Top 10 questions to ask during preoperative assessment

Question	Tips
Have you or your family member had problems with anesthesia?	Examples: MH, pseudocholinesterase deficiency, difficult airway, allergies to typical anesthetic medications, unexpected postoperative admission, prolonged intubation, severe PONV
What prescriptions and over-the-counter medications do you take?	More than five drugs should trigger an in-person anesthesia preoperative evaluation Literature suggests that >5 drugs increases the risk of morbidity and mortality in ambulatory surgery [1, 2]
Are you dependent on others for eating, dressing, or bathing?	Frailty is associated with increased perioperative morbidity in the ambulatory surgeries, independent of age, type of anesthesia, and other comorbidities. Local or MAC decreases this risk [3–5] Lack of ability to perform ADL should be considered as an increase in ASA score [6]
Have you been hospitalized in the last 30 days?	Hospital admission is associated with significant morbidity and mortality within 30 days [7, 8]
Have you had a myocardial infarction in the last 60 days?	Not a candidate for elective surgery [9]
Have you had cardiac catheterization or received a coronary stent within the last 6 months?	Bare metal stent recommendation: 30 days DES: 6 months before elective surgery
Do you have a pacemaker or an implantable cardiac defibrillator?	ICD check within 6 months; pacemaker within 1 year [10]
Have you had a stroke in the last 9 months?	Not a candidate for elective surgery [11]
Are you on dialysis?	Timing is important

MH, malignant hyperthermia; PONV, postoperative nausea and vomiting; MAC, monitored anesthesia care; ADL, activities of daily living; ASA, American Society of Anesthesiologists; DES, drug-eluting stent; ICD, implantable cardioverter–defibrillator.

•*Medications* – patients should continue taking medications as per their usual schedule, especially cardiovascular, bronchodilating, chronic pain, anxiety, and anticonvulsant agents. Angiotensin-converting enzyme (ACE) inhibitors, angiotensin receptor blockers, and diuretics are frequently held in the morning of surgery to avoid refractory hypotension; this decision must be made on a case-to-case basis, as patients with CHF or uncontrolled HTN, or who will undergo procedures under regional block (e.g., cataract surgery), may benefit from continuing these agents. Management of insulin and hypoglycemic agents is summarized in Table 27.2.

•*Premedication* – use of premedication must be assessed on a patient-by-patient basis. There are benefits to the use of low-dose anxiolytics when indicated, in terms of sedation, decreased anxiety, optimization of intraoperative hemodynamic stability, and decreased postoperative side effects, without prolonging recovery from anesthesia. Midazolam remains the most common anxiolytic used for premedication in the ambulatory setting and, at doses of $10–20$ μg kg^{-1}, can improve the fast-tracking process by decreasing anxiety-related complications, as well as improve patient comfort level and satisfaction. Patients at risk of aspiration benefit from prophylaxis with a nonparticulate antacid such as sodium citrate/citric acid (Bicitra, 30 mL orally before procedure), an H2 receptor antagonist (ranitidine 50 mg intravenously (IV) before procedure), and especially for patients with diabetic gastroparesis, metoclopramide (10 mg IV before surgery).

Table 27.2 Recommendations for perioperative management of oral hypoglycemic agents and insulin

	Day before surgery	Day of surgery
Insulin pump	No change	No change
Long-acting insulins	No change	75–100% of morning dose
Intermediate-acting insulins	No change with daytime dose; 75% of dose if taken in the evening	50–75% of morning dose
Short-acting insulin	No change	Hold the dose
Oral hypoglycemic agents	No change	Hold the dose

Source: Okocha O, Gerlach R, Sweitzer B. Preoperative evaluation for ambulatory anesthesia: what, when, and how? *Anesthesiol Clin.* 2019;37:195–213.

Anesthesia Management

The choice of anesthetic has an impact at multiple levels: efficiency of work-flow at the ASC; recovery time from anesthesia; and patient's ability to resume activities after an ambulatory procedure. Therefore, anesthesiologists play a pivotal role in improving perioperative efficiency, enhancing rapid recovery from anesthesia, enabling early discharge from the facility, and rapid resumption of activities of daily living by the patient.

- *General anesthesia* – for many procedures, the use of anesthetic techniques, such as regional blocks and monitored anesthesia care (MAC), is not feasible and general anesthesia might be the best choice. Selection of agents that facilitate a fast recovery and decrease perioperative complications is important.

  ○ *Propofol* – due to its rapid onset of action and redistribution, with fast recovery, propofol is the ideal choice for induction of general anesthesia in the ambulatory setting. It has a low rate of side effects compared to other agents. Because of its favorable profile, propofol can also be used as an agent for maintenance of anesthesia, especially for patients at high risk of postoperative nausea and vomiting (PONV).

  ○ *Volatile anesthetics* – the low-solubility agents sevoflurane and desflurane are preferred for general anesthesia, because recovery from these agents is relatively fast. More rapid emergence from anesthesia has been observed with desflurane compared to sevoflurane; however, no difference in the late recovery phase has been observed between these two agents. Volatile agents increase the risk of PONV, which can be minimized by use of prophylactic drugs, including a combination of dexamethasone (4–8 mg IV) and a 5-HT receptor antagonist such as ondansetron (4 mg IV).

  ○ *Neuromuscular blocking agents* – when muscle relaxation is required for optimal surgical conditions or endotracheal intubation, the intermediate-acting muscle relaxants rocuronium and vecuronium are the best choices. These agents, more specifically rocuronium, can be effectively reversed by sugammadex. Quantitative monitoring of the train-of-four must be performed to ensure full reversal and decrease the risk of respiratory complications in PACU. Succinylcholine can also be used for intubation, keeping in mind that myalgias can occur as a side effect and that this agent is a trigger for malignant hyperthermia.

  ○ *Opiates* – several complications result from the use of opiates. A multimodal approach to analgesia will result in decreased need for opiates and a lower rate of complications associated with their use. Remifentanil infusion is becoming a popular choice for maintenance of anesthesia, but it offers no benefit for postoperative analgesia. Carefully titrated long-acting opiates, such as morphine and hydromorphone, along with nonsteroidal antiinflammatory drugs (NSAIDs) and acetaminophen, can be used to ensure optimal analgesia postoperatively.

- *MAC* – use of IV sedation, in combination with infiltration of the surgical site with local anesthesia or a PNB, is the most common way that MAC is performed and can facilitate a rapid recovery compared to general anesthesia. Close monitoring of respiratory depression is very important to avoid complications. The most frequently used sedative for MAC is propofol as a continuous infusion at a rate of 25–100 µg/(kg min). When other sedatives, such as midazolam or fentanyl, are used, the risk of respiratory depression is increased and careful titration of any additional sedation is imperative.

- *Regional anesthesia* – the two major types of regional anesthesia that are used at ASCs include PNBs and neuraxial blocks. The benefits of regional anesthesia are a faster recovery time, without the side effects or complications of general anesthesia, and excellent analgesia. Use of peripheral nerve catheters also allow for an extended benefit of pain control at home and decreased use of opioids.

  - *Neuraxial blocks*:
    - Subarachnoid blocks – fast onset with reliable results, commonly used for pelvic, perineal, and lower extremity surgery. Duration of procedure should not exceed duration of the spinal block. Complications include hypotension, postdural puncture headache, urinary retention, and transient radicular irritation.
    - Epidural anesthesia – when used with a catheter, it allows for titration of additional local anesthesia for procedures of uncertain duration. Complications include epidural hematoma, hypotension, and accidental dural puncture.
  - *PNBs* – ideal for surgeries involving the extremities. Table 27.3 summarizes the most commonly used blocks for ambulatory surgery.

Postoperative Care

Patients are admitted to PACU after they have emerged from anesthesia. Traditionally, patients will go to phase I PACU, but for patients who are alert, awake, and oriented, with minimum pain and no nausea or vomiting,

Table 27.3 Must-know regional blocks for ambulatory surgical procedures

Type of block	Indications	Upper extremity		
		Local	Tips and tricks	Complications/challenges
Cervical paravertebral	Shoulder surgery	Ropivacaine 0.5% 10–15 mL	Target C6 (biceps twitch)	Phrenic nerve palsy, vascular injury
Interscalene	Shoulder surgery, proximal humerus, lateral third of clavicle	Ropivacaine 0.5% 10–15 mL	C6 usually is split at this location; diaphragm hemiparesis may not be tolerated in patients with moderate to severe lung disease; numbness in the thumb indicates a good working block	Feeling of dyspnea (education), posterior shoulder pain, accidental vascular injury (transverse cervical artery, branch of inferior thyroid artery, vertebral artery)
Supraclavicular	Surgery in upper arm below the shoulder (mid-distal humerus down to the hand)	Ropivacaine 0.5% 20–25 mL	The 3-in-1 method (corner pocket, middle trunk, upper trunk) decreases the incidence of hemidiaphragmatic paresis. Tilt the probe towards the chest and find the rib protecting the lower trunk	Onset of surgical block is 20–30 minutes; watch vascular targets (use color Doppler)
Infraclavicular	Surgery in upper arm below the shoulder	Ropivacaine 0.5% 20–25 mL	The proximal approach can have three cords adjacent to each other	Difficult in morbidly obese patients, pneumothorax, vascular injury
Axillary	Surgery at the elbow or below	Ropivacaine 0.5% 20–25 mL	Compressible area if vascular injury – therefore, good for patients with anticoagulation and scanning the arm, as well as twitching helpful to identify the independent nerves	Challenges: have to remember to anesthetize the musculocutaneous nerve

Truncal blocks

Type of block	Indications	Local	Tips and tricks	Complications/challenges
PEC I	Breast surgery (subpectoral implants, breast augmentation)	Ropivacaine 0.5% 10–15 mL	Local anesthetic between pectoralis major and pectoralis minor. Place the probe as for a traditional infraclavicular block	For major breast surgery, additional nerve blocks will be needed
Serratus	Breast surgery, rib fracture, chest wall	Ropivacaine 0.5% 20–30 mL	Blocks lateral cutaneous branches of T2–9, intercostobrachial nerve, and long thoracic and thoracodorsal nerves. Between latissimus dorsi and serratus in T4 posterior axillary crease	Challenges: avoid the thoracodorsal artery when placing the block
PVB	Breast, hernia, axillary dissection, cholecystectomy, appendectomy	Ropivacaine 0.5% 10 mL per couple of levels	1 cm past transverse process at thoracic level, 2 cm past transverse process in lumbar area. Use of ultrasound helpful. Decreased risk of sympathetic block, lower risk of bleeding in anticoagulated patients	Challenges: obese patients, risk of pneumothorax
TAP	Cesarean section, inguinal hernia, abdominal incisions	Ropivacaine 0.5% 15–20 mL on each side	Hernia repair – targets ilioinguinal and iliohypogastric	Target pain distribution. Can do subcostal, ilioinguinal/hypogastric, and lateral or posterior

Table 27.3 (cont.)

	Truncal blocks		
Type of block	Indications	Local	Complications/challenges
Rectus sheath	Umbilical hernia, midline laparotomy	Ropivacaine 0.5% 20 mL (10 mL on each side)	Rectus sheath extends laterally; use Doppler to prevent gastric vascular injury
			Challenges: do not go below the umbilicus or risk placing where the posterior rectus sheath disappears (arcuate line) and risk peritoneal spread. No visceral pain control, only somatic

	Lower extremity		
Type of block	Indications	Local	Complications/challenges
Femoral	Knee surgery, Femur fracture, anterior thigh surgery	Ropivacaine 0.5% 15–20 mL	If you get the sartorius twitch, remember to move lateral and deeper with your needle
Adductor	Knee surgery, TKA, distal femur	Ropivacaine 0.5% 10–15 mL	Challenges: high-volume block can lead to higher incidence of motor block
			Decreased incidence of motor blockade
Obturator	Knee, medial thigh, or hip surgery	Ropivacaine 0.2–0.5% 10 mL	Will cause motor weakness
			For hip surgery, go proximal and do subpectineus obturator
LFC	Knee surgery, THA	Ropivacaine 0.5% 5–10 mL	Make sure you are below the ASIS
			Useful for incisional pain or skin grafting

Block	Indication	Local anesthetic	Technique	Challenges
Sciatic	Knee surgery, ankle surgery, posterior thigh or leg surgery	Ropivacaine 0.5% 15–20 mL	In morbidly obese patients, using twitch monitor, in addition to ultrasound, helps	Will cause significant motor weakness
Popliteal	Tibial/fibula surgery, ankle surgery, Achilles tendon	Ropivacaine 0.5% 15–20 mL	Place needle in between the tibial and the common peroneal in same sheath	Challenges: motor weakness, difficult needle movement to learn
Saphenous	Ankle surgery	Ropivacaine 0.5% 10 mL	Can be blocked at the femoral triangle, adductor canal, medial femoral condyle, or medial malleolus	Partial quadriceps weakness can be achieved if done proximally and in bigger volumes
iPACK	TKA, ACL, posterior knee surgery	Ropivacaine 0.5% 20 mL	Curvilinear probe helps visualize a wider area, block proximal to concyles. Calculate the distance from skin to target, and insert the needle at equal distance from probe. Careful with saphenous vein if doing a medial approach	Challenges: challenging due to depth and distance between popliteal artery and femur
PENG	Hip arthroscopy	Ropivacaine 0.2–0.5% 20 mL	Targets: obturator, accessory obturator, and femoral nerve branches to the hip. No motor weakness. Curvilinear probe	Challenges: inadequate volume, can violate the joint capsule

PVB, paravertebral block; TAP; transversus abdominis plane; TKA, total knee arthroplasty; LFC, lateral femoral cuteneous; THA, total hip arthroplasty; ASIS, anterior superior iliac spine; iPACK, infiltration between the popliteal artery and the capsule of the knee; ACL, anterior cruciate ligament; PENG, pericapsular nerve group:

and who can otherwise sit up without assistance, they can go directly to phase II PACU. These patients have typically received MAC, with or without PNB. Management of PACU issues is important in optimizing timing and patient condition upon discharge, and addressing these issues begins during the preoperative care phase.

- *Pain* – unsatisfactory pain control not only can delay discharge from PACU, but also can delay resumption of activities of daily living. Excessive reliance on narcotics will result in increased side effects (nausea, vomiting, respiratory depression, urinary retention, and ileus). On the other hand, relying exclusively on agents such as NSAIDs might not be enough to achieve pain relief. A multimodal approach to analgesia involves use of multiple modalities for pain control, with the goal of achieving synergistic effects and reducing side effects from any particular medication, thus improving recovery and patient outcomes after ambulatory procedures. This includes infiltration of local anesthesia in the surgical site, PNBs, acetaminophen, NSAIDs and cyclooxygenase 2 (COX-2) inhibitors, α2-agonists, ketamine, gabapentin, and pregabalin. If the patient experiences severe pain in PACU, it is advisable to treat immediately with an opiate IV. Oxycodone is effective in treating moderate pain, and if not given ahead of time, ibuprofen and acetaminophen can be administered once the patient is awake.

- *PONV* – major risk factors for PONV are female gender, nonsmoker status, a history of PONV or motion sickness, pelvic procedures, and use of volatile agents or opiates. Use of multiple prophylactic agents should be considered for patients with at least two risk factors. Ondansetron and other 5-HT antagonists, dexamethasone, transdermal scopolamine, and droperidol (its use has declined since a black box warning was issued by the Food and Drug Administration (FDA)) are effective as prophylactic agents. Consideration also must be given to minimizing the use of volatile agents and opiates, and using total intravenous anesthesia (TIVA) for patients at high risk of PONV. Appropriate IV hydration is also important to minimize the risk of PONV.

- *Discharge criteria* – patients can be safely discharged home once their mental status is back to baseline, vital signs are stable, ambulation is achieved, pain and nausea/vomiting are well controlled, and there are no signs of surgical complications. Ability to tolerate oral intake and voiding are not mandatory for patients who had surgeries that are low risk for these complications, with instructions to seek care if they cannot tolerate oral intake or void 6–8 hours after discharge.

- *Unanticipated admission* – rate of unanticipated admission is <1% for ASCs. Uncontrolled nausea and vomiting, uncontrolled pain, and bleeding from the surgical site are common causes for unanticipated admission. The

Table 27.4 Key elements for fast-tracking after elective ambulatory anesthesia

Period	Details
Preoperative period	Stabilize coexisting diseases; encourage prehabilitation exercise program and smoking cessation. Minimize patient anxiety and discomfort. Ensure adequate hydration by replacing fluid deficits. Appropriate use of prophylactic therapies to prevent postoperative complications (e.g., nausea, vomiting, pain)
Intraoperative period	Utilize anesthetic techniques that optimize surgical conditions, while ensuring rapid recovery with minimal side effects. Administer local anesthesia via peripheral nerve blocks or wound infiltration. Apply multimodal analgesia and antiemetic prophylaxis. Minimize use of nasogastric tubes and avoid excessive fluid administration
Postoperative period	Allow patients who fulfill discharge criteria to be fast-tracked (i.e., discharged earlier from recovery units). Ensure adequate pain control during the postdischarge period, utilizing nonopioid analgesics to minimize the need for opioid-containing analgesics. Encourage early ambulation and resumption of normal activities of daily living

Source: Adapted from Whit P, Eng M. Fast-track anesthetic techniques for ambulatory surgery. *Curr Opin Anaesthesiol*. 2020;552. Original Table 27.4.

ASC needs to have a contingency plan for inpatient or extended stay admission for patients who cannot be discharged after reasonable measures have been taken in the PACU.

Table 27.4 summarizes key aspects to safely and effectively fast-tracking patients after ambulatory surgical procedures.

Human Resources Management in Ambulatory Surgery Centers

ASC costs are significantly lower compared to hospital outpatient costs for the same procedure, which translates into an increasing number of ambulatory surgical procedures to be scheduled at ASCs. Because of lower costs, ASCs must manage budgets carefully. Part of these expenses are those related to human resources (HR). ASC leadership must assess these variables and create a balance between case volume and staffing levels, while optimizing scheduling to maintain proper operating room utilization and, at the same time, maintaining a culture of safety. HR management (HRM) is an approach to bring the right people to an organization and mobilize them to accomplish its goals. This approach requires determining what qualifications are required for each position, recruitment of qualified staff, training and development of employees, and a system to assess job performance, with adequate rewards to attract and retain high-performing staff. For ASCs, an HR manager needs to have, and communicate, a clear vision for the future of the ASC, so the hired staff are aligned with that vision and those goals. Strategic HRM involves formulating and implementing HR strategies and implementation tactics that are in alignment and reinforce the organization's mission and future direction. In healthcare, strategic HR can be achieved by putting the orientation focus on patient demands (excellent patient care and satisfaction), with a commitment to employee development. HR add value to any organization, but the need for professional development of staff is also fundamental to carrying its mission successfully. Therefore, ASC leaders need to identify approaches to improving performance and patient satisfaction, and to reward employee success. They need to work with employees effectively, and be knowledgeable about all systems and practices at the organization, so a skilled and motivated workforce, with clearly outlined roles and responsibilities at the time of hiring, can be put together. HRM for ASCs can be very challenging for ASCs that do not directly employ all staff (as opposed to hospitals), and many staff members, including healthcare professionals, and representatives from equipment companies are involved in patient care at the facility.

Sexual Harassment

With a high rate of sexual harassment in healthcare organizations, and with more than a third of female physicians and nurses perceiving they have experienced sexual harassment, ASCs need to have policies and procedures for reporting sexual harassment and carrying out investigations of misconduct. Sexual harassment in the workplace has a negative impact not only on individuals, but also on the organization at all levels. Organizations where discrimination is ingrained in the culture discourage victims from reporting incidents of sexual harassment, or have inadequate systems to address these complaints. Developing an organizational culture that fosters a climate of dignity and integrity, where gender discrimination is forcefully opposed, and implementing a safe system for individuals to report grievances, followed by enforcement of a code of conduct and implementation of an effective sexual harassment policy, can effectively protect the rights of ASC employees, as well as the business interests of the employer.

Workplace Diversity and Cultural Competence

The United States has been growing more diverse year after year, and the assumption would be that our fundamental institutions as well would grow more diverse. However, despite the growing demographic change in the United States, minorities are still underrepresented in healthcare leadership positions, with minorities representing 31% of patients nationally, but only 14% of hospital board members, 12% of executive leadership positions, and 17% of first- and mid-level management positions. *"Missing Persons: Minorities in the Health Professions"* is a report from the Sullivan Commission on diversity in the healthcare workforce, which states that "The fact that the nation's health professions have not kept pace with changing demographics may be an even greater cause of disparities in health access and outcomes than the persistent lack of health insurance for tens of millions of Americans." Lack of diversity in healthcare results in disparities in health access and outcomes, to the detriment of the communities we serve. Cultural competence encompasses the knowledge, skills, and behavior required from a healthcare professional to optimally care for patients from many different cultural and ethnic backgrounds. Different systems of belief and other culturally and ethnically determined factors influence how patients experience illness, seek medical advice, and respond to treatment plans, and the outcome of care is therefore also dependent on these factors. ASCs can be active agents in creating a more diversified and culturally competent team of providers, where the outcome of care improves by addressing these factors.

Privileging and Credentialing

Credentialing is the process through which ASCs ensure the qualifications and license of their practitioners. It protects patients and ASCs by minimizing the risk of medical errors secondary to unqualified providers. Therefore, ASCs need to be diligent in their credentialing processes and have a robust set of policies and procedures with this purpose. However, ASCs may have less oversight. In 2014, half of the organizations surveyed were not in compliance with the standard of privileging. ASCs that receive Joint Commission accreditation are those that prove they provide the highest level of performance and service to their patients. Because of the complexity in maintaining updated and complete information for credentialing, outsourcing credentialing might be a cost-effective function if the ASC does not have enough staff to manage this workload.

Further Reading

Boezaart AP. *Primer for Regional Anesthesia Anatomy: Macroanatomy, Microanatomy, and Sonoamatomy*, 3rd ed. RAEducation.com LLC; 2018.

Brennan M, Rajan N. HR issues: sexual harassment, workplace diversity, cultural sensitivity, privileging, credentialing, denying privileges, difficult conversations. *Manual of Practice Management for Ambulatory Surgery Centers*. 2020;16:239–52.

Kopp SL, Horlocker TT. Regional anaesthesia in day-stay and short-stay surgery. *Anaesthesia*. 2010;65 Suppl 1:84–96.

References

1. Mathis M, Naughton N. Patient selection for day case-eligible surgery. *Anesthesiology*. 2013;119:1310–21.

2. Lermitte J, Chung F. Patient selection in ambulatory surgery. *Curr Opin Anaesthesiol.* 2005;18:598–602.

3. Bryson G, Chung F. Patient selection in ambulatory anesthesia – an evidence based review (parts I and II). *Can J Anesth.* 2004:51(8):768–94.

4. Visnjevac O, Davari-Farid S. The effect of adding functional classification to ASA status for predicting 30-day mortality. *Anesth Analg.* 2015;121(1):110–16.

5. Lee JH. Anesthesia for ambulatory surgery. *Korean J Anesthesiol.* 2017;70 (4):398–406.

6. White P, Eng M. Fast-track techniques for ambulatory surgery. *Curr Opin Anaesthesiol.* 2007;20:545–57.

7. Park S, Warren L. Ambulatory anesthesia. In: PF Dunn, T Alston, K Baker, *et al.* eds. *Clinical Anesthesia Procedures of the Massachusetts General Hospital,* 7th ed. Philadelphia, PA: Lippincott Williams & Wilkins; 2007, pp. 563–69.

8. Okocha O, Gerlach R, Sweitzer B. Preoperative evaluation for ambulatory anesthesia: what, when, and how? *Anesthesiology Clin.* 2019;37:195–213.

9. Ardon AE, *et al.* Regional anesthesia for ambulatory anesthesiologists. *Anesthesiol Clin.* 2019;37(2):265–87.

10. Mulroy MF, McDonald SB. Regional anesthesia for outpatient surgery. *Anesthesiol Clin North Am.* 2003;21(2):289–303.

11. Klein SM, *et al.* Peripheral nerve block technique for ambulatory surgery. *Anesth Analg.* 2005;101(6):1663–76.

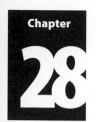

Chapter

28

Chronic Pain Medicine

Ken P. Ehrhardt, Devin S. Reed, Mark Motejunas, and Ken Candido

Epidemiology, Patient History, and Physical Examination

Chronic neck pain and low back pain are highly prevalent medical conditions that cause considerable pain, disability, and economic burden [1, 2]. Cervicalgia has an annual prevalence exceeding 30%, with an estimated half of these individuals experiencing some degree of chronicity, making it the fourth leading cause of disability in the United States [1]. The lifetime prevalence of low back pain is estimated at 60–70%, affecting people of all ages, but the highest likelihood is in the fifth or sixth decade of life. This contributes to the highest number of disability-adjusted life years in the United States in 2010 [2–4]. Furthermore, low back pain is the leading cause of disability worldwide, according to a 2010 study of Global Burden of Disease [5].

The causes of low back pain can be due to muscular strain, cartilaginous deterioration, spinal cord nerve compression, intervertebral disc herniation, traumatic injury, or many other pathologic conditions. A 2018 meta-analysis demonstrated with level 1 data that obesity is a major risk factor for developing low back pain in men and women [6]. Other risk factors include age, fitness level, job-related factors, and psychological components [7]. There is loss of bone strength, intervertebral disc volume, and muscle elasticity with age [7, 8]. A weak back and weak core muscles do not properly support the spine. Jobs requiring heavy lifting can lead to injury; however, desk work can also contribute to pain from poor posture over prolonged periods [4, 7]. Anxiety and depression can influence one's perception of pain, whereas chronic pain can also perpetuate negative mood and depression [7].

A thorough pain history is essential in order to generate an accurate diagnosis and treatment plan for each specific patient. Characterization and location of the pain in quality and distribution can differentiate somatic versus neurogenic origin. Somatic pain will be described typically as having a dull, aching quality from nociceptors in tendons, ligaments, and bones. Radicular pain is often described as burning and shooting, with potential paresthesias, and will often radiate along dermatomal distributions. This is caused by irritation of a nerve root by compression or surrounding inflammation. Concerning symptoms, such as weakness, gait or grip disturbances, and bladder or bowel incontinence, are crucial to identify for early surgical decompression. A complete review of systems for back pain can identify referred pain from more malignant retroperitoneal sources such as aortic aneurysms, pelvic organs, gastrointestinal etiology, neoplasms, or infections [7, 8]. Understanding inciting events and psychosocial factors about the pain is important and can be predictive of chronicity and disability.

Coupling a patient's history of present illness with a skilled physical examination can help delineate contributing sources, identify "red flags" signifying serious pathology, and direct a cost-effective management plan [1]. Examining the patient is useful to identify obvious structural abnormalities or asymmetry, as well as attention to gait and possible use of assistive devices. Assessing the range of motion is important. One should also assess palpable focal tenderness, strength of isolated muscle groups, dermatomal sensation, deep tendon reflexes, and signs of upper motor neuron injury [8, 9]. Specific diagnostic maneuvers, such as straight leg raise, facet loading, and FABER testing, can provide increased specificity to help the clinician narrow down their differential diagnosis [8].

Laboratory Testing, Imaging, and Diagnoses

Further investigation of chronic back pain, whether cervical or lumbar, is often necessary to identify or rule out certain pathologies. Blood tests are not routinely necessary but could be ordered to identify signs of inflammation or arthritis, such as erythrocyte sedimentation rate or C-reactive protein levels. Blood tests can also show signs of infection, such as leukocytosis, or markers of cancer such as smear testing under microscopy. Additionally, metabolic panels are ordered to assess kidney and liver function when prescribing medications for relief of both somatic pain and neuropathic pain. Calcium and alkaline phosphatase levels can be used if suspecting conditions that affect bone metabolism, such as in osteoporosis or Paget's disease.

Physicians should order imaging for patients with chronic persistent pain or new weakness in order to better assess pathology. Initially, imaging has limited utility in chronic low back pain because most patients harbor nonspecific findings [11]. There is lack of evidence supporting improvement from early imaging in patients with nonspecific pain without "red flags," so imaging should be delayed at least 1–2 months while implementing conservative treatment modalities [8]. These "red flags" are patients who are older than 50 years with new symptoms, constitutional symptoms, or a history of malignancy, infectious concerns, or new neurologic findings on examination [9]. Initial conservative modalities consist of either physical therapy, massage therapy, acupuncture, or chiropractic maneuvers, or over-the-counter analgesics, such as acetaminophen and ibuprofen. Imaging should begin with plain radiographs; however, these lack specificity without correlating exam findings because degenerative changes in cervical and lumbar spine are common in people over 30 years old [9]. CT or MRI are indicated where there are concerns of malignancy, infection, cord compression, or disc herniations. CT better identifies bony pathology; MRI is superior at evaluating soft tissues. After chronic pain patients have failed conservative therapy, physicians normally order an MRI scan without contrast, as it can provide additional information and images of the intervertebral discs and spinal canal that plain X-rays and CT cannot. An MRI scan with contrast is generally ordered for patients with a history of neurosurgery with hardware in their spine or for patients with infection or malignancy high on their differential.

A skilled interventional pain physician needs to synthesize the information provided by these various imaging modalities with the patient's history, as well as with a thorough physical examination, in order to properly diagnose the root cause of the patient's chronic pain. The most common pain diagnoses include degenerative disc disease, intervertebral disc herniation, spinal stenosis, facet joint arthropathy, and sacroiliac (SI) joint arthropathy.

The vertebral bodies are interconnected by intervertebral discs and supported by longitudinal ligaments anteriorly and posteriorly. Intervertebral discs comprise a central gelatinous nucleus pulposus, ringed by a fibrosis annulus. Discogenic pain develops by two mechanisms. The first is due to loss of disc height as the nucleus pulposus degenerates with advancing age or trauma resulting in reactive formation of osteophytes. This diagnosis is called degenerative disc disease. The second cause is due to protrusion of the nucleus pulposus posteriorly, causing direct compression of nerve roots, which is called intervertebral disc herniation. This most often occurs in the lumbar spine due to the posterior longitudinal ligament being thinnest at L2–5 [12].

Spinal stenosis occurs with advancing age, resultant of cumulative spinal changes that lead to progressive narrowing of the spinal canal. This pain is characteristically worsened with exercise or standing, and relieved with rest or sitting in anterior flexion. This pain often radiates from the low back into the buttocks and thighs, unilaterally or bilaterally, and can also present as neurogenic claudication. Stenosis of the neural foramen, resulting in unilateral radicular pain in a dermatomal distribution along the shoulder, arm, thigh, or leg, is classically referred to as neural foraminal stenosis. Diagnosis for both of these conditions can be confirmed by MRI, CT, or myelography [12].

Degenerative forces lead to pain at the zygapophysial joints, also known as facet joints, exhibiting a pain prevalence of 15–45% of chronic low back pain [12]. This pain is often near the midline, radiating into the shoulder in the cervical region and the buttock or thigh in the lumbar region. Facet loading, which is a physical examination maneuver involving hyperextension and lateral rotation of the facet joints, will reproduce the pain and provide insight to the physician that facet arthropathy is the most likely cause of the patient's pain. Facet joint pain can be treated with a local anesthetic injection surrounding the medial branch of the posterior spinal ramus or by an intraarticular injection into the facet joints [12].

The SI joint is the largest axial joint in the human body, linking the spine and pelvis, and can be influenced by pathologies in both the hip and the spine. SI joint arthropathy often affects the iliac side first where cartilage is the thinnest, then progresses to the sacral side [12]. This pain will be situated over the joint line and radiates to the buttocks or low back, provoked by prolonged standing or stair climbing. On physical examination, the affected SI joint is generally tender to palpation. Multiple provocative tests are used to elicit SI joint pain, including the FABER or Patrick's test, thigh thrust test, SI joint compression test, and Gaenslen's test.

Basic Pain Procedures

Epidural steroid injections (ESIs) are the most common procedure in pain medicine. They provide symptomatic relief for radicular pain associated with nerve root compression or discogenic etiology, and pain relief for claudication from mild to moderate spinal stenosis. Clinical improvement is thought to be due to resolution of inflammatory edema. Under fluoroscopic guidance and sterile conditions for the interlaminar approach, a needle is advanced into the epidural space using a loss of resistance technique targeted to the location of the patient's pain or pathology. Once the needle is engaged into the ligamentum flavum, the lateral view or contralateral oblique view is obtained, taking care to prevent insertion of the needle into the subdural or intrathecal space. Once loss of resistance is obtained, contrast is injected to ensure that the needle is not intravascular or intrathecal and indeed in the epidural space covering the expected pathology. The greatest benefit of pain relief is often achieved when medication is deposited as close as possible to the irritated nerve [13]. Cervical epidural steroid injections are higher risk than lumbar epidural steroid injections because the cervical region has increased vasculature, smaller epidural space, and closer proximity to the spinal cord. When cervical epidural steroid injections are done, often C7–T1 is targeted because, in general, it has the largest epidural space-to-cord ratio in the cervical region.

Transforaminal epidural steroid injections are also a good treatment for chronic radicular pain along a particular dermatomal pattern. They are thought to provide a more concentrated local distribution for radicular symptoms caused by the exiting nerve root irritation but can require multiple levels for optimal outcome. Considered relatively safe in the lumbar region, cervical transforaminal ESIs present higher vascular risks, most notably to the vertebral artery.

Caudal ESIs are commonly used to treat patients with lumbar radicular pain who have had previous lumbar neurosurgery, since the pain physician is unable to access the epidural space by the traditional lumbar approach. For this procedure, the epidural space is entered through the sacral hiatus with either a spinal or an epidural needle. The needle should not be advanced higher than the level of S3 in order to decrease the risk of dural puncture. Generally, higher volumes of injectate are used for this procedure and some physicians target the affected nerve root by advancing a catheter through the epidural needle to ensure the medication is deposited in the correct location. There is no agreed-upon volume or composition of injectate used for ESIs. However, in general, total volumes typically are 2–10 mL, depending on the specific location (cervical, lumbar, or caudal), and vary in composition with corticosteroid alone or a mixture of local anesthetic or saline [13]. Many will choose to use a nonparticulate corticosteroid (such as dexamethasone) to minimize the risk of spinal cord infarction or stroke [13].

The zygapophysial (facet) joints are innervated by the medial branches of the posterior rami of that level and the superior-level dorsal spinal nerve. Intraarticular facet joint injections can be done under fluoroscopy by injecting corticosteroid, with or without local anesthetic, into the joint. According to *Bonica's Management of Pain* (4th ed.), intraarticular facet injections have never been validated or shown to have therapeutic validity, yet they are still commonly used for patients by physicians in many chronic pain practices [14].

Medial branch blocks are diagnostic for facetogenic pain. If these blocks are positive for pain relief in a series of injections, patients are then typically treated with medial branch radiofrequency ablation to provide longer relief. Cervical medial branch blocks are normally performed unilaterally to mitigate the risk of vertigo, a potential side effect of the procedure. Medial branch blocks are typically provided at multiple levels during diagnosis, as a single block would provide minimal benefit. For medial branch blocks, the needle trajectory is perpendicular to the nerve, while maximal radiofrequency or neurolysis is achieved with parallel needle-to-nerve orientation. During medial branch blocks, contrast can be used to rule out venous uptake of anesthetic, minimizing a false negative diagnosis and giving a high confidence of concordant response.

Historically, chemical neurotomy with phenol or alcohol provided non-selective neuronal destruction via Wallerian degeneration. Cryoneurotomy has also been performed, utilizing compressed carbon dioxide through an electrode to freeze sections of the medial branch nerves [15]. Thermal lesions by radiofrequency ablation are most common today due to their safety and efficacy profile [15]. High-frequency alternating current administered through an insulated needle causes oscillation of intracellular ions, resulting in coagulation of the nerve at multiple sites, which provides a mean of 6- to 18-month relief [15].

SI joint pain contributes to a substantial proportion of patients with chronic low back pain. SI joint injections are both diagnostic and therapeutic for this type of pain. SI joint injections introduce a corticosteroid, plus or minus local anesthetic, into the joint to quell inflammation in the joint capsule or surrounding ligamental insertions. A needle is advanced from a medial point towards the inferior SI joint, under fluoroscopy, aiming for 1–2 cm superior to the inferior aspect. While SI joint injection with local anesthetic or steroid can provide reasonable short-term relief, the systematic evaluation of this duration of pain relief is heterogenous [16]. There is a limited, but growing, amount of evidence suggesting platelet-rich plasma injections may also provide durable relief for this type of pain [17].

Advanced Pain Procedures

As the field of pain medicine has evolved over time, physicians are more frequently treating their patients with advanced surgical procedures when conservative therapy, medications, and less invasive procedures have failed the patient. Since 1968, physicians have been using spinal cord stimulation (SCS) to treat persistent chronic pain that has failed with less invasive interventions. The first implantable SCS was developed in 1984, and the first rechargeable implantable pulse generator was developed in 2004 [18]. The basic understanding of SCS is thought to be the gate control theory. Stimulation of the large A-beta fibers of the spinal cord causes paresthesias at conventional frequency (50 Hz) and is thought to close the "gate" to pain transmitted to the small pain fibers, A-delta and C fibers [18]. New stimulation systems differ from conventional stimulation and are thought to be superior at treating different types of pain without generating uncomfortable paresthesias. This includes high-frequency stimulation, which can occur with up to 10 kHz, and burst stimulation, which is 500 Hz per burst pulsed at 40 Hz [18]. Studies have indicated that these newer stimulation frequencies treat patients by a different mechanism of action than traditional SCS. The field of SCS is constantly evolving by using different programs and frequencies to relieve pain and stimulate the spinal cord, although the full mechanism of action is unknown.

The most common indications for SCS are postlaminectomy syndrome, also known as failed back surgery syndrome, failed neck surgery, complex regional pain syndrome (CRPS), ischemic pain due to peripheral vascular disease, and peripheral neuropathies. Other indications that are not as common include postherpetic neuralgia, intractable angina, postthoracotomy syndrome, chronic urogenital pain syndromes, and chronic mesenteric ischemia [18]. When patients are offered SCS to treat these conditions, the physician explains the risks and benefits to the patients. Patients must also pass a psychological assessment test to evaluate the probability of successful outcome with SCS. This assessment gauges whether the patient has any psychological factors that may interfere with successful SCS [18]. If the patient passes this assessment, the physician goes forward with the spinal cord stimulator trial. The trial period, which generally lasts 3–10 days, is used to determine whether SCS will decrease pain and improve quality of life [18]. The trial is performed as an outpatient sterile procedure by the interventional pain physician. The lead is placed percutaneously with a sterile epidural needle into the epidural space. The lead is then secured to the skin once it is verified to be in the correct position under fluoroscopy. The patient uses an external battery for the pulse generator and should keep a log of their pain scores, functional status, and overall quality of life during the trial period [18].

If the patient has a successful spinal cord stimulator trial, the patient is scheduled for a permanent implantation of the device. A successful trial generally means the patient had both >50% pain relief and >50% improvement in quality of life during the trial. During permanent implantation of the spinal cord stimulator, the leads are again placed in the epidural space at the same spinal levels that were effective for the patient during the trial. The leads should be anchored to the supraspinous ligament to prevent lead migration. A subcutaneous pocket is then created for the implantable pulse generator (IPG), and the leads are tunneled through the subcutaneous tissue to the IPG and connected [18]. The most common sites for the subcutaneous pocket are the buttock and the abdomen.

Unfortunately, like all surgical procedures, side effects do occur during spinal cord stimulator placements. The most common side effects are infection and lead migration. Less common side effects are lead fracture, IPG failure, epidural hematoma, and seromas [18]. Fever and increased pain at the surgery sites are signs of infection. If this is the case, the leads must be removed and antibiotics must be prescribed in order to help prevent seeding of the infection to the spinal cord. In general, complication rates are low and decrease with advancing technology and increasing number of studies of SCS. Proper patient selection is the most obvious factor to ensure successful SCS.

Vertebroplasty and kyphoplasty are also advanced procedures that help treat vertebral compression fractures secondary to both osteoporosis and neoplastic lesions, including multiple myeloma and metastatic disease [19]. For both of these procedures, the fractured vertebral body is filled with various polymers or acrylic-based cement [19]. For both procedures, the trocar introducer is placed using either a transpedicular or a parapedicular approach. Kyphoplasty differs from vertebroplasty because the kyphoplasty procedure first involves inflation of a balloon in the vertebral body to create a space, so that the cement can be injected under lower pressure [19]. Vertebroplasty involves injecting the cement once the trocar is in the target space in the vertebral body directly, without a cavity created by a balloon, which creates a higher-pressure injection. Advantages of kyphoplasty over vertebroplasty are less chance of cement extravasation and a greater chance of restoring vertebral height, which, in turn, can improve pulmonary function [19].

With constant advances in medicine, more and more patients will be living longer and unfortunately will likely be suffering from chronic pain. To match this growing patient population, there are numerous investigations into new technologies, such as new stimulation frequencies for SCS, the development of peripheral nerve stimulation, and various other forms of minimally invasive treatment procedures to help treat this growing population. As physicians, we cannot underestimate the importance of the patient–physician relationship in providing our patients both empathy and hope for a better quality of life. Tailoring our approach and treatments to each specific patient is imperative to achieving successful outcomes.

References

1. Cohen SP. Epidemiology, diagnosis, and treatment of neck pain. *Mayo Clin Proc.* 2015;90:284–99.

2. Ferguson SA, Merryweather A, Thiese MS, *et al.* Prevalence of low back pain, seeking medical care, and lost time due to low back pain among manual material handling workers in the United States. *BMC Musculoskelet Disord.* 2019;20:243.

3. Vos T, Flaxman AD, Naghavi M, *et al.* Years lived with disability (YLDs) for 1160 sequelae of 289 diseases and injuries 1990–2010: a systematic analysis for the Global Burden of Disease Study 2010. *Lancet.* 2012;380:2163–96.

4. Shmagel A, Foley R, Ibrahim H. Epidemiology of chronic low back pain in US adults: data from the 2009–2010 National Health and Nutrition Examination Survey. *Arthritis Care Res.* 2016;68:1688–94.

5. Hoy D, March L, Brooks P, *et al.* The global burden of low back pain: estimates from the Global Burden of Disease 2010 study. *Ann Rheum Dis.* 2014;73:968–74.

6. Zhang T-T, Liu Z, Liu Y-L, Zhao J-J, Liu D-W, Tian Q-B. Obesity as a risk factor for low back pain. *Clin Spine Surg.* 2018;31:22–7.

7. National Institute of Neurological Disorders and Stroke. Low back pain fact sheet. Available from: www.ninds.nih.gov/Disorders/Patient-Caregiver-Education/Fact-Sheets/Low-Back-Pain-Fact-Sheet.

8. Last AR, Hulbert K. Chronic low back pain: evaluation and management. *Am Fam Physician.* 2009;79:1067–74.

9. Teichtahl AJ, McColl G. An approach to neck pain for the family physician. *Aust Fam Physician.* 2013;42(11):774–7.

10. Murgatroyd DF, Casey PP, Cameron ID, Harris IA. The effect of financial compensation on health outcomes following musculoskeletal injury: systematic review. *PLoS One.* 2015;10:e0117597.

11. Don AS, Carragee E. A brief overview of evidence-informed management of chronic low back pain with surgery. *Spine J.* 2008;8:258–65.

12. Mcguirk BE, Bogduk N. Chronic low back pain. In: JC Ballantyne, SM Fishman, JP Rathmell, eds. *Bonica's Management of Pain*, 4th ed. Baltimore, MD: Lippincott, WIlliams & Wilkins; 2010, pp. 1105–19.

13. Bogduk N. Epidural steroid injections. In: JC Ballantyne, SM Fishman, JP Rathmell, eds. *Bonica's Management of Pain*, 4th ed. Baltimore, MD: Lippincott, WIlliams & Wilkins; 2010, pp. 1423–36.

14. Curatolo M, Bogduk N. Diagnostic and therapeutic nerve blocks. In: JC Ballantyne, SM Fishman, JP Rathmell, eds. *Bonica's Management of Pain*, 4th ed. Baltimore, MD: Lippincott, WIlliams & Wilkins; 2010, pp. 1401–23.

15. Govind J, Bogduk N. Neurolytic blockade for noncancer pain. In: JC Ballantyne, SM Fishman, JP Rathmell, eds. *Bonica's Management of Pain*, 4th ed. Baltimore, MD: Lippincott, WIlliams & Wilkins; 2010, pp. 1467–84.

16. Hansen H, Manchikanti L, Simopoulos TT, *et al.* A systematic evaluation of the therapeutic effectiveness of sacroiliac joint interventions. *Pain Physician.* 2012;15: E247–78.

17. Singla V, Batra YK, Bharti N, Goni VG, Marwaha N. Steroid vs. platelet-rich plasma in ultrasound-guided sacroiliac joint injection for chronic low back pain. *Pain Pract.* 2017;17:782–91.

18. Benyamin R, Vallejo R, Cedeño DL. Spinal cord stimulation. In: L Manchikanti, AD Kaye, FJE Falco, JA Hirsch, eds. *Essentials of Interventional Techniques in Managing Chronic Pain.* Cham: Springer International Publishing; 2018, pp. 659–70.

19. Hameed H, Hameed M, Cohen SP. Vertebroplasty and kyphoplasty. In: H Benzon, SN Raja, SM Fishman, S Liu, SP Cohen, RW Hurley, eds. *Essentials of Pain Medicine*, 4th ed. Philadelphia, PA: Elsevier; 2018, pp. 639–46.

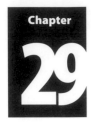

Chapter 29

Acute Pain Management

Farees Hyatali, Karina Gritsenko, and Kay Lee

Introduction

Pain is defined by the International Association for the Study of Pain (IASP) as "An aversive sensory and emotional experience typically caused by, or resembling that caused by, actual or potential tissue injury." Acute pain is defined as a normal, predicted physiologic response to an adverse chemical, thermal, or mechanical stimulus, which generally resolves within 1 month. There are a variety of techniques for the treatment of acute pain – via interventional procedures (such as peripheral nerve blocks and neuraxial interventional techniques), anesthetics, and analgesic and adjuvant medications. In this current opioid crisis era, most clinicians have adopted a multimodal approach to acute pain management to reduce the risk of opioid addiction, which generally includes a combination of interventional procedures, as well as administration of analgesics. This chapter deals with the comprehensive management of acute pain.

Anesthetics, Analgesics, and Adjuvants

Local Anesthetics

Local anesthetics have been commonly used in modern anesthesia practice in order to provide surgical anesthesia or analgesia in the perioperative period. Commonly used local anesthetic agents include chloroprocaine, lidocaine, mepivacaine, ropivacaine, and bupivacaine. They are generally administered via perineural, intrathecal, epidural, and intravenous (in the case of lidocaine) routes. They work by blocking the sodium channels on nerves, resulting in reduced propagation of nerve conduction, ultimately leading to both motor and sensory block. In addition, adjuncts to local anesthesia, such as epinephrine and dexmedetomidine, can prolong the duration of nerve blockade and will be discussed in further detail later in this chapter.

Recently, novel formulations of local anesthetics have allowed them to have a prolonged effect. These drugs were created in an effort to reduce both postoperative and, to a larger extent, total perioperative opioid use, with the aim to reduce the risk of postoperative opioid dependence and abuse. Liposomal bupivacaine was introduced with a lipid shell surrounding bupivacaine, which allows a slow release of bupivacaine, thus resulting in a delayed onset, but theoretically in prolonged nerve blockade. It was initially marketed to provide between 24 and 72 hours of pain relief. However, this has had a varied response among patients. Currently, this drug is only approved by the Food and Drug Administration (FDA) for interscalene brachial plexus blocks and field blocks. However, many clinicians have used this drug for off-label uses. More novel than this is HTX-011, a polymer of meloxicam and bupivacaine, with laboratory studies showing both drugs having a synergistic effect between the two drugs and possibly providing up to 72 hours of postoperative pain relief after surgery. Currently, this drug is undergoing clinical trials and has been used for buniectomy, herniorrhaphy, and total knee arthroplasty, and has been shown to reduce perioperative opioid requirements and reduced postoperative pain scores, when compared to the control.

Overdose of local anesthetics via epidural and intrathecal use can lead to a high block, resulting in hypotension and bradycardia, with possible cardiopulmonary collapse. If local anesthetics are administered in large enough quantities, local anesthetic systemic toxicity (LAST) may occur, especially if accidental intravascular administration occurs. Signs and symptoms of LAST include tinnitus, altered mental status, malignant ventricular arrhythmias, and respiratory depression, with severe cases leading to cardiopulmonary collapse. The American Society of Regional Anesthesia and Pain Medicine (ASRA) has a protocol for LAST and LAST-related events. Of all the local anesthetics listed, bupivacaine and ropivacaine are the most cardiotoxic of these. Care must be taken to avoid accidental intravascular administration.

Lidocaine, due to its short half-life and high hepatic extraction ratio and rapid clearance, is currently the only local anesthetic that can be administered via continuous intravenous infusion. Intravenous infusions of lidocaine have been used to reduce perioperative opioid consumption in patients who have difficulties in pain management, such as those with chronic pain syndromes and patients with a history of opiate abuse. Lidocaine infusion may be started pre-, intra-, or postoperatively, with continuous monitoring throughout the duration of the infusion for signs and symptoms of LAST.

Opiates

Opiates used for acute perioperative pain management include morphine, hydromorphone, fentanyl, buprenorphine, methadone, remifentanil, sufentanil, alfentanil, and ketamine. These medications can be administered via oral, intravenous, sublingual, intramuscular, and rectal administration. All of these medications provide excellent analgesia. However, numerous unwanted side effects, as well as significant abuse potential, have prevented successful management of perioperative pain due to secondary sequelae and patient dissatisfaction. Adverse side effects include nausea, vomiting, sedation, opioid-induced respiratory depression, opioid-induced constipation, opioid-induced pruritus, and urinary retention.

Morphine is the most commonly used opiate and was one of the first opiates utilized in clinical practice. It can be administered via numerous routes, with intravenous, intramuscular, and intrathecal, as well as oral, routes being the most popular. It is fast-acting and provides effective analgesia for patients. Intrathecal administration, especially in parturients, provides post-operative analgesia for cesarean sections for up to 24 hours and can also be used in intrathecal pumps in providing chronic pain management in cancer patients. Oral formulations are used to treat chronic pain, especially cancer pain in patients who have severe intractable pain.

Methadone is generally administered to patients who have a history of opiate abuse and are attempting to overcome their addiction. In addition, it can also be used as part of an anesthetic plan to reduce perioperative pain. This drug is generally administered orally or intravenously. Administration of methadone in particular can prolong the QTc interval and can lead to torsades de pointes, which may result in ventricular tachycardia and fibrillation in patients with a history of prolonged QT interval.

Remifentanil may be used as a continuous intravenous infusion at a low rate with a patient-controlled bolus, as part of patient-controlled analgesia (PCA) for acute pain management, in particular for parturients who are not candidates for neuraxial analgesia. Remifentanil is unique of all the opiates in that it has a very short half-life and a context-sensitive half-time of approximately 10 minutes, resulting in complete clearance of the opiate from blood. This is due to the fact that it is metabolized by red blood cell esterases which rapidly break down the drug in the bloodstream.

Sufentanil may be given by neuraxial administration or via an intravenous route (as a bolus or continuous infusion) for acute pain management. It is an excellent adjuvant in local anesthetic solutions for neuraxial analgesia, and has also been used as an adjuvant to prolong the duration of a spinal anesthetic when used for surgical anesthesia. However, it is associated with opioid-induced pruritus, nausea, and vomiting when used as an intrathecal adjuvant. Sufentanil when used as an infusion has a longer context-sensitive half-time, when compared to remifentanil, and care must be taken with regard to administration of large doses of this medication.

Ketamine is another commonly used analgesic in the perioperative period. It can be administered mainly via the intravenous (bolus or continuous infusion), intramuscular, oral, sublingual, and intranasal routes, and has its action on the N-methyl-D-aspartate (NMDA) receptor as an NMDA antagonist. Its use in pain management is generally by continuous infusion, as it reduces the perioperative consumption of opiates in patients, and is generally employed in patients who have difficulties in pain management, such as those who have chronic pain conditions, as well as patients with a history of opiate abuse.

Buprenorphine is another medication used in the perioperative period in patients with a history of opiate abuse. It is generally combined with naloxone to produce buprenorphine/naloxone (naloxone added to reduce the abuse potential of this drug). It is a partial opioid agonist that provides a ceiling effect with regard to analgesia and does not produce as much respiratory depression compared to more potent opiates. This drug is commonly used for withdrawal of opiates in those who have a history of opiate abuse and is generally administered as an oral formulation and, in some instances, as a transdermal patch for this purpose. In addition, it can be combined within local anesthetic solutions as an adjuvant due to the fact that it possesses some local anesthetic properties by blocking voltage-gated sodium channels and can thus be administered via the epidural or intrathecal route.

Meperidine is an opioid with an atropine-like structure with local anesthetic-like properties. Meperidine has been used intrathecally to prolong the duration of spinal anesthesia. However, it has unpleasant side effects, including opioid-induced pruritus, constipation, sedation, nausea, and vomiting. When compared to other commercially available opioids used as adjuvants in intrathecal local anesthetic solutions, meperidine has a greater rate of side effects. Currently, meperidine is most commonly used in the postoperative care unit for the treatment of postoperative shivering. In addition, intrathecal meperidine is associated with a decreased rate of postoperative shivering.

Tramadol is an opiate with both serotonin and norepinephrine reuptake inhibitor properties that can be given via oral, intravenous, intramuscular, and intrathecal administration. Side effects include increased risk of seizures in those with a history of seizures and increased risk of serotonin syndrome (especially in patients who take medications that increase serotonin levels). Intrathecal administration of tramadol, when compared to intrathecal fentanyl, for parturients undergoing cesarean section results in a prolonged duration of spinal block and a reduced incidence of shivering.

Hydrocodone has also been used for acute pain management, especially in the perioperative period. It is a powerful analgesic that is prescribed orally; it provides pain relief for a few hours and should be administered with care. Hydrocodone is generally combined with acetaminophen and is used as part of a multimodal pain regimen. Care must be taken in patients with compromised liver function, as well as in patients who have also been taking acetaminophen separately from this medication, as this can lead to liver toxicity.

Hydromorphone is another powerful analgesic used to treat moderate to severe pain, most commonly given via the intravenous and intramuscular, as well as oral, routes. Hydromorphone has a quick onset and a short duration of action, making it effective for titration in the perioperative period. Intravenous use is most commonly given in the perioperative period either in divided doses administered by healthcare personnel or as a patient-controlled infusion. It is used as part of a multimodal pain regimen, as the drug has significant side effects with a high risk of abuse potential.

Nonsteroidal Antiinflammatory Agents

These medications inhibit the cyclooxygenase (COX) enzymes, of which there are two main types related to pain – COX-1 and 2. These medications work by reducing inflammatory mediators that provide nociceptive pain. They provide excellent analgesia, especially when incorporated within a multimodal analgesia regimen. It must be noted that these particular agents have a ceiling effect with regard to analgesia. Side effects include nausea, vomiting, gastrointestinal bleeding, increased risk of cardiovascular disease (especially in COX-2-selective nonsteroidal antiinflammatory drugs (NSAIDs)), platelet dysfunction, and increased risk of bleeding and renal dysfunction. Most clinicians tend to avoid these medications in patients who have had a history of gastrointestinal bleeding and renal disease, in order to prevent worsening of the disease. As mentioned earlier in this chapter, meloxicam, an NSAID, has been combined with bupivacaine to produce an extended duration of analgesia.

Adjunct Medications

Alpha-2 Agonists

Dexmedetomidine and clonidine are two α2-agonists used in the perioperative period and can provide analgesia when utilized as part of a multimodal analgesic regimen for acute pain management. These medications can be administered via intranasal (dexmedetomidine), oral (clonidine), intravenous, perineural, and intrathecal routes. They act via receptors in the locus ceruleus in the brain and the dorsal horn in the spinal column, which reduces central perception of pain. These medications also reduce the release of norepinephrine, resulting in decreased sympathetic outflow. Side effects include xerostomia, nausea, vomiting, bradycardia, hypotension, and sedation. Dexmedetomidine, when given as a rapid bolus, may produce bradycardia with hypertension due to an α agonist effect on the vasculature, resulting in increased vascular tone. Clonidine, which may be used to treat essential hypertension, may produce rebound hypertension in the event of acute discontinuation.

Dexmedetomidine also is used in chronic withdrawal syndromes, as it can help patients withdrawing from opiates and alcohol via reduction in the sympathetic outflow that can occur as a result of withdrawal of these medications.

Epinephrine

Epinephrine is a common adjuvant used in local anesthetic solutions and can be administered via perineural, epidural, or intrathecal routes. Epinephrine is generally combined with lidocaine (or mepivacaine or bupivacaine) in order to create a dense block for surgical anesthesia. It also results in increased onset of block (in the case of lidocaine with epinephrine) and prolonged duration of the block (in perineural, intrathecal, and epidural routes). All these factors promote the use of lidocaine with epinephrine solutions in emergent cesarean sections to provide quick, effective, reliable surgical anesthesia. This is due to the fact that epinephrine causes vasoconstriction of the vasa nervorum that provide blood supply to the nerves and reduces blood flow to them, resulting in decreased uptake at the nerves. This has led to some controversy, as some laboratory studies have shown that epinephrine compromises the perfusion of nerves secondary to this vasoconstriction.

Epinephrine is also combined in local anesthetic solutions to allow an increased dose of local anesthetic with epinephrine to be administered without reaching levels of systemic toxicity (lidocaine 7 mg kg^{-1}, bupivacaine 3 mg kg^{-1}), as compared to solutions which do not have epinephrine (lidocaine 4 mg kg^{-1}, bupivacaine 2.5 mg kg^{-1}).

Furthermore, epinephrine is used as a marker of possible intravascular injection of local anesthetic agents. When combined with a local anesthetic, 10–15 μg of epinephrine administered intravascularly can produce an increase in the heart rate of >10 bpm from baseline or a systolic blood pressure of 15 mmHg or greater suggesting intravascular administration. This alerts the clinician that there is possible intravascular administration of local anesthetic and caution must be taken to prevent further such administration.

Steroids

In clinical practice, steroids have been used to prolong the duration of neuraxial as well as peripheral nerve blockade. For neuraxial anesthesia and analgesia, preservative-free dexamethasone and methylprednisolone are commonly used. For peripheral nerve blocks, preservative-free dexamethasone, when administered by intravenous injection or perineural administration, prolongs the duration of peripheral nerve blockade (motor blockade greater than sensory blockade). It is imperative that the steroid solution be free of preservative due to possible arachnoiditis (when administered intrathecally) and neuritis (when administered perineurally). In addition, in diabetic patients, dexamethasone has been shown to increase blood glucose levels; however, this has not been shown to be clinically significant in meta-analyses.

Gabapentinoids

Gabapentinoids are orally administered medications used to treat neuropathic pain. Gabapentin and pregabalin are the most commonly used in clinical practice, with the former being more popular than the latter. They produce centrally mediated analgesia by producing calcium channel blockade, leading to reduced propagation of nerve conduction. Side effects include nausea, vomiting, peripheral edema, dizziness, ataxia, and tremor. Caution must be taken in patients with kidney disease, as gabapentin can accumulate in renal dysfunction. Initially, gabapentin was used in multiple Enhanced Recovery After Surgery (ERAS) protocols, in particular in knee and hip replacement protocols. However, more recent meta-analyses have shown that gabapentin does not produce as much analgesia as initially thought and the risks of side effects weighed against benefits may prove to be more in favour of the former, rather than of the latter.

Selective Norepinephrine Reuptake Inhibitors

These drugs reduce the reuptake of norepinephrine and serotonins, and have their site of action at the locus ceruleus in the brain. They have been shown to be a useful adjunct in reducing both acute and chronic pain (used more frequently for chronic pain management). In particular, they have been useful in treating pain related to fibromyalgia and neuropathic pain, with venlafaxine. Side effects include nausea, vomiting, sweating, sexual dysfunction, dizziness, headache, and increased suicidal thoughts. Selective norepinephrine reuptake inhibitors (SNRIs) are contraindicated in patients who are currently taking monoamine oxidase inhibitors. Preexisting diseases, such as hypertension and coronary artery disease, should be managed prior to starting SNRIs, as these drugs can worsen symptoms and increase the progression of such diseases.

Tricyclic Antidepressants

These medications work by blocking sodium channels, resulting in reduced nerve transmission. These drugs have been used successfully in neuropathic pain, in particular in diabetic neuropathy and fibromyalgia. Of all tricyclic antidepressants (TCAs), amitriptyline has been shown to be the most successful as an adjunct in the treatment of diabetic neuropathic pain. Side effects of these medications include, but are not limited to, blurred vision, sedation, xerostomia, cardiac arrhythmias (especially widened QRS), and urinary retention. Treatment is with activated charcoal and sodium bicarbonate.

Magnesium

Magnesium has been used as an adjuvant in pain management via inhibition of NMDA receptors and calcium channels, ultimately resulting in an antinociceptive effect. It is generally given as an intravenous infusion and needs continuous monitoring, as magnesium toxicity is a serious, albeit rare, complication. It can also be given as an adjunct in local anesthetic solutions for regional anesthesia, especially in intravenous regional anesthesia, where a prolongation of the nerve block is desired.

Magnesium toxicity can manifest ranging from reduced deep tendon reflexes to cardiac conduction abnormalities and respiratory compromise. These risks are increased in patients who have renal dysfunction, as well as hypocalcemia.

Capsaicin

Capsaicin is a compound extracted from chilli peppers that has had some moderate success as an adjunct to pain. Its mechanism of action is related to stimulation of the transient receptor potential vanilloid subtype 1 (TRPV1) found on C fibers and Aδ fibers, which ultimately results in reduction and eventual depletion of substance P, a nociceptive neurotransmitter involved in pain and heat sensation. This medication is applied topically as a patch to the affected area, causing pain reduction. In some reports, it has been shown to provide up to 12 weeks of pain relief.

Interventional Procedures

Peripheral Nerve Blocks

Injections of local anesthetic, with or without adjuvant medications (such as dexamethasone, clonidine, dexmedetomidine, and epinephrine), can provide effective pain management in the perioperative period. Peripheral nerve blocks can be performed either as a single injection of local anesthetic with or without adjuvants, or as a continuous infusion of local anesthetic solution with or without adjuvant medications. Furthermore, these nerve blocks can be performed with either a nerve stimulator (where the nerve or nerve plexus is stimulated by a needle with a continuous electric current, and an injection of local anesthetic performed when the needle is deemed to be near the nerve or nerve plexus) or via an ultrasound-guided approach (where the needle is visualized directly under ultrasound guidance). Currently, the latter approach is preferred, as it allows the proceduralist to directly visualize the spread of local anesthetic around the nerve or nerve plexus, theoretically reducing the risk of intravascular and intraneural injection due to direct visualization, and ultimately reducing the risk of complications, compared to nerve stimulator-guided peripheral nerve blocks. Adjuvants are added to prolong the duration of the block in order to ultimately reduce the need for perioperative opioid consumption.

The selection of each nerve block is related to where the pain is located or, in the event that the block is administered prior to surgery, to the location of anticipated pain.

Table 29.1 lists the most common nerve blocks performed, the type of pain blocked, the dermatomes involved, and the surgical indication for each.

Table 29.1 Most common nerve blocks and their indications in the clinical practice of anesthesia

Peripheral nerve block	Type of pain blocked	Nerves blocked	Surgical indication
Interscalene	Somatic pain	C5–7	Shoulder surgery
Supraclavicular	Somatic pain	C5–T1	Upper extremity surgery
Infraclavicular	Somatic pain	C5–T1	Upper extremity surgery
Superior trunk	Somatic pain	C5–7	Shoulder surgery
Axillary	Somatic pain	C5–T1	Upper extremity surgery
Pectoral I and II	Somatic pain	T1–4	Chest wall surgery
Serratus anterior plane	Somatic pain	T2–5	Chest wall surgery
Transversus thoracis plane	Somatic and visceral pain	T2–6	Thoracic surgery, rib fractures
Paravertebral	Somatic and visceral pain	T1–L5	Thoracic and abdominal surgery
Transversus abdominis plane	Somatic pain	T10–L1	Lower abdominal surgery
Quadratus lumborum	Somatic and visceral pain	T10–L1	Lower abdominal surgery, hip and proximal femur
Erector spinae plane	Somatic and visceral pain	C7–L5	Thoracic and abdominal surgery, hip and proximal femur
Fascia iliaca	Somatic pain	L2–5	Hip and proximal femur
Lumbar plexus	Somatic pain	L1–5	Hip, femur, and lower leg
Femoral	Somatic pain	L2–4	Hip, femur, and lower leg
Obturator	Somatic pain	L2–4	Hip and femur
Sciatic (classic)	Somatic pain	L4–S3	Hip, femur, and lower leg
Sciatic (infragluteal)	Somatic pain	L4–S3	Hip, femur, and lower leg

Table 29.1 (cont.)

Peripheral nerve block	Type of pain blocked	Nerves blocked	Surgical indication
Sciatic popliteal	Somatic pain	L4–S3 (does not include the posterior cutaneous nerve of the thigh)	Lower extremity surgery
Adductor canal	Somatic pain	L3–4	Lower extremity surgery
Infiltration between the popliteal artery and capsule of the knee (iPACK)	Somatic pain	Small sensory nerves of the obturator nerve and sciatic nerve	Knee surgery

Contraindications to peripheral nerve blockade include patient refusal, infection over the procedure site, and true allergy to local anesthetics.

Neuraxial Interventional Techniques

Neuraxial interventional techniques can be a useful tool in acute pain management in the perioperative period to reduce the total consumption of opioids. Current techniques include epidural, spinal, and combined spinal epidural, performed in various parts of the neuraxis. Of all these techniques, epidural analgesia performed at the thoracic and lumbar levels are the most popular.

Thoracic epidural analgesia provides analgesia for the thoracic and upper to mid-abdominal dermatomes, and is useful for acute perioperative pain management in surgeries performed in thoracic and upper, as well as mid-abdominal, areas. Lumbar epidural analgesia provides analgesia for lower extremity dermatomes (see Table 29.2 for various uses of these techniques).

Spinal anesthesia is commonly employed for surgical anesthesia of the lower extremities and lower abdomen, and adjuvant medications, added to local anesthesia, such as dexmedetomidine, opiates, and clonidine, have reduced the need for postoperative opiate consumption due to potentiation of the local anesthetics. In addition, dilute local anesthetic infusions administered through epidural analgesia tend to have a small concentration of opiates (usually fentanyl, hydromorphone, and sufentanil) due to the synergistic effect of opiates on the substantia gelatinosa in the spinal cord, leading to reduction in the perception of pain.

Table 29.2 Comparison of thoracic and epidural analgesia for surgery and their surgical indications

Neuraxial technique	Type of pain blocked	Nerves blocked	Surgical indications
Thoracic epidural	Somatic and visceral	T1–12	Thoracic trauma (traumatic rib fractures), thoracic surgery (video-assisted thoracoscopic surgery, thoracotomy, esophagectomy, mastectomy, sternotomy), mid-abdominal surgeries (gastrectomy, Whipple procedure, hepatic surgery), lower abdominal surgeries (colectomy, abdominal perineal resection)
Lumbar epidural	Somatic and visceral	L1–5	Hip, lower extremity, orthopedic, and vascular surgeries

Side effects of neuraxial anesthesia include, but are not limited to, nausea, vomiting, urinary retention, and lower extremity weakness (especially in the case of lumbar epidural). If opiates are added to the local anesthesia administered via these routes, opioid-induced pruritus can also occur. In addition, the choice of using these techniques must be weighed against their possible side effects, as some ERAS protocols recommend patients ambulate without difficulty after surgery. As such, lumbar epidurals have recently fallen out of favour in lower extremity surgical procedures due to the unwanted side effect of lower extremity weakness, which can delay successful and effective physical therapy.

Contraindications to neuraxial interventional techniques include patient refusal, hemodynamic instability, true allergy to local anesthetic drugs, and active anticoagulation (guided by the anticoagulation guidelines from ASRA).

Conclusion

It is imperative that a pain management regimen, focusing on a multimodal approach involving various drugs, adjuvants, and interventional techniques, be implemented in order to reduce the risk of opioid dependence. One must consider the benefits and risks of each method of acute pain management and tailor the management to the patient, by considering their comorbidities, in order to provide safe and effective care.

Further Reading

Anand P, Bley K. Topical capsaicin for pain management: therapeutic potential and mechanisms of action of the new high-concentration capsaicin 8% patch. *Br J Anaesth.* 2011;107(4):490–502.

Batra RK, Krishnan K, Agarwal A. Paravertebral block. *J Anaesthesiol Clin Pharmacol.* 2011;27:5–11.

Desai N, Albrecht E, El-Boghdadly K. Perineural adjuncts for peripheral nerve block. *BJA Educ.* 2019;19:276–82.

Do SH. Magnesium: a versatile drug for anesthesiologists. *Korean J Anesthesiol.* 2013;65(1):4–8.

Grosu I, Lavand'homme P. Use of dexmedetomidine for pain control. *F1000 Med Rep.* 2010;2:90.

Kandil E, Melikman E, Adinoff B. Lidocaine infusion: a promising therapeutic approach for chronic pain. *J Anesth Clin Res.* 2017;8(1):697.

Schwenk ES, Viscusi ER, Buvanendran A, *et al.* Consensus guidelines on the use of intravenous ketamine infusions for acute pain management from the American Society of Regional Anesthesia and Pain Medicine, the American Academy of Pain Medicine, and the American Society of Anesthesiologists. *Reg Anesth Pain Med.* 2018;43(5):456–66.

Subedi A, Biswas BK, Tripathi M, Bhattarai BK, Pokharel K. Analgesic effects of intrathecal tramadol in patients undergoing caesarean section: a randomised, double-blind study. *Int J Obstet Anesth.* 2013;22(4):316–21.

Thobhani S, Scalercio L, Elliott CE, *et al.* Novel regional techniques for total knee arthroplasty promote reduced hospital length of stay: an analysis of 106 patients. *Ochsner J.* 2017;17(3):233–8.

Verret M, Lauzier F, Zarychanski R, *et al.* Perioperative use of gabapentinoids for the management of postoperative acute pain: a systematic review and meta-analysis. *Anesthesiology.* 2020;133:265–79

Wongrakpanich S, Wongrakpanich A, Melhado K, Rangaswami J. A comprehensive review of non-steroidal anti-inflammatory drug use in the elderly. *Aging Dis.* 2018;9:143–50.

Yu S, Wang B, Zhang J, Fang K. The development of local anesthetics and their applications beyond anesthesia. *Int J Clin Exp Med.* 2019;12:13203–20.

Anesthetic Emergencies

Eric Fried and Aaron Reagan

Introduction to the Emergent Patient

Many anesthetic emergencies can be avoided with constant vigilance. However, the most effective way to prevent an anesthetic emergency is through preparedness. Adopting a methodological approach to verifying drugs and dosages and ensuring that syringes are well labeled can prevent many emergencies. Preparedness is key because equipment will malfunction, difficult airways will be encountered, and emergencies will occur; however, multistep preparations can make all the difference during stressful situations. This chapter provides an overview of the intraoperative management of anesthetic emergencies, including a brief discussion of Advanced Cardiac Life Support (ACLS) as it applies in the operating room, and a guide to assessing an unstable intraoperative patient, and concludes with a survey of various intraoperative emergencies [1].

Advanced Cardiovascular Life Support

Circulation, Airway, and Breathing

Any intraoperative emergency can quickly become an intraoperative cardiac arrest. Accordingly, the anesthesiologist must be familiar with ACLS, especially as it applies to the operating room [2].

ACLS was initially developed for the resuscitation of patients found unresponsive, in contrast to patients in the operating room where the cardiac arrest is both witnessed, and sometimes predicted. Therefore, ACLS should be modified in the operating room, as discussed by Moitra *et al.* [2].

Although the management of cardiac arrest is similar both in and outside the operating room, there are unique considerations for the surgical patient. In contrast to the various causes of cardiac arrest outside the operating room, intraoperative cardiac arrests frequently stem from induced bradycardias, hypoxemia, and hypovolemia, whereas etiologies such as transmural myocardial infarctions (MIs) from plaque rupture are relatively uncommon [2].

Because many intraoperative emergencies require resuscitation, it is important to be aware of the priorities during resuscitation: circulation, airway, breathing. During an intraoperative emergency that has degraded into a cardiac arrest, the anesthesiologist must first assess the patient's circulation. If the patient is pulseless, chest compressions should be initiated immediately at a rate of 100–120 compressions per minute. If end-tidal carbon dioxide ($ETCO_2$) is present via an endotracheal tube (ETT), the anesthesiologist should target chest compressions to an $ETCO_2$ >10 mmHg, to ensure adequate circulation. Chest compression depth should be the lesser of 2 inches or one-third the anterior–posterior diameter of the patient [1]. While a noninvasive cuff can be used initially, an arterial line is preferred to allow for closer monitoring. The anesthesiologist should assess the ECG rhythm as soon as possible to identify whether there is a perfusing rhythm or if the rhythm should be cardioverted or defibrillated. Every anesthesiologist should be comfortable identifying arrhythmias and their individual management.

Once circulation is assessed, the anesthesiologist should turn to the airway and begin ventilation. The provider must assess the adequacy of ventilation and establish an advanced airway if noninvasive ventilation is inadequate. If an ETT is indicated, chest compressions should not be interrupted for >10 seconds at a time. Once an advanced airway is placed, a rate of one breath every 6–8 seconds should be administered, with caution to avoid hyperventilation [3].

Beyond the standard American Society of Anesthesiologists' (ASA) monitors, there are multiple monitoring modalities available to the anesthesiologist during an emergency. Perhaps the most important from a diagnostic perspective is the ultrasound, which allows the anesthesiologist to diagnose a number of conditions, including pulmonary pathologies (pneumothoraces, pleural effusions, hemothoraces), abdominal pathologies such as hemorrhage, and cardiac pathologies (acute valvulopathies, pericardial effusions, MI, ventricular failure). Another important monitoring modality is an arterial catheter, which is critical to trending and correcting blood gas abnormalities, monitoring blood pressure, and identifying/treating electrolyte abnormalities that may contribute to lethal arrhythmias.

After stabilization, obtaining additional information in the form of labs and imaging is of prime importance and the patient will need to be transported to either the postanesthesia care unit (PACU) or the intensive care unit (ICU). If the patient's surgery took place at an outpatient surgical facility, the facility may need to arrange for an ambulance to transport the patient to a nearby hospital.

Extracorporeal Cardiopulmonary Resuscitation

Patients presenting with sudden cardiac arrest or respiratory impairment refractory to conventional medical therapy may be candidates for extracorporeal membrane oxygenation (ECMO). However, there are currently no guidelines for when ECMO is indicated. The American Heart Association (AHA) recognizes that there is insufficient evidence to recommend the routine use of extracorporeal cardiopulmonary resuscitation (eCPR) for patients with cardiac arrest [4]. Accordingly, the use of ECMO during ACLS depends on institution-specific processes and procedures.

Intraoperative Emergencies Related to Anesthesia Practice

As previously mentioned, the initial response to intraoperative emergencies that progress to cardiac arrest is resuscitation. To help ensure a successful outcome, however, requires the anesthesiologist to address the underlying condition that precipitated the cardiac arrest. Below in Table 30.1 are a

Table 30.1 Hs and Ts adapted for anesthesia

Hs and Ts	Examples
Hypovolemia	Hemorrhage, anaphylaxis
Hypoxemia	Bronchospasm, laryngospasm, hemoptysis, pulmonary edema, main stem intubation, kinked endotracheal tube
Hydrogen ion	Malignant hyperthermia, shock, metabolic acidosis, renal failure
Hypothermia	Cold fluid administration, low ambient temperature, liver failure
Hyperthermia	Serotonin syndrome, thyroid storm, malignant hyperthermia, neuroleptic malignant syndrome, infection
Hypoglycemia	Insulin overdose, prolonged NPO time, abrupt discontinuation of TPN, liver failure, metabolic disease
Hypokalemia	Metabolic alkalosis, hyperventilation, excessive diuretic
Hyperkalemia	Inappropriate succinylcholine use, beta-blocker overdose, medication error, renal failure, hypoventilation
Pneumothorax	Iatrogenic, infectious, traumatic
Thrombus (PE)	DVT/PE, hypercoagulable state, air, fat
Thrombus – coronary	Acute coronary syndrome, air embolism
Toxins	Anaphylaxis/anaphylactoid or transfusion reaction, local anesthetic toxicity
Tamponade	Postoperative/iatrogenic, uremic pericarditis, infectious, malignant

NPO, nil *per os*; TPN, total parenteral nutrition; PE, pulmonary embolism; DVT, deep vein thrombosis.

few of the Hs and Ts discussed specifically in regard to the practice of anesthesiology.

Hypovolemia

Hemorrhage

(See also Chapter 13.) Despite excellent surgical technique and appropriate anticipation and preparation for intraoperative blood loss, mistakes happen, vessels are transected, and highly vascular organs are perforated. Hypovolemia reduces cardiac output and blood pressure, and if it is not recognized and treated, it can precipitate hemodynamic instability and cardiac arrest. Massive hemorrhage may require the activation of a massive transfusion protocol (MTP), defined as the allocation of four or more red blood cell units within 1 hour [5]. Early military research in this field stemmed from studies on the use of whole blood; however, today, a more common ratio of 1:1:1 of packed red blood cells, fresh frozen plasma, and whole blood-derived platelets continues to be used across the majority of trauma centers [6]. Research into the field of transfusion protocols, timing of triggering the MTP, and use of supplemental agents, such as antifibrinolytics or other factor derivatives, is ongoing, but each individual institution has its own transfusion triggers and protocols. Much of recent data focus not on the ratio of blood components, but on individualizing each MTP using data from rotational thromboelastometry (ROTEM) to predict which components are deficient and determine when normal coagulation has been achieved in order to minimize excessive transfusions [7, 8].

Hypoxia

Hypoxia and respiratory failure are frequent occurrences in monitored anesthesia care due to use of sedatives, hypnotics, and narcotics without a secured airway. The primary treatment for hypoxia in this setting is noninvasive and includes the use of jaw thrust, chin lift, oral/nasal airway, and placement of a supraglottic airway or an ETT. If hypoxia persists after the airway is secured, further investigation is required since the patient may be experiencing an issue other than airway obstruction, such as hypoxic delivery of oxygen, hypoventilation, shunt, ventilation/perfusion mismatch, or diffusion impairment.

Management of the difficult airway will be discussed in Chapter 2.

"H^+" Acidosis

Malignant hyperthermia (MH) is typically caused by an autosomal dominant mutation in RYR1 (ryanodine receptor, or less commonly, CACNA1S). MH susceptibility may also be inherited with various myopathies [9]. Exposure to triggering agents (volatile anesthetics and succinylcholine) results in the release of calcium from the sarcoplasmic reticulum of primarily myocytes, leading to a hypercatabolic and hypermetabolic state. Signs and symptoms include tachycardia, hyperthermia, hypercarbia, muscle rigidity, and metabolic acidosis. Treatment includes the following: removing the triggering agent, utilizing a charcoal filter (with hourly replacement), and replacing the ventilator circuit while maintaining high oxygen flow and minute ventilation to accommodate increased production of carbon dioxide [10]. If it is not possible to cancel the procedure, total intravenous anesthesia should be utilized. Dantrolene should be administered and repeated as frequently as necessary until $PaCO_2$, heart rate, and muscle rigidity are reduced. Bicarbonate should be considered for base excess (BE) <-8. Active cooling should be utilized. Dysrhythmias should be treated with caution, and calcium channel blockers should be avoided. Potassium levels should be monitored and hyperkalemia should be promptly treated. After the patient is stabilized, creatine kinase levels should be monitored (as they are a presumptive sign of rhabdomyolysis and myoglobinuria) [11].

Tension Pneumothorax

A pneumothorax is a collection of air or fluid between the parietal and visceral pleura, resulting in the compression of pulmonary and/or vascular systems. Tension pneumothorax refers specifically to a one-way inlet allowing for an acute compromise of the thoracic anatomical structures. A pneumothorax may present as an intraoperative emergency with hemodynamic instability and difficulty ventilating. Causes of a pneumothorax include penetrating chest trauma, iatrogenic injury during central line placement or peripheral nerve block, any other procedures near the lungs, or rupture of bullae. Alternatively, the accumulation of fluids (blood, lymph, or malignant effusions) may result in a hemothorax, chylothorax, or large pleural effusion, and cardiopulmonary resuscitation (CPR) causing rib fractures and perforation of the pleura [12]. A pneumothorax may present with dyspnea, pleuritic chest pain, tachycardia, tachypnea, and, in the case of tension pneumothorax, acute hemodynamic collapse. Identification of a pneumothorax in an anesthetized patient is more challenging, but the diagnosis should be considered when there is hemodynamic instability during abdominal or thoracic surgeries, elevated airway pressure, deviation of the trachea from the midline, decreased breath sounds, jugular venous distension, elevated airway pressures, loss of lung sliding on lung ultrasound, loss of comet tails or B-lines, and the presence of A-lines on ultrasound [13]. Treatment involves needle decompression. If needle decompression on the second mid-clavicular line is not effective, decompression on the fourth or fifth mid-axillary line (just cranial to the ribs) may be attempted. If neither of these relieves the obstruction, then conversion to open thoracotomy may be indicated. Regardless, tube thoracostomy should be performed following these maneuvers.

"Thrombosis"/Embolism

Emboli of various etiologies can occur intraoperatively or postoperatively, and cause hemodynamic instability. In this section, we briefly go through the commonly encountered emboli in anesthesia.

Pulmonary emboli (PEs) are divided into either massive or submassive, depending on the presence of hemodynamic instability. Clinically, only a massive PE is likely to be apparent to the anesthesiologist. Mechanistically, a blood clot, amniotic fluid, or fat embolism gets dislodged from the venous system and becomes wedged in the pulmonary vascular tree, increasing right ventricular (RV) afterload and causing RV dilation and reduced function, ultimately resulting in reduced cardiac output and potentially cardiogenic shock. Diagnosis depends on recognition of clinical signs and risk factors such as recent major surgery, high body mass index, use of contraceptive pills, immobility, etc. Treatment depends on the severity and stability of the patient and must take into consideration the risks and benefits of various treatment options. Treatment generally includes systemic anticoagulation, catheter-based thrombolysis, and an open-heart embolectomy.

Venous air emboli (VAEs) can occur in almost any procedure but is commonly seen in craniotomies, especially in the sitting position [14]. VAEs occur when room air is entrained with the venous system (typically when venous access is above the heart). Hemodynamic collapse can occur by obstructing the right ventricular outflow tract (RVOT), for which 100–300 mL of air is generally required [15]. Detection depends on the device utilized, but transesophageal echocardiography (TEE) is the most sensitive and capable of detecting 0.02 mL kg^{-1}. Clinically, there is an acute drop in $ETCO_2$ and arterial oxygen saturation, as dead space increases, dysrhythmias occur, and RV strain is seen on imaging. If VAE is suspected, the surgical field should be flooded with saline to minimize further entrainment. To maintain oxygenation and facilitate reabsorption of the entrained air, 100% oxygen should be administered. Aspiration from a pulmonary artery (PA) catheter may aid in reducing the volume of obstructing air by as much as 50%, and bilateral jugular venous compression should be applied to increase venous pressure, allowing for detection of sites of air entrainment and interrupting ongoing VAEs. Positional changes, such as left lateral decubitus and the Trendelenburg position, to decrease RVOT obstruction may be beneficial. The best treatment of VAEs is prevention, which can be achieved by meticulous line placement, patient positioning, and liberal use of bone wax, as the intramedullary venous system may be a possible source of VAEs [16].

Acute Coronary Syndrome

Acute coronary syndrome (ACS) refers to ST-segment myocardial infarction (STEMI), nonST-segment myocardial infarction (NSTEMI), and unstable angina. The Revised Cardiac Risk Index was created to identify patients most likely to have a major adverse cardiac event (MACE), including cardiac arrest, MI, or death, after surgery [17]. For the anesthesiologist, the diagnosis of myocardial injury under anesthesia may be complicated by the lack of usual presenting signs and symptoms. Intraoperative diagnosis is often made after observing hemodynamic instability, with ECG changes consistent with NSTEMI or STEMI if available; ultrasonography may demonstrate regional wall motion abnormalities consistent with myocardial ischemia, or PA catheters may demonstrate worsening myocardial function. In the event of intraoperative ACS, the primary goal is to optimize cardiac oxygen supply and demand, reducing the heart rate with a beta-blocker if hemodynamically stable and ensuring adequate blood pressure to ensure coronary perfusion. Pending no contraindication, anticoagulation should be initiated, and troponin and CK-MB labs obtained. A 12-lead ECG should be performed and the cardiology service should be consulted. If deemed appropriate, the patient should be taken to the cardiac catheterization lab for coronary angiography and possible intervention as soon as possible [18].

"Toxin"

Anaphylaxis, defined by the European Academy of Allergy and Clinical Immunology, as severe or life-threatening systemic hypersensitivity of multiple organ systems, often involving severe asthma and hypotension, is most commonly due to immunoglobulin E (IgE)-mediated release of histamine, tryptase, immunoglobulin G (IgG), complement, or immune complexes [19, 20]. Common intraoperative triggering agents include both depolarizing and nondepolarizing neuromuscular blocking agents (47.1%), latex (20%), and antibiotics (18%) [21]. Comparatively, anaphylaxis to sugammadex occurred with approximately the same incidence as with neuromuscular blocking agents [22]. Due to profound capillary leak and vasodilation causing hypotension and relative hypovolemia [23], anaphylaxis commonly presents with skin changes (urticaria, wheals, angioedema involving the face and oropharynx), hypotension, and hypoxia under general anesthesia. Treatment includes epinephrine, intravenous fluids, and removing the offending agent. Secondary treatment includes administration of steroids and histamine (H1 and H2) antagonists, such as diphenhydramine and famotidine, respectively. A serum tryptase level may be sent immediately to confirm the diagnosis of anaphylaxis [24].

Although blood product transfusion is often necessary, there are many potentially serious transfusion reactions that can occur, and thus the risks and benefits should be weighed before every transfusion. There are two transfusion reactions that may present as emergencies: hemolytic transfusion reactions and transfusion-associated anaphylaxis. The classic triad of a hemolytic transfusion reaction is fever, flank pain, and hematuria. Patients under general anesthesia will not demonstrate flank pain and may not demonstrate fever, and thus the first clue may be hematuria from hemolysis. Other common signs in the awake patient are chills, rigors, dyspnea, anxiety, and pain at the infusion site. If a hemolytic transfusion reaction is suspected, a direct Coombs' test can confirm the presence of an antibody to a major blood antigen (i.e., ABO mismatch). Other supporting tests include elevated levels of lactate dehydrogenase (LDH), creatinine, potassium, and hyperbilirubinemia, along with decreased haptoglobin levels. The suspected bag of blood product, along with a sample of the patient's blood, should be sent to the blood bank to confirm the possibility of a clerical error. Treatment for transfusion reactions is supportive, including halting the transfusion.

Anaphylaxis to blood components (most often platelets) [25], typically seen in those with an immunoglobulin A (IgA) deficiency, occurs when the patient is deficient in IgA and develops antibodies to IgA. It is recommended to administer washed blood products if the patient has known IgA antibodies, so the antibodies may be removed. The diagnosis of an anaphylactic transfusion reaction is established by demonstrating an IgA antibody in the patient's serum. See the anaphylaxis section of this chapter for diagnosis and management.

Local Anesthetic Systemic Toxicity

Local anesthetic systemic toxicity (LAST) will be covered separately in Chapter 7. In brief, LAST results from toxic plasma levels of local anesthetics, which can lead to altered mental status, seizures, and cardiac arrest. Unlike the other anesthetic emergencies discussed in this chapter, ACLS for LAST is different. LAST commonly results in cardiac arrhythmias and hemodynamic instability, but its management has unique considerations. Intralipid should be administered early. Local anesthetics, such as lidocaine, are frequently used for ventricular arrhythmias but should be avoided due to preexisting systemic toxicity. Furthermore, if LAST results in hemodynamic instability and cardiac arrest, epinephrine boluses should be minimized [26]. Ultimately, ECMO or cardiopulmonary bypass may be the only effective supportive treatment for LAST.

Tamponade

Cardiac tamponade is a clinical diagnosis referring to hemodynamic compromise from a large, hemodynamically significant pericardial effusion. Tamponade presents with clinical signs consistent with the equilibration of pressures in all four cardiac chambers due to a large effusion that limits expansion of the chambers. Large effusions are commonly caused by infectious, inflammatory, or malignant etiologies, trauma causing hemopericardium, myocardial contusion, or iatrogenic causes as occurs after cardiac surgery or percutaneous procedures [27]. The diagnosis is supported by the following clinical signs: jugular venous distension, hypotension, tachycardia, pulsus paradoxus, and a low-voltage ECG with electrical alternans [28]. Management of these patients includes ensuring euvolemia, which often requires the administration of volume to ensure that the heart is full, maintaining an elevated heart rate due to limited stroke volume, and maintaining afterload and systemic vascular resistance [28]. Invasive monitoring with an arterial line should be obtained for hemodynamic monitoring. Maintenance of spontaneous ventilation is preferred in these patients since positive pressure ventilation can precipitate further hemodynamic collapse [29]. Prior to induction, preparations should be made for rapid drainage of the effusion if hemodynamic collapse occurs with induction of anesthesia and initiation of positive pressure ventilation. Treatment includes evacuation of the pericardial effusion, via a drain or a pericardial window, and source control.

Summary

Anesthesiologists are occasionally faced with intraoperative emergencies that require rapid assessment of the clinical situation, differential diagnosis formation, and immediate action to prevent deterioration of the emergency into cardiac arrest. This chapter has reviewed many of the different anesthetic emergencies that an anesthesiologist might encounter and their management.

Review Questions

1. A patient arrives at an outpatient surgical facility for a procedure that is performed under monitored anesthesia care. The patient is brought into the operating room; standard monitors are placed, and the patient is induced. Shortly after induction, the blood pressure cannot be measured and the SpO_2 waveform disappears. A pulse cannot be palpated, and advanced cardiovascular life support (ACLS) is initiated. Unfortunately, the patient ultimately dies. According to the Anesthesia Patient Safety Foundation Closed Claims Project database for anesthesiologist-related lawsuits for death or brain damage, what is the most common cause of intraoperative death?

2. With a similar clinical presentation to malignant hyperthermia, which "toxin" can present with hypertension, arrhythmias, and elevated end-tidal carbon dioxide, and can be unmasked in the intraoperative period?

Answers

1. Death was the most common claim associated with monitored anesthesia care, and respiratory depression accounted for the greatest percentage (almost a quarter of claims). Oversedation, complicated by hypoxemia and hypercarbia, was the primary reason for respiratory depression. Cardiac events were the second most common [30].

2. The decompensated, severe form of hyperthyroidism is termed thyroid storm, which can occur with or without preexisting hyperthyroidism. It is triggered by trauma, myocardial infarction, surgery, or infection [31]. In some cases, acute exposure to excess iodine (such as iodinated contrast) may result in iodine-induced hyperthyroidism. For the anesthesiologist, presenting signs and symptoms include cardiac arrhythmias, hyperthermia, and hypertension. Increased thyroid hormone levels are common in thyroid storm. Treatment should be initiated promptly, targeting all steps of thyroid hormone formation, release, and action. These include antithyroid drugs, potassium iodide, beta-blockers, and glucocorticoids [32].

References

1. Panchal AR, Berg KM, Kudenchuk PJ, *et al.* 2018 American Heart Association focused update on advanced cardiovascular life support use of antiarrhythmic drugs during and immediately after cardiac arrest: an update to the American Heart Association Guidelines for Cardiopulmonary Resuscitation and Emergency Cardiovascular Care. *Circulation.* 2018;138(23):e740–9. [See Figure 2.]

2. Moitra VK, Gabrielli A, Maccioli GA, O'Connor MF. Anesthesia advanced circulatory life support. *Can J Anaesth.* 2012;59(6):586–603.

3. Sutherasan Y, Vargas M, Brunetti I, Pelosi P. Ventilatory targets after cardiac arrest. *Minerva Anestesiol.* 2015;81(1):39–51.

4. Panchal AR, Berg KM, Hirsch KG, *et al.* 2019 American Heart Association focused update on advanced cardiovascular life support: use of advanced airways, vasopressors, and extracorporeal cardiopulmonary resuscitation during cardiac arrest: an update to the American Heart Association Guidelines for Cardiopulmonary Resuscitation and Emergency Cardiovascular Care. *Circulation.* 2019;140(24):e881–94.

5. Hayter MA, Pavenski K, Baker J. Massive transfusion in the trauma patient: continuing professional development. *Can J Anaesth.* 2012;59(12):1130–45.

6. Eckel AM, Hess JR. Transfusion practice in trauma resuscitation. *South Med J.* 2017;110(8):554–8.

7. Unruh M, Reyes J, Helmer SD, Haan JM. An evaluation of blood product utilization rates with massive transfusion protocol: before and after thromboelastography (TEG) use in trauma. *Am J Surg.* 2019;218(6):1175–80.

8. Gonzalez E, Moore EE, Moore HB, *et al.* Goal-directed hemostatic resuscitation of trauma-induced coagulopathy: a pragmatic randomized clinical trial comparing a viscoelastic assay to conventional coagulation assays. *Ann Surg.* 2016;263 (6):1051–9.

9. De Wel B, Claeys KG. Malignant hyperthermia: still an issue for neuromuscular diseases? *Curr Opin Neurol.* 2018;31(5):628–34.

10. Cieniewicz A, Trzebicki J, Mayzner-Zawadzka E, Kostera-Pruszczyk A, Owczuk R. Malignant hyperthermia – what do we know in 2019? *Anaesthesiol Intensive Ther.* 2019;51(3):169–77.

11. Rosenberg H, Davis M, James D, Pollock N, Stowell K. Malignant hyperthermia. *Orphanet J Rare Dis.* 2007;2:21.

12. Childs SG. Tension pneumothorax: a pulmonary complication secondary to regional anesthesia from brachial plexus interscalene nerve block. *J Perianesth Nurs.* 2002;17(6):404–10; quiz 410–12.

13. Blaivas M, Lyon M, Duggal S. A prospective comparison of supine chest radiography and bedside ultrasound for the diagnosis of traumatic pneumothorax. *Acad Emerg Med.* 2005;12: 844–9.

14. Palmon SC, Moore LE, Lundberg J, Toung T. Venous air embolism: a review. *J Clin Anesth.* 1997;9(3):251–7.

15. Yeakel AE. Lethal air embolism from plastic blood-storage container. *JAMA.* 1968;204:267–9.

16. Sato S, Toya S, Ohira T, Mine T, Greig NH. Echocardiographic detection and treatment of intraoperative air embolism. *J Neurosurg.* 1986;64(3):440–4.

17. Schonberger RB, Haddadin AS. The anesthesia patient with acute coronary syndrome. *Anesthesiol Clin.* 2010;28(1):55–66.

18. Margolis AM, Kirsch TD. Tube thoracostomy. In: JR Roberts, ed. *Roberts and Hedges' Clinical Procedures in Emergency Medicine and Acute Care*, 7th ed. Philadelphia, PA: Elsevier; 2019, pp. 196–220.

19. Dhami S, Panesar S, Roberts, *et al.*; EAACI Food Allergy and Anaphylaxis Guidelines Group. Management of anaphylaxis: a systematic review. *Allergy.* 2014;69:168–75.

20. Johansson SG, Hourihane JO, Bousquet J, *et al.* A revised nomenclature for allergy. An EAACI position statement from the EAACI nomenclature task force. *Allergy.* 2001;56:813–24.

21. Dong SW, Mertes PM, Petitpain N, Hasdenteufel F, Malinovsky JM ; GERAP. Hypersensitivity reactions during anesthesia. Results from the ninth French survey (2005–2007). *Minerva Anestesiol.* 2012;78(8):868–78.

22. Miyazaki Y, Sunaga H, Kida K, *et al.* Incidence of anaphylaxis associated with sugammadex. *Anesth Analg.* 2018;126(5):1505–8.

23. Takazawa T, Mitsuhata H, Mertes PM. Sugammadex and rocuronium-induced anaphylaxis. *J Anesth*. 2016;30(2):290–7.

24. Schwartz LB, Metcalfe DD, Miller JS, Earl H, Sullivan T. Tryptase levels as an indicator of mast-cell activation in systemic anaphylaxis and mastocytosis. *N Engl J Med*. 1987;316:1622–6.

25. Gilstad CW. Anaphylactic transfusion reactions. *Curr Opin Hematol*. 2003;10 (6):419–23.

26. El-Boghdadly K, Pawa A, Chin KJ. Local anesthetic systemic toxicity: current perspectives. *Local Reg Anesth*. 2018;11:35–44.

27. O'Connor CJ, Tuman KJ. The intraoperative management of patients with pericardial tamponade. *Anesthesiol Clin*. 2010;28(1):87–96.

28. Khanna S, Maheshwari K. Hemopericardium and acute cardiac tamponade. *Anesthesiology*. 2018;128:1006.

29. Spodick DH. Acute cardiac tamponade. *N Engl J Med*. 2003;349(7):684–90.

30. Bhananker SM, Posner KL, Cheney FW, Caplan RA, Lee LA, Domino KB. Injury and liability associated with monitored anesthesia care: a closed claims analysis. *Anesthesiology*. 2006;104(2):228–34.

31. Leung AM. Thyroid emergencies. *J Infus Nurs*. 2016;39(5):281–6.

32. Alkhuja S, Pyram R. In the eye of the storm: iodinated contrast medium induced thyroid storm presenting as cardiopulmonary arrest. *Heart Lung*. 2013;42(4):267–9.

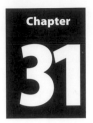

Chapter 31

Trauma Anesthesia

Amanda Frantz, Meghan Brennan, and Corey Scher

Trauma Patient Evaluation

A primary survey is performed immediately on admission to evaluate and treat life-threatening injuries such as hemorrhage, airway, and brain injuries. Hemorrhage leads to 40% of trauma-related deaths, particularly in the first 24 hours. Thromboelastography (TEG), rotational thromboelastometry (ROTEM), complete blood count, fibrinogen, prothrombin time (PT), activated partial thromboplastin time (aPTT), and international normalized ratio (INR) should be obtained to evaluate coagulation targeted to obtain clot stability [1]. It is also essential to measure renal and liver function, as both affect coagulation and drug elimination [2].

Hemostasis and the Coagulation Cascade

The vascular endothelium is designed to regulate blood flow and plays an active role in hemostasis to induce thrombosis and activate the coagulation cascade. Intact vasculature is lined by the endothelial glycocalyx (EGC), a supportive layer of glycoproteins, glycosaminoglycans, and proteoglycans. It supports vascular permeability, fluid homeostasis, immunomodulation, and hemostasis [3, 4]. Hemostasis is achieved by activating the cascade of the intrinsic and extrinsic pathways, platelet activation, and disruption of the vascular endothelium.

Primary hemostasis is initiated by tissue trauma exposing the vascular endothelium and disrupting the EGC. Sheer stress on the endothelium results in increased release and binding of circulating von Willebrand factor (vWF) on its surface to glycoproteins on the exterior of platelets. After binding to the endothelium, platelets release hormones and proinflammatory substances, inducing platelet aggregation and initial clot formation.

The clotting cascade is set in motion by the extrinsic pathway, commonly known as the tissue factor (TF) pathway, and the intrinsic pathway, also known as the contact activation pathway (CAP). Trauma and the resultant exposure of TF lining the vasculature lead to binding and activation of factors V and VII, further propagating the coagulation cascade. Factor VII encounters TF, forming a complex that initiates the extrinsic pathway via conversion of factors IX and X to their activated forms.

Fibrinogen, an acute phase glycoprotein synthesized in the liver, is the precursor to fibrin, a key factor in the coagulation cascade. Activated factors IXa and Xa generate thrombin, which converts fibrinogen into fibrin, leading to further clot propagation and stabilization [5, 6]. Fibrin is necessary for clot strength and stability, prevention of fibrinolysis, and promotion of platelet aggregation [7].

The CAP begins with collagen exposure on the basement membrane of damaged blood vessels, forming another elaborate complex with factor XII and other inflammatory markers and progressing towards the common pathway. Minimal fibrin is formed via this route; therefore, it is less important for secondary hemostasis [5]. Both coagulation routes converge into the common pathway, which is initiated by factor X.

Coagulopathy in Trauma

Coagulopathy in trauma patients is multifactorial. Extrinsic factors are activated in traumatic brain injury, acidosis, inflammation, hypothermia, and consumptive coagulopathies. Traumatic injury, hypoperfusion, and tissue damage result in trauma-induced coagulopathy (TIC). This condition affects approximately 25–30% of trauma patients and is directly related to the Injury Severity Score (ISS) [8]. Risk factors for the development of TIC include a base deficit <-6 mEq L^{-1}, temperature $<35°C$, prehospital crystalloid administration, and head injuries (Glasgow Coma Scale score <6) [4, 9, 10]. TIC occurs at the onset of traumatic injuries, as patients exhibit prolonged PT and partial thromboplastin times immediately following the event prior to the start of resuscitation [8]. These patients have higher transfusion requirements, longer hospital lengths of stay, higher incidences of organ dysfunction, and up to four times higher overall mortality risks [4]. The mechanisms behind TIC are not fully understood but likely stem from a combination of tissue injury and the resulting endothelial and EGC dysfunction causing an impaired coagulation response, combined with a hyperfibrinolytic state.

Tissue injury, sympathetic upregulation, inflammation, and hypoperfusion result in disruption and breakdown of the vascular endothelium and EGC [8, 11–13]. Consumptive coagulopathy is directly proportional to the amount of tissue injured, and can worsen factor depletion and exaggerate hypofibrinogenemic states [14]. EGC breakdown leads to an increase in cellular expression of glycoproteins, thrombomodulin (TM), and endothelial protein C receptors. With less extensive injury, there is local release of thrombin, which binds to TM. The thrombin–TM complex then binds to, and activates, protein C. In severe trauma, there is a large systemic, rather than local, release of thrombin. This creates more thrombin–TM complexes to accelerate activated protein C (APC) activity, which has multiple pathways to function as an anticoagulant. The rapid rise in APC leads to coagulopathies by inactivating factors Va and VIIa, which aid in clot formation [3, 15, 16].

Severe trauma leads to a hyperfibrinolytic state due to initial upregulation of plasmin through thrombin release, as well as tissue ischemia. This state results in an increased release of tissue plasminogen activator. APC additionally inactivates plasminogen activator inhibitor-1, leading to an overall increase in plasmin and subsequent fibrinolysis [3, 16]. Trauma patients with elevated APC levels have been found to have higher fibrinolytic activity, lower fibrinogen levels, higher transfusion rates, longer hospitalizations, and higher mortality [10, 16]. An early treatment of hyperfibrinolysis is use of tranexamic acid (TXA), a lysine analog that functions as an antifibrinolytic in patients who are bleeding, preventing clot breakdown by inhibiting plasmin. The CRASH-2 trial found no evidence of increased thromboembolic events with the use of antifibrinolytics in trauma and a decrease in blood loss with a reduced need for blood product transfusions [17]. The recommended dosing for TXA in the trauma patient varies from a fixed dose of 1 g every 8 hours. Other guidelines promote weight-based doses ranging from 2.5 to $100 \, \text{mg} \, \text{kg}^{-1}$, with varying administration periods ranging from 1 to 12 hours [2, 17]. Two other drugs that function in this class of antifibrinolytics are aminocaproic acid and aprotinin [17].

Another source of coagulopathy is "auto-heparinization" that occurs in severe traumatic injuries. Damaged vasculature leads to shedding and release of endogenous heparin sulfates that make up the EGC [11–13]. "Auto-heparinization" has been documented in TEG and ROTEM studies seen with prolonged reaction time (R-time) or clotting time (CT).

The combination of hemodilution, hypothermia, and acidosis are referred to as the trauma triad. Acidosis, defined as a pH of <7.2, hypothermia with temperatures lower than 36°C, and hemodilution from prehospital crystalloid administration frequently occur together and contribute to this coagulopathic phenomenon. Mild hypothermia of 34–36°C typically does not result in clinically significant coagulation derangements. However, when a patient's temperature is lower than 32–34°C, thrombin generation, fibrinogen production, and platelet function are reduced and bleeding risk becomes clinically significant [9, 14, 18]. Effects of hypothermia may not be evident on viscoelastic testing, as samples are warmed to 37°C. To combat hypothermia, trauma rooms should be warmed, with readily available fluid warmers and forced air warming devices. Correction of these metabolic or respiratory derangements is necessary for coagulation enzymes to function properly, using ventilator adjustments on intubated patients, as well as administration of medications containing bicarbonate to raise the pH. Crystalloid resuscitation-induced coagulopathy occurs due to further injury and breakdown of the EGC, existing clots, hemodilution, and immunomodulation [9]. Dilutional coagulopathy is inversely proportional to clot strength, factor availability, and time to initiation of clot formation [14]. Balanced crystalloid solutions are recommended because large volumes of normal saline create hyperchloremic metabolic acidosis [9].

Hypercoagulability of Trauma

After an initial TIC, patients are at risk of becoming hypercoagulable and are at higher risk of thromboembolic events. Up to 80% of trauma patients may develop deep vein thrombosis (DVT), and up to 20% may form pulmonary embolism. Some may be hypercoagulable on admission, which can be detected with a short TEG R-time, elevated TEG maximum amplitude (MA), and alpha angle. Contributing factors include endothelial injury, upregulation of inflammatory factors, increased platelet and factor activation, venous stasis, and a shift to a hypofibrinolytic state after the initial trauma [19]. Risk increases as the ISS increases, as well as with head injuries, pelvic and lower extremity fractures, age, longer surgical procedures, and prolonged immobilization [20, 21]. Patients are at an increased risk of thromboembolic events as long as 3 months after the initial traumatic injury [21].

Pharmacologic prophylaxis is the most effective preventative measure against thromboembolic events in trauma patients. Unless there is a contraindication, low-molecular weight heparin is currently recommended by the Eastern Trauma Association for DVT prophylaxis because it is associated with the lowest mortality from thromboembolic events [21]. Unfractionated heparin and fondaparinux, a factor Xa inhibitor, have also been proved for use in DVT prophylaxis in trauma patients. Mechanical prophylaxis with graduated compression stockings, pneumatic compression stockings, and vena cava filters can be used in conjunction with pharmacologic prophylaxis or as a substitute in cases where patients cannot receive pharmacologic prophylaxis [21].

Anticoagulation

Anticoagulants are prescribed for patients with thrombotic diseases, mechanical heart valves, and stent placement, and for treatment of acute or chronic venous thrombosis and stroke prevention in patients with atrial fibrillation. If the patient also suffers traumatic injuries, these medications lead to increased blood loss. In addition to evaluating injuries, it is essential to obtain the patient's medical history, identify the disease process necessitating anticoagulation, and determine the timing of their last medication dose to appropriately weigh the risks and benefits of anticoagulation reversal [2].

The varying pharmacokinetics of each anticoagulant, in combination with the patient's bleeding risk and medical comorbidities, determine whether a reversal agent or a specific blood product is required. For example, in a patient with a recent cardiac stent taking dual antiplatelet medications, platelet administration may increase the risk of stent thrombosis. If their bleeding risk from trauma is low, reversal is likely not indicated; however, it may be lifesaving if they suffer significant traumatic injuries or head injuries. In addition to antiplatelet medications blocking cyclooxygenase 1 and 2 and preventing platelet aggregation, factor inhibition can range from vitamin K antagonists (VKAs) to direct oral anticoagulants (DOACs). These medications impede specific components of the coagulation cascade, such as direct thrombin or factor Xa inhibitors. Warfarin is a commonly used VKA that was prescribed for prophylaxis against stroke in 2010 to over 30 million patients with atrial fibrillation [5]. DOACs are now more commonly used than VKAs due to reduced risk of life-threatening bleeds and ease of perioperative management [22].

Patients taking these medications will have abnormal diagnostic labs. A prolonged aPTT is indicative of drugs or other coagulopathies affecting factors of the intrinsic pathway. Factor II inhibitors, such as dabigatran, can also prolong aPTT times [5]. The extrinsic pathway, measured with PT and INR, is affected by warfarin and factor Xa inhibitors, such as rivaroxaban. Drug-specific assays, such as antifactor Xa, cannot be obtained within the time needed to treat a trauma patient during primary resuscitation [5, 22].

TEG and ROTEM

TEG (TEG® analyzer 5000 and TEG® 6s, Haemonetics Corporation, Boston, MA) and ROTEM (ROTEM® analyzer systems, Instrumentation Laboratory, Bedford, MA) are point-of-care whole blood functional assay tests of clot formation that guide goal-directed blood product and factor replacement. TEG and ROTEM provide rapid results and have been proven effective at identifying trauma-related coagulopathies [23]. Both tests measure phases of clot formation and degradation, producing electric signals that are transformed into the graph shown in Figure 31.1.

TEG R-time in minutes is the time from test start to clot formation and the strength that produces a 2-mm amplitude reading. R-time is related to initial clot formation and is prolonged in deficiencies of factors II, VII, VIII, X, and XII. R-time is best corrected with administration of fresh frozen plasma (FFP), prothrombin complex concentrate (PCC), or factor concentrates. TEG K-time, in minutes, is the time from onset of R-time to the time of clot formation and strength producing a 20-mm amplitude reading. K-time is related to continued clot formation and strength. A prolonged K-time is best corrected with administration of cryoprecipitate or fibrinogen concentrate (FC) [24]. The TEG alpha angle, reported in degrees, is a measurement of clot strength related to fibrinogen cleavage and fibrin cross-linking. If the angle is below the normal range, it is best to replace with cryoprecipitate or FC. The TEG MA is a measurement of the maximum clot strength [25]. The MA contains 80% platelets and 20% fibrinogen.

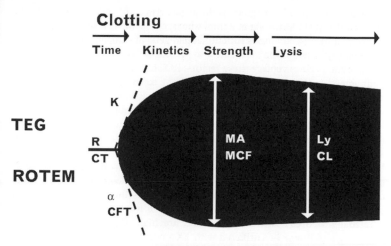

Figure 31.1 Schematic thromboelastography (TEG, upper part)/rotational thromboelastometry (ROTEM, lower part) trace, indicating commonly reported variables: reaction time (R)/clotting time (CT), clot formation time (K, CFT), alpha angle (α), maximum amplitude (MA)/maximum clot firmness (MCF), and lysis (Ly)/clot lysis (CL). Source: Reprinted under CC BY 2.0 (https://creativecommons.org/licenses/by/2.0/) from Johansson PI, Stissing T, Bochsen L, *et al*. Thrombelastography and tromboelastometry in assessing coagulopathy in trauma. *Scand J Trauma Resusc Emerg Med*. 2009;17:45.

If the MA is below normal, platelets are usually the problem. TEG lysis is measured at 30 minutes (LY30) and reported as a percentage of clot fibrinolysis. If this factor is elevated, it is best corrected with antifibrinolytics such as TXA or, less frequently, aminocaproic acid. TEG studies may also be completed in patients who have received heparin, using heparinase to correct the anticoagulant. Platelet mapping TEGs are available to assess coagulation and platelet function if there is a concern for platelet inhibition from antiplatelet medications [26].

ROTEM measures and reports parameters similar to those of TEG. ROTEM CT is the time in seconds from the start of the test to the time when the clot reaches an amplitude of 2 mm. In general, an increased time indicates a factor deficiency [27]. Prolonged EXTEM CT can be corrected with plasma, unless volume restriction is necessary. PCCs are used in that scenario.

ROTEM clot formation time (CFT) is the time in seconds from the start of the clot reaching 2 mm to when it reaches 20 mm. CFT is related to the speed and strength of clot formation, and may be best corrected with plasma, cryoprecipitate, or PCC. If CFT is short, it may indicate a hypercoagulable state [25]. ROTEM alpha angle, measured in degrees, is the angle between 0° and the tangent to the point on the ROTEM tracing at 2 mm, which reflects the rate of clot formation.

The alpha angle requires functional platelets, fibrinogen, and factor VIII. If the angle is high, it may indicate a hypercoagulable state. A low value may indicate the need to replace these factors. ROTEM amplitude of 10 (A10), in millimeters, is the amplitude of the ROTEM tracing measured 10 minutes after CT. A low value indicates a problem with clot formation and strength, which may be corrected with platelets or products containing fibrinogen [27]. ROTEM maximum clot firmness (MCF), in millimeters, is the MA of the ROTEM tracing during the test. Similar to A10, MCF reflects clot formation and strength, and can be corrected with fibrinogen-containing products. ROTEM lysis index 30 (LI30) is the clot lysis rate, measured as a percentage, calculated 30 minutes after CT by using the amplitude firmness at that time divided by MCF. ROTEM maximum lysis (ML) is the maximum clot lysis during the test, which is calculated as the MA of the ROTEM measured as a percentage of MCF. If both parameters are high, increased fibrinolysis is occurring and it may be corrected with TXA administration [18, 25].

Reversal of Anticoagulation

Warfarin reversal depends on the presence of a life-threatening bleed and INR level. Vitamin K is administered to reverse the effects of warfarin, with peak effects 4–6 hours after intravenous administration. If bleeding is not present, the oral route can be used, with INR levels decreasing 24 hours after administration [5]. Warfarin inhibits vitamin K epoxidase, which depletes factors II, VII, IX, and X and downregulates the production of proteins C and S [5]. Irrespective of the anticoagulation status, during a life-threatening bleed, the trauma patient should be appropriately resuscitated with blood products and other intravascular fluids to provide supportive care. FFP contains all clotting factors, as well as vWF, fibrinogen, and other proteins. The INR of FFP is 1.5 and no clinical benefits have been shown with an INR of 1.7 or less, with a slow onset of action of 13–48 hours after its administration [5].

Blood product transfusions carry the risk of infectious pathogens, transfusion-related acute lung injury (TRALI), transfusion-associated circulatory overload (TACO), and allergic reactions [6]. By administering vitamin K coagulation factors through either three or four PCCs, many of the above complications can be avoided, with an onset of action within 10–30 minutes. Use of FFP to reverse VKAs provides a transient benefit when PCC is not available [28].

Current recommendations for reversal of various agents are in flux due to innovative recombinant factor development and lack of comparison trials to evaluate full efficacy, compared to allogeneic transfusion, in the trauma cohort. Table 31.1 reviews the current recommendations of various anticoagulants and their reversal strategies.

Table 31.1 Anticoagulant recommendations and reversal strategies

Drug name	Mechanism of action	Elimination half-ife	Route of administration	Reversal agent	Mechanism of action of reversal
Fondaparinux	Pentasaccharide, factor Xa inhibitor	17–21 hours	Oral, IV, SC	Andexanet, recombinant factor VIIa[a], aPCC[b], ciraparantag	Recombinant factor Xa binder or factor VIII inhibitor bypassing activity
Heparin	Binds to, and activates, antithrombin III, indirect thrombin inhibitor	1 hour	IV, SC	Protamine	Neutralizes factor Xa activity
Coumadin	Vitamin K epoxidase inhibitor	40 hours	Oral	Vitamin K (oral or IV), PCC	Supplies substrate for blocked factors, while PCC directly supplies factors
Enoxaparin Dalteparin	Form a complex with antithrombin III to inhibit factor Xa and indirectly factor II	3–6 hours	SC	Protamine (60% reversal)	Neutralize factor Xa activity
Dabigatran	Direct thrombin (factor IIa) inhibitor	13 hours	Oral	Idarucizumab, PCC, aPCC[b], hemodialysis	Monoclonal antibody that binds free dabigatran and bound factor IIa complex
Bivalirudin	Direct thrombin (factor IIa) inhibitor	25 minutes	IV	None	Off-label use of FEIBA and aPCC
Argatroban	Direct thrombin (factor IIa) inhibitor	45 minutes	IV	None	Off-label use of FEIBA and aPCC

Table 31.1 (cont.)

Drug name	Mechanism of action	Elimination half-life	Route of administration	Reversal agent	Mechanism of action of reversal
Rivaroxaban Apixaban Edoxaban Betrixaban	Competitive, reversible factor Xa inhibitors	5–9 hours 12 hours 10–14 hours	Oral	Andexanet alfa, PCC, aPCC, activated charcoal	All with minimal evidence of efficacy
Aspirin	COX-1 and COX-2 inhibitor	20 minutes	Oral	DDAVP, platelets for neurosurgical intervention	Increases the release of endogenous factor VIII to enhance platelet adhesion
Clopidogrel Prasugrel Ticlopidine	Irreversible inhibitors of P2Y12 ADP receptor on platelets	6–8 hours 2–15 hours 12 hours	Oral	DDAVP	Increase the release of endogenous factor VIII to enhance platelet adhesion
Ticagrelor	Reversible inhibitor of P2Y12 ADP receptor	7 hours	Oral	DDAVP	Increases the release of endogenous factor VIII to enhance platelet adhesion
Dipyridamole	Reversible adenosine reuptake inhibitor	10 hours	Oral	DDAVP	Increases the release of endogenous factor VIII to enhance platelet adhesion

[a] Not FDA approved.

[b] Activated PCC → factor VII inhibitor bypassing activity (FEIBA).

IV, intravenous; SC, subcutaneous; aPCC, activated prothrombin complex concentrate; PCC, prothrombin complex concentrate; COX-1, cyclooxygenase 1; COX-2, cyclooxygenase 2; ADP, adenosine diphosphate.

Transfusion in Trauma

Massive transfusion protocols (MTPs) and transfusion guidelines vary by institution but are used to reduce overall need for transfusion, complications related to transfusion, and blood product waste [1]. For major hemorrhage, the American College of Surgeons Trauma Quality Improvement Program recommends 1:1:1 or 1:2:1 for packed red blood cells (PRBCs), plasma, and platelets, respectively. Plasma derivatives used in transfusion medicine are FFP, thawed plasma, solvent detergent plasma, and plasma frozen within 24 hours [28]. With a 1:1 ratio of FFP to PRBCs in the massive transfusion group, current evidence shows that use of nonfactor-specific allogeneic transfusions can promote hemostasis and improve platelet function due to extensive EGC damage [28]. FFP can be used to replace albumin, coagulation factors, immunoglobulins, and lipids, along with other proteins, to promote thrombus formation. Military studies have advocated for higher ratios of cryoprecipitate with MTPs, with a limiting factor of 30 minutes of thawing time to administration of transfusion [28]. Recommended point-of-care testing using TEG, ROTEM, or FIBTEM A10, along with the Clauss assay, in the actively bleeding patient enables assessment of overall coagulation and functional fibrinogen levels [1, 6].

Guidelines for administration of blood products and factor concentrates are based on expert consensus due to a lack of prospective trials. Early fibrinogen administration in the bleeding trauma patient is key to successfully treating TIC and other coagulopathies in the early resuscitation phase. Fibrinogen can be replaced with plasma, FC, or cryoprecipitate [16]. Plasma contains approximately 2 g L^{-1} of fibrinogen; cryoprecipitate contains 10–20 g L^{-1}, and FC contains 20 g L^{-1} [6]. The goal is contested, but most studies target serum fibrinogen levels of 1.5–2.0 g L^{-1} in the bleeding trauma patient [6, 7, 29]. Other European pilot studies, including the early fibrinogen concentrate therapy for major haemorrhage in trauma (E-FIT 1) pilot trial, have increased the goal to >2 g L^{-1} in major hemorrhage patients, without an increase of thromboembolic events [29]. If fibrinogen levels are <1.5 g L^{-1} or qualitative studies show decreased fibrinogen on admission, the patient has a higher risk of a need for large volumes of blood products and increased mortality [6]. While the critically low concentration threshold is debated in the trauma population, goals have been increased from 1.0 g L^{-1} as an acceptable level.

In certain instances, using plasma to achieve target fibrinogen levels can lead to volume overload [6, 29]. Cryoprecipitate is an allogeneic blood derivative used to increase fibrinogen levels, and also contains factors VIII and XIII, fibronectin, immunoglobulins, and vWF [16]. It is outside of mainstream transfusion therapy to use FC solely to correct levels; however, it bypasses the time needed to crossmatch and thaw products, as well as decreases the risk of viral transmission to 1 in 31,000 doses due to the pasteurization process [6].

FC can be stored at room temperature for up to 5 years and contains 1 g of fibrinogen, as well as albumin and L-arginine [14]. Institutions in Europe have begun to use FC early in MTPs to minimize allogeneic blood administration, to reduce the likelihood of the patient developing TRALI, TACO, acute respiratory distress syndrome, viral infections, and other MTP-related injuries [6]. In the E-FIT 1 study, a double-blinded randomized controlled trial, 6 g of FC was administered, alongside typical transfusion guidelines, and an increase of 0.9 g L^{-1} within the trauma patient population was noted, compared to a decrease of 0.2 g L^{-1} in the placebo group [29]. There was no increase in thrombotic events in the experimental arm [29]. Military studies have found a decrease in mortality with high fibrinogen-to-red blood cell transfusion ratios, compared to low ratios [6]. A Cochrane review of FC use in other high blood loss events, such as postpartum hemorrhage or cardiopulmonary bypass surgery, revealed only four studies and one randomized controlled trial. The results were mixed and no conclusions could be made as to the benefit of using cryoprecipitate, compared to FC, outside of the trauma population [14].

References

1. Foster JC, Sappenfield JW, Smith RS, Kiley SP. Initiation and termination of massive transfusion protocols: current strategies and future prospects. *Anesth Analg*. 2017;125:2045–55.

2. Thomas S, Makris M. The reversal of anticoagulation in clinical practice. *Clin Med (Lond)*. 2018;18:314–19.

3. Chignalia AZ, Yetimakman F, Christiaans SC, *et al.* The glycocalyx and trauma: a review. *Shock*. 2016;45:338–48.

4. Brohi K, Singh J, Heron M, Coats T. Acute traumatic coagulopathy. *J Trauma*. 2003;54:1127–30.

5. Yee J, Kaide CG. Emergency reversal of anticoagulation. *West J Emerg Med*. 2019;20:770–83.

6. Grottke O, Mallaiah S, Karkouti K, Saner F, Haas T. Fibrinogen supplementation and its indications. *Semin Thromb Hemost*. 2020;46:38–49.

7. Levy JH, Goodnough LT. How I use fibrinogen replacement therapy in acquired bleeding. *Blood*. 2015;125:1387–93.

8. Brohi K. Prediction of acute traumatic coagulopathy and massive transfusion – is this the best we can do? *Resuscitation*. 2011;82:1128–9.

9. Simmons JW, Pittet J-F, Pierce B. Trauma-induced coagulopathy. *Curr Anesthesiol Rep*. 2014;4:189–99.

10. Davenport RA, Brohi K. Cause of trauma-induced coagulopathy. *Curr Opin Anaesthesiol*. 2016;29:212–19.

11. Moore EE, Moore HB, Chapman MP, Gonzalez E, Sauaia A. Goal-directed hemostatic resuscitation for trauma induced coagulopathy: maintaining homeostasis. *J Trauma Acute Care Surg*. 2018;84:S35–40.

12. Ostrowski SR, Johansson PI. Endothelial glycocalyx degradation induces endogenous heparinization in patients with severe injury and early traumatic coagulopathy. *J Trauma Acute Care Surg*. 2012;73:60–6.

13. Astapenko D, Benes J, Pouska J, Lehmann C, Islam S, Cerny V. Endothelial glycocalyx in acute care surgery – what anaesthesiologists need to know for clinical practice. *BMC Anesthesiol*. 2019;19:238.

14. Jensen NH, Stensballe J, Afshari A. Comparing efficacy and safety of fibrinogen concentrate to cryoprecipitate in bleeding patients: a systematic review. *Acta Anaesthesiol Scand*. 2016;60:1033–42.

15. Brohi K, Cohen MJ, Ganter MT, Matthay MA, Mackersie RC, Pittet JF. Acute traumatic coagulopathy: initiated by hypoperfusion: modulated through the protein C pathway? *Ann Surg*. 2007;245:812–18.

16. Davenport RA, Guerreiro M, Frith D, *et al*. Activated protein C drives the hyperfibrinolysis of acute traumatic coagulopathy. *Anesthesiology*. 2017;126:115–27.

17. Roberts I, Shakur H, Coats T, *et al*. The CRASH-2 trial: a randomised controlled trial and economic evaluation of the effects of tranexamic acid on death, vascular occlusive events and transfusion requirement in bleeding trauma patients. *Health Technol Assess*. 2013;17:1–79.

18. Watts DD, Trask A, Soeken K, Perdue P, Dols S, Kaufmann C. Hypothermic coagulopathy in trauma: effect of varying levels of hypothermia on enzyme speed, platelet function, and fibrinolytic activity. *J Trauma*. 1998;44:846–54.

19. Gonzalez E, Moore EE, Moore HB. Management of trauma-induced coagulopathy with thrombelastography. *Crit Care Clin*. 2017;33:119–34.

20. Toker S, Hak DJ, Morgan SJ. Deep vein thrombosis prophylaxis in trauma patients. *Thrombosis*. 2011;2011:505373.

21. Ruskin KJ. Deep vein thrombosis and venous thromboembolism in trauma. *Curr Opin Anaesthesiol*. 2018;31:215–18.

22. Cuker A, Burnett A, Triller D, *et al*. Reversal of direct oral anticoagulants: guidance from the Anticoagulation Forum. *Am J Hematol*. 2019;94:697–709.

23. Baksaas-Aasen K, Van Dieren S, Balvers K, *et al*. Data-driven development of ROTEM and TEG algorithms for the management of trauma hemorrhage: a prospective observational multicenter study. *Ann Surg*. 2019;270:1178–85.

24. Gonzalez E, Moore EE, Moore HB, *et al*. Goal-directed hemostatic resuscitation of trauma-induced coagulopathy: a pragmatic randomized clinical trial comparing a viscoelastic assay to conventional coagulation assays. *Ann Surg*. 2016;263:1051–9.

25. Whiting D, DiNardo JA. TEG and ROTEM: technology and clinical applications. *Am J Hematol.* 2014;89:228–32.

26. Haemonetics. Introducing TEG 6s – White Paper. Available from: https://pdf.medi calexpo.com/pdf/haemonetics/introducing-teg-6s-white-paper/78504-152619.html.

27. Korpallová B, Samoš M, Bolek T, *et al.* Role of thromboelastography and rotational thromboelastometry in the management of cardiovascular diseases. *Clin Appl Thromb Hemost.* 2018;24:1199–207.

28. Nair PM, Rendo MJ, Reddoch-Cardenas KM, Burris JK, Meledeo MA, Cap AP. Recent advances in use of fresh frozen plasma, cryoprecipitate, immunoglobulins, and clotting factors for transfusion support in patients with hematologic disease. *Semin Hematol.* 2020;57:73–82.

29. Curry N, Foley C, Wong H, *et al.* Early fibrinogen concentrate therapy for major haemorrhage in trauma (E-FIT 1): results from a UK multi-centre, randomised, double blind, placebo-controlled pilot trial. *Crit Care.* 2018;22:164.

Chapter 32

Perioperative Cognitive Disorders

Catherine Price, Sarah McCraney,
Margaret E. Wiggins, Carlos Hernaiz
Alonso, Catherine Dion, Franchesca Arias,
Kristin Hamlet, and Patrick Tighe

Abnormal Cognitive Aging

Abnormal cognitive aging includes unexpected changes in cognition or memory functions. Changes can present either acutely or gradually. Within the *Diagnostic and Statistical Manual of Mental Disorders*, fifth edition (DSM-5) by the American Psychiatric Association (APA) [1], abnormal cognitive profiles are divided into Mild Neurocognitive Disorder and Major Neurocognitive Disorder (also known as dementia).

Diagnostic criteria for Mild Neurocognitive Disorder are based on either self-reported, or objective evidence of, mild cognitive decline from a previous level of performance [1]. Cognitive changes can occur within any cognitive domain, including complex attention, executive functioning, learning and memory, language, perceptual–motor, or social cognition. Furthermore, the changes in cognition do not interfere with the capacity for independent functioning, cannot occur exclusively in the context of delirium, and cannot be explained by any other mental disorder [1]. The commonly used term mild cognitive impairment (MCI) represents a prodromal state of cognitive change prior to the development of dementia, or most traditionally Alzheimer's disease (AD). MCI is subsumed under the DSM-5 Mild Neurocognitive Disorder diagnosis [2].

Diagnostic criteria for Major Neurocognitive Disorder, or dementia, by contrast, involve evidence of significant decline from a previous level of performance in one or more of the previously mentioned cognitive domains. Such decline may be evident from: (1) concerns expressed by the individual or a knowledgeable informant; or (2) objective and substantial impairment in cognitive performance on neuropsychological testing that did not occur in the context of delirium [1]. Contrary to MCI, cognitive impairment must interfere with the individual's ability to function independently. Major Neurocognitive Disorder is further organized into three severity levels, based on the stage of functional impairment: mild, moderate, and severe. Major Neurocognitive Disorder, mild, refers to subtle difficulties with instrumental activities of daily living such as housework and managing money. Major Neurocognitive Disorder, moderate, describes impairment with feeding, dressing, and other basic activities of daily living. Major Neurocognitive Disorder, severe, refers to a state of total reliance on others to complete basic and instrumental activities of daily living.

Considering Abnormal Cognitive Aging Profiles in Preoperative Settings

Although it is often assumed that the neurotoxic effects of sedative/hypnotic anesthetic agents are fully reversible, there appears to be diminished capacity for returning to their baseline in older adults [3]. Various factors contribute to this age-related increased vulnerability, including changes in the aging brain such as increased free radical buildup (due to fewer scavenging agents), accumulation of prion-like proteins, increased brain atrophy, and diminished oxidative phosphorylation [3]. Individuals with preoperative mild or major neurocognitive disorders/neurodegenerative disorders present with additional challenges regarding increased sensitivity to pharmaceuticals acting on the central nervous system (CNS) [4].

Understanding brain–behavioral–anesthetic interactions, particularly for those with mild/major neurocognitive disorder and neurodegenerative diseases, is especially prudent, given our current population challenges. By 2050, people aged 65 and older will reach 1.6 billion worldwide [5]. Our healthcare system will face greater numbers of individuals with early- to late-stage AD [6] and other neurodegenerative disorders who require procedures with anesthesia due to comorbid health-related conditions (e.g., cardiac) or who desire operations for improved quality of life (e.g. joint replacement) [7]. Low- and high-risk operations are performed annually on more than half a million individuals aged 65 and older, and with population aging, this number will likely increase [7]. Meanwhile, many older adults may be relatively unaware of, or even deny, their cognitive impairments or neurodegenerative symptoms.

Preoperative markers of mild to major neurocognitive disorder predict postoperative cognitive complications, including delirium and mortality [8, 9]. Individuals with AD and related dementias, as well as other neurodegenerative disorders, such as Parkinson's disease (PD), have greater risks in perioperative settings [10]. For example, cognitive and psychiatric deficiencies associated with dementia interfere with a patient's ability to comply with medical recommendations and navigate complex environments independently [11]. Furthermore, cholinergic system response to anesthesia [12] and inflammatory responses [13] are hypothesized to be atypical for individuals with AD [14, 15] and PD [16]. Preoperative indicators of cognitive reserve and brain integrity (e.g., reduced entorhinal thickness, greater white matter disease burden, larger ventricular size) predict differences in intraoperative anesthesia EEG responses in the brain [17, 18] and pre-/postfunctional and structural brain changes [19–21].

Older adults with mild or major neurocognitive disorder involving AD or PD profiles also present with increased anesthetic challenges due to alterations in physiology that affect both the pharmacokinetics and pharmacodynamics of drugs [22, 23]. Interestingly, mechanisms underlying general anesthesia (GA) have reciprocally been suggested to cause neurodegenerative changes similar to those seen in AD. A review article by Vutskits *et al.* (2016) detailed experiments showing underlying mechanisms that suggest a role of GA exposure in both elderly and postnatal brains leading to lasting morphofunctional CNS changes [24]. For example, various in vitro and in vivo rodent experiments have elucidated mechanisms that link GA-induced apoptosis to increased generation and aggregation of amyloid β [25–27]. Anesthetics have also been linked to increased tau hyperphosphorylation [28], another dominant pathologic feature of AD. This effect was exacerbated in Mapt transgenic mouse models encoding the gene for tau [29]. These in vitro and in vivo experiments found that dexmedetomidine increased tau phosphorylation and aggregation in mice, as well as impaired spatial reference memory.

Another characteristic pathologic finding in AD is the degeneration of the cholinergic CNS. Elderly rats exposed to repeated intravenous (IV) anesthesia with pentobarbital exhibited altered cholinergic binding, relative to controls, due to reduced cerebral cortex cholinergic receptors [30]. Postoperative elevations in AD pathology following anesthesia have also been demonstrated in humans [31]. One such experiment revealed elevated cerebrospinal fluid (CSF) levels of tau and amyloid β_{1-42}, a form of amyloid β consistently implicated in AD pathophysiology, 1 week after coronary artery bypass graft (CABG) surgery under GA [31]. These findings suggest that anesthesia may induce neurologic changes in the elderly, resembling those found in AD, with important implications for a patient population with increased susceptibility not only to neurocognitive diseases, but also to postoperative cognitive impairment.

Studies in individuals diagnosed with PD have shown that these individuals may, in fact, be more sensitive to gamma-aminobutyric acid (GABA)-activating agents and that this mechanism may play a role in anesthetic exacerbation of motor symptoms. In a study by Calon *et al.* (2002), postmortem observation of individuals with PD demonstrated increased $GABA_A$ receptor concentration in the globus pallidus internus (GP_i) of dyskinetic PD compared to nondyskinetic individuals [32]. There is also evidence suggesting that anesthetics may affect neuronal activity of the subthalamic nucleus (STN), as propofol was found to inhibit the STN in individuals with advanced PD under consideration for deep brain stimulation implantation [33]. Because the STN has been demonstrated to play a role in inhibiting corticothalamic projections responsible for movement [20], decreased output from the STN facilitates movement, as evidenced by individuals with STN lesions who exhibit ballism and choreiform movements [34]. Taken together, these studies suggest possible mechanisms underlying an increased risk of anesthesia-induced dyskinesia in PD. Furthermore, a study by Jamsen *et al.* (2014) found that individuals diagnosed with PD undergoing total knee or hip replacement surgery had prolonged hospitalization, increased risk of recurrent dislocation in the first postoperative year, and poor long-term prognosis, compared to their counterparts without PD who underwent the same procedures [35]. Previous work has demonstrated that relative to healthy controls, individuals diagnosed with PD show a significant decline in cognitive function after anesthesia and surgery, compared to baseline functioning [22]. Retrospective studies and single case reports have shown that individuals with neurodegenerative disorders, such as PD, have greater rates of postoperative delirium and cognitive decline [36].

Nevertheless, individuals with mild and major neurocognitive disorders showing prodromal to severe signs of AD and other neurodegenerative disorders receive preoperative care that is comparable to their cognitively intact counterparts, without taking into account their additional needs [15]. For these reasons, the benefit–risk ratios for procedures can be misrepresented to individuals with compromised cognition, inadequately identifying the potential for surgical anesthesia to exacerbate neurodegeneration, and thereby precluding informed decision-making [37]. Insight into a patient's preoperative cognitive status in medical settings can identify individuals who may benefit from prerehabilitation, additional preoperative support when preparing for surgery, and increased monitoring during and after surgery [38–40]. A discussion on preexisting cognitive vulnerabilities may help patient–caregiver dyads make informed healthcare decisions [41].

For many of these reasons, there has been a call to action for preoperative identification of mild and moderate neurocognitive disorders, awareness of AD and related dementias, and improved understanding of brain mechanisms of change to facilitate options for intervention [42]. Anesthesiologists who are knowledgeable in cognitive–behavioral profiles can therefore improve patient outcomes, appreciating how individuals with predisposing cognitive impairment require fewer precipitating factors (such as anticholinergics, anesthesia, pain, infection) for delirium onset [43]. For theoretical discussions on this topic, a review published in 1993 on the "threshold theory" summarizes how individuals remain at a critical threshold until various "stressors" overwhelm their remaining cognitive reserve capacity and accelerate symptom manifestation of disease [44].

The effects of anesthesia on older adults and the pharmacologic vulnerabilities of the aging brain are also topics that are increasingly surfacing within the anesthesiology community, including the American Board of Anesthesiology (ABA) Initial Certification in Anesthesiology. Trainees are expected to demonstrate knowledge of geriatric anesthesia, including pre- and postjunctional mechanisms of the cholinergic system, the neurotransmitter being heavily implicated in AD pathology. There are also sections addressing neurologic consequences of anesthesia, including confusion, delirium, cognitive dysfunction, and failure to emerge from anesthesia.

Identifying Characteristics of Preoperative Cognitive Disorders

Anesthesiologists can identify characteristics of preoperative cognitive disorders, even if a disorder is not formally diagnosed on the medical chart. The Society for Perioperative Assessment and Quality Improvement (SPAQI), in collaboration with experts in preoperative neuropsychology, anesthesiology, and geriatric medicine, drafted a two-part statement to detail the rationale for evaluating cognition preoperatively, and provided a succinct list of instruments designed to screen cognitive functioning in fast-paced settings [45, 46]. Part I introduces the most common neurodegenerative disorders affecting older adults and lists the common signs and symptoms associated with each of those disorders. Part II of this statement: (1) describes factors that must be considered when selecting cognitive screening tools; (2) summarizes a review of the literature on existing cognitive screening tools and lists available cognitive screening tools with demonstrated utility within primary care and preoperative settings; and (3) provides a workflow diagram to assist clinicians with decision-making [45].

Cognitive screening tests assess selected neurocognitive domains and are interpreted using prespecified cutoff scores [47]. While administration of a cognitive screening tool does not substitute for a thorough neuropsychological assessment, this approach is highly desirable in clinical environments with high throughput. A handful of cognitive screening instruments have been used in preoperative settings. The average administration time for cognitive screening tools previously used in preoperative settings is 5 minutes, and administration time ranges from 1 to 10 minutes.

Studies have shown that these screenings identify symptoms of mild to major neurocognitive disorders in 19–33% of older adults scheduled for elective surgical procedures [48, 49] and predict cognitive and noncognitive complications after surgery and anesthesia [9]. Most screenings include variants of short traditional neuropsychological/neurologic tools, that is, three-word memory, counting backwards from 100 by 7, spelling the word 'WORLD' backwards such as in the Mini-Cog [50] or the Mini-Mental State Examination [51], and clock drawing to command and copy [52]. Routine inclusion of preoperative cognitive screening for the risk of dementia and delirium is in its infancy. We are only beginning to learn how to integrate educational and cognitive screening into busy clinical settings, and to appropriately report and implement cognitive/memory screening data for perioperative management. Very few hospitals include cognitive screening of older adults as a routine component of their preoperative evaluation. Even fewer hospitals collaborate with neuropsychologists and geriatricians for more integrated pre- and postoperative care.

The University of Florida Health System has established a cognitive screening program for adults aged 65 and older with a planned surgical procedure [53]. Individuals who present to a presurgical clinic and "fail" a preadmission cognitive/memory screen are immediately referred to a team of neuropsychologists and geriatric medicine physicians [41, 47]. The purpose of this follow-up assessment is to identify modifiable risk factors for negative postoperative outcomes, including anticholinergic burden or polypharmacy, to provide the anesthesia–surgical team with potential considerations regarding the patient's cognitive impairment, and to provide recommendations for inpatient geriatric medicine follow-up and closer inpatient and home-based delirium monitoring for both the patient and the care team. Individuals at risk of negative postoperative cognitive outcomes are then educated (along with their families when available) on perioperative risks, thus improving the quality of patient-centered care (e.g., see [41] and [54]). Patient reports are available to the anesthesiology and surgery team prior to the surgical procedure, so that anesthesiologists and surgeons can tailor their care based on the patient's preoperative profile, when possible. For individuals deemed to be at elevated risk and who are inpatient following surgery, perioperative follow-up teams monitor for delirium and inform the patients and families about the possibility of longer hospitalization and discharge to a nursing facility, rather than home.

This form of integrated care provides a more patient-centered approach but does also require close collaboration between multiple medical providers from the patient's care team, including those from anesthesiology, neuropsychology, and geriatric medicine. Prospective studies across various surgical types are needed to further address and understand the interactions and relationships between preoperative cognitive impairment and the type/depth of anesthesia, invasiveness of the surgical procedure, biomarker changes, and patient outcomes. Addressing cognition within the preoperative environment is relevant to predicting risk or documenting the baseline cognitive status.

Until the efficacy for such programs is shown across multiple hospitals, cognitive screening by anesthesiologists is a viable option. In addition, cognitive screening training workshops have been provided at various International Anesthesia Research Society meetings. We encourage a review of the resources listed in published articles, to contact the American Society of Anesthesiologists' Brain Health Initiative, or to contact the University of Florida's Perioperative Cognitive Anesthesia Network (PeCAN) program for more information on available screening resources.

Labeling Postoperative Cognitive Disorders

In 2018, clinicians and researchers aimed to develop a terminology for classifying postoperative cognitive status changes in the general population [55]. They recommended an umbrella term of "perioperative neurocognitive disorders" be used to identify cognitive changes or impairments observed or reported during the pre- or postoperative period [55]. Regarding delirium, "postoperative delirium" should be recognized as a specific category that is consistent with the current DSM-5 terminology and that has appropriate specifiers. It is suggested that "postoperative delirium" be defined as occurring in the hospital up to 1 week after surgery or until discharge (whichever is first) and meeting DSM-5 diagnostic criteria [55]. For cognitive changes identified within a postoperative setting, the terms "delayed neurocognitive recovery" and mild or major neurocognitive disorder are used, depending on the timeline and severity [55]. Clinical diagnosis is best associated with team members such as neuropsychologists, geriatric physicians, and neurologists.

Multidisciplinary Consideration for Identification of Perioperative Cognitive Disorder and Care

Perioperative care is a team effort, with every individual helping to maximize positive patient outcomes [46, 54]. Through the integration of neuropsychology, geriatric medicine, anesthesiology, surgery, and primary care, individuals can receive optimal care centered around their needs, with increased importance placed on brain health. In this multidisciplinary team, neuropsychologists are uniquely trained to provide psychometrically grounded and standardized information about a patient's neurocognitive function, thereby providing recommendations to the perioperative care team regarding cognition risk, diagnostic differentials, and potential postoperative complications. Anesthesiology team members may then use available neurobehavioral data to supplement decision-making within the perioperative environment. Geriatric medicine providers provide postoperative care intervention options and can leverage preoperative neurobehavioral status data for postoperative differential diagnoses and care intervention planning. Primary care providers, ideally the most accessible to the patient's family, can provide comprehensively informed follow-up care, as needed. Finally, the patient's caregivers are a fundamental member of the care team, as they are responsible for helping to communicate with the patient and provide postoperative care.

Future Directions for Perioperative Cognitive Disorders

Our healthcare system faces an extensive gap in evidence-based anesthesia-focused care for adults with preoperative cognitive disorders and in evidence-based approaches for postoperative cognitive disorder intervention.

Anesthesiologists are at the forefront of this effort, as they are the clinicians most vigilant to behavioral change before, during, and after surgical anesthesia procedures. We encourage anesthesiologists to remain alert to perioperative brain–behavioral profiles, particularly in adults at risk of neurodegenerative disorders. This involves an appreciation for preoperative cognitive disorders via chart review, behavioral observation, and rapid pre-/postcognitive screening. Clinical observations and scientific hypothesis generation regarding these profiles and intraoperative monitoring procedures are necessary. Sound scientific studies addressing preoperative disorders and intraoperative responses are needed. This will improve future trainees' awareness of disorders and eventually lead to evidence-based approaches to anesthesia. Multidisciplinary team integration within the perioperative setting will provide stabilization for complex patient care and treatment options.

References

1. American Psychiatric Association. *Diagnostic and Statistical Manual of Mental Disorders*, 5th ed. Washington, DC: American Psychiatric Publishing; 2013.

2. Petersen RC, Smith GE, Waring SC, Ivnik RJ, Tangalos EG, Kokmen E. Mild cognitive impairment: clinical characterization and outcome. *Arch Neurol.* 1999;56(3):303–8.

3. Cottrell JE, Hartung J. Anesthesia and cognitive outcome in elderly patients: a narrative viewpoint. *J Neurosurg Anesthesiol.* 2020;32(1):9–17.

4. Burton DA, Nicholson G, Hall GM. Anaesthesia in elderly patients with neurodegenerative disorders: special considerations. *Drugs Aging.* 2004;21(4):229–42.

5. He W, Goodkind D, Kowal P; US Census Bureau. An Aging World: 2015. Washington, DC: US Government Publishing Office; 2016. Available from: www.census.gov/content/dam/Census/library/publications/2016/demo/p95-16-1.pdf.

6. Hebert LE, Scherr PA, Bienias JL, Bennett DA, Evans DA. Alzheimer disease in the US population: prevalence estimates using the 2000 census. *Arch Neurol.* 2003;60(8):1119–22.

7. Williams SN, Wolford ML, Bercovitz A. Hospitalization for total knee replacement among inpatients aged 45 and over: 2000–2010. *NCHS Data Brief.* 2015;210:1–8.

8. Oresanya LB, Lyons WL, Finlayson E. Preoperative assessment of the older patient: a narrative review. *JAMA.* 2014;311(20):2110–20.

9. Price CC, Garvan C, Hizel L, Lopez MG, Billings FT. Delayed recall and working memory MMSE domains predict delirium following cardiac surgery. *J Alzheimers Dis.* 2017;59(3):1027–35.

10. Aminoff MJ, Christine CW, Friedman JH, *et al.* Management of the hospitalized patient with Parkinson's disease: current state of the field and need for guidelines. *Parkinsonism Relat Disord.* 2011;17(3):139–45.

11. Ala TA, Simpson G, Holland MT, Tabassum V, Deshpande M, Fifer A. Many caregivers of persons with memory loss or Alzheimer's disease are unaware of the abilities of their persons with AD to recall their drugs and medical histories. *Dementia (London)*. 2020;19(7):2354–67.

12. Pratico C, Quattrone D, Lucanto T, *et al*. Drugs of anesthesia acting on central cholinergic system may cause post-operative cognitive dysfunction and delirium. *Med Hypotheses*. 2005;65(5):972–82.

13. Whittington RA, Planel E, Terrando N. Impaired resolution of inflammation in Alzheimer's disease: a review. *Front Immunol*. 2017;8:1464.

14. Baranov D, Bickler PE, Crosby GJ, *et al*. Consensus statement: first international workshop on anesthetics and Alzheimer's disease. *Anesth Analg*. 2009;108 (5):1627–30.

15. Silbert B, Evered L, Scott DA, Maruff P. Anesthesiology must play a greater role in patients with Alzheimer's disease. *Anesth Analg*. 2011;112(5):1242–5.

16. Bohnen NI, Albin RL. The cholinergic system and Parkinson disease. *Behav Brain Res*. 2011;221(2):564–73.

17. Giattino CM, Gardner JE, Sbahi FM, *et al*. Intraoperative frontal alpha-band power correlates with preoperative neurocognitive function in older adults. *Front Syst Neurosci*. 2017;11:24.

18. Hernaiz Alonso C, Tanner JJ, Wiggins ME, *et al*. Proof of principle: preoperative cognitive reserve and brain integrity predicts intra-individual variability in processed EEG (Bispectral Index Monitor) during general anesthesia. *PLoS One*. 2019;14(5):e0216209.

19. Huang H, Tanner J, Parvatancni H, *et al*. Impact of total knee arthroplasty with general anesthesia on brain networks: cognitive efficiency and ventricular volume predict functional connectivity decline in older adults. *J Alzheimers Dis*. 2018;62 (1):319–33.

20. Browndyke JN, Berger M, Harshbarger TB, *et al*. Resting-state functional connectivity and cognition after major cardiac surgery in older adults without preoperative cognitive impairment: preliminary findings. *J Am Geriatr Soc*. 2017;65(1):e6–12.

21. Hardcastle C, Huang H, Crowley S, *et al*. Mild cognitive impairment and decline in resting state functional connectivity after total knee arthroplasty with general anesthesia. *J Alzheimers Dis*. 2019;69(4):1003–18.

22. Price CC, Levy SA, Tanner J, *et al*. Orthopedic surgery and post-operative cognitive decline in idiopathic Parkinson's disease: considerations from a pilot study. *J Parkinsons Dis*. 2015;5(4):893–905.

23. Roberts DP, Lewis SJG. Considerations for general anaesthesia in Parkinson's disease. *J Clin Neurosci*. 2018;48:34–41.

24. Vutskits L, Xie Z. Lasting impact of general anaesthesia on the brain: mechanisms and relevance. *Nat Rev Neurosci.* 2016;17(11):705–17.

25. Xie Z, Culley DJ, Dong Y, *et al.* The common inhalation anesthetic isoflurane induces caspase activation and increases amyloid beta-protein level in vivo. *Ann Neurol.* 2008;64(6):618–27.

26. Zhen Y, Dong Y, Wu X, *et al.* Nitrous oxide plus isoflurane induces apoptosis and increases beta-amyloid protein levels. *Anesthesiology.* 2009;111(4):741–52.

27. Dong Y, Zhang G, Zhang B, *et al.* The common inhalational anesthetic sevoflurane induces apoptosis and increases beta-amyloid protein levels. *Arch Neurol.* 2009;66 (5):620–31.

28. Le Freche H, Brouillette J, Fernandez-Gomez FJ, *et al.* Tau phosphorylation and sevoflurane anesthesia: an association to postoperative cognitive impairment. *Anesthesiology.* 2012;116(4):779–87.

29. Whittington RA, Virag L, Gratuze M, *et al.* Dexmedetomidine increases tau phosphorylation under normothermic conditions in vivo and in vitro. *Neurobiol Aging.* 2015;36(8):2414–28.

30. Hanning CD, Blokland A, Johnson M, Perry EK. Effects of repeated anaesthesia on central cholinergic function in the rat cerebral cortex. *Eur J Anaesthesiol.* 2003;20 (2):93–7.

31. Palotas A, Reis HJ, Bogats G, *et al.* Coronary artery bypass surgery provokes Alzheimer's disease-like changes in the cerebrospinal fluid. *J Alzheimers Dis.* 2010;21(4):1153–64.

32. Calon F, Di Paolo T. Levodopa response motor complications–GABA receptors and preproenkephalin expression in human brain. *Parkinsonism Relat Disord.* 2002;8 (6):449–54.

33. Raz A, Eimerl D, Zaidel A, Bergman H, Israel Z. Propofol decreases neuronal population spiking activity in the subthalamic nucleus of Parkinsonian patients. *Anesth Analg.* 2010;111(5):1285–9.

34. Krauss JK, Borremans JJ, Nobbe F, Mundinger F. Ballism not related to vascular disease: a report of 16 patients and review of the literature. *Parkinsonism Relat Disord.* 1996;2(1):35–45.

35. Jamsen E, Puolakka T, Peltola M, Eskelinen A, Lehto MU. Surgical outcomes of primary hip and knee replacements in patients with Parkinson's disease: a nationwide registry-based case-controlled study. *Bone Joint J.* 2014;96-B(4):486–91.

36. Newman JM, Sodhi N, Dalton SE, *et al.* Does Parkinson disease increase the risk of perioperative complications after total hip arthroplasty? A nationwide database study. *J Arthroplasty.* 2018;33(7S):S162–6.

37. Arora SS, Gooch JL, Garcia PS. Postoperative cognitive dysfunction, Alzheimer's disease, and anesthesia. *Int J Neurosci.* 2014;124(4):236–42.

38. Calkins MP. From research to application: supportive and therapeutic environments for people living with dementia. *Gerontologist.* 2018;58:S114–28.

39. Mohanty S, Rosenthal RA, Russell MM, Neuman MD, Ko CY, Esnaola NF. Optimal perioperative management of the geriatric patient: a best practices guideline from the American College of Surgeons NSQIP and the American Geriatrics Society. *J Am Coll Surg.* 2016;222(5):930–47.

40. Prizer LP, Zimmerman S. Progressive support for activities of daily living for persons living with dementia. *Gerontologist.* 2018;58:S74–87.

41. Arias F, Bursian AC, Sappenfield JW, Price CC. Delirium history and preoperative mild neurocognitive disorder: an opportunity for multidisciplinary patient-centered care. *Am J Case Rep.* 2018;19:1324–8.

42. Crosby G, Culley DJ, Hyman BT. Preoperative cognitive assessment of the elderly surgical patient: a call for action. *Anesthesiology.* 2011;114(6):1265–8.

43. Marcantonio ER. Delirium in hospitalized older adults. *N Engl J Med.* 2017;377 (15):1456–66.

44. Satz P. Brain reserve capacity on symptom onset after brain injury: a formulation and review of evidence for threshold theory. *Neuropsychology.* 1993;7(3):273–95.

45. Arias F, Wiggins M, Urman RD, *et al.* Rapid in-person cognitive screening in the preoperative setting: test considerations and recommendations from the Society for Perioperative Assessment and Quality Improvement (SPAQI). *J Clin Anesth.* 2020;62:109724.

46. Wiggins M, Arias F, Urman RD, *et al.* Common neurodegenerative disorders in the perioperative setting: recommendations for screening from the Society for Perioperative Assessment and Quality Improvement (SPAQI). *Perioper Care Oper Room Manag.* 2020;20:100092.

47. Block CK, Johnson-Greene D, Pliskin N, Boake C. Discriminating cognitive screening and cognitive testing from neuropsychological assessment: implications for professional practice. *Clin Neuropsychol.* 2017;31(3):487–500.

48. Amini S, Crowley S, Hizel L, *et al.* Feasibility and rationale for incorporating frailty and cognitive screening protocols in a preoperative anesthesia clinic. *Anesth Analg.* 2019;129(3):830–8.

49. Culley DJ, Flaherty D, Reddy S, *et al.* Preoperative cognitive stratification of older elective surgical patients: a cross-sectional study. *Anesth Analg.* 2016;123 (1):186–92.

50. Borson S, Scanlan JM, Chen P, Ganguli M. The Mini-Cog as a screen for dementia: validation in a population-based sample. *J Am Geriatr Soc.* 2003;51(10):1451–4.

51. Folstein MF, Robins LN, Helzer JE. The Mini-Mental State Examination. *Arch Gen Psychiatry.* 1983;40(7):812.

52. Libon DJ, Malamut BL, Swenson R, Sands LP, Cloud BS. Further analyses of clock drawings among demented and nondemented older subjects. *Arch Clin Neuropsychol.* 1996;11(3):193–205.

53. Wiggins ME, Hernaiz C, Fahy BD, Price CC. Cognitive change and elective surgeries with anesthesia: considerations for neuropsychologists and the growing field of perioperative cognitive medicine. In: DJ Libon, M Lamar, RA Swenson, KM Heilman, eds. *Vascular Disease, Alzheimer's Disease, and Mild Cognitive Impairment: Advancing an Integrated Approach.* New York, NY: Oxford University Press; 2020, pp. 433–57.

54. Hamlet KM, Pasternak E, Rabai F, Mufti M, Hernaiz Alonso C, Price CC. Perioperative multidisciplinary delirium prevention: a longitudinal case report. *A A Pract.* 2021;15(1):e01364.

55. Evered L, Silbert B, Knopman DS, *et al.* Recommendations for the nomenclature of cognitive change associated with anaesthesia and surgery–20181. *J Alzheimers Dis.* 2018;66(1):1–10.

Chapter 33

Acute Pain Management in the ICU

Farees Hyatali, Franciscka Macieiski, Harish Bangalore Siddaiah, and Alan David Kaye

Introduction

Pain in the critically ill patient is often underreported and misdiagnosed. Contributing factors include such patients not being able to express themselves due to invasive respiratory support or altered mental function. Pain management in the intensive care unit (ICU) can be challenging due to the severity of illness of critically ill patients. The benefits and risks of pain management techniques and medications should be weighed against the severity of the patient's illness and their comorbidities, as well as the side effects of each technique and medication.

Regional Anesthesia

Peripheral Nerve Blocks

Regional anesthesia in the form of peripheral nerve blocks has been used to decrease postoperative pain in the ICU. Peripheral nerve blocks have the benefit of being associated with less strict anticoagulant guidelines prior to performing the block and fewer side effects, while providing safe and effective analgesia. These blocks can be performed via a single injection or a continuous catheter-based technique.

Fascial plane blocks, such as the pectoralis (PECS) I and II blocks and the erector spinae block (ESPB), as well as the serratus anterior plane block (SAPB), have been used for rescue analgesia in cardiac surgical patients who have had severe postsurgical pain, and can also improve lung function by reducing splinting from severe thoracic pain.

Patients who have had sternal fractures, sternotomies, and rib fractures have also benefited from ultrasound-guided transversus thoracis plane block (TTPB), which can also decrease pain scores and ultimately improve lung function by reducing splinting secondary to severe pain.

Neuraxial Analgesia

Patients who have suffered rib fractures, as well as those undergoing thoracic and upper and mid-abdominal surgeries, can benefit from neuraxial analgesia, in particular, thoracic epidural analgesia.

Benefits include reduced pain scores, improved pulmonary function, increased gastric motility, decreased risk of deep vein thrombosis (DVT), which may assist in early extubation in patients who are intubated, reduced time to initial bowel movement, and reduced morbidity and mortality.

Side effects of neuraxial anesthesia include, but are not limited to, nausea, vomiting, urinary retention, and lower extremity weakness (especially in the case of lumbar epidural). If opiates are added to the local anesthetic administered via these routes, opioid-induced pruritus can also occur. In addition, the choice of using these techniques must be weighed against their possible side effects.

Contraindications to neuraxial interventional techniques include patient refusal, hemodynamic instability, true allergy to local anesthetic drugs, and active anticoagulation (guided by the anticoagulation guidelines from the American Society of Regional Anesthesia).

Analgesics

Opiates

Opiates used for acute perioperative pain management include morphine, hydromorphone, fentanyl, buprenorphine, methadone, remifentanil, sufentanil, alfentanil, and ketamine. These medications can be administered via the oral, intravenous, sublingual, intramuscular, and rectal routes. All of these medications provide excellent analgesia; however, many have unwanted side effects, as well as significant abuse potential. Adverse side effects include nausea, vomiting, sedation, opioid-induced respiratory depression, opioid-induced constipation, opioid-induced pruritus, and urinary retention. In addition, they can result in hypoventilation and hypercarbia, and can lead to cardiopulmonary compromise in critically ill patients, which may result in these patients requiring respiratory support or prolonged intubation in some of these patients.

Methadone is generally administered to patients who have a history of opiate abuse and are attempting to overcome their addiction. In addition, it can also be used as part of an anesthetic plan to reduce perioperative pain. This drug is generally administered orally or intravenously. Administration of methadone, in particular, can prolong the QTc interval and can lead to torsades de pointes, which may result in ventricular tachycardia and fibrillation in patients with a history of prolonged QT interval. A careful review of medications must be performed prior to reducing the risk of increasing the QTc interval.

Remifentanil may be used as a continuous intravenous infusion at a low rate, with a patient-controlled bolus, as part of patient-controlled analgesia (PCA) for acute pain management. Remifentanil is unique of all the opiates in that it has a very short half-life and a context-sensitive half-time of approximately 10 minutes, resulting in complete clearance of the opiate from blood. This is due to the fact that it is metabolized by red blood cell esterases which rapidly break down the drug in the bloodstream.

Sufentanil may be administered via the neuraxial or intravenous route (as a bolus or a continuous infusion) for acute pain management. It is an excellent adjuvant in local anesthetic solutions for neuraxial analgesia and has also been used as an adjuvant to prolong the duration of a spinal anesthetic when used for surgical anesthesia; however, it is associated with opioid-induced pruritus, nausea, and vomiting when used as an intrathecal adjuvant. Sufentanil, when used as an infusion, has a longer context-sensitive half-time when compared to remifentanil, and care must be taken with regard to administration of large doses of this medication.

Buprenorphine is another medication used in the perioperative period in patients with a history of opiate abuse. It is generally combined with naloxone to produce buprenorphine/naloxone (naloxone added to reduce the abuse potential of this drug). Buprenorphine is a partial opioid µ-agonist and a kappa antagonist with a half-life of approximately 37 hours. When buprenorphine is administered, the drug provides a ceiling effect with regard to analgesia and does not produce as much respiratory depression compared to more potent opiates. This drug is commonly used for withdrawal of opiates in those who have a history of opiate abuse and is generally administered as an oral formulation and, in some instances, as a transdermal patch for this purpose. It has also been approved for pain management. In addition, it can be combined with local anesthetic solutions as an adjuvant, given that it possesses some local anesthetic properties by blocking voltage gated sodium channels, and can thus be administered via the epidural or intrathecal routes. In this regard, buprenorphine can be effective in treating drug cravings in opioid-dependent patients in the ICU.

Meperidine is an opioid with an atropine-like structure and local anesthetic-like properties. Meperidine has been used intrathecally to prolong the duration of spinal anesthesia; however, it has unpleasant side effects of opioid-induced pruritus, constipation, sedation, nausea, and vomiting. When compared to other commercially available opioids used as adjuvants in intrathecal local anesthetic solutions, meperidine has a greater rate of side effects. Currently, meperidine is most commonly used in the ICU for treatment of postoperative shivering, as well as shivering in patients undergoing hypothermia after sudden cardiac arrest. It can also be used to provide analgesia; however, other agents, such as fentanyl, can provide superior analgesia in comparison.

Tramadol is an opiate with both serotonin and norepinephrine reuptake inhibitor properties that can be administered via the oral, intravenous, intramuscular, and intrathecal routes. Side effects include increased risk of seizures in those with a history of seizures and increased risk of serotonin syndrome (especially in patients who take medications that increase serotonin levels). It can be considered as an analgesic agent in the ICU; however, there are other agents that can provide better quality of analgesia.

Nonsteroidal Antiinflammatory Agents

Nonsteroidal antiinflammatory drugs (NSAIDs) inhibit the cyclooxygenase (COX) enzymes, of which there are two main types related to pain: COX-1 and 2. COX-2-mediated effects include pain, inflammation, and fever. These medications work by reducing inflammatory mediators, which provide nociceptive pain. They provide excellent analgesia, especially when incorporated within a multimodal analgesia regimen. It must be noted that these particular agents have a ceiling effect with regard to analgesia. Side effects include nausea, vomiting, gastrointestinal bleeding, increased risk of cardiovascular disease (especially in COX-2-selective NSAIDs, of which celecoxib is the only one still available), platelet dysfunction, and increased risk of bleeding and renal dysfunction, and these must be considered prior to administration in critically ill patients.

Adjuvants

Dexmedetomidine

Dexmedetomidine, a selective α2-agonist, has been used for sedation; however, in relation to local anesthetic properties, it has been used as an adjuvant to pain management. It is given as an infusion (0.2–2 μg/(kg hr)) and has been used in order to decrease opioid requirements in patients. Dexmedetomidine can be used as a sole analgesia agent or as an adjuvant in order to decrease opioid requirements. It can also be added to peripheral nerve blocks and neuraxial anesthetics to prolong their duration and reduce opiate consumption in critically ill patients.

Lidocaine

Lidocaine infusions have been used as an adjuvant to pain management as it decreases opioid requirements for these patients. Lidocaine has antinociceptive and antiinflammatory properties. It acts on sodium channels and reduces neuronal transmission. It is especially useful in patients who have contraindications.

The infusion is generally administered at 0.5–3 mg/(kg hr), and care must be taken to avoid systemic toxicity, especially in patients who suffer from cardiac and renal failure, as the metabolites of lidocaine may accumulate in these patients and can cause systemic toxicity.

The acid–base status and rate of injection, e.g., bolus or infusion, as well as the dose, of lidocaine, factors that influence the plasma concentration of free lidocaine, altered plasma protein levels, and hepatic or renal function are major factors in determining the patient's risk of toxicity. In patients who are critically ill, their metabolism may be altered, leading to an accumulation of lidocaine and its metabolites, resulting in an increased risk of systemic toxicity.

Careful monitoring must be used by using standard American Society of Anesthesiologists (ASA) monitors while the infusion is being administered, in order to monitor for signs and symptoms of local anesthetic toxicity, such as seizures or cardiac arrhythmias. If local anesthetic toxicity is suspected, a serum lidocaine level should be obtained and equipment and medications needed to treat local anesthetic toxicity should be available, including lipid emulsion.

Ketamine

Ketamine infusions have been used as an adjuvant for pain management in the ICU, and numerous studies have demonstrated its efficacy, with limited side effects. It is an N-methyl-D-aspartate (NMDA) receptor antagonist and results in a dissociative state when given at anesthetic doses (generally 0.35 mg kg^{-1} as a single bolus, followed by an infusion of 0.1–1 mg/(kg hr). Subanesthetic doses of ketamine have been used to decrease intraoperative and postoperative pain requirements, and have recently been a popular adjuvant in the ICU in order to decrease opioid requirements.

Further Reading

1. Kaushal B, Chauhan S, Saini K, *et al*. Comparison of the efficacy of ultrasound-guided serratus anterior plane block, pectoral nerves II block, and intercostal nerve block for the management of postoperative thoracotomy pain after pediatric cardiac surgery. *J Cardiothorac Vasc Anesth*. 2019;33(2):418–25.

2. Yalamuri S, Klinger RY, Bullock WM, Glower DD, Bottiger BA, Gadsden JC. Pectoral fascial (PECS) I and II blocks as rescue analgesia in a patient undergoing minimally invasive cardiac surgery. *Reg Anesth Pain Med*. 2017;42(6):764–6.

3. Fujii S, Roche M, Jones PM, Vissa D, Bainbridge D, Zhou JR. Transversus thoracis muscle plane block in cardiac surgery: a pilot feasibility study. *Reg Anesth Pain Med*. 2019;44(5):556–60.

4. Krishna SN, Chauhan S, Bhoi D, *et al*. Bilateral erector spinae plane block for acute post-surgical pain in adult cardiac surgical patients: a randomized controlled trial. *J Cardiothorac Vasc Anesth*. 2018;33(2):368–75.

5. Alford DP, Compton P, Samet JH. Acute pain management for patients receiving maintenance methadone or buprenorphine therapy. *Ann Intern Med*. 2006;144 (2):127–34. [Published correction appears in: *Ann Intern Med*. 2006;144(6):460.]

6. Weibel S, Jelting Y, Afshari A, *et al*. Patient-controlled analgesia with remifentanil versus alternative parenteral methods for pain management in labour. *Cochrane Database Syst Rev*. 2017;4(4):CD011989.

7. Budd K. The role of tramadol in acute pain management. *Acute Pain*. 1999;2 (4):189–96.

8. Ho KY, Gwee KA, Cheng YK, Yoon KH, Hee HT, Omar AR. Nonsteroidal anti-inflammatory drugs in chronic pain: implications of new data for clinical practice. *J Pain Res*. 2018;11:1937–48.

9. Schwenk ES, Viscusi ER, Buvanendran A, *et al*. Consensus guidelines on the use of intravenous ketamine infusions for acute pain management from the American Society of Regional Anesthesia and Pain Medicine, the American Academy of Pain Medicine, and the American Society of Anesthesiologists. *Reg Anesth Pain Med*. 2018;43(5):456–66.

10. Dunn LK, Durieux ME. Perioperative use of intravenous lidocaine. *Anesthesiology*. 2017;126(4):729–37.

11. Jung S, Ottestad E, Aggarwal A, Flood P, Nikitenko V. 982: Intravenous lidocaine infusion for management of pain in the intensive care unit. *Crit Care Med*. 2020;48(1):470. Available from: https://journals.lww.com/ccmjournal/Fulltext/ 2020/01001/982__INTRAVENOUS_LIDOCAINE_INFUSION_FOR_MANAG EMENT.943.aspx.

12. Habibi V, Kiabi FH, Sharifi H. The effect of dexmedetomidine on the acute pain after cardiothoracic surgeries: a systematic review. *Braz J Cardiovasc Surg*. 2018;33 (4):404–17.

Chapter 34

Infection Control
for the Anesthesia Provider

Tamara Lawson

Introduction

A newly acquired infection that a patient contracts during the course of receiving medical care is known as a healthcare-associated infection (HAI). These nosocomial infections are a serious source of morbidity and mortality for patients receiving care in hospitals, nursing homes, rehabilitation facilities, and surgery centers. HAIs include central line-associated bloodstream infections, catheter-associated urinary tract infections, ventilator-associated infections, and surgical site infections (SSIs). It is estimated that each day, 1 in every 31 patients in the United States is diagnosed with at least one of these nosocomial infections. Annually, approximately 2 million patients are diagnosed with a HAI in the United States, with 90,000 cases resulting in death [1, 2]. SSIs account for upward of 20% of all HAIs. Not only do they lead to an increase in the length of hospital stay, but they also are associated with increased readmission rates and the development of multidrug-resistant infections and drive up the cost of care. This contributes to an increase in healthcare costs of between 3.5 and 10 billion dollars per year [3, 4]. Just as staggering is the knowledge that it is estimated that up to 60% of SSIs are preventable. There are numerous factors that contribute to these infections. In recent years, there has been an increased awareness of the role that anesthesia providers can play in mitigating the risk of HAIs. Vigilant adherence to infection control measures is paramount to reducing perioperative HAIs [5].

Standard Precautions

The anesthesia provider plays an integral role in perioperative infection control. The cornerstone to the delivery of safe care in the perioperative environment is consistent observation of standard precautions, with special emphasis on hand hygiene, environmental disinfection, and safe medication handling [6].

Utilization of clean scrubs, surgical head coverings, face masks, and eye protection represents the minimum level of protection for anesthesia providers in sterile procedural environments, to minimize the transfer of infectious material between staff and patients. Clean, comfortable-fitting surgical scrubs and head coverings contribute to infection control by containing shed skin and hair cells of the provider. It is estimated that with average activity, an individual may lose 10,000 enucleated cells/minute (600,000 cells/hour) from the outermost layer of skin, of which up to 10% carry bacteria [6, 7]. Use of face masks is recommended to limit microbial shedding by the wearer [5, 6]. In addition, together with use of eye protection, these items form an effective barrier that protects the wearer from splash contamination of fluids in procedural areas.

Escalation of personal protective equipment (PPE) may be required, based on a patient's comorbidities. Timely identification of a patient's infectious status and application of appropriate isolation measures are paramount to minimizing contraction risk. These transmission-based precautions include contact, droplet, and airborne precautions.

Transmission-Based Precautions

See reference [8].

Standard

- Apply to all patients, regardless of their diagnosis or presumed infection status.
- PPE may include gloves, plastic apron/gown, mask, face shield/eye protection – based on risk of exposure to bodily fluids.

Airborne

- N95 mask or powered air-purifying respirator (PAPR).
- Source control with face mask for patient.
- Monitored air pressure room.
- Examples: coronavirus disease 2019 (COVID-19), tuberculosis, varicella, rubeola.

Droplet

- Surgical mask if within 3 feet of patient.
- Source control with face mask for patient.
- Private room.
- Examples: influenza, meningitis, mumps, pneumonia.

Contact

- Gloves, gown.
- Source control with face mask for patient.

- Private room.
- Examples: methicillin-resistant *Staphylococcus aureus* (MRSA), *Clostridium difficile*.

Hand Hygiene

Numerous studies have implicated provider hands as a source of perioperative contamination and transmission of infectious microorganisms [9–11]. In the course of caring for a patient, anesthesia providers touch, handle, and manipulate multiple instruments and surfaces within their workspace. This high-task density work environment presents challenges in consistently practicing real-time hand hygiene and other infection control measures [12]. Deliberate focus on hand hygiene during an anesthetic case can mitigate the spread of HAIs.

In response to the global issue of HAIs, the World Health Organization (WHO) has suggested *5 Moments for Hand Hygiene* [9]:

1. Before touching a patient
2. After touching a patient
3. Before clean/aseptic procedures
4. After exposure to body fluids
5. After touching a patient's surroundings.

These are the minimum recommended hand hygiene events. Providers should consider also thoroughly cleaning their hands before/after entering a procedure room, when their hands are visibly soiled, and prior to touching the anesthesia workstation [5, 9]. Artificial nails and chipped nail polish have been found to support microorganism growth after handwashing when compared to natural nails. As a result, it is recommended that providers keep their nails clean, short, and free of chipped polish. Jewelry should also be removed [10, 11].

Time spent on periprocedural hand hygiene is key to limiting the role that anesthesia providers play as vectors of cross-contamination of patients and the surgical environment.

- *Routine handwash* [9] – utilized for cleaning visibly soiled and transient microorganisms, using water and antimicrobial soap:
  o Apply to all surfaces of the hands/fingers for a minimum of 20–40 seconds.
  o Should be done at the start and end of every work day.
- *Antiseptic handwash* – to remove transient microorganisms and to reduce resident flora, using water and antimicrobial soap:
  o Apply to all surfaces of the hands/fingers for a minimum of 20–40 seconds.

- *Antiseptic handrub* – to remove or destroy transient microorganisms and reduce resident flora:
  - o For hands that are not visibly soiled.
  - o Alcohol-based.
  - o Apply to all surfaces of the hands/fingers until the hands are dry.
  - o Frequently throughout patient care actions.
  - o Apply before and after changing gloves.
- *Surgical antisepsis* – to remove or destroy transient microorganisms and to reduce resident flora, using water and antimicrobial soap:
  - o Apply to all surfaces of the hands/fingers up to the forearms for 2–6 minutes.
  - o Before performing invasive patient procedures.

Strategic placement of hand sanitizer dispensers throughout the anesthesia work area has been shown to significantly increase the frequency of provider-initiated hand hygiene events in the course of anesthesia [5, 13].

Cleaning/Disinfection

High-level cleaning and disinfection of soiled and high-touch surfaces in the anesthesia work area is essential before and after each procedural case. Institutions should establish cleaning protocols for environmental disinfection of equipment, based on manufacturer's recommendations. There are multiple studies demonstrating contamination of the operating room environment as a source of HAIs [14–16]. Observational data have demonstrated the significant levels of contamination that collects in procedural rooms [10, 11, 13, 14]. Hand hygiene alone cannot fully eliminate SSIs. Robust, strict cleaning protocols, in conjunction with hand hygiene and other mitigation strategies, are necessary. Studies using culturing techniques and fluorescent markers have shown the role providers play in transferring biological matter between patients and frequently touched equipment in the perioperative setting [12, 16, 17]. Thorough cleaning of accessible, high-touch surfaces, such as the anesthesia machine, anesthesia work area, computer keyboard, and monitor, contributes significantly to infection risk reduction.

SSI reduction starts with the initial operating room design and workflow. This includes minimizing use of unnecessary equipment in order to reduce the surface areas that require disinfection. In addition, institutions may consider the potential benefit of using disposable workstation covers or plastic covers in their mitigation strategy. At this time, data supporting a significant advantage for their routine use have not been established [18], but the incorporation of disposable covers may be a useful adjunct in an infection control strategy.

Disposal of medical waste material should be undertaken in accordance with local and national guidelines. Each institution should provide a safe method for collection, storage, and removal of all types of hospital waste, including general, infectious, hazardous, and radioactive material.

Airway Management

Optimizing oxygenation, ventilation, and airway protection must be paired with infection control measures that mitigate HAI transmission. An important aspect of airway management is minimizing contamination of operating room surfaces with oral secretions from the patient. Double gloving during intubation, extubation, and tube manipulation may mitigate cross-contamination of anesthesia from high-touch surfaces by providers [5, 19]. To be effective, after completion of successful airway instrumentation, the outer layer of gloves can be removed prior to touching the airway machine or other items in the workspace. The clean second pair of gloves will be ready for all urgent tasks, such as hand bagging and auscultation of breath sounds. At the earliest opportunity, the anesthesia provider should remove this second pair of gloves in order to perform thorough hand hygiene with alcohol rub or handwashing. Other important strategies include frequent hand hygiene, designation of separate clean versus dirty areas in the workspace, and cleaning of any visible or known contaminated surfaces.

To minimize HAIs, it is imperative that airway equipment is sterile and readily available for patient use. Many facilities have adapted to single-use direct laryngoscopes and videoscopes. Alternatively, standard reusable direct laryngoscopes and video laryngoscopes can be cleaned using high-level disinfection or sterilization techniques, in accordance with the manufacturer's instructions. Care must be taken to ensure that the cleaning process of these instruments is validated and reliable [20]. A breach in the integrity of instrument handling can have devastating effects [20–22]. For example, there are documented reports of *Pseudomonas aeruginosa* infection outbreaks associated with poorly cleaned laryngoscope blades.

Medication Handling

Another important source of potential perioperative HAIs is inconsistent aseptic handling of parenteral medications. When preparing and administering medications, anesthesia providers must observe strict aseptic technique. Consistent with other infection control measures, hand hygiene is the first step in aseptic medication preparation. Medications should only be handled by clean, gloved hands working in a disinfected work area [23–25].

It is important to note that vials and ampoules of medications that are drawn up by anesthesia providers are typically *not* sterile. This includes the rubber stopper and the neck of the medication vials. As a result, providers must carefully disinfect the vial prior to accessing with a sterile needle. These vials can serve as a source of HAIs. This has been documented in numerous studies [23–25].

Preferentially, single-dose vials of medications should be used when possible. If multidose vials must be employed, the vial should be restricted for single patient use. With each entry into the vial, a new sterile syringe and needle should be used. Medication syringes that are used to administer multiple doses during the course of a procedure should be capped after each use. Without proper handling, these needleless syringes pose a source of potential bacterial contamination. The cap should completely cover the Luer lock connector on the syringe.

Injection ports are a common source of HAIs and special care needs to be taken with these to reduce the risk of contamination throughout the perioperative period [25, 26]. Prior to accessing, a port needs to be disinfected with either an alcohol wipe or use of a previously applied isopropyl alcohol-containing cap. If the cap is used, the manufacturer's recommended dwell time should be observed. For alcohol disinfection, it is important for providers to remember to scrub the port for 10–15 seconds followed by time to dry [26]. In the dynamic operating room environment, this additional time needed for alcohol wipe disinfection may be incompatible with the demands of swift patient care. Use of isopropyl alcohol-containing caps may be an effective part of an infection control strategy that permits the port to be continuously immediately available for use (see Figure 34.1).

Invasive Procedures

Anytime the skin barrier is broken, there is an increased risk of microorganism transmission. In this section, the infection control considerations for anesthesia providers will be discussed for both regional anesthesia procedures and intravascular access.

Skin Preparation

Prior to any invasive procedure, a patient's skin needs to be cleaned with an appropriate skin preparation agent. A surgical skin preparation agent should be:

1. Nonirritating
2. Fast-acting
3. Possess a broad spectrum of antimicrobial properties
4. Substantially reduce transient microorganisms
5. Have cumulative, persistent activity.

It is recommended to use an antiseptic agent such as chlorhexidine gluconate or iodophors containing alcohol for skin preparation. Single-use

Intraoperative aseptic medication management and administration

- Use clean, gloved hands.
- Alcohol-disinfect rubber stopper/ampoule.
- Single-use new syringe and needle.
- Preferably use single-dose vials. All vials for only one patient.
- Multidose vials to be used for only one patient. If accessed more than once for a single patient, disinfect with alcohol and use a new needle and syringe each time.
- Minimize time between drawing up medication and administration.
- Prefilled syringes are for single patient use.
- Clean patient injection port prior to medication administration.
- Recap port when not in use. Consider use of alcohol-containing cap.

Invasive procedures

- Hand hygiene.
- Use of appropriate personal protective equipment.
- Disinfection of insertion site.
- Nontouch technique/maintenance of sterile barrier precautions.
- Use sterile dressings.

Anesthetic considerations for patients with COVID-19 or suspected COVID-19 infection

- Plan
  - Frequent communication and coordinatec care.
  - Avoid elective surgery/procedures.
  - Avoid emergent intubation/cesarean sections when possible.
  - Minimize patient movement within hospital.
  - Designate location for care with airborne precautions.

- **Personal protective equipment**
  - Fit tested N95 mask or powered air-purifying respirator.
  - Eye protection/face shield.
  - Careful attention to proper donning/doffing technique. Consider assigning an observer.

- **Airway management**
  - Utilize lowest oxygen flows preferably via oxygen mask versus nasal cannula with surgical mask.
  - Prepare anesthesia equipment and medications.
  - Utilize a heat and moisture exchange filter (HMEF).
  - Intubation by experienced provider with good first-pass success.
  - Preoxygenate for a minimum of 5 minutes with tight seal.
  - Use rapid sequence induction and avoid bag–mask ventilation if possible.
  - Use disposable products, including video laryngoscope blade if possible.
  - Double-glove and resheathe laryngoscope blade.
  - Recover patient in operating room or airborne precaution room.

- **Transport**
  - Minimize patient route of travel through hospital.
  - Communicate and coordinate any patient transport in advance.
  - Patient to wear a surgical mask or oxygen mask if supplemental oxygen needed.
  - For intubated patients, use of a HMEF.

Figure 34.1 Anesthetic principles of infection control.

individual packets are associated with decreased bacterial growth. Chlorhexidine is a broad-spectrum antiseptic with a fast onset and a long duration of action that causes minimal skin irritation. Depending on the concentration, it has both bacteriostatic and bactericidal activity. The agent binds to protein present on the skin surface, releasing slowly, which leads to its prolonged effect. The iodophor povidone iodine is a widely used antiseptic that possesses a broad microbicidal activity, with a rapid onset, but with minimal residual activity. Isopropyl alcohol as a skin prep in 60–90% solution has the fastest onset, but no residual effect. The combination of chlorhexidine with alcohol or povidone iodine with alcohol, when not contraindicated, offers the benefit of immediate onset with persistent action.

For neonates, particularly those under 2 months old, use of a chlorhexidine-containing solution for skin preparation should be based on clinical judgment and institutional protocol. If there is a contraindication to chlorhexidine, povidone–iodine or alcohol may be used. Unless contraindicated, skin preparation solutions should contain alcohol [27, 28].

Regional Anesthesia

Regional anesthesia procedures are a potential route of entry and source of exposure to microorganisms. Infections after peripheral nerve blocks or neuraxial anesthesia are rare occurrences. Anesthesia providers must be vigilant in observing aseptic practices for all regional procedures (see Figure 34.2). This includes completion of hand hygiene and use of a face mask, a head cap, sterile gloves, and an ultrasound probe cover. Consider the use of a surgical gown when a catheter is inserted. On completion of the procedure, a sterile occlusive

	Skin prep in alcohol[1]	Sterile gloves	Mask	Sterile gown	Sterile drape	Filter on injection/gtt
Single-shot peripheral nerve block	◆				◊	
Single-shot neuraxial	◆	◆			◆	
Continuous peripheral nerve catheter	◆	◆	◆	◊	◆	◆
Continuous neuraxial catheter	◆	◆	◆	◊	◆	◆
Long-term implanted device/ catheter	◆	◆	◆	◆	◆	◆
Peripheral venous catheter	◆					◊
Arterial line	◆	◆	◆		◆	
Central venous catheter/ Swan–Ganz	◆	◆	◆	◆	◆	◊

Figure 34.2 Invasive procedures – infection control. ◆ recommended; ◊, consider. For skin prep in alcohol, use chlorhexidine in alcohol or povidone iodine in alcohol.

dressing should be placed over the catheter site. Anytime the catheter is redressed, a sterile technique should be observed [28, 29]. Catheters should be monitored daily for signs of infection, and removed when no longer clinically necessary or if there is any concern of infection.

Peripheral Intravenous Access, Arterial Vascular Access, and Central Venous Catheter

Initiation of intravenous access is often necessary when access is nonexistent or inadequate in the course of an anesthetic case. Catheter-related bloodstream infections (CRBSIs) and other complications have been well documented. Even peripheral intravenous catheters are not without potential risks [28]. Aseptic precautions help to mitigate the risk of inadvertent transmission of provider skin flora or contamination of the insertion site or catheter [29–33]. Thus, for all catheter insertion events, hand hygiene should be performed before and after palpating catheter insertion sites (see Figure 34.2).

Peripheral Intravenous Access

- For peripheral venous catheter insertion, clean the skin with an antiseptic (70% alcohol, tincture of iodine, an iodophor, or chlorhexidine gluconate).
- Palpation of the insertion site should not be performed after the application of antiseptic, unless an aseptic technique is maintained.
- For insertion of peripheral intravascular catheters, use clean gloves.
- Use either sterile gauze or sterile, transparent, semipermeable dressing to cover the catheter site.

Arterial Line

- Sterile gloves should be worn for insertion of arterial catheters.
- If using an ultrasound machine for vascular access, a sterile ultrasound probe cover is required.
- Prepare and clean the skin with a >0.5% chlorhexidine preparation with alcohol. If there is a contraindication to chlorhexidine, tincture of iodine, an iodophor, or 70% alcohol can be used as alternatives.
- Use sterile drape.
- Use new sterile gloves prior to dressing changes on central access sites.

Central Venous Catheter/Peripherally Inserted Central Catheter (PICC)/Swan–Ganz

- Full sterile barrier precautions, including use of a cap, mask, sterile gown, sterile gloves, and sterile drape, are indicated.

- Skin preparation with a >0.5% chlorhexidine preparation with alcohol. If there is a contraindication to chlorhexidine, tincture of iodine, an iodophor, or 70% alcohol can be used as alternatives.

- Catheters coated with antibiotics or a combination of chlorhexidine and silver sulfadiazine may be considered for selected patient populations at increased risk of infection. A positive association between the use of antibiotic-coated catheters and a reduction in catheter colonization has been observed when compared with controls. Findings are equivocal for CRBSIs.

- Site selection should be based on clinical need and access availability. In adults, upper body central access sites are preferred due to decreased risk of catheter colonization and bacteremia.

- Replace catheter site dressing if the dressing becomes damp, loosened, or visibly soiled.

- Use a sterile sleeve for all pulmonary artery catheters.

- Chlorhexidine-impregnated dressings with an FDA-cleared label that specifies a clinical indication for reducing CRBSI or catheter-associated bloodstream infection (CABSI) are recommended to protect the insertion site of short-term nontunneled central venous catheters.

Other Measures

There are additional perioperative measures that have been positively associated with reducing a patient's risk of HAI. Decolonization of *Staphylococcus aureus*, treatment of remote site infections, smoking cessation, maintenance of normothermia, and timely antibiotic prophylaxis have all been shown to improve HAI rates in select patient populations [32–34]. Achieving and maintaining glycemic control throughout the perioperative period have also been tied to decreased patient morbidity and infection rates. Early identification of patients at increased risk in the perioperative setting is important to effectively target interventions. Risk factors such as immunosuppression, advanced age, length of hospital stay, multiple comorbidities, mechanical ventilatory support, recent invasive procedures, the presence of indwelling devices, and the need for intensive care level care all place patients at higher risk of a HAI [32, 33]. Preoperative optimization has been demonstrated to have a positive impact on HAI in surgical patients. Establishment of a multidisciplinary perioperative optimization strategy has been demonstrated to result in positive patient outcomes in surgical patients. For instance, the integration of Enhanced Recovery After Surgery (ERAS) protocols has demonstrated improved outcome measures, including for SSIs [35].

Monitoring

Quality assessment of these measures are an important aspect of an infection mitigation strategy. Communication of expected provider actions, through education and training, provides a foundation for provider compliance. Use of checklists, direct observation, video monitoring, and electronic, automated feedback are helpful tools in the adaption and maintenance of infection control-centered behaviors. Regular monitoring and feedback to providers are important because they help to foster a sense of urgency and emphasize the importance of these best practices, while eliminating deficits in performance that negatively impact infection control measures. Measuring and frequent reporting on the benefits resulting from adopted infection control behaviors also help improve sustained provider compliance [32, 33].

COVID-19

COVID-19 is an infectious disease caused by a novel coronavirus – severe acute respiratory syndrome coronavirus 2 (SARS-CoV-2). This pandemic has infected over 46 million people worldwide, resulting in over 1.2 million deaths [35]. This highly infectious viral infection is transmitted via aerosolized particles and surface contamination. As a result, special precautions must be taken when caring for a patient with known or suspected COVID-19 infection.

Personal Protective Equipment

All anesthesia providers caring for COVID-19 patients should use airborne-precaution PPE to minimize the risk of disease contamination during close patient contact and aerosolizing procedures [36–38]:

- N95 mask, with fit tested, *National Institute for Occupational Safety and Health (NIOSH)-approved N95 filtering face piece respirator or higher, or a PAPR*
- Eye protection (goggles or face shield)
- Isolation gown
- Gloves.

Hand hygiene is important before donning, and after doffing, PPE. Extreme caution should be used when removing and disposing of PPE to avoid self-contamination. Use of trained observers (TOs) is highly recommended to ensure each provider is using equipment correctly [37].

Elective procedures and surgeries should be avoided in patients with known or suspected infection. Utilization of a negative pressure isolation room is recommended. When the use of a positive pressure environment is required, the number of providers present during aerosolizing procedures should be minimized. Traffic in and around the room should be limited to essential movement only, thereby minimizing exposure of additional individuals to potentially harmful COVID-19 contamination [36–39].

The procedural or operative room should be cleared of extraneous equipment that is not needed for the planned procedure [36, 40]. Emergency equipment should be immediately available outside of the treatment area. Use of plastic covers and drapes should be considered to protect equipment surfaces in the operating room. In addition, only sufficient personnel wearing appropriate PPE to care for the patient safely should be present in the room.

Anesthetic Management of COVID-19-Positive Patients

The type of anesthesia employed should be based on individual patient factors and the planned operative procedure [36–40]. For cases requiring regional and monitored anesthesia care, patients should wear a surgical mask throughout the duration of the procedure. Peripheral nerve blocks and neuraxial anesthesia are not considered aerosol-generating procedures; thus, regular contact and droplet-precaution PPE can be used. However, consideration for use of N95 masks or a PAPR may be necessary with prolonged close contact in a closed setting.

For patients requiring supplemental oxygen, the lowest flows necessary should be used to minimize dispersion of droplets and generation of aerosols. A surgical mask can be placed over a nasal cannula or preferentially an oxygen mask can be used at the minimum flows necessary to maintain oxygen saturation.

For any case requiring general anesthesia, the internal components of the anesthesia machine should be protected. A viral filtration efficiency (VFE) of 99.99% is recommended to prevent transmission of SARS-CoV-2 from the patient to the anesthesia machine. Preferably a viral heat and moisture exchange filter (HMEF) is used between the breathing circuit and the patient's airway, with the ability to sample from the machine side of the filter. A second filter at the expiratory limb should be considered as an adjunct to protect the machine from any viral particles that may pass through the primary filter. It also amplifies the effectiveness of the first filter. Depending on the design of the anesthesia machine, filtration of the gas sampling line may be necessary. For systems that lead to the scavenging system, a separate filter is not needed; if returned to the breathing circuit, then a high VFE filter is necessary.

Pediatric patients weighing <20 kg and those unable to tolerate additional dead space should have the high-efficiency particulate absorbing (HEPA) filter placed at the expiratory limb of the breathing circuit. A filter with a smaller internal volume can be used. Alternatively, a filter can be placed on the inspiratory limb, and a separate 0.2-μm filter placed at the gas sampling line.

Preoxygenate the patient for at least 5 minutes. Ensure a tight seal or use a two-hand "vice-grip" of the mask on the patient's face. Preferentially do not bag–mask the patient. This produces patient aerosols and spreads droplets. If mask ventilation is needed, maintain a tight mask seal and use small-volume breaths to keep airway pressures <20 mmHg.

The anesthesia provider performing the intubation should be experienced and highly competent, with good first-pass success. Use of double gloves, as with nonCOVID-19 intubations, will mitigate surface contamination when the outer layer is removed following intubation. When appropriate, consider a rapid sequence induction with medications to minimize the time to intubation. Use of a video laryngoscope is recommended to avoid placement of the operator's face close to the patient's airway. Direct laryngoscopy (DL) with a disposable laryngoscope (the latter removes the need for sterilization and cleaning of airway equipment) can also be utilized. Unless indicated, fiberoptic intubations should be avoided. There is an increased risk of aerosolization of viral particles with this procedure. Preferentially disposable airway equipment should be used to minimize the items for high-level decontamination.

Once intubated, inflate the cuff fully *before* bagging, to avoid droplets.

Keep the HEPA filter in place and consider clamping the endotracheal tube if disconnecting from, or switching, the circuit to minimize contamination of the environment with patient aerosols.

During both intubation and extubation, the number of providers in the room should be limited to those necessary to care safely for the patient. Each institution will determine the appropriate time interval needed to elapse prior to return of other personnel to the operating room following aerosolizing procedures. This will be based upon the frequency of air exchanges, the size of the room, and individual facility factors.

Preparation for extubation of a COVID-19-positive patient should include mitigation strategies to reduce aerosolization. Preemptively, providers need to consider administration of antiemetics, lidocaine, opioids, and/or dexmedetomidine to prevent vomiting or coughing. Upon extubation, the patient's nose and mouth should be covered by either the circuit mask or an oxygen face mask. The patient should be recovered in the operating room or transferred to a designated negative pressure isolation room (see Figure 34.1).

Transport of COVID-19-Positive Patients and Patients under Investigation (PUIs)

Transport routes for COVID-19 patients should be minimized and planned in advance [37–41]. Exposure to other patients and personnel should be avoided.

For intubated patients or those receiving aerosolizing procedures during transport, consider involving hospital security to clear hallways and to hold elevators. Communicate with the receiving nursing units in advance to streamline the handoff process and to avoid unplanned exposure. A HEPA filter must remain in use during transport of intubated patients. Providers in contact with the patient during transport should avoid touching medical facility surfaces. Another team member or other hospital personnel should be available to open doors and elevators. Nonintubated patients should wear a surgical mask if transport is required within the medical facility.

After the patient has been transported out of the operating environment, the room should remain empty for a period of time. This will be institution-specific and will vary based on the number of air exchanges per hour and the room dimensions. A terminal deep cleaning should follow, as recommended by the Centers for Disease Control and Prevention (CDC) and local hospital protocols.

COVID-19-Positive and PUI Obstetric Patients

Peripartum COVID-19 infection presents unique challenges for the hospital team caring for these patients [42]. As with nonparturient patients, it is recommended that the number of providers interacting with these patients is limited. These patients should be cared for in designated airborne-precaution labor and operating rooms. Anesthesia equipment and supplies brought into the patient room, such as an epidural kit and medications, should be limited to items needed for immediate use. The most experienced anesthesia provider should perform procedures to minimize the need for catheter replacement or for a blood patch due to inadvertent dural puncture. For these patients, neuraxial anesthesia is still the preferred anesthetic for an operative delivery. Early and frequent communication between the obstetric, anesthesia, and nursing teams is imperative to minimize delays in patient care and to mitigate transmission of infection to staff. Crash cesarean sections should be avoided when possible. It is highly recommended that all personnel in the operating room don airborne-precaution PPE in acknowledgment of the risk of conversion to general anesthesia or of vomiting during the course of a cesarean section.

References

1. Centers for Disease Control (CDC). Public health focus: surveillance, prevention, and control of nosocomial infections. *MMWR Morb Mortal Wkly Rep.* 1992:41:783–7.

2. Centers for Disease Control and Prevention. 2018 National and state healthcare-associated infections progress report. 2019. Available from: www.cdc.gov/hai/data/archive/2018-HAI-progress-report.html.

3. Shepard J, *et al.* Financial impact of surgical site infections on hospitals: the hospital management perspective. *JAMA Surg.* 2013;148:907–14.

4. Stone PW. Economic burden of healthcare-associated infections: an American perspective. *Expert Rev Pharmacoecon Outcomes Res.* 2009;9:417–22.

5. Munoz-Price, L., *et al.* Infection prevention in the operating room anesthesia work area. *Infect Control Hosp Epidemiol.* 2019;40:1–17.

6. American Society of Anesthesiologists. Guidelines for surgical attire. 2019. Available from: www.asahq.org/standards-and-guidelines/guidelines-for-surgical-attire.

7. Hambraeus A. Aerobiology in the operating room – a review. *J Hosp Infect.* 1988;11:68–76.

8. Centers for Disease Control and Prevention. Transmission-based precautions. Available from: www.cdc.gov/infectioncontrol/basics/transmission-based-precautions.html.

9. World Health Organization. WHO guidelines on hand hygiene in healthcare. 2009. Available from: www.who.int/publications/i/item/9789241597906.

10. Baillie JK, *et al.* Contamination of anaesthetic machines with pathogenic organisms. *Anaesthesia.* 2007;62:1257–61.

11. Loftus RW, *et al.* The dynamics of *Enterococcus* transmission from bacterial reservoir commonly encountered by anesthesia providers. *Anesth Analg.* 2015;120:827–36.

12. Sharma A, *et al.* Perioperative infection transmission: the role of the anesthesia provider in infection control and healthcare-associated infections. *Curr Anesthesiol Rep.* 2020;10(3):1–9.

13. Koff MD, *et al.* Reduction in intraoperative bacterial contamination of peripheral intravenous tubing through the use of a novel device. *Anesthesiology.* 2009;110:978–85.

14. Loftus RW, *et al.* The epidemiology of *Staphylococcus aureus* transmission in the anesthesia work area. *Anesth Analg.* 2015;120:807–18.

15. Loftus RW, *et al.* Transmission dynamics of gram-negative bacterial pathogens in the anesthesia work area. *Anesth Analg.* 2015;120:819–26.

16. Jefferson J, *et al.* A novel technique for identifying opportunities to improve environmental hygiene in the operating room. *AORN J.* 2011;93:358–64.

17. Munoz-Price LS, *et al.* Decreasing operating room environmental pathogen contamination through improved cleaning practices. *Infect Control Hosp Epidemiol.* 2012;33:897–904.

18. Biddle CJ, *et al.* Assessing a novel method to reduce anesthesia machine contamination: a prospective, observational trial. *Can J Infect Dis Med Microbiol.* 2018;2018:1905360.

19. Birnbach DJ, *et al.* Double gloves: a randomized trial to evaluate a simple strategy to reduce contamination in the operating room. *Anesth Analg.* 2015;121:1209–14.

20. Schaffzin J, *et al.* The hospital epidemiologist's perspective on the anesthesia operating room work area. *Anesthesia Patient Safety Foundation.* 2019;34:37–9.

21. Rutala WA, Weber DJ. Disinfection and sterilization in health care facilities: an overview and current issues. *Infect Dis Clin North Am.* 2016;30:609–37.

22. Muscarella LF. Reassessment of the risk of healthcare acquired infection during rigid laryngoscopy. *J Hosp Infect.* 2008;68:101–7.

23. Centers for Disease Control and Prevention. Safe injection practices to prevent transmission to patients. 2007. Available from: www.cdc.gov/injectionsafety/ip07-standardprecaution.html.

24. Loftus RW, *et al.* Transmission of pathogenic bacterial organisms in the anesthetic work area. *Anesthesiology.* 2008;109:399–407.

25. Gargiulo DA, *et al.* Anaesthetic drug administration as a potential contributor to healthcare associated infections – a perspective simulation based evaluation of aseptic technique in administration of anaesthetic drugs. *BMJ Qual Safe.* 2012;21:826–34.

26. Moureau NL, Flynn J. Disinfection of needless connector hubs: clinical evidence systematic review. *Nurs Res Pract.* 2015;2015:796762.

27. Association of Surgical Technologists. AST standards of practice for skin prep of the surgical patient. 2008. Available from: www.ast.org/uploadedFiles/Main_Site/Content/About_Us/Standard_Skin_Prep.pdf

28. [No authors listed]. Practice advisory for the prevention, diagnosis, and management of infectious complications associated with neuraxial techniques: an updated report by the American Society of Anesthesiologists Task Force on Infectious Complications Associated with Neuraxial Techniques and the American Society of Regional Anesthesia and Pain Medicine. *Anesthesiology.* 2017;126:585–601.

29. Schulz-Stubner S, *et al.* Infection control in regional anesthesia. Available from: www.nysora.com/topics/complications/infection-control-regional-anesthesia/.

30. Zhang Li, *et al.* Infection risks associated with vascular catheters. *J Infect Prev.* 2016;17:207–13.

31. O'Grady NP, *et al.* Guidelines for the prevention of intravascular catheter-related infections. *Clin Infect Dis.* 2011;52(9):e162–93.

32. Joint Commission International. Evidence based principles and practices for preventing surgical site infections. 2018. Available from: https://store.jointcommissioninternational.org/evidence-based-principles-and-practices-for-preventing-surgical-site-infections-toolkit/.

33. Berríos-Torres SI, *et al.* Centers for Disease Control and Prevention guideline for the prevention of surgical site infection. *JAMA Surg.* 2017;152:784–91.

34. World Health Organization. Global guidelines for the prevention of surgical site infection. 2016. Available from: www.ncbi.nlm.nih.gov/pubmedhealth/PM H0095752/pdf/PubMedHealth_PMH0095752.pdf.

35. Gronnier C, *et al*. Influence of Enhanced Recovery Pathway on surgical site infection after colonic surgery. *Gastroenterol Res Pract*. 2017;2017:9015854.

36. World Health Organization. Weekly epidemiological update – 3 November 2020. 2020. Available from: www.who.int/publications/m/item/weekly-epidemiological-update—3-november-2020.

37. Centers for Disease Control and Prevention. Infection control guidance for healthcare professionals about coronavirus (COVID-19). 2020. Available from: www.cdc.gov/coronavirus/2019-ncov/hcp/infection-control.html.

38. Caputo KM, *et al*. Intubation of SARS patients: infection and perspectives of healthcare workers. *Can J Anaesth*. 2006;53(2):122–9.

39. Centers for Disease Control and Prevention. Interim infection prevention and control recommendations for healthcare personnel during the coronavirus disease 2019 (COVID-19) pandemic. Atlanta, GA: Centers for Disease Control and Prevention; 2022.

40. Lockhart SL, *et al*. Personal protective equipment (PPE) for both anesthesiologists and other airway managers: principles and practice during the COVID-19 pandemic. *Can J Anaesth*. 2020;67(8):1005–15.

41. Zucco L, *et al*. Perioperative considerations for the 2019 novel coronavirus (COVID-19). Rochester, MN: Anesthesia Patient Safety Foundation; 2020.

42. Bauer ME, *et al*. Obstetric anesthesia during the COVID-19 pandemic. *Anesth Analg*. 2020;131:7–15.

Chapter 35

Coagulation

Kenneth Flax and Erica Fagelman

Introduction

Understanding of coagulation and coagulopathy is essential to the practice of anesthesia. This begins with preoperative assessment and planning. A detailed history is the first step. Laboratory testing can reveal abnormalities that may have otherwise gone undetected, as many disorders are asymptomatic until unmasked by the stress of surgery. Some of these disorders may be inherited or acquired, and their presentation and treatment must be considered. Intimate familiarity of this topic allows the anesthesiologist to adequately prepare for coagulopathy and thrombotic events in the perioperative environment.

Coagulation begins with vascular endothelial injury. The first step in the coagulation cascade is platelet aggregation. After injury, exposed von Willebrand factor (vWF) binds to circulating platelets, resulting in platelet activation and thromboxane generation. Platelet activation results in conformational change, allowing for further binding of vWF and fibrinogen. As more circulating platelets become bound and activated, cross-linking of vWF and fibrinogen results in a platelet plug. The activated platelet surface, now as part of a stable structure, can allow for initiation of the humoral coagulation cascade [1].

When performing a preoperative assessment for a patient in whom you expect existing coagulopathy, or if there is an elevated risk of developing coagulation issues intraoperatively, it is important to focus on the patient's bleeding and clotting history [1]. This is also crucial to discuss prior to surgery involving a significant degree of expected blood loss with a high likelihood of blood product transfusion. The anesthesiologist must conduct a thorough review of the patient's medical and surgical history, and perform relevant parts of the physical examination, in addition to the standard components of a preoperative assessment. Questions regarding the patient's family history and the presence of any coagulation disorders are also helpful, as some are inherited. It is important to include assessment for renal and hepatic dysfunction, as impairments in these organ systems may produce coagulopathy [1]. A thorough review of the patient's medication list will reveal any nonsteroidal antiinflammatory drugs (NSAIDs) (including aspirin), antiplatelet therapy, or anticoagulation that may produce an elevated bleeding risk and potentially pose a contraindication to particular surgical procedures. Asking the patient about any prior history of blood transfusion is helpful in identifying an increased risk of antibodies to particular blood antigens. In some cases, patients may have rare antibodies that make it challenging to locate sufficient crossmatched blood. Standard laboratory tests (including, but not limited to, complete blood count (CBC), comprehensive metabolic panel (CMP), coagulation studies, type and screen (T+S)) may help to unmask some of these issues. It can also be useful to probe about bleeding history with particular questions that address bleeding disorders, outside the realm of our standard preoperative laboratory tests (ex: minor mucosal bleeding and von Willebrand's disease (vWD)) [1].

Screening questions often start with the patient's medical history, and should be directed at assessing whether the patient has any known coagulation disorders or any renal or hepatic dysfunction, whether there is a positive family history, and whether the patient has undergone any significant bleeding challenge in the past, including the results of that encounter. A patient with renal dysfunction (acute or chronic) may exhibit some degree of uremic platelet dysfunction. A patient suffering from end-stage liver disease (or fulminant hepatic failure) may exhibit coagulopathy in the form of deficient coagulation factor production and thrombocytopenia. Take note of any significant blood loss, especially requiring transfusion, during any prior routine procedures. The overall assessment of a patient's coagulation status becomes increasingly important in preparation for major surgery with significant expected blood loss and a high likelihood of transfusion. This will also influence the intravenous access and invasive monitoring planned for the procedure.

If the patient is taking any form of NSAID, aspirin, antiplatelet therapy, or anticoagulation, it is important to be familiar with guidelines for reversal and discontinuation prior to surgery [1]. This will often require a multidisciplinary discussion involving the surgeon, anesthesiologists, and the patient's primary care physician (often a cardiologist). Depending on the location and type of surgery, the surgical team may permit the patient to remain on some "blood-thinning" medications, if the risk of discontinuing these is greater than that of significant surgical bleeding (such as recent percutaneous coronary intervention (PCI) with stent placement, recent cerebrovascular accident (CVA), etc.).

Although typical preoperative laboratory values can be quite revealing, it remains crucial to perform pertinent parts of the physical examination when assessing the patient's coagulation status. The patient may exhibit oozing at their mucosal surfaces, extensive ecchymosis, joint deformation, or jaundice indicating possible liver disease, or they may develop hematuria, with significant thrombocytopenia [1]. The patient may report a history of hematoma formation out of proportion to any trauma they have incurred. Perhaps the patient is a female who has given birth, and reports a history of significant blood product transfusion in the absence of obstetric complications.

Prior to major surgery, the patient will often undergo some form of preoperative medical workup, including a visit with their primary provider and laboratory tests, and often additional cardiac workup (ECG, transthoracic echocardiography (TTE), stress test) in patients with a history of cardiac disease or with cardiac risk factors. Standard blood work should include CBC, CMP, coagulation studies (prothrombin time (PT), activated partial thromboplastin time (aPTT), international normalised ratio (INR)). Collectively, these values can provide abundant information about the presence of coagulopathy, the likelihood of major bleeding, the risk of clotting, and the likelihood of transfusion. Also, blood bank testing should include T+S. If this screen is positive, it indicates the patient has antibodies present and more time is required for the blood bank to investigate the nature of the antibody and whether or not it is clinically significant [1].

Preoperative Management of Antiplatelets and Anticoagulants

Antiplatelet and anticoagulation medications are often prescribed for post-procedural management of vascular stents, coronary artery disease, or a primary coagulation disorder, and it is important to be familiar with their properties. When patients are scheduled for surgery, a review of their medication list should identify any drugs of this class. It is essential to understanding why the patient is prescribed the medication and whether or not these medications should be held prior to surgery [2]. This decision may depend on the potential for significant blood loss, the condition for which the patient is prescribed the medication, emergent versus scheduled surgery, the type of surgery being performed, assessment of bleeding and thromboembolic risk, and the necessary duration of discontinuation, among other reasons.

In the event that anticoagulants or antiplatelet medications need to be discontinued, the patient should be educated on the proper time to stop the medication preoperatively. Multidisciplinary discussion may be warranted to decide when it is safe for the patient to resume their medication postoperatively. Medications such as warfarin require discontinuation well in advance (4–7 days prior), and it may be prudent to repeat coagulation labs to ensure the INR reflects adequate warfarin reversal prior to surgery (often target INR <1.5) [2]. When holding warfarin, there is the option to "bridge" the patient to an anticoagulant with a shorter half-life, such as enoxaparin, so that the patient does not need to be without anticoagulation for as long a period of time. Many of the newer oral anticoagulants have a shorter half-life and therefore require less time to reverse. There are also antidotes for some of these medications, making them essentially immediately reversible. Heparin and low-molecular-weight heparin (LMWH) have relatively short half-lives and require discontinuation 4–6 hours, and 24 hours, prior to surgery, respectively [2]. Reversal of heparin and LMWH can be monitored with partial thromboplastin time (PTT), and protamine is also available for immediate reversal if necessary.

Antiplatelet drugs include aspirin, P2Y12 inhibitors, and glycoprotein 2b/3a inhibitors. In order to monitor the reversal of these medications, platelet function testing with platelet aggregation studies is the most reliable and considered the gold standard. Many of these medications will also affect thromboelastography (TEG) values and require ample time for reversal, with even longer half-lives in patients with renal dysfunction. Although there is a large range of half-lives within this class of medications, abciximab requires the longest time for reversal and typically discontinuation 2 weeks prior to surgery [2].

Direct thrombin inhibitors and direct Xa inhibitors comprise the last two major classes of anticoagulation. The most commonly used direct thrombin inhibitors are bivalirudin (intravenous) and dabigatran (oral), and the most common direct Xa inhibitors are rivaroxaban and apixaban (both administered orally). Direct thrombin inhibitors do not have specific antidotes but are removable by dialysis, and this method has been employed in patients who are actively bleeding. With advance notice, these medications require no more than a few days of discontinuation prior to surgery. Direct Xa inhibitors, on the other hand, are not removable by dialysis. Their reversal may be monitored with antiXa levels, and they too require a few days of discontinuation prior to surgery [1].

Laboratory Testing

Laboratory tests can provide information about individual components in the coagulation cascade. A CBC informs about the starting hematocrit and the need for red blood cell transfusion, whereas a platelet count informs about the need for platelet transfusion. PT can evaluate the extrinsic and common pathways of coagulation [1]. In this test, the patient's plasma is mixed with thromboplastin and calcium, and a clotting time is determined. These values are standardized across institutions using the INR, to account for differing thromboplastins used. PT can be prolonged due to warfarin, vitamin K deficiency, inherited or acquired factor deficiencies, or inhibitors. The PTT measures the intrinsic and common pathways, including prothrombin and fibrinogen. The patient's plasma is mixed with an activating agent such as silica, calcium, and phospholipid. The PTT can be prolonged due to heparin, factor deficiencies, inhibitors such as factors VIII and IX, anticoagulant or lupus antibody, and vWD [2].

These standard laboratory tests are limited in their ability to guide the decision to transfuse blood products such as fresh frozen plasma (FFP), platelets, and cryoprecipitate, because they do not reliably predict a patient's risk of bleeding. Viscoelastic testing, invented in 1948, analyzes a developing clot from whole blood. Real-time results can be used to treat specific deficits in the clotting cascade of a patient. Why do conventional coagulation tests (CCTs) fail to capture this picture? The PT/INR is measured from plasma and correlates poorly with clotting time. Plasma lacks certain activators, as well as the presence of pro- and anticoagulants present in whole blood. Tissue factor expressed on cells such as monocytes also affects actual clotting and will not be a component of PT/INR. The strength of the clot is determined by platelets and fibrinogen. Due to this tight interplay, the direct platelet count is not a reliable measure of a patient's ability or tendency to clot and whether the clot will be strong. Viscoelastic testing such as TEG and rotational thromboelastometry (ROTEM) can provide a global picture of coagulation and fibrinolysis over time, thereby providing valuable and evidence-based guidance for therapy [5, 6].

Intraoperative Management

Often patients may develop surgical bleeding secondary to the development of intraoperative coagulopathy. There are a variety of tests available to monitor and treat this, but only some provide immediate results. These patients may represent those who had normal coagulation prior to surgery or may include patients with preexisting coagulopathy who have not received thorough preoperative management and preparation. Often, these patients are undergoing cardiac surgery, and the coagulopathy results, in part, from cardiopulmonary bypass (CPB) [1]. Many cirrhotic patients undergoing liver transplantation will also exhibit significant derangements in coagulation, with the possibility for both bleeding and/or thrombosis.

CPB is known for causing platelet dysfunction during cardiac surgery, as a result of inappropriate platelet activation and agglutination, as platelets come in contact with the nonbiological material contained in the CPB circuit [1]. In addition to the deleterious effect of CPB on platelet function, many of the patients undergoing cardiac surgery have been prescribed antiplatelet agents after suffering acute coronary syndrome (ACS). Due to uncertainty regarding the timing of surgery, these agents may continue to exert their effects intraoperatively and cause further platelet dysfunction. However, not all antiplatelet medications have the same effect, and clopidogrel has been shown to have a significant deleterious effect on platelets, leading to more postoperative bleeding and reoperation when compared to aspirin alone [1]. Therefore, ideally, clopidogrel should be discontinued 3 days prior to cardiac surgery when possible. In cases where there is insufficient notice to discontinue clopidogrel, transfusion of platelets may be considered. Administration of DDAVP may also be helpful in scenarios where a patient is hemorrhaging and there is a high suspicion for platelet dysfunction after CPB [1].

Orthotopic liver transplantation (OLT) is often associated with intraoperative hemorrhage, and these patients tend to have deranged coagulation at baseline and live along a spectrum that involves the tendency to bleed and clot. Throughout the phases of OLT, coagulation progressively worsens and reaches a nidus during the anhepatic phase, when there is no functioning liver to clear substances such as tissue plasminogen activator (tPa). Upon reperfusion of the donor organ, an influx of tPa is reintroduced into the bloodstream and can create a hyperfibrinolytic state. In the event that hyperfibrinolysis is severe and causing hemorrhage, antifibrinolytic agents such as tranexamic acid may be considered. After successful transplantation, the new organ will start to replenish procoagulant factors before anticoagulant factors, and this may be why acute hepatic artery thrombosis occurs most commonly during this time period. In patients with a history of cirrhosis complicated by hepatorenal syndrome, there may be a component of uremic platelet dysfunction, and DDAVP can be considered to address this.

Postoperative Management of Coagulopathy

Coagulopathy postoperatively can lead to significant postoperative bleeding, which is associated with more surgical re-exploration, hemodynamic instability and prolonged hypotension with poor tissue perfusion, increased blood product transfusion, and overall increased morbidity and mortality. When managing coagulopathy intraoperatively, it is important to ensure adequate hemostasis prior to leaving the operating room. A patient with deranged coagulation that is not addressed will continue to bleed once out of the operating room. This significantly increases the likelihood that they will require re-exploration for continued bleeding, which may manifest as increased surgical drain output, hemodynamic instability, and/or continued blood product transfusion requirement [1]. Additional reasons for postoperative coagulopathy may include hypothermia, obesity, complex surgery, and long CPB time in cardiac surgery.

If postoperative coagulopathy is treated early, it may reduce the chances that the patient will need to return to the operating room. When this is suspected, it is prudent to send laboratory tests and identify any components of coagulation in which the patient is deficient. Ideally, point-of-care testing will provide the quickest results. However, if this is not available, sending coagulation tests, including fibrinogen, and a CBC may provide helpful results [5].

Common Bleeding Disorders

Hemophilia A, B (also known as Christmas disease), and C are characterized by deficiencies in clotting factors VIII, IX, and XI, respectively. The clinical manifestation of this disease varies significantly and depends on whether the patient has a mild or severe case. In milder cases, the patient tends to have factor activity level >5% of normal, whereas in severe cases, the patient may have factor activity levels <1% of normal [2]. Physical signs of the disease may appear as early as in the first few weeks of life (often circumcision), and certainly by the time the patient starts to walk, the development of spontaneous hemarthroses should raise high suspicion for severe hemophilia. In milder cases, a lack of significant symptoms can make it difficult to diagnose. Further investigation into the patient's coagulation status may be prompted by the incidental finding of a prolonged PTT on routine blood work, or bleeding out of proportion to surgery, or trauma incurred by the patient [2].

Perioperative management of hemophilia is focused on replacement of deficient factors, either preemptively prior to surgery to prevent major bleeding or in treatment of active bleeding. Depending on the site of bleeding, there are different factor activity levels that should be achieved in order to establish adequate hemostasis [2]. For example, an intracranial bleed warrants much more significant factor repletion than bleeding associated with a dental procedure. As an anesthesiologist, it is important to familiarize yourself with these treatments and how to properly administer them. However, consulting a hematology service for pre- and postoperative management of hemophilia, as well as guidance on proper dosing of factor replacement, is advised.

vWD (types 1, 2, and 3) is the most common of all inherited bleeding disorders and is inherited in an autosomal dominant pattern. Patients with vWD may have either an abnormally low quantitative value or a qualitative defect with decreased circulating amounts of normal vWF molecules. Unlike hemophilia, vWD typically presents with skin and mucosal bleeding such as epistaxis or bleeding gums while brushing teeth. Clinical manifestation of vWD is not sufficient to diagnose the condition, and there are specific laboratory tests that can aid in its diagnosis. Blood work should include evaluation for vWF antigen and assaying for vWF activity [2].

Type 1 vWD is characterized by low quantitative levels of vWF (partial, not complete, deficiency). Type 2 vWD, on the other hand, is characterized by a quantitative defect and reduced number of normal vWF molecules. Lastly, type 3 vWD, the most severe, is diagnosed when the patient has severe vWF deficiency. While some of these varieties may have similar clinical manifestations, it is important to distinguish the type of vWD present, as it may influence the way you navigate treatment [2].

There are a few different treatment options for vWD, including desmopressin, vWF-containing concentrates, and antifibrinolytic therapy. DDAVP is useful in treating type 1 vWD, and typically these patients have a good response. Sometimes, DDAVP will also be effective in treating type 2 vWD. However, it will have no effect on patients with type 3 vWD. This is because DDAVP works by encouraging the expression of vWF on platelets; it is ineffective in type 3 vWD because the patient has complete deficiency of vWF [2].

vWF transfusion, in the form of purified concentrates, is available for treatment of type 3 vWD and those patients with type 1 and 2 vWD who do not respond to DDAVP therapy. Transfusion is aimed at targeting roughly 100% of normal levels, but this determination does also depend on the severity of bleeding and the type of surgery required [2].

Lastly, antifibrinolytic agents also are available for treatment of vWD. This class of medication includes medications such as aminocaproic acid and tranexamic acid. These medications may also be administered in addition to DDAVP or vWF concentrate [2]. By decreasing clot lysis, overall clot integrity will improve and persist, and ultimately reduce overall bleeding.

Common Clotting Disorders

Antithrombin III (AT-III) deficiency is inherited in an autosomal dominant fashion and is a major cause of venous thromboembolism (VTE). Typically, antithrombin is present in circulation to inactivate thrombin, along with many other coagulation factors. In the absence of antithrombin III, thrombin and the other coagulation factors will predominate, significantly increasing the patient's risk of thrombosis. Antithrombin III is also the site of action for heparin, and patients with this deficiency may present as heparin nonresponders. This disorder is typically diagnosed with a plasma functional assay, which has the ability to detect and diagnose all subtypes of AT-III deficiency. There are many mechanisms by which patients can acquire AT-III deficiency, including end-stage liver disease, acute thrombosis, burns, and extracorporeal membrane oxygenation (ECMO) [2].

Protein C deficiency is another clotting disorder that is inherited in an autosomal dominant fashion and is characterized by type 1 and 2 deficiencies, which are quantitative and qualitative, respectively. Typically, protein C acts in areas of intact endothelium to prevent clot extension, and a deficiency of this anticoagulant factor will lead to excessive clot formation. Interestingly, protein C levels in any given individual will vary on a daily basis [2]. Despite this, patients who are heterozygotes for this mutation tend to have protein C levels that are 35–65% of normal, with levels >65% being considered "normal." There are various causes of acquired protein C deficiency, which tend to include disseminated intravascular coagulation (DIC), acute thrombosis, young age (associated with lower levels; level increases to normal with age), and vitamin K deficiency [2].

Protein S deficiency also has an autosomal dominant inheritance and is classified as type 1 (quantitative) and type 2 (qualitative), similar to protein C deficiency. Unlike protein C, protein S has no independent role as an anticoagulant and, in its unbound form, acts as a cofactor for activated protein C. When testing for protein S deficiency, quantitative assays are performed to assess for the amount of free protein S, as this is the functionally active form [2]. Typically, free protein S levels of <33% of total protein S content are correlated with clot formation and tend to represent mutations in its gene. Similarly to protein C deficiency, one can develop acquired protein S deficiency and causes of this include acute thrombosis, cirrhosis, oral contraceptive therapy, and nephrotic syndrome [2].

Factor V Leiden mutation represents one of the most common inherited clotting disorders, and results from a mutation in the factor V gene which makes factor V more resistant to inactivation. Typically, in patients with this disorder, factor V will stay active for longer than normal, leading to increased thrombin generation. Patients who are heterozygous for this condition tend to have only a slightly increased risk of VTE when compared to those who are homozygous. Typically, patients with factor V Leiden mutation will initially present with deep vein thrombosis (DVT) or pulmonary embolism (PE) [2].

Antiphospholipid antibody syndrome (APLS) is characterized by thrombosis and the presence of one or more of the antiphospholipid antibodies (anticardiolipin, antiB2-glycoprotein, and lupus anticoagulant). There have been many instances of healthy individuals transiently having detectable quantities of these antibodies, in the absence of any thrombosis. For this reason, diagnosis requires the clinical manifestation of thrombosis to be present. Patients with these antibodies are at higher risk of developing recurrent thromboses, and many times, indefinite anticoagulation may be indicated, even if this is complicated by bleeding [2]. APLS often presents itself similarly to the other clotting disorders mentioned here. However, recurrent and late losses of multiple fetuses in women of childbearing age should raise high suspicion.

Prothrombin gene mutation tends to affect patients of European descent and is almost never found in other patient populations. This gene mutation results in the accumulation of prothrombin RNA, which leads to roughly 30% increase in the amount of circulating prothrombin protein. This, in turn, leads to increased thrombin formation, such as in factor V Leiden disorder. Patients with this gene mutation tend to form DVTs and rarely form arterial thrombi [2].

Anticoagulation in the Perioperative Period

Many patients are prescribed anticoagulation in the perioperative period. One should determine if it is still indicated. If this is unclear, it is prudent to reach out to the prescribing provider to obtain more information. Also, the type of procedure for which the patient is presenting will play a role in management. The consequence of perioperative bleeding often depends on the location of surgery. For example, a small amount of bleeding in a neurosurgical procedure or ophthalmologic surgery can be devastating.

If the decision is made to interrupt a patient's anticoagulation, the next step is to determine which medication the patient is on and how long it requires for reversal. Any patient with a history of anticoagulation use should be counseled preoperatively on their increased risk of surgical bleeding if this is deemed to be the case. Also, when the perioperative plan involves interrupting anticoagulation, the patient should be educated on their risk of thrombosis. Patients with a recent thrombotic event are at higher risk of recurrence, and ideally any elective surgery should be postponed until 3–6 months after the event [2]. It has been suggested that patients who suffer from hereditary thrombophilias are also at increased risk, especially in the setting of anticoagulation disruption. On the other hand, patients with an isolated thrombosis event, especially when provoked, are at relatively low risk of thrombosis with a brief interruption in anticoagulation, and can be counseled as such [2].

In addition to the perioperative management of venous thrombosis, anesthesiologists must be familiar with the risk factors for arterial thrombus formation and how to manage these patients and their medications perioperatively. Often patients with risk factors for coronary artery disease are placed on aspirin for primary prevention, and this may be interrupted for a brief period of time, with fairly low risk. More careful consideration must be made, however, in patients for whom aspirin is being used as secondary prevention and/or in those with coronary stents [2]. Patients who are prescribed anticoagulation for atrial fibrillation also require risk stratification. Patients who suffer from atrial fibrillation undergo assessment to determine their risk of stroke, using the CHADS-VASC score, which assesses the 1-year risk of a thromboembolic event in a patient with non-valvular atrial fibrillation. If a patient has one to two comorbidities listed in this score (or more), such as congestive heart failure or a history of CVA, the patient is deemed high risk and they should be considered for anticoagulation. The risk of a thromboembolic event in any patient with atrial fibrillation should be weighed against the risk of bleeding if the planned procedure is to be performed without interrupting anticoagulation. Although the CHADS-VASC score is useful, it does not reflect the inherent risk in holding anticoagulation for a short period of time in a patient with atrial fibrillation [2].

Patients with artificial heart valves represent another large group of patients who may present for noncardiac surgery. Additional considerations in these patients involve the type and location of the artificial heart valve. For example, patients with a manufactured mechanical valve typically require lifelong anticoagulation, and replaced aortic valves are typically associated with less thrombosis than artificial mitral valves [2].

In complex scenarios where the risk–benefit analysis is unclear regarding interruption of a patient's anticoagulation, it is prudent to consult additional sources. First and foremost, communication with the prescribing practitioner, whether it be a cardiologist, a hematologist, or a primary care physician, etc., should always be conducted. The surgical team also must be involved in these discussions. The proceduralist can clarify the exact planned procedure, the expected blood loss, and whether or not this can (or should) be performed on anticoagulation, or sometimes whether the procedure should be deferred.

References

1. Nguyen A, DasGupta A, Wahed A, Cruz MI. *Management of Hemostasis and Coagulopathies for Surgical and Critically Ill Patients: An Evidence-Based Approach.* Amsterdam: Elsevier; 2017.

2. Kitchens CS, Kessler CM, Konkle BA, Garcia DA. *Consultative Hemostasis and Thrombosis*, 4th ed. Philadelphia, PA:Elsevier; 2019.

3. Luddington RJ. Thrombelastography/thromboelastometry. *Clin Lab Haematol.* 2005;27(2):81–90.

4. Wikkelsø A, Wetterslev J, Møller AM, Afshari A. Thromboelastography (TEG) or thromboelastometry (ROTEM) to monitor haemostatic treatment versus usual care in adults or children with bleeding. *Cochrane Database Syst Rev.* 2016;8:CD007871.

5. Mallett SV. Clinical utility of viscoelastic tests of coagulation (TEG/ROTEM) in patients with liver disease and during liver transplantation. *Semin Thromb Hemost.* 2015;41(5):527–37.

6. Mackman N, Tilley RE, Key NS. Role of extrinsic pathway of blood coagulation in hemostasis and thrombosis. *Arterioscleros Thromb Vasc Biol.* 2007;27:1687–93.

Index